PLEASE ENTER ON LOAN SLIP:

AUTHOR: FEWKES

TITLE: ILLUSTRATED ATLAS OF CUTANEOUS SURGERY

ACCESSION NO:

Illustrated Atlas of
CUTANEOUS SURGERY

Jessica L. Fewkes, MD
Assistant Professor
Department of Dermatology
Harvard Medical School
Boston, Massachusetts

Mack L. Cheney, MD, FACS
Assistant Professor
Department of Otolaryngology
Harvard Medical School
Boston, Massachusetts

Sheldon V. Pollack, MD
Associate Professor of Medicine
Division of Dermatology
University of Toronto
Toronto, Ontario, Canada

Forewords by
Richard Fabian and Thomas B. Fitzpatrick

J.B. Lippincott Company • Philadelphia
Gower Medical Publishing • New York • London

Distributed in the USA and Canada by:
JB Lippincott Company
East Washington Square
Philadelphia, PA 19105
USA

Gower Medical Publishing
101 Fifth Avenue
New York, NY 10003
USA

Distributed in the UK, Europe, and the rest of the world by:
JB Lippincott Company
Middlesex House
34-42 Cleveland Street
London, W1P 5FB

Distributed in Japan by:
Nankodo Co, Ltd
42-6, Hongo, 3-Chome,
Bunkyo-Ku
Tokyo 113 Japan

Library of Congress Cataloging-in-Publication Data
Fewkes, Jessica L. (Jessica Lynn), 1948-
   Illustrated atlas of cutaneous surgery / Jessica L. Fewkes,
Sheldon V. Pollack, Mack L. Cheney.
      p.   cm.
   Includes bibliographical references.
   ISBN 0-397-44676-4 (hardcover):$95.00
   1. Skin—Surgery—Atlases. I. Pollack, Sheldon V. II. Cheney,
Mack L. (Mack Lowell), 1955-   . III. Title.
   [DNLM: 1. Skin—surgery—atlases.   WR 17 F432i]
   RD520.F49 1991
   617.4'77059—dc20
   DNLM/DLC
   for Library of Congress   91-9919
                                                   CIP

British Library Cataloguing in Publication Data
Fewkes, Jessica L. *1948-*
   Illustrated atlas of cutaneous surgery.
   1. Humans. Skin. Surgery
   I. Title II. Pollack, Sheldon V. *1949-* III. Cheney, Mack
L. *1955-*
   617.477059

   ISBN 0-397-44676-4

Project Editor: Joy Noel Travalino
Art Director: Jill Feltham
Interior Design: Jessica Stockholder, Paul Fennessy
Cover Design: Paul Fennessy
Illustration Supervisor: Alan Landau
Illustrators: Alan Landau, Gary Welch

Printed in Hong Kong
Produced by Mandarin Offset

10 9 8 7 6 5 4 3 2 1

To the many teachers who permitted us to participate in their pursuits of learning and to the multitude of students who have guided us in ours.

To our families for their untiring support, patience, and love during our pursuit of academic excellence:

Rene and Lili Camille Mugnier
Penny, Jessica, and Adam Pollack
Wendy, Luke, and Jenna Cheney

Forewords

The skin is a vital organ without which the human body perishes and, like all other organs, it is subject to its frailties. It yields to disease emerging within the body or to that evolving from its own substance. The results of such affliction, unchecked, are pain, suffering, mutilation, humiliation, or even death. Aside from the myriad physiologic functions provided by the skin, the character and aesthetic structure of the individual are wrapped in its embrace.

Surgery of the skin has evolved as a subspecialty that gathers the skills, knowledge, and complex decision-making techniques of an ever-widening group of disciplines including general surgery, otolaryngology, general plastic surgery, oral-maxillofacial surgery, and dermatologic surgery. No one specialty claims or should claim total domination, as each contributes to the growing body of knowledge and expertise that guides our understanding of this important organ as well as its surgical manipulation.

The ILLUSTRATED ATLAS OF CUTANEOUS SURGERY by Drs Fewkes, Pollack, and Cheney is a melting pot of basic surgical reasoning and techniques from the dermatologic as well as the reconstructive surgeon. As with any Atlas, it is a work that reflects the vision of its authors and as such is limited in complexity to the techniques and decision-making patterns that each considers to be the foundation on which cutaneous surgery rests.

It is logically organized, beginning with preparation, materials, and basic treatment techniques, and progresses to intermediate and advanced surgical techniques. Each of 34 chapters is condensed into a concise narrative that defines the principles of a disease or technique and the rationale for therapy, and gives a detailed description of the procedures relating to the chapter theme. Complications and alternative therapies are cited when needed.

The illustrations and color photographs are outstanding, detailed, clear, and exacting. Preoperative, postoperative, and intraoperative details meld with those operative pearls that often ensure surgical success. The suggested readings at the end of each chapter are modest but highly selective.

For the student and resident, this Atlas will provide the basic principles needed for a foundation in the study of cutaneous surgery. For the surgical specialist, its detailed methodology will serve as a valuable tool for reference and review. In the prolific world of medical publishing, this work should make its mark.

Richard L Fabian, MD
Director Head and Neck Surgery
Massachusetts Eye and Ear Infirmary
& Massachusetts General Hospital
Boston

In the past two decades, there has been a forceful attack on the major primary cancers arising in the skin—malignant melanoma, squamous cell carcinoma, and basal cell carcinoma. For example, detailed descriptions of the clinical features of *early* malignant melanoma and the massive efforts of public education regarding the detection of early melanoma have dramatically increased the 5-year overall survival rate from 53% in 1962 to 89% in 1990. This is by far the best improvement in the 5-year survival rates of any of the major serious cancers, and malignant melanoma is indeed a major cancer, with 32,000 new cases reported in the United States in 1990.

For skin cancers that are not melanomas, there have been advances in surgical approaches, the most important of which is the widespread use of Mohs' micrographic, or histographic, surgery. Mohs' surgery is but one of many cutaneous surgical approaches that are now being used to treat the skin. The realm of cutaneous surgery, by virtue of the background and training of its practitioners, brings together the collective experience of dermatologists and dermatologic surgeons, plastic and reconstructive surgeons, head and neck surgeons, pathologists, and anesthesiologists. The combined efforts of these various physicians have created a large body of techniques that are being used to treat diseases and deformities of the skin and to enhance its cosmetic appearance—following trauma, the deleterious effects of sunlight, or natural aging.

This new ILLUSTRATED ATLAS OF CUTANEOUS SURGERY adds a dimension not available in previous texts—a step-wise, procedural approach that is illustrated with over 850 color photographs and drawings (a necessity for teaching a manual skill). Furthermore, it is an authoritative work written by two experienced dermatologic surgeons in collaboration with an experienced head and neck reconstructive surgeon. By assembling many techniques and principles into a single volume, the authors present a broadened view of cutaneous surgery. It is all here: fundamentals, from anesthesia to wound infections; descriptions, drawings, and color photographs of specific procedures, including complex excisions, facial scar revision, sclerotherapy, tissue expansion, flaps, grafts, nail surgery, among others; and advanced techniques, including Mohs' micrographic surgery, carbon dioxide laser surgery, dermabrasion, chemical peels, punch hair transplants, and new methods of cultured epidermal autografts, which have proven so successful in the treatment of indolent ulcers.

This new Atlas—clearly written, richly illustrated, and informative—supplements the several excellent books already available on cutaneous surgery, including standard texts and reference manuals. There is no doubt that it will serve to educate both dermatologists and dermatologic surgeons as well as head and neck surgeons and other practitioners interested in cutaneous surgery.

Thomas B Fitzpatrick, MD, PhD, DSc (hon)
Edward C Wigglesworth Professor, *emeritus*
  and *former* Chairman, Department of
  Dermatology
Harvard Medical School
Boston, Massachusetts

Preface

Enthusiasm for this project, and indeed its conception, was founded upon the perceived need for a thorough yet concise visual reference work to address the major aspects of cutaneous surgery from a clinical and practical point of view. This Atlas is our attempt to provide such a work, in presenting a foundation of visual and textual information upon which the physician interested in a variety of techniques in cutaneous surgery can build.

The format for this Atlas has been carefully constructed to provide the reader with a discussion of the basic principles of surgery followed by a practical approach to a wide range of clinical problems and surgical options. The Atlas seeks to address the needs of many levels of experience, from the beginner to the advanced student of cutaneous surgery, and from the resident to the practitioner seeking to broaden his or her clinical range. Aside from its purely practical purpose of providing a basis upon which technique can be learned, we hope that the Atlas can also serve as an educational tool to enable physicians to have greater knowledge of specific procedures in discussing surgical options with their patients. The Atlas is divided into four sections. The first two sections cover the basic principles and techniques upon which the more intermediate and advanced techniques in cutaneous surgery are based. The third section covers intermediate techniques and the fourth section covers advanced techniques. The presentation of clinical and intraoperative color photographs and illustrations is accompanied by extensive descriptive information to enable the reader to obtain as complete an understanding as possible of the procedure under discussion. A list of suggested readings at the end of each chapter seeks to enable the reader to further his or her knowledge by obtaining additional information on a particular topic.

As a group, we bring varied clinical backgrounds to this Atlas. Dr Fewkes is currently Co-Director of Mohs' and Cutaneous Surgery at the Massachusetts General Hospital in Boston; Dr Pollack is formerly Director of Dermatologic Surgery at Duke University Medical Center in Durham, North Carolina (1979 to 1990) and currently is Director of Cutaneous Surgery at the University of Toronto, Division of Dermatology, in Toronto, Ontario, Canada; Dr Cheney is presently Director of Facial Plastic and Reconstructive Surgery at the Massachusetts Eye and Ear Infirmary in Boston. We hope that the breadth of our experience and training speaks to the diversity of physicians who have an interest in surgery of the skin. Indeed, the field of cutaneous surgery is a "melting pot," and the broad range of its practitioners' backgrounds has enhanced the development of techniques and procedures that are used to treat diseases of the skin and to provide acceptable options for the full aesthetic and functional reconstruction of cutaneous defects and the appropriate management of cosmetic complaints.

Jessica L Fewkes, MD
Sheldon V Pollack, MD
Mack L Cheney, MD

Contents

Section Three
Intermediate Techniques

Section Four
Advanced Techniques

SECTION ONE

PATIENT PREPARATION AND MATERIALS

chapter 1

INTRODUCTION

The cutaneous surgeon handles a broad range of treatment options for the largest organ of the body, the skin. From the removal of benign or malignant skin diseases, to the repair of skin when it has been injured, to the improvement of its appearance, the techniques available to the cutaneous surgeon are many. In applying these techniques, the practitioner of cutaneous surgery combines elements of otolaryngology, dermatology, surgery, ophthalmology, and plastic surgery. Cutaneous surgery is thus unique in that it encompasses many different specialties.

Because of the way in which most cutaneous surgical procedures are performed, in an outpatient setting under local anesthesia, and because of the visibility of the operative result, routine aspects of surgery take on special significance. These aspects, including patient preparation, physical plant, and the relationship between patient and physician, are the subject of this chapter.

PATIENT PREPARATION

Patient preparation is an important aspect of cutaneous surgery and should be considered a part of it. It begins with a consultation between patient and physician at a time prior to the scheduled procedure. First, the surgeon must ascertain the accuracy of the diagnosis and the appropriateness of the planned pro-cedure. For example, the surgeon may be presented with a referral for excision of a large malignant lesion not previously sampled by biopsy, whose removal will leave a significant scar. The surgeon may feel that it is better to document the malignancy before proceeding with the excision. Similarly, the surgeon may be faced with a controversial biopsy report that has been provided by a pathol-

---

FIGURE 1.1
SPECIAL CATEGORIES TO BE COVERED IN MEDICAL HISTORY

1. Infectious diseases, eg, hepatitis
2. Cardiac disease
   a. pacemaker
   b. valve disease/replacement
   c. history of rheumatic fever
3. Bleeding disorders
4. Hypertension
5. Medications
   a. monoamine oxidase inhibitors
   b. anticoagulants, including aspirin
   c. anti-inflammatory agents
   d. propranolol hydrochloride
6. Prostheses

7. Allergies
   a. tapes/adhesives
   b. iodine or other topical antiseptics
   c. topical antibacterials
   d. anesthetic agents
8. Prophylaxis
9. Epilepsy
10. Alcohol use
11. Tobacco use
12. Keloid formation
13. Glaucoma
14. Pregnancy

ogist with whom he or she is unfamiliar. In such a case, the surgeon may elect to have the tissue sample reexamined.

Once the surgeon is comfortable with the diagnosis and choice of procedure, the surgery itself should be explained completely to the patient, along with a discussion of alternative modes of treatment. The risks and benefits of the procedure should be explained, as well as the preoperative and postoperative requirements and how the patient must plan to meet those requirements. For example, without such guidance, a patient may arrive on the morning of surgery for removal of a lesion on the lower leg with plans to leave the following day on a long and active vacation. Similarly, a patient whose job requires a great deal of talking may fail to arrange for adequate time off from work for removal of a skin cancer on the upper lip. Surgical complications are fewer when an understanding is reached between physician and patient as to the procedure and its perioperative requirements. In this regard, the presurgical consultation and/or a written explanation of the procedure is essential.

MEDICAL HISTORY

The preoperative consultation also provides the surgeon with an opportunity to obtain from the patient a detailed medical history. In addition to a complete review of systems,

special attention should be paid to certain categories (Figure 1.1). A consultation with the internist or specialist caring for the patient may be done and can help the surgeon to determine such factors as whether anticoagulant medications may be stopped 5 to 7 days before surgery, whether prophylaxis should be considered for the patient, and whether the patient has any special preoperative or postoperative needs. For example, the use of epinephrine in the local anesthetic for a patient with cardiac disease and/or arrhythmias may be contraindicated, or there may be concerns over a patient's emotional stability and/or support system relative to a planned procedure.

INFORMED CONSENT

Informed consent is a critical issue today. The patient must give his or her informed consent to the procedure. This may be done at the time of the preoperative consultation or immediately prior to the procedure. The consent form should be read by the patient, his or her questions answered, and any issues specific to the patient, such as pregnancy or any preexisting neural deficits, noted on the form. The patient, or responsible adult on behalf of the patient, must be of legal age, which may vary from state to state.

At a minimum, a consent for cutaneous surgery should include the possibility of bleeding, infection, pain, scarring, incomplete removal of abnormal tissue, recurrence of abnormal tissue, and nerve damage (Figure 1.2). It is especially important to inform the patient that there will be a scar, as patients often are not expecting one. In addition to the consent, it is often helpful to obtain the patient's permission for use of photographs taken in connection with the procedure (see Figure 1.2).

The patient also may be provided with printed preoperative and postoperative instructions, which the surgeon can distribute during the consultation or at the time of surgery along with other pertinent information. Patients will greatly appreciate having a written reference should they not remember the physician's exact instructions pertaining to the procedure, as is sometimes the case.

PHYSICAL PLANT

Once the necessary paperwork is completed, attention may turn toward preparation of the surgical suite. The comfort of the physician and the patient is of paramount importance. The surgeon may perform the procedure sitting or standing, although there must be as little strain as possible placed on his or her back. This usually requires that the surgeon be positioned in fairly close proximity to the surgical site, with the patient placed on an adjustable table that elevates as a unit and also allows independent movement of the patient's torso, head, and feet. The table should be narrow enough so that the surgeon can be comfortable when operating on a lesion in the patient's midline. It should also allow the patient to be placed in Trendelenburg's position. The patient may need extra support under his or her knees or back. Table tops with thin paper coverings may be slippery and angling the table back a little may help the patient feel more secure.

Good lighting is another essential feature. Overhead track lighting with multiple sources is ideal as it removes the lighting apparatus completely from the operating field while permitting light to illuminate it regardless of the head positions of the surgical team. Cool halogen bulbs are a tremendous advantage. Single spot lights, attached either to a pole on the operating table or to a movable stand, also work well. They are less expensive than track lighting although they are somewhat more cumbersome. The lighting should be positioned so that it does not shine directly into the patient's eyes.

A sink should also be available, and emergency equipment must be positioned in close proximity to the operating suite. Also necessary are a suction machine and a cautery machine. For the setup of instruments to be used during the procedure, Mayo stands placed near the operating table or attached to it on a pole are most useful.

The room itself should be used as much as possible for surgery, to the exclusion of other procedures. There should be adequate ventilation and relatively little floor traffic. Patients with obvious contamination of wounds (impetigo, viral infections) or with colonized skin (eczema, psoriasis) are best not examined in surgical rooms, although if such examination is unavoidable, the room should be cleansed thoroughly before a surgical procedure is performed. This involves the wiping off of all surfaces with a disinfectant and airing out of the room.

ASPECTS OF THE PATIENT/PHYSICIAN RELATIONSHIP

As noted earlier, most cutaneous surgery is performed under local anesthesia, often in an office surgical suite. Because of this fact, and because in many cases the patient has the opportunity to respond immediately to the results of surgery, a unique relationship exists between physician and patient. Beforehand, the surgeon should plan to spend a fair amount of time explaining to the patient the procedure and its possible sequelae, such as persistent erythema following a deep chemi-

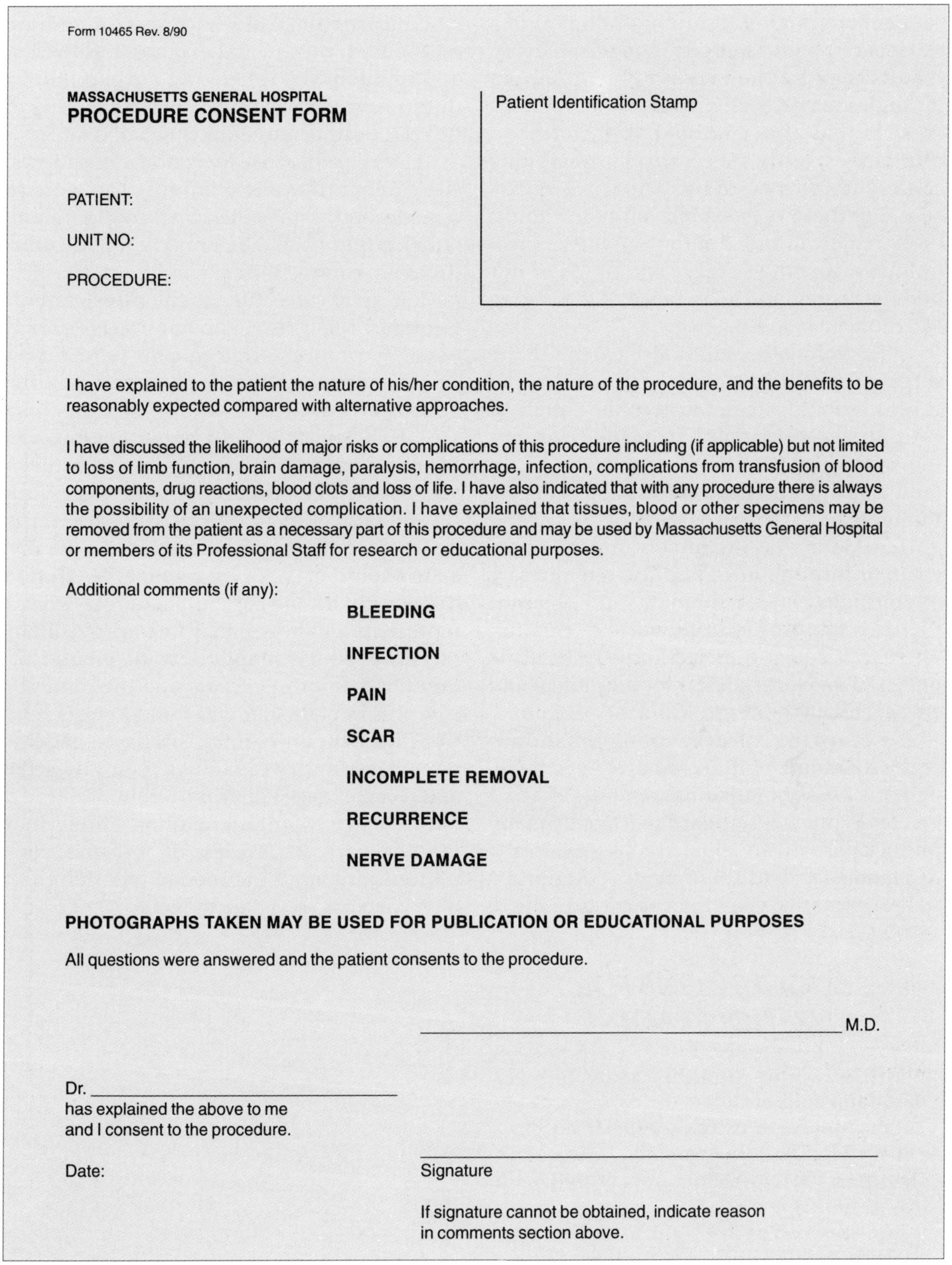

Form 10465 Rev. 8/90

MASSACHUSETTS GENERAL HOSPITAL
PROCEDURE CONSENT FORM

Patient Identification Stamp

PATIENT:

UNIT NO:

PROCEDURE:

I have explained to the patient the nature of his/her condition, the nature of the procedure, and the benefits to be reasonably expected compared with alternative approaches.

I have discussed the likelihood of major risks or complications of this procedure including (if applicable) but not limited to loss of limb function, brain damage, paralysis, hemorrhage, infection, complications from transfusion of blood components, drug reactions, blood clots and loss of life. I have also indicated that with any procedure there is always the possibility of an unexpected complication. I have explained that tissues, blood or other specimens may be removed from the patient as a necessary part of this procedure and may be used by Massachusetts General Hospital or members of its Professional Staff for research or educational purposes.

Additional comments (if any):

    BLEEDING

    INFECTION

    PAIN

    SCAR

    INCOMPLETE REMOVAL

    RECURRENCE

    NERVE DAMAGE

PHOTOGRAPHS TAKEN MAY BE USED FOR PUBLICATION OR EDUCATIONAL PURPOSES

All questions were answered and the patient consents to the procedure.

_____ M.D.

Dr. _____
has explained the above to me
and I consent to the procedure.

Date: _____

Signature

If signature cannot be obtained, indicate reason
in comments section above.

FIGURE 1.2 An example of the procedure consent form in current use at Massachusetts General Hospital. All of the specific complications noted under "Additional comments" are a modification to the form made by the Department of Dermatologic Surgery at Massachusetts General Hospital for use by them only.

cal peel or scarring following removal of a skin cancer. With some techniques, satisfying results may be months away as scars go through a remodeling process or dermabraded skin reassumes normal skin tones. In other cases, truly successful surgical outcomes may be marred by recurrence of disease. For these reasons, the surgeon should be extremely mindful of the patient's expectations regarding surgery and of his or her understanding and acceptance of the course of treatment and recovery.

These considerations also extend to the surgery itself. Throughout the procedure, the surgeon should attempt to keep the patient at ease. Strategies for doing so include conversing with the patient during the procedure (and also minimizing conversation with the nurse or assistant to the exclusion of the patient); the playing of soft music from a radio or through head phones; a temperate operating room environment; and pleasant pictures hanging on the walls or ceiling. These techniques, if used effectively, have the potential to reduce anxiety for the patient and stress for both the surgeon and the patient.

Following surgery, patients should receive adequate follow-up care. Normally, patients are seen for suture removal at 1 to 2 weeks. While not standard practice by many physicians, patients should be seen again at 3 to 6 months and also at 12 months. At the initial preoperative visit, the patient is likely to be concerned mainly with the immediate postoperative result and diagnosis. However, at 3 to 6 months following surgery, other questions may arise such as those having to do with postoperative scarring and cosmesis.

A frequent cause for concern in patients, scars generally take 6 months to 1 year to remodel and assume their final configuration. During that time, they may vary in color, firmness, contractibility, and discomfort. The patient who can return to the physician for guidance regarding a postoperative scar is usually a more satisfied one who better understands the nature and timetable of the healing process.

Honesty is the most important factor in the relationship between cutaneous surgeon and patient. The cutaneous surgeon's work by and large is available for all to see. If the patient is unhappy with the outcome, the surgeon should make every reasonable effort to discuss it with the patient, including what it represents and how it may be improved. The physician who is straightforward about treatment outcomes in general and the patient's concerns in particular will build a closer relationship with the patient. Similarly, patients who feel that they can talk to their physician and receive honest answers rarely will find it necessary to complain to others about their medical care. Regardless of outcome, such patients are more inclined to feel that their physician has served them well.

SUGGESTIONS FOR FURTHER READING

Bennett RG. Office Surgical Facility. In: Fundamentals of Cutaneous Surgery. St Louis, Mo: C V Mosby Co;1988:181-193.

Goldwyn R. The Patient and the Plastic Surgeon. Boston, Mass: Little, Brown & Co Inc;1981.

Tobin HA. Office surgery: the surgical suite. J Dermatol Surg Oncol. 1988;14:247-255.

chapter 2

SUTURE MATERIALS AND INSTRUMENTS

The choice of proper suture materials, in combination with correct needle type and appropriate instrumentation, is important in enabling the cutaneous surgeon to achieve the best possible long-term, soft-tissue result. Suture materials vary in terms of their handling, strength, and retention and have been designed with specific surgical needs in mind. The personal preference of the surgeon also plays a role in the selection of suture materials.

Sutures are divided into two broad categories: absorbable and nonabsorbable. Absorbable sutures have a limited life in soft tissue whereas nonabsorbable sutures are retained permanently. A further subdivision is that of monofilament versus multifilament. Monofilament suture is made of a single strand of material, which gives it smooth handling properties. However, there is some associated knot slippage, which can be reduced by careful knot placement. Multifilament suture, by contrast, consists of several filaments twisted or braided together, an arrangement that enhances its tying capabilities and also reduces knot slippage. It does, however, permit the harboring of microorganisms.

The size and tensile strength of all suture materials are standardized. Size denotes the diameter of the material, which, stated numerically, decreases with the number of zeros listed. The most common suture sizes for cutaneous surgical procedures are between 3-0 (000) and 6-0 (000000), with 3-0 and 4-0 used for subcutaneous closure and 5-0 and 6-0 used for cutaneous closure. The tensile strength, by definition, is the amount of tension or pull expressed in pounds that a suture strand can withstand before it breaks. It is related to the type of suture material and to its size, with the larger suture materials exhibiting the greater tensile strength.

ABSORBABLE SUTURES

The *United States Pharmacopeia (USP)* defines an absorbable suture as (1) a sterile strand of material that is prepared from collagen derived from healthy mammals, or (2) a synthetic polymer that is capable of being absorbed by living mammalian tissue. Figure 2.1 lists the common types of absorbable sutures and gives the basic raw material from which each is manufactured.

In terms of performance, the important characteristics of absorbable sutures are how long they retain their tensile strength and their absorption rate. Absorption rates can be influenced by body temperature and by the presence of infection, both of which can result in more rapid absorption of sutures. Absorbable sutures should be avoided in situations in which long-term tension control will be required for adequate closure of the wound.

Absorbable surgical gut sutures are classified either as plain or chromic, both of which are monofilament sutures made of highly purified collagen from the submucosa of sheep. Chromic gut suture is processed to provide greater resistance to absorption and in certain patients may elicit a local soft-tissue response. Plain gut suture retains its maximum tensile strength for approximately 7 days, while chromic gut suture retains its maximum strength for 10 to 14 days. *Dexon*, a braided suture composed of polyglycolic acid, was originally introduced as an uncoat-

FIGURE 2.1
TYPES OF ABSORBABLE SUTURES

SUTURE	RAW MATERIAL
surgical gut	submucosa of sheep intestine
Dexon	polyglycolic acid
Vicryl	copolymer of glycolide
PDS	polyester of *p*-dioxane

ed suture (Dexon "S") but has since been modified with a coating of Poloxamer 188, which provides the newer suture (Dexon Plus) with improved soft-tissue handling characteristics. Dexon retains approximately 65% of its tensile strength for 14 days. It is absorbed faster than PDS but persists longer than Vicryl. It is used for subcutaneous soft-tissue closure.

Vicryl is a synthetic absorbable multifilament suture that retains its maximum strength for 14 to 21 days and therefore is good for tissue support over a longer period of time than that provided by surgical gut. *PDS* is a monofilament synthetic absorbable suture that retains its maximum strength for

35 to 45 days and offers long-term tissue support. Absorption of PDS can be expected to be complete after approximately 180 days (Figure 2.2).

NONABSORBABLE SUTURES

By *USP* definition, nonabsorbable sutures are strands of material that are resistant to degradation by living, mammalian tissue. Figure 2.3 lists several nonabsorbable sutures and the basic material from which each is manufactured. *Surgical silk* is a commonly used multifilament nonabsorbable suture material, which historically for many surgeons has

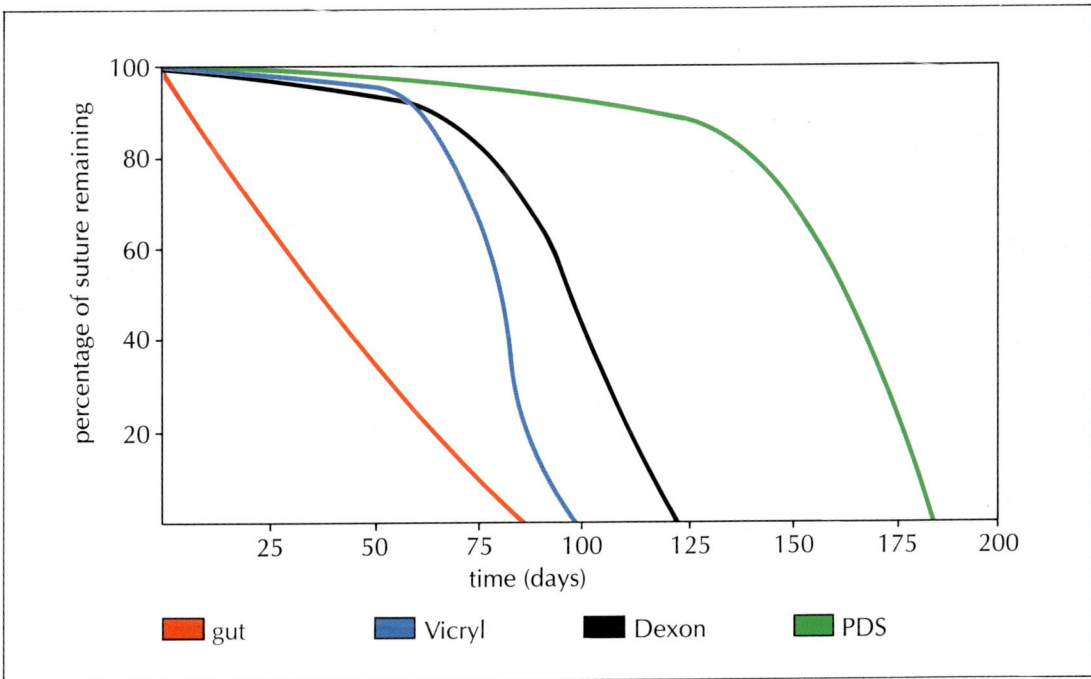

FIGURE 2.2 Graph showing percentage of absorbable suture material remaining over time.

represented the highest standard of performance, particularly in terms of its handling
properties. It does, however, elicit a moderate
tissue reaction if left in place for more than 4
to 5 days and therefore is useful in the closure
of wounds in rapidly healing areas such as
the head and neck, mucosal surfaces, and the
eyelids.

Surgical stainless steel wire sutures represent optimal strength and minimal tissue
reaction in wound closure. They are used in
areas where long-term tension control is
needed, such as in cartilage graft stabilization
and in auricular repairs. Many surgeons dis-
like wire however because it is difficult to tie.

Nylon (Ethilon) suture, a synthetic monofilament suture, has a high tensile strength
and its tissue reaction is extremely low. Because it is a monofilament suture its tying
properties are good, although careful knot
placement is essential to prevent slippage.
Although traditionally used for external cutaneous closure, nylon also is well suited for
the subcutaneous closure of wounds in
which there is an unusual degree of tension.
Polypropylene (Prolene) suture is extremely
inert in tissue, thereby causing minimal tissue reaction. Due to its relative biologic inert-
ness, it is recommended for use in locations
where the least possible tissue reaction is
desired, such as in the head and neck area. A
synthetic monofilament suture, it holds a
knot better than do other monofilament
sutures although careful attention to knot
tying must be given to avoid the complication
of slippage, which is largely avoided with
multifilament suture. Also, because of the
lack of reaction to it in tissue, polypropylene
is well suited for use as a running subcuticular (pull-out) suture.

Ethibond is a braided strand of polyester
fibers coated with polybutilate. The coating
is very adherent to the suture fibers and acts
as a lubricant to improve the passage of the

FIGURE 2.3
TYPES OF NONABSORBABLE SUTURES

SUTURE	RAW MATERIAL
surgical silk	raw silk spun by silkworms
surgical stainless steel	iron, nickel, & chromium alloy
nylon (Ethilon)	polyamide polymer
polypropylene (Prolene)	polymer of propylene
Ethibond	polyester fibers

suture material through the tissue. Both the polyester suture material and the polybutilate coating are inert and should elicit minimal tissue reaction. However, in clinical use, some erythema is always noted around sutures left in place for more than 7 days, which rapidly fades after suture removal and leaves no residual mark. A table comparing the commonly used suture materials discussed in this chapter is presented in Figure 2.4.

FIGURE 2.4
COMPARISON OF COMMONLY USED SUTURE MATERIALS

SUTURE MATERIAL	ABSORPTION PROFILE*	STRENGTH	HANDLING	KNOT SECURITY	TISSUE REACTION
surgical gut	70-90 days	fair	fair	good	moderate
Dexon "S"	90-120 days	good	fair	good	minimal to moderate
Dexon Plus	90-120 days	good	good	fair	minimal to moderate
Vicryl	75-90 days	good	fair	good	minimal to moderate
PDS	150-180 days	excellent	fair to good	fair	minimal
surgical silk	long-term†	good	excellent	excellent	moderate to high
surgical stainless steel	permanent	excellent	poor	fair	minimal
nylon	long-term†	excellent	good	fair	minimal
polypropylene	permanent	excellent	fair to good	fair	minimal
Ethibond	long-term	excellent	good	good	moderate

*Time in days at which suture material is completely absorbed

†While this suture is classified as nonabsorbable, some degradation over time can be expected for sutures left in place.

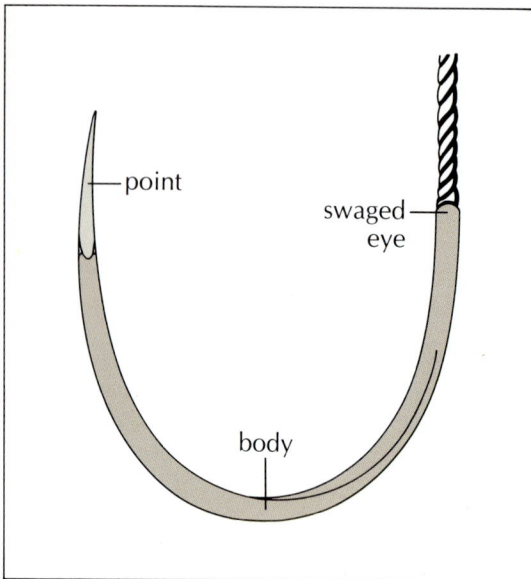

FIGURE 2.5
Schematic drawing showing basic needle components, including the point, the body, and the eye. Shown here is a needle with a flat body and a tapered point. The eye is swaged, with the suture thread attached to it.

Needle Shape		Clinical Applications
straight		nasal cavity oral cavity skin
¼ circle		microsurgical procedures
⅜ circle		fascia perichondrium periosteum muscle
½ circle		muscle nasal cavity oral cavity skin subcutaneous fat

FIGURE 2.6 Schematic drawing showing the basic needle body shapes used in cutaneous surgery, with common clinical applications.

BASIC NEEDLE DESIGN

All surgical needles have three basic components: the eye, the body, and the point (Figure 2.5). Approximately 80% of sutures in use today are "swaged," with the suture material attached to the needle at the eye. Nonswaged needles are used when the surgeon needs to customize the suture material and needle type, using a combination that is not commercially available. Nonswaged needles have either a drilled hole in the end of the needle for insertion of the suture material or a hollow lumen through which the suture is placed.

The *body*, or shaft, of the needle is the area at which it is grasped by the needle holder. The cross-sectional configuration of the needle body varies so that round, triangu-lar, or flat-sided needles may be selected. Additionally, the longitudinal shape of the needle body may be straight, half curved (¼ circle), or fully curved (⅜ circle or ½ circle), with the choice of body shape relating to the specific surgical requirements (Figure 2.6).

The *point* of the needle extends from its extreme tip to the maximum cross section of its body. The sharpness of the needle point, in association with the shape and size of its body, is important. The basic needle types are conventional cutting, reverse cutting, tapered, and blunt (Figure 2.7).

Conventional cutting needles and reverse cutting needles are useful for skin sutures that pass through relatively thick soft tissue. Conventional cutting needles are unsuitable for the suturing of thin or friable tissue such as oral mucosa in that inadvertent

Point		Body	Soft-Tissue Application
◬	conventional cutting	▢	cutaneous surgery
▽	reverse cutting	▽	cutaneous surgery oral mucosa
⊙	tapered	▢	muscle nerve subcutaneous fat or fascia
○	blunt	▢	mucosal repair compromised tissue repair

FIGURE 2.7 Schematic drawing showing the configuration of the commonly used needle body shapes and point designs that can be utilized for various soft-tissue closure objectives.

cutting of the tissue may result. Reverse cutting needles, by contrast, are safer when used in more delicate tissues because of the location of the cutting surface. Tapered needles are characterized by a body that tapers to a sharp point at the tip. They are preferred in situations in which the smallest possible hole in the tissue is desired and produce minimal tissue damage. They are used primarily in soft, easily penetrated tissues such as muscles, fascia, or subcutaneous tissue. The blunt point needle is used to dissect through friable tissue. It has a tapered body with a rounded blunt point, which pushes rather than cuts through the tissue. Its use in cutaneous surgery is minimal, limited to its occasional use for the closure of very friable mucosal tissue or irradiated tissue.

    The cutaneous surgeon should also be familiar with the nomenclature used for the marketing of needles. According to one manufacturer's system, four different types of needles commonly used in cutaneous surgery are identified as *FS* ("for skin"), *PS* ("plastic surgery"), *PC* ("precision cosmetic"), and *P* ("plastic"). All of these needles are reverse cutting needles, except for PC, which is a conventional cutting needle. Apart from their cutting edge, these needles differ in terms of their caliber (measured at the swaged end), their needle curvature length, and their sharpness. Needle nomenclature is unique to each manufacturer (Figure 2.8A,B).

INSTRUMENTS

Proper instrument selection is equally important to the surgical repair of soft-tissue defects, with instruments that are commonly used in general surgery too large and cumbersome for the fine detail of careful skin suturing. Therefore special instruments are necessary. The needle holder is designed to grasp and securely maintain the body of the

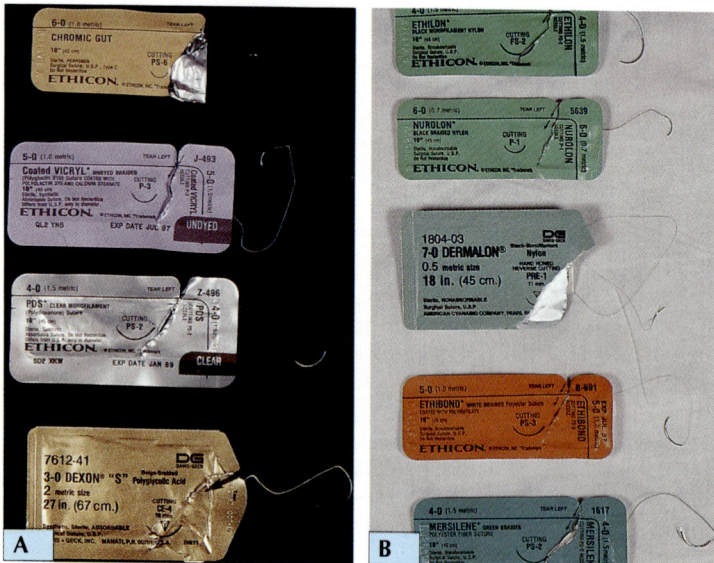

FIGURE 2.8 (A) Four packages of absorbable suture with various needle types: (top to bottom) 6-0 chromic gut on a PS-6 needle (suture not shown), 5-0 Vicryl on a P-3 needle, 4-0 PDS on a PS-2 needle, and 3-0 Dexon on a CE-4 needle. Note that the larger suture is usually attached to a larger needle. (B) Some examples of nonabsorbable suture with various needle types: (top to bottom) 4-0 Ethilon on an FS-2 needle, 6-0 Nurolon on a P-1 needle, 7-0 Dermalon on a PRE-1 needle, 5-0 Ethibond on a PS-3 needle, 4-0 Mersilene on a PS-2 needle.

suture needle and to facilitate suture tying. The most commonly used needle holder for soft-tissue repair is the *Webster needle holder*, which handles 4-0 to 7-0 suture well. Its flat platforms are less traumatic to the suture than are the grooves or teeth on the occlusal platforms of other needle holders. The *Gillies needle holder* also is useful although due to its asymmetric design usually requires some experience before it can be handled properly. The curve of the Gillies needle holder, as well as its built-in suture scissors, can enable efficient suture tying (Figure 2.9).

Soft-tissue forceps are used for the handling of tissue. They are available with either toothed or smooth tips. In most situations, forceps with teeth are less traumatic than are smooth forceps, which tend to crush soft tissue. In the former category, *Brown-Adson forceps* are useful for the handling of large, heavy tissues such as those encountered in the closure of scalp, neck, lip, and cheek wounds. Their rows of sharp teeth provide secure traction and the grasping platform is useful for facilitating the passage of the suture needle through the tissue. For the handling of more

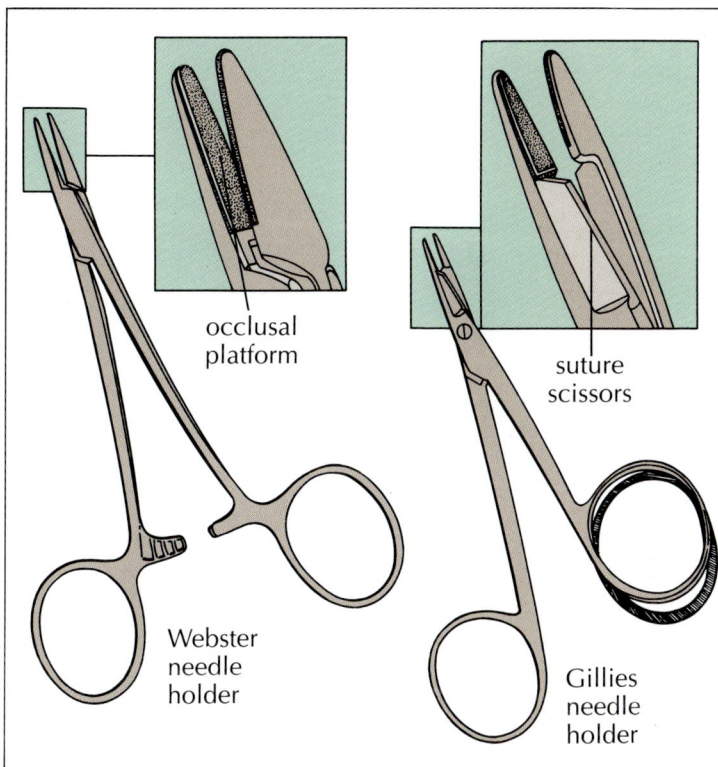

occlusal platform

suture scissors

Webster needle holder

Gillies needle holder

FIGURE 2.9 *At left,* a Webster needle holder, with inset showing occlusal platform. *At right,* a Gillies needle holder, with inset showing occlusal platform and suture scissors.

delicate tissues, such as those of the eyelid, nose, or ear, *Castroviejo forceps* are recommended, with the platform behind their teeth useful for manipulation of the delicate needle found with fine suture material (Figure 2.10). For the handling of thin tissue, many very fine forceps exist, such as *Bishop-Harmon forceps*, *Foerster forceps*, and *fine iris forceps*. The preference of the surgeon for any of these types may depend on the hand size of the surgeon, the tissue being worked on, and the surgeon's training.

Every effort should be made to use delicate skin hooks to retract soft-tissue flaps. Double, single, and scleral hooks are available and each has a place in proper soft-tissue management (Figure 2.11). Double hooks are used for larger tissue flaps; single hooks for

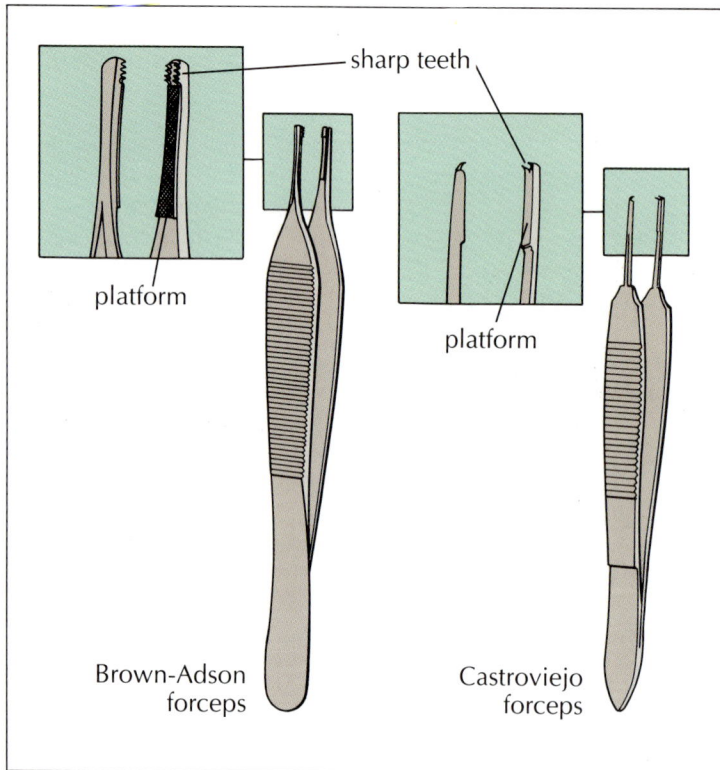

sharp teeth

platform

platform

Brown-Adson forceps

Castroviejo forceps

FIGURE **2.10** *At left,* Brown-Adson forceps are useful for the handling of large, heavy tissues. *At right,* Castroviejo forceps are useful for the manipulation of more delicate tissues, such as those of the eyelid, nose, or ear.

smaller tissue flaps and to direct cutaneous tension favorably to facilitate undermining; and scleral hooks are used with delicate tissue flaps where thin skin is encountered.

In addition, to minimize soft-tissue trauma, the surgeon must insist on sharp, well-maintained scissors. *Metzenbaum scissors*, because of their design advantages including a gently curved blade, blunt tip, and long contact area, are useful in developing local flaps and in cutting thick, less delicate tissue. *Delicate suture scissors*, by design, have sharp points, a shorter contact area, and straight blades and therefore are useful for finer struc-

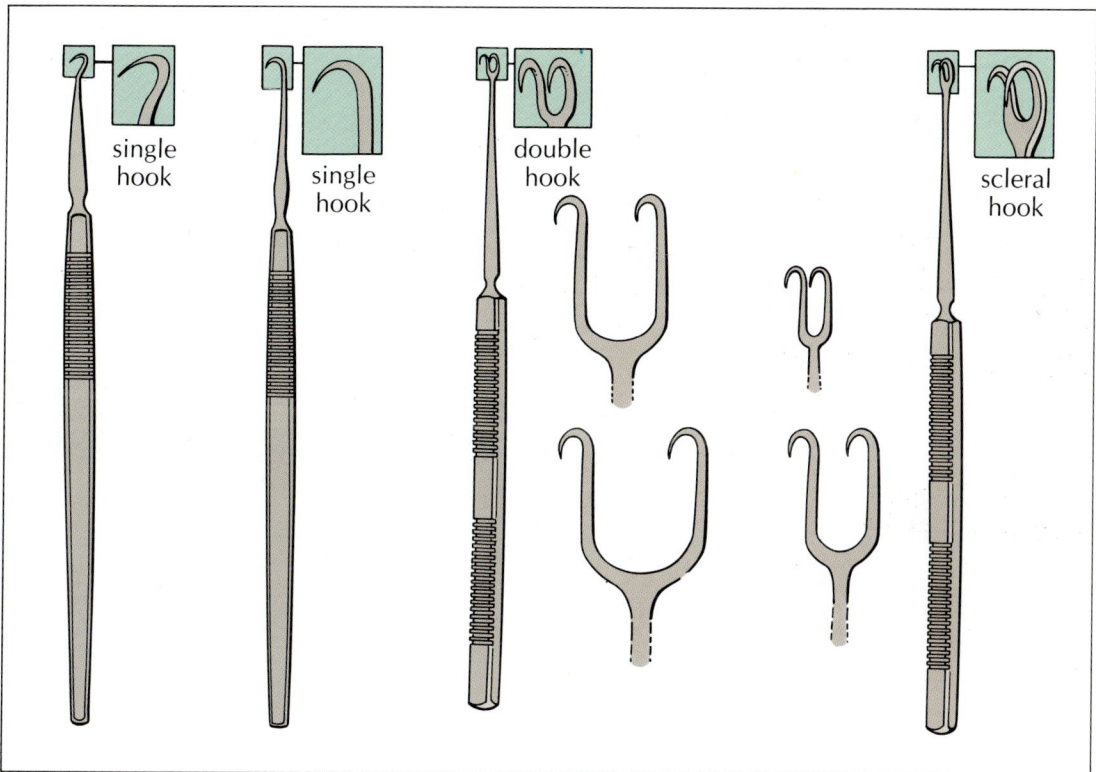

single hook

single hook

double hook

scleral hook

FIGURE 2.11 From left to right, a variety of single, double, and scleral hooks are shown.

tures and for performing detailed and accurate soft-tissue tailoring (Figure 2.12). In addition to suture scissors for fine tissue cutting, there are *Stevens tenotomy scissors*, *fine iris scissors*, and *Gradle scissors*, all of which do the same job. The choice of instrument is mainly dependent on the preference of the surgeon and his or her experience with any one type.

Castroviejo calipers (Figure 2.13) are designed to allow the surgeon to make accurate measurements of soft-tissue defects, lesions, and proposed local flaps for reconstruction. The calipers are easily adjusted for appropriate measurement, which then can be "locked in" for future reference.

The scalpel blades used most commonly in soft-tissue surgery are #15, #10, and #11 (Figure 2.14). The #15 blade is most commonly used for initial incisions and in some cases for soft-tissue undermining. The #10 blade is a larger blade, whose purpose in soft-tissue surgery is to incise heavy tissues such as scalp and cervical skin. The #11 blade is used for detailed cutting around flaps and for tailoring.

For approximating wound edges in superficial lacerations and incisions, for minimizing tension across a surgical incision in the immediate postoperative period, and for long-term control of tension across the surgical incision following suture removal, Steri-Strips are useful (Figure 2.15; see also Figure 15.5D).

For general soft-tissue surgery, the surgeon's tray might include the following: one Webster needle holder, one Gillies needle

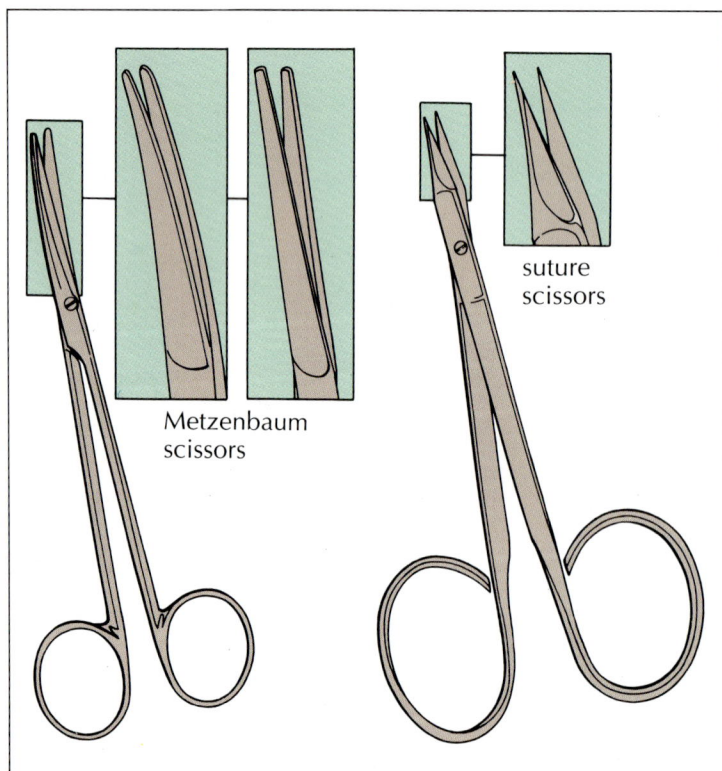

suture scissors

Metzenbaum scissors

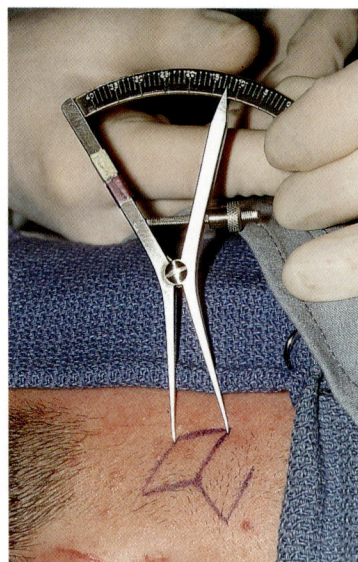

FIGURE 2.13 Castroviejo calipers allow the surgeon to make accurate measurements of soft-tissue defects, lesions, and proposed local flaps for reconstruction.

FIGURE 2.12 *At left,* Metzenbaum scissors are useful for developing local flaps and for the cutting of thick, less delicate tissues. *At right,* delicate suture scissors are useful for the accurate tailoring of finer structures.

holder, one pair of Metzenbaum scissors, one pair of delicate suture scissors, two Castroviejo forceps, two Brown-Adson forceps, two single hooks, two double hooks, two scleral hooks, one pair of suture scissors, scalpel handles, scalpel blades, and one pair of Castroviejo calipers. This setup is useful for a variety of plastic reconstructive techniques (Figure 2.16). For other types of cutaneous surgical procedures, such as simple and complex excisions, Mohs' surgery, nail surgery, biopsy, or other excisional techniques, an alternative setup may be preferred (Figure 2.17). With regard to additional techniques described throughout this Atlas, such as electrosurgery, cryosurgery, curettage, or der-

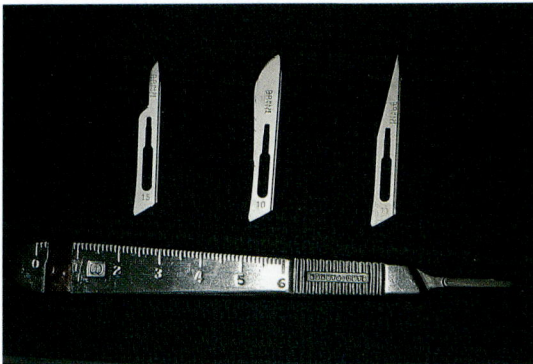

FIGURE 2.14 Commonly used blades in cutaneous surgery include #15, #10, and #11. They are interchangeable with a standard Bard-Parker scalpel handle.

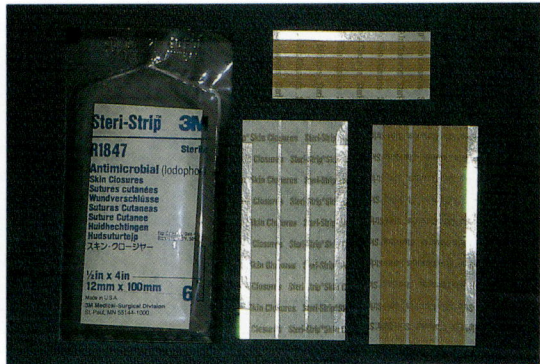

FIGURE 2.15 Steri-Strips are available in a variety of sizes and colors and are useful to facilitate the long-term control of tension across surgical incisions and traumatic lacerations.

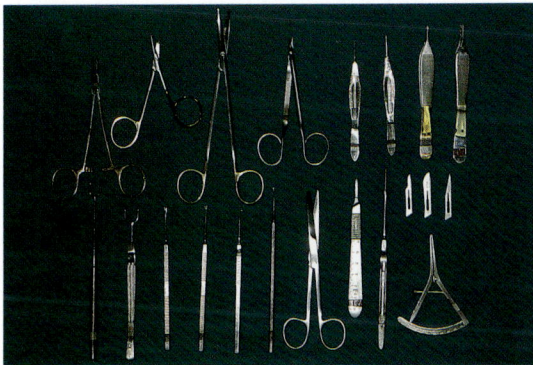

FIGURE 2.16 This soft-tissue surgical tray includes (top row) a Webster needle holder, a Gillies needle holder, Metzenbaum scissors, delicate suture scissors, two Castroviejo forceps, and two Brown-Adson forceps; (bottom row) single hooks, wide double hooks, two scleral hooks, suture scissors, two scalpel handles, scalpel blades, and Castroviejo calipers.

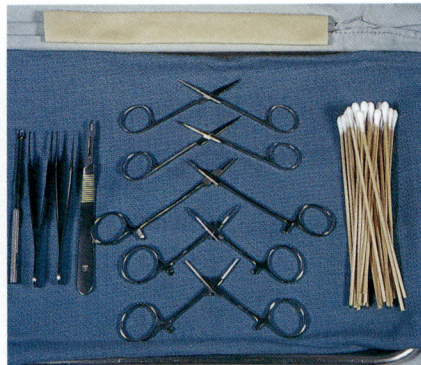

FIGURE 2.17 Basic instrument tray used in cutaneous surgery. Included are the following: (left to right) a double-pronged skin hook, Brown-Adson forceps, smooth Adson forceps, scalpel handle with #15 blade; (top to bottom) Penrose drain for use as sterile sleeve for electrocautery unit, suture scissors, straight fine iris scissors, Webster needle holder, and curved and smooth mosquito hemostats; (right) cotton-tipped applicators to blot small areas.

mabrasion, specific surgical instruments and materials are described as they relate to the particular surgical procedure.

STERILIZATION OF INSTRUMENTS

General guidelines regarding the sterilization of instruments are presented here. All new or nonsterile surgical instruments should be washed meticulously in warm soapy water, rinsed thoroughly, and dried. The instruments should then be placed in breathable, peel-open packages that should be dated and sealed. The packages are commercially supplied along with rolls of tape that change color to indicate the completion of sterilization, and a piece of this tape should be placed in each package to be sterilized. If a gas sterilizer is used, tip protectors may be used instead of plastic packages.

All instruments are then placed in the sterilizer unit on appropriate sterilizer trays and the manufacturer's instructions for proper use of the sterilizer unit followed. Once sterilization is complete, instruments are sorted into appropriate surgical sets, which are then wrapped in surgical towels, appropriately labeled, and placed in a designated clean area that contains only sterilized instruments. Individual instruments and packages that have been sterilized by gas remain as such for 1 year, whereas steam-sterilized instruments are good for 1 month following sterilization.

SUGGESTIONS FOR FURTHER READING

Bennett RG. Fundamentals of Cutaneous Surgery. St Louis, Mo: C V Mosby Co;1988: 274-309.

Clark DE. Surgical suture materials. Contemporary Surgery. 1980; 17:33-48.

Grande DJ, Neuburg M. Instrumentation for the dermatologic surgeon. J Dermatol Surg Oncol. 1989;15:288-297.

Sabiston DC Jr, ed. Davis-Christopher Textbook of Surgery. The Biological Basis of Modern Surgical Practice. 11th ed. Philadelphia, Pa: Saunders, 1977.

Trier WC. Considerations in the choice of surgical needles. Surg Gynecol Obstet. 1979;149:84-94.

Van Winkle W Jr, Hastings JC. Considerations in the choice of suture materials for various tissues. Surg Gynecol Obstet. 1972;135:113-126.

chapter 3

ANTISEPSIS

Antisepsis is the process by which micro-organisms are eliminated on living tissue. It is a process that is centuries old and dates back to times when the cleansing of wounds with wine or beer was standard medical practice. However, little advancement was made in the reduction of wound infection until Ignaz Semmelweis in the mid-19th century advocated routine hand washing for medical personnel. Joseph Lister, approximately 20 years later, considered the probability that microorganisms in and about a wound were responsible for wound infections. By suggesting that they be killed by using phenol, he thus advocated specific elimination of pathogenic microorganisms. He is considered the father of antisepsis, also called listerism.

Antiseptic principles did not arise for use only in operating theaters, but also for use in nurseries and critical care units. They were mostly ignored in outpatient settings. The majority of cutaneous surgery is now done in the physician's office or in an ambulatory care setting. There, in the absence of a standard and familiar operating room routine, the onus is on the physician to adhere strictly to appropriate antiseptic technique.

Asepsis, by contrast, refers to the prevention of wound infection by eliminating the introduction of new microbes into the area by medical personnel, instruments, or the surgical suite. Lister also was a major advocate of this concept, and by the end of the 19th century surgeons were beginning to wear gloves, gowns, and masks and to sterilize instruments for invasive procedures. The practice of hand washing before examining patients remained controversial. Even today, it is not practiced routinely by all physicians. Similarly, not all cutaneous surgeons routinely don gloves for minor office procedures, such as biopsies or electrodesiccation and curettage. Since hands may be the most important route of contamination, gloves are recommended for all contacts with a patient, not only for protection of the patient and surgical wound but also for protection of the physician. The same is true of caps, masks, protective eye wear, and gowns (Figure 3.1A–C). For those allergic to sterile gloves, hypoallergenic brown gloves often alleviate the problem. Nonsterile gloves may be used for the injection of anesthesia or for routine examination of patients. Protective covering that becomes torn or wet should be replaced, as it no longer provides an effective barrier.

CUTANEOUS FLORA

Human skin harbors microorganisms. The majority of these are either gram-positive aerobes, such as *Staphylococcus epidermidis* and micrococci, gram-positive anaerobes, such as *Propionibacterium acnes*, and fungi such as *Candida* species and *Pityrosporum* species. *Staphylococcus aureus*, *Klebsiella* species, *Enterobacter* species, and *Proteus* species also may be found in some individuals. These organisms are considered to be members of the resident flora that live on a person's skin, which rarely cause problems. While they are ubiquitous, they are more concentrated in the axilla, groin, and scalp areas. Because they seem to be anchored firmly to epidermal elements, they are more difficult to remove with antiseptics than are transient flora. Similarly, up to 20% live in hair follicles or in other nooks and crannies on the skin surface, and therefore are not accessible to surface scrubbing.

Transient bacteria include *S. aureus*, *Streptococcus* species, *Clostridium perfringens*, *Escherichia coli*, *Klebsiella* species, *Enterobacter* species, *Proteus* species, *Pseudomonas* species, and others. They are introduced to the skin from an outside source, and because they may live in surface debris or in dust particles on the skin they are more easily washed off than are resident flora.

ANTISEPTICS

A number of preparations are available that serve to decrease the number of microorganisms on the skin. They do not, however, create a totally sterile surgical field since, as noted earlier, the resident flora on the skin is not 100% accessible to these preparations, and transient microbes can always be brought in by circulating personnel, through open doors, or through ventilation systems.

The ideal solution should be inexpensive, broad spectrum, nonirritating, non-allergenic, have a rapid onset with sustained activity, and resist easy contamination. Alcohol, usually 70% isopropyl, has a rapid onset but covers only gram-positive organisms and has no sustained action. However, it has been shown that a 10-second wipe with 70% isopropyl alcohol probably reduces aerobic

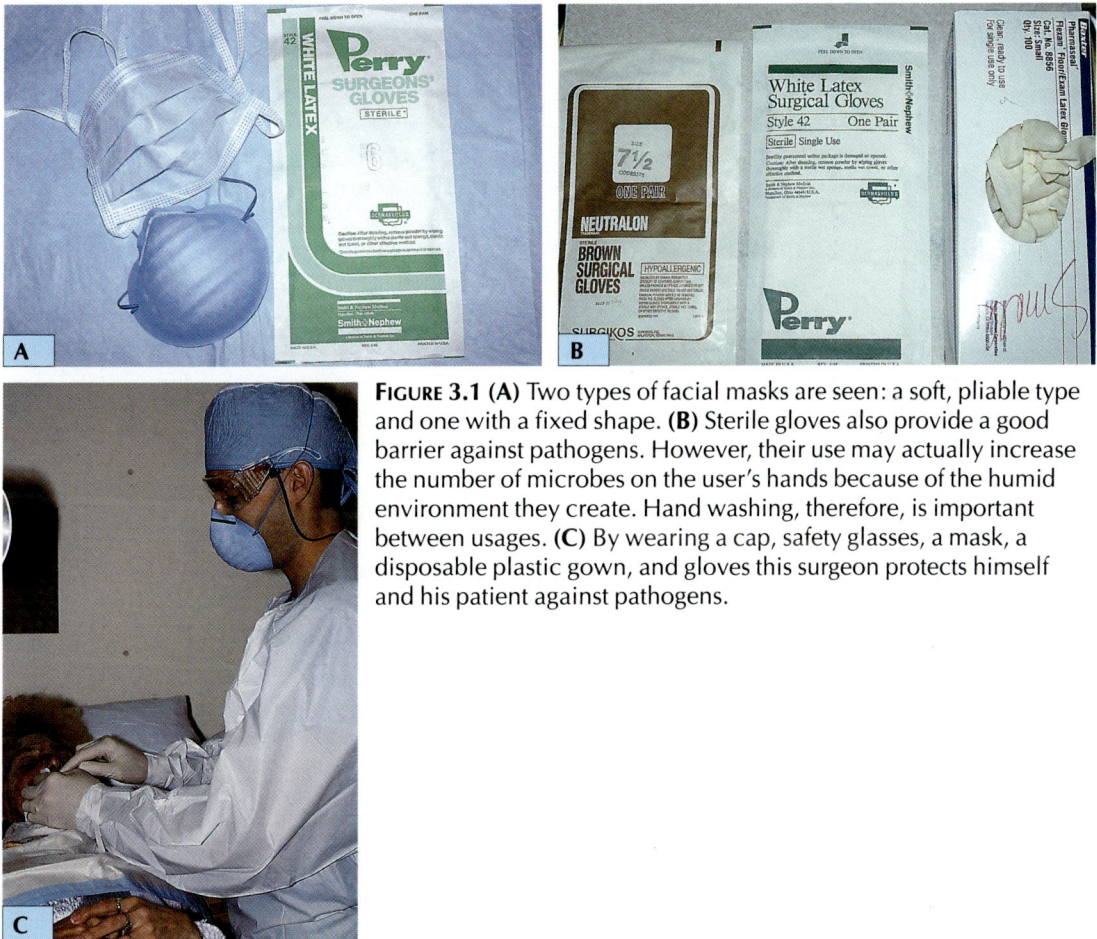

FIGURE 3.1 (A) Two types of facial masks are seen: a soft, pliable type and one with a fixed shape. (B) Sterile gloves also provide a good barrier against pathogens. However, their use may actually increase the number of microbes on the user's hands because of the humid environment they create. Hand washing, therefore, is important between usages. (C) By wearing a cap, safety glasses, a mask, a disposable plastic gown, and gloves this surgeon protects himself and his patient against pathogens.

bacteria by 75%, and therefore it is commonly used to reduce microbes just before an area is injected with anesthetic (Figure 3.2A,B). An antiseptic with more sustained action is then used to prepare the surgical site.

Iodine is an excellent antiseptic for the preparation of skin in that it is broad spectrum and fast acting. Many patients, however, are sensitive to it and therefore it is recommended with caution. Iodine also may be conjugated with organic compounds to form iodophors, which are fast acting, broad spectrum, and have sustained activity, especially if they are not washed off. Iodophors such as povidone-iodine (Betadine) are popular and are associated with less toxicity, staining, and sensitivity. However, since the release of iodine—the active component of the compound—is variable, its effectiveness is decreased. In addition, these compounds may interfere with wound healing.

Hexachlorophene is another antiseptic that was used frequently because of its good gram-positive action and sustained activity. It is a phenol, as was the first antiseptic recommended by Lister 100 years earlier. Unfortunately, it is absorbed through the skin and may be teratogenic and toxic to tissue.

Chlorhexidine (Hibiclens) is the most frequently used surgical scrub and preoperative site cleanser. It is effective against both gram-positive and gram-negative organisms, it is fast acting, and it has significant sustained activity. It is contraindicated for use around the eyes and ears, as it may cause irritation in the former and middle ear damage in the latter. For routine hand washing, the manufacturers recommend a 15-second gentle scrub, and for preoperative skin preparation, two 2-minute scrubs, each dried with a sterile towel.

Because contamination of all of the above preparations has been reported, long-term use of multiple-dose containers is not advised. The use of single-dose pledgets may help to avoid contamination (Figures 3.3 and 3.4).

ANTISEPTIC TECHNIQUE

Once the room is cleansed and the instruments are sterilized, the patient is prepped and draped. This commonly used phrase

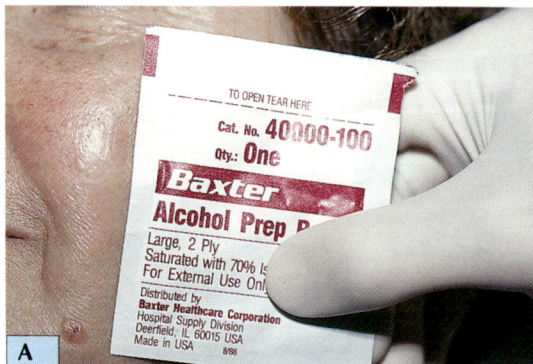

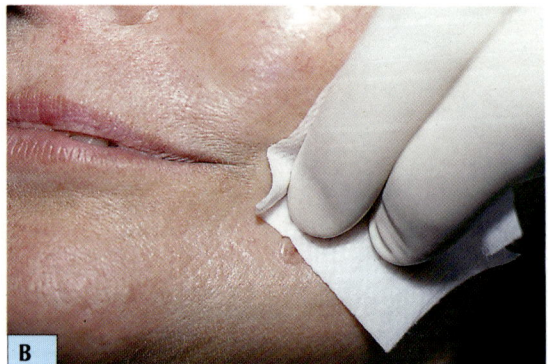

FIGURE 3.2 (A) Handy, prepackaged alcohol wipes are used to prepare the area for injection with anesthetic. (B) The skin immediately surrounding the lesion, through which the needle will pass, should be cleansed with the wipe.

refers to the culmination of a long series of events, beginning with evaluation of the patient for susceptibility to infection. Host factors such as immunocompetence are important, as is the presence or absence of potential pathogens on or about the patient. Evidence of pustules or folliculitis near the surgical site or other sign of infection is justification for postponement of the surgery. The patient can be instructed to wash the area regularly with an antiseptic soap before the rescheduled date of surgery. However, washing with one of these preparations for a short period of time probably will not serve to decrease resident flora enough to select for pathogenic organisms.

Once the procedure begins, the area is cleansed for 10 seconds with an alcohol wipe before injection of the anesthetic. Then an antiseptic with more sustained action is used, which should be applied to the area in concentric circles, starting centrally and working toward the periphery with increasingly wider circles. The applicator should never be brought back over an area that has already been cleansed. Depending on the preparation

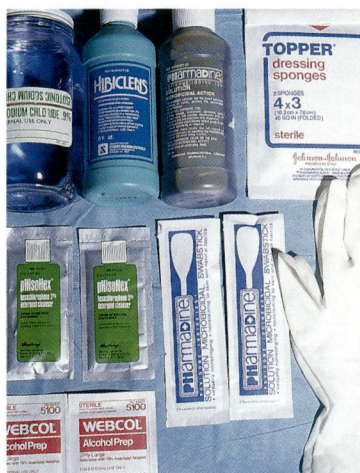

FIGURE 3.3 Various antiseptics are shown, including (top row) sterile sodium chloride, chlorhexidine (Hibiclens), an iodophor, sterile gauze for application; (middle row) pillow packages of hexachlorophene, individually packaged iodophor swabs, gloves for the operator; (bottom row) 70% isopropyl alcohol wipes.

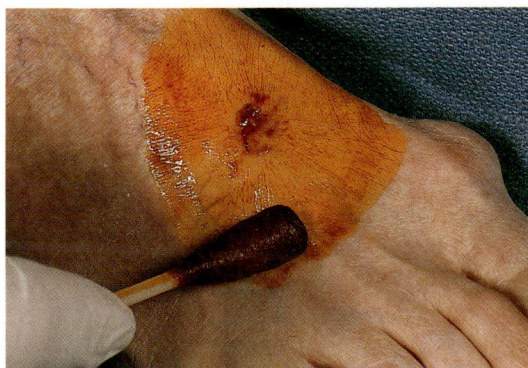

FIGURE 3.4 Individually packaged cotton swabs saturated with an iodophor are handy to use and avoid leakage, spillage, and contamination through the repeated use of large bottles and sterile cotton gauze.

used, the area can be patted dry or left as is (Figure 3.5A,B).

A drape is then placed over the area to isolate antiseptically prepared skin from unprepared skin. Drapes may be plastic or paper and most usually have a self-adhesive backing to secure them in place (Figure 3.6). Cloth drapes (Figure 3.7), by contrast, can be molded to the operative site but they also introduce the possibility of slippage. Since cloth drapes are not fixed to the perioperative skin, blood may ooze under the cloth down onto the patient or onto the patient's clothing. For working specifically on the face, an opaque drape may be used as it allows the surgeon to see contours and nearby structures easily during surgery (Figure 3.8). To avoid the problem of distortion during surgery, some surgeons prefer to prep and drape the entire face. A sterile water solution may be used to cleanse the face, with a more potent antiseptic reserved for the operative site.

If the area is hairy, it is preferable to leave it as is. Studies have shown increased infection rates associated with preoperative shaving. The longer in advance of the procedure that it is done, the higher the rate of infection. Snipping of the hair with scissors is associated with a somewhat lower infection rate, although the most effective measure is no hair removal at all with adequate antiseptic preparation. Depilatories also may be used but they are similar to clipping in their association with increased wound infection. They also may be irritating to the patient's skin and, if done far in advance of surgery to allow for reduction of inflammation, may actually increase the chances of infection.

FURTHER PRECAUTIONS

The infection rate in any outpatient facility should be actively monitored and if infections do occur their source should be found. Operating rooms as well as personnel should be cultured. Nasal passages and subungual debris may be hiding places for pathogens. Antiseptic solutions too should be cultured and instrument sterilization techniques reviewed. As an added precaution, personnel with an active severe dermatitis like hand eczema may harbor many bacteria and probably should not participate in surgery.

In summary, many factors are involved in the prevention of wound infection. The

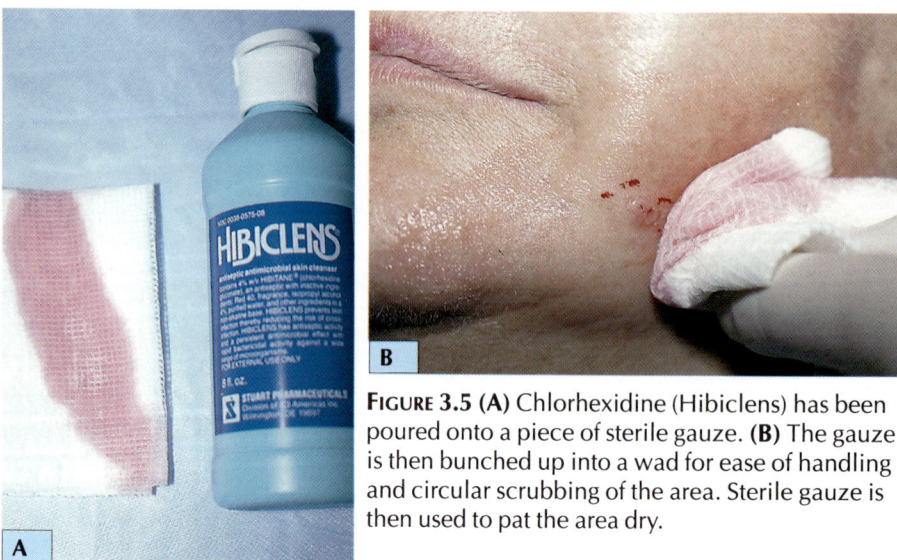

FIGURE 3.5 (A) Chlorhexidine (Hibiclens) has been poured onto a piece of sterile gauze. **(B)** The gauze is then bunched up into a wad for ease of handling and circular scrubbing of the area. Sterile gauze is then used to pat the area dry.

operating room should be clean with adequate ventilation and minimal walk-through traffic. Health care personnel should routinely wash hands before and after each patient contact and should protect themselves and the patient by wearing gloves, masks, eye shields or eyeglasses, and gowns. As stated earlier, these barriers should always be in good condition and should be replaced if they are torn or wet. Good operative technique must be followed by gentle handling of tissues and use of a drape as a barrier between antiseptically prepared skin and the unprepared cutaneous surface. Lastly, all wound infections must be critically analyzed by staff and a source or an explanation found. In short, a microorganism-controlled environment must be as readily accessible to the outpatient or to the patient undergoing an office procedure as it is to patients undergoing surgery in hospital operating room suites.

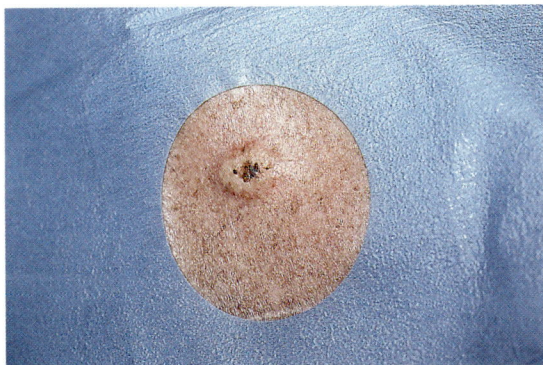

FIGURE 3.6 This adhesive-backed non-opaque drape comes in various sizes with different-sized fenestrations.

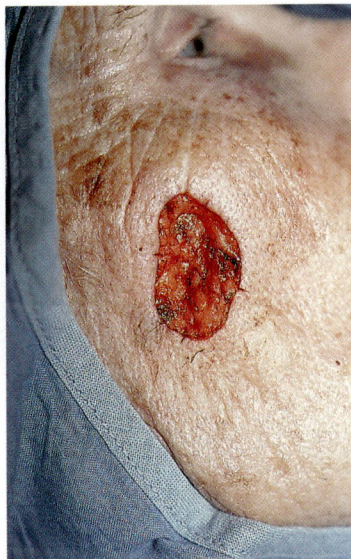

FIGURE 3.7 A cloth drape is used to expose a larger surface area, enabling the surgeon to view the entire cosmetic unit. The entire area of exposure has been prepped.

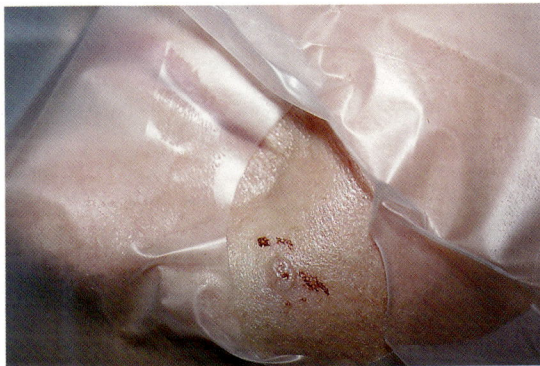

FIGURE 3.8 A clear plastic drape is used to cover the jowl area, allowing the surgeon to visualize all surrounding landmarks. Note how the upper pole of the opening has been folded over itself to make the opening smaller. Only prepared skin must be exposed.

SUGGESTIONS FOR FURTHER READING

Bennett RG. Microbiologic considerations in cutaneous surgery. In: Bennett RG. Fundamentals of Cutaneous Surgery. St Louis, Mo: C V Mosby Co; l988:136-178.

Craven DE, Moody B, Connolly MG, et al. Pseudo bacteremia caused by povidone-iodine solution contaminated with *Pseudomonas cepacia*. N Engl J Med. 1981;305:621-623.

Dzubow LM, Halpern AC, Leyden JJ, et al. Comparison of preoperative skin preparations for the face. J Am Acad Dermatol. 1988;19:737-741.

Kaul AF, Jewett JF. Agents and techniques for disinfection of the skin. Surg Gynecol Obstet. 1981;152:677-685.

Sebben JE. Surgical Preparation. In: Roenigk RK, Roenigk HH Jr, eds. Dermatologic Surgery. Principles and Practice. New York, NY: Marcel Dekker Inc;1989:11-40.

Sebben JE. Avoiding infection in office surgery. J Dermatol Surg Oncol. 1982;8: 455-458.

Seropean R, Reynolds BM. Wound infections after preoperative depilatory versus razor preparation. Am J Surg. 1971;121:251-254.

Steere AC, Mallison GF. Hand washing practices for the prevention of nosocomial infections. Ann Intern Med. 1975;83:683-690.

SECTION TWO

FUNDAMENTALS OF TREATMENT

chapter 4

LOCAL ANESTHESIA

The modern age of anesthesia began in 1846 in the still existing Ether Dome at Massachusetts General Hospital, when the first operation using ether was done before an assembled audience. Before that time, the most frequently used anesthetic came in the form of four large men holding down the patient. Alternatives to this were a blow to the head or mild strangulation, alcohol, or various opiates. These methods were a bit extreme for small operations and carried high mortality rates associated with the induction of anesthesia alone. But surgery at that time was considered a treatment of last resort for even the most serious of illnesses. Few people electively sought removal of cutaneous lesions or enhancement of physical features by surgical methods.

Once ether had been introduced and surgical procedures could be performed painlessly, attitudes toward cutaneous surgery were free to change. Also at this time, antisepsis was being introduced, thus decreasing mortality from postoperative infection. Surgical technique was improving. What was needed now was an anesthetic that could provide local control over sensation for use in smaller procedures. In 1884, Sigmund Freud and Karl Koller introduced cocaine hydrochloride as such a drug. It rapidly caught on and would expand the horizons of surgery.

MECHANISM OF ACTION

Local anesthesia is defined as the production of nerve-conduction blockage in a circumscribed area. The mechanism by which local anesthetics accomplish nerve blockage is by changing the permeability of the sodium ion at the cell membrane. The action potential for a particular sensation cannot be generated and conducted down the nerve. Blockage is not 100% and does not affect all nerves. Instead, the various types of nerve fibers are blocked differentially.

Of the three main groups of nerves—A, B, and C—group A nerves are the largest. This group is further divided into alpha, beta, delta, and gamma nerves, again based on size and conduction velocity. The smaller diameter C group and the delta nerves of the A group are those most susceptible to anesthesia and carry pain and temperature sensations, which are the first to be numbed. Next to go are touch and deep pressure sensations carried by medium beta fibers. If some of these fibers remain unaffected, patients may continue to feel some pressure during an operation and should be forewarned of this possibility. Otherwise, thinking that they have not been anesthetized adequately, patients may remain ill at ease throughout a procedure. Some of the larger group A alpha motor nerves also may be numbed temporarily, and patients should be forewarned of this too. Usually, once the anesthetic wears off, full motor control is regained (Figure 4.1).

ANESTHETICS

The ideal anesthetic should be nonirritating, nonallergenic, cause no permanent damage to nerves, have low systemic toxicity, and be of short onset but of long enough duration to last throughout the procedure. Cocaine was the first local anesthetic to be used in modern medicine. However, it was associated with

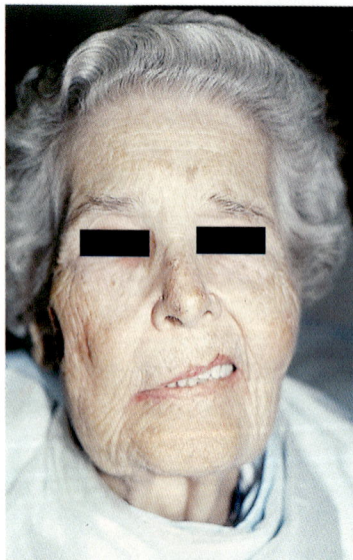

FIGURE 4.1 At the conclusion of surgery on the right lateral cheek, this patient's attempt at smiling elevated only her left upper lip (teeth showing). Knowing of the loss of sensation, the patient was careful when drinking hot liquids and eating and was not alarmed at her loss of motor control.

serious systemic toxicity. A synthetic substitute was eagerly sought, and, in 1905, Einhorn synthesized procaine hydrochloride, an ester of *p*-aminobenzoic acid (PABA). This prototypical drug was used widely until 1943 when Lofgren synthesized lidocaine. An amide-linkage drug, it eliminated the main drawback of the esters, which was their high rate of allergic reaction. Lidocaine hydrochloride is now the most widely used local anesthetic. The ester–amide classification still separates the major local anesthetics in use today (Figure 4.2).

In addition to cocaine and procaine, other examples of esters are tetracaine hydrochloride and chloroprocaine hydrochloride.

These drugs are metabolized in the plasma. Procaine is relatively short acting; without the addition of epinephrine, its duration on average is approximately 30 minutes. Tetracaine, by contrast, averages 180 minutes' duration. Because of its high toxicity, it is not used as an injectable anesthetic but only as a topical one (Figure 4.3). Both procaine and tetracaine have a slow onset of action.

The amide-linkage group is characterized by lidocaine. Because the amides are metabolized in the liver, they must be evaluated carefully for use in patients with significant liver disease. Lidocaine and mepivacaine hydrochloride average 90 minutes' duration without the addition of epinephrine. Epi-

---

FIGURE 4.2
CLASSIFICATION OF LOCAL ANESTHETICS

ESTERS	AMIDES
cocaine HCl	lidocaine (Xylocaine) HCl
procaine (Novocaine) HCl	mepivacaine (Carbocaine) HCl
tetracaine (Pontocaine) HCl	bupivacaine (Marcaine) HCl
chloroprocaine (Nesacaine) HCl	etidocaine (Duranest) HCl
	prilocaine (Citanest)

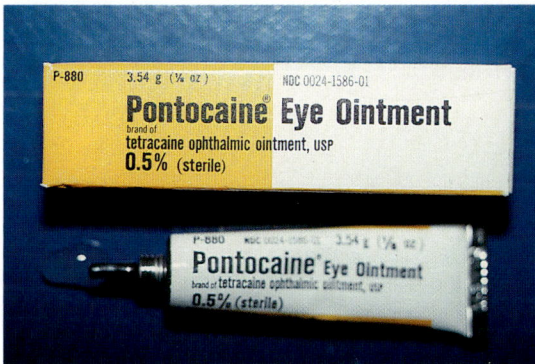

FIGURE 4.3 Tetracaine (Pontocaine) is commonly used as an ophthalmic ointment to numb the eye before the use of a corneal shield or a chalazion clamp. It is important to remember that this drug is a PABA derivative with its inherent allergic potential.

nephrine, if added, may double their duration. Bupivacaine hydrochloride (Figure 4.4) and etidocaine hydrochloride average 200 minutes' duration, and since epinephrine increases their duration only minimally, they are marketed without it. These drugs may be used whenever epinephrine is contraindicated. Lidocaine and etidocaine have the fastest onset of action of the amides. Bupivacaine is relatively slow acting.

With the exception of cocaine, all of the anesthetics are vasodilators. Therefore, epinephrine is added to many of these agents to prolong their action and to reduce systemic absorption of the drug by keeping it at the site of injection. Epinephrine also affords some hemostasis during the procedure. However, it may take up to 15 minutes for the epinephrine to work, although an anesthetic such as lidocaine will rapidly anesthetize the area. If hemostasis is crucial, a 15-minute delay should occur between injection of the anesthetic and the onset of surgery.

A drawback to the use of epinephrine is that once the drug's effects have begun to abate, vessels that have not been cauterized or tied off may bleed. If such bleeding occurs under a flap or graft or if it results in hematoma formation, the integrity of the surgical closure may be jeopardized. Following the

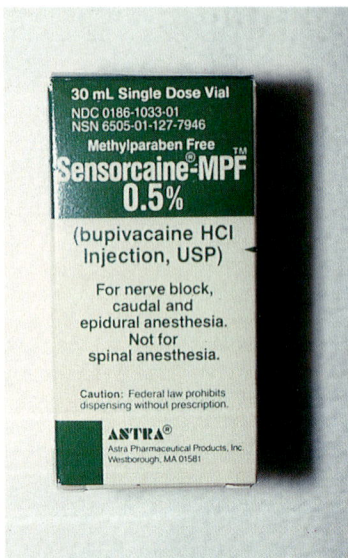

FIGURE 4.4 This is one marketed brand of bupivacaine hydrochloride, a slow-acting but long-lasting amide-linkage anesthetic. It is commonly used for long procedures and nerve blocks. Note how the package states that it is free of methylparaben, which is one of the preservatives felt to be the cause of some "allergic" reactions to the amides.

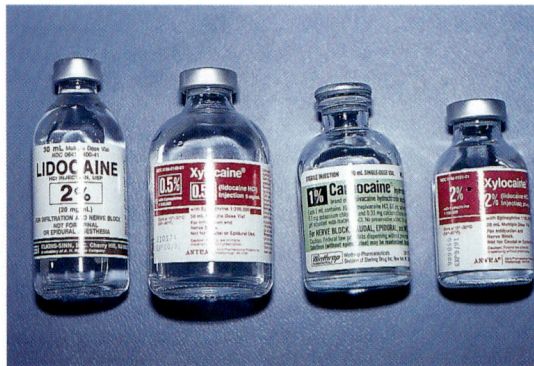

FIGURE 4.5 The solutions that contain epinephrine have red labels. Note that lidocaine hydrochloride is marketed without (2% plain) or with (0.5% and 2%) epinephrine at concentrations of 1:100,000 or 1:200,000. It is important to know the concentrations of both drugs to be able to calculate the maximum recommended dosages. Mepivacaine (Carbocaine) hydrochloride (green label) is a long-acting amide, marketed with or without epinephrine. In this example it is shown without it.

procedure, the surgeon should keep the patient in the office long enough to check for bleeding and/or should apply a pressure dressing to the area to avoid these potential complications.

Epinephrine should not be used on digits or on the penis. It is also contraindicated for use in patients taking monoamine oxidase inhibitors, tricyclic antidepressants, and phenothiazines. Furthermore, it should be used with caution and in the smallest possible amounts in patients taking propranolol hydrochloride as well as certain antihypertensives, digitalis, or amphetamines (Figure 4.5). Patients with peripheral vascular disease, acute angle-closure glaucoma, hyperthyroidism, unstable mental status, and pregnancy also should be considered candidates for the use of a local anesthetic without epinephrine.

ADVERSE EFFECTS

The ester group is derived mainly from PABA. Drugs in this group should not be used in patients who are sensitive to PABA or to its cross-reacting drugs, the sulfur derivatives. Also, as these drugs are metabolized by pseudocholinesterase, they are contraindicated in patients in whom this enzyme may be lacking.

Allergic reactions also may be seen with lidocaine, although such reactions are rare and may be due to preservatives in the solution rather than to the anesthetic itself. To ferret out these drug sensitivities, serial titration and challenge testing may be done. Cross reactions with other medications may occur, such as amphetamines, phenothiazines, some antihypertensives, Dilantin, and diazepam.

At the site of injection, anesthetics can cause pain, swelling, bruising, and hematoma formation. Necrosis and inflammation also may occur, though rarely. Systemically, these agents affect mainly the central nervous and cardiovascular systems. Side effects pri-

marily are dose related. High dosages may occur by exceeding the recommended limits for a particular drug, by inadvertent injection into the vascular system, or by use in a patient who cannot adequately metabolize the drug. Package inserts should be checked by the surgeon for all medications that he or she uses routinely, to gain familiarity with each maximum dosage.

For the most commonly used drug, lidocaine, the dosage in a healthy adult, when epinephrine is added, should not exceed 7 mg/kg of body weight or a total of 500 mg (50 mL of a 1% solution) in a 70-kg man. If epinephrine is not added, the maximum dosage is reduced to 4.5 mg/kg of body weight or a total of 300 mg of lidocaine for the same man.

At low doses of an anesthetic (1 to 5 mg/mL), the patient may experience lightheadedness, tinnitus, numbness of the lips, and a metallic taste. With increasing concentrations, these symptoms may progress to tremors and slow speech, which may precede actual seizures at doses of 8 to 15 mg/mL. Cardiovascular effects such as tachycardia, elevated blood pressure, or chest pain usually are due to the addition of epinephrine. However, at high doses of the drug, myocardial depression can occur, leading to cardiovascular collapse.

Vasovagal reactions to the use of local anesthetics are not uncommon. The patient usually reports such a reaction as a drug allergy. It is best to treat it as such or to verify the allergic response using a challenge test. Alternatives to be used are Phenergan, diphenhydramine hydrochloride, or even normal saline. Patients properly informed in advance of the surgery about a drug's potential side effects may be spared some of the anxiety of uncertainty and feel more relaxed. Other techniques used to relax the patient during surgery include talking to him or her during the procedure, keeping his or her mind otherwise occupied, keeping all instruments out of sight, and working quickly and efficiently. If the patient's chief complaint regarding local anesthetics is that of palpitations, one of the longer acting drugs can be used as they do not contain epinephrine. Other available alternatives include liquid nitrogen or one of the refrigerant sprays such as Frigiderm (Freon 114). With a quick freeze to the area, Frigiderm will desensitize it long enough to enable needle insertion or snip or shave removal of a small lesion. Some surgeons routinely premedicate all patients using sublingual Valium.

TECHNIQUE

LOCAL INFILTRATION

To produce localized anesthesia, the anesthetic is injected around the nerve endings that supply the operative site. A Luer-Lok syringe is used to prevent the needle from popping off during injection due to a build-up of pressure (Figure 4.6). This is especially important when small-bore needles, such as 30-gauge needles, are used. These needles are recommended for cutaneous injections as they cause the least amount of pain. Larger

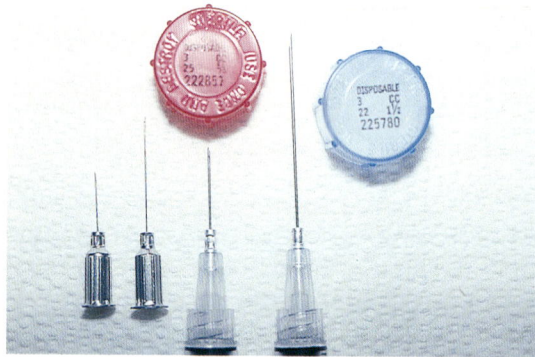

FIGURE 4.7 From left to right, a ½-inch 30-gauge needle, a 1-inch 30-gauge needle, a ⅝ -inch 25-gauge needle, and a 1½-inch 22-gauge needle are shown.

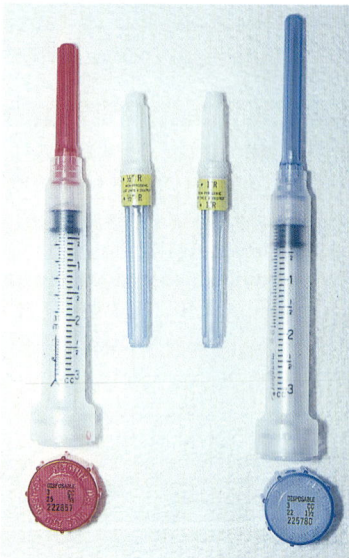

FIGURE 4.6 Luer-Lok syringes (3 mL) with large-bore needles such as a 22-gauge needle (blue) or a 25-gauge needle (red) are used to draw up the solution from a multiple-dose vial. A 30-gauge needle (white) can then be placed on the syringe for injection. Syringes of 1, 3, and 5 mL are good for injection. Larger syringes will cause too much back-up pressure when small-bore needles are used.

(22- or 25-gauge) needles may be used for infiltration of very large areas, perhaps after a wheal has been raised using a 30-gauge needle. Needles also come in different lengths. To anesthetize large areas, needles of 1 to 1½ inches are preferable to ½-inch needles (Figure 4.7). The surgeon should keep in mind that the 1-inch 30-gauge needle is very flexible and somewhat unsteady.

The needle should be placed in the dermis for injection, and a wheal should be raised (Figure 4.8). If the needle is placed in the epidermis instead, the skin will assume a peau-d'orange appearance (Figure 4.9). Anes-

thesia of deeper tissues occurs more slowly. If the injection is made directly into fat, the anesthetic will dissipate more quickly and there will be an increased chance of injection into a vessel. To avoid injection directly into a blood vessel and high systemic doses, the surgeon should aspirate when injecting the operative site.

Before insertion of the needle, it is important that the surgeon alert the patient to the impending injection as well as to the possibility of discomfort. The amount of discomfort felt will vary according to the site, the amount of anesthetic used, and the speed at

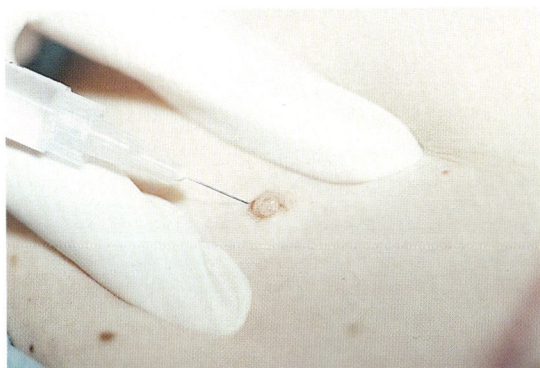

FIGURE 4.8 A small amount of anesthetic, properly placed in the dermis and injected with a 30-gauge ½-inch needle, raises the area gently. If the anesthetic is placed too deeply, no elevation occurs. Because the anesthetic diffuses centrifugally, reinjection of the area is not necessary to obtain adequate anesthesia around the lesion. Note that the area of blanched skin does not correspond completely to the area of anesthetized skin and therefore should not be used as an indicator of such.

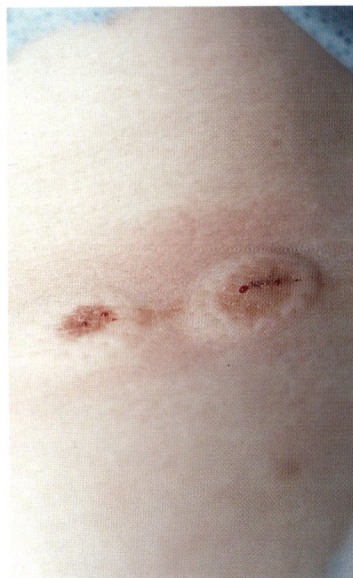

FIGURE 4.9 Prominent hair follicles are seen in what is called peau d'orange, which occurs when the anesthetic is injected into epidermis. The resulting expansion of the skin causes increased discomfort to the patient, along with slower numbing of the deeper skin layers.

which it is injected. A slow, steady injection causes the least amount of discomfort (Figure 4.10). Pain also may be decreased somewhat by buffering the solutions with sodium bicarbonate to alkalize them. This is because the drugs, being weak bases with low solubility in water, are marketed as their salts, which are acidic. A less painful injection also is reported to occur from mixing of the epinephrine into the anesthetic freshly each day, in contrast to the use of commercially available mixtures.

For the injection of small lesions, one needle puncture should suffice (Figure 4.11 A,B). As the injection may distort the site, any landmarks or margins critical to the surgical procedure should be marked beforehand. For larger lesions, a longer needle may help to spread the anesthetic. If reinsertion of the needle is necessary, it should always be advanced into an area that already has been numbed by the anesthetic (Figure 4.12A–C). If prolonged anesthesia is necessary, lidocaine, which has a rapid onset, can be used

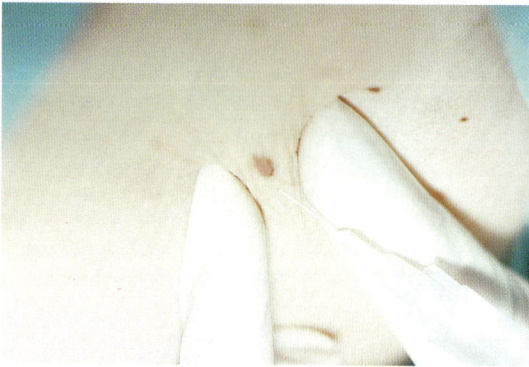

FIGURE 4.10 Pinching of the skin with the fingers as the anesthetic is injected helps to decrease the patient's sensation of pain.

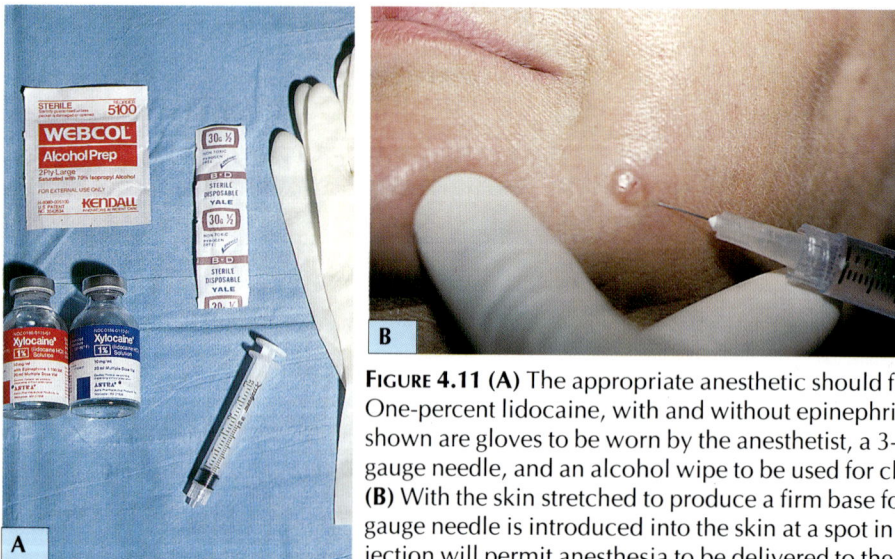

FIGURE 4.11 (A) The appropriate anesthetic should first be selected. One-percent lidocaine, with and without epinephrine, is shown. Also shown are gloves to be worn by the anesthetist, a 3-mL syringe, a 30-gauge needle, and an alcohol wipe to be used for cleansing of the area. (B) With the skin stretched to produce a firm base for stability, a 30-gauge needle is introduced into the skin at a spot in which a single injection will permit anesthesia to be delivered to the entire surgical site.

initially, followed by a long-acting anesthetic such as bupivacaine, which can be infiltrated into areas needing anesthesia for longer than 1 hour.

NERVE BLOCKS

Variations of the infiltration technique are ring or field blocks and nerve blocks. For lesions such as cysts, it is easier to place a ring of anesthesia around the lesion rather than to inject the lesion itself. This prevents distortion of the area and of the lesion. A nerve block is intended to block the nerves before they reach the area. It anesthetizes a larger area using a smaller amount of anesthetic and usually lasts longer than simple infiltration. Caution should be exercised in the numbing of large nerve trunks so that the needle does not damage the nerve. Anesthetic should not be injected at the foramen where the major nerves supplying the face exit through the bone. There is too great a chance of causing injury to the nerve with the needle or of causing pressure on the nerve from the injection of fluid into a confined space. Similar consid-

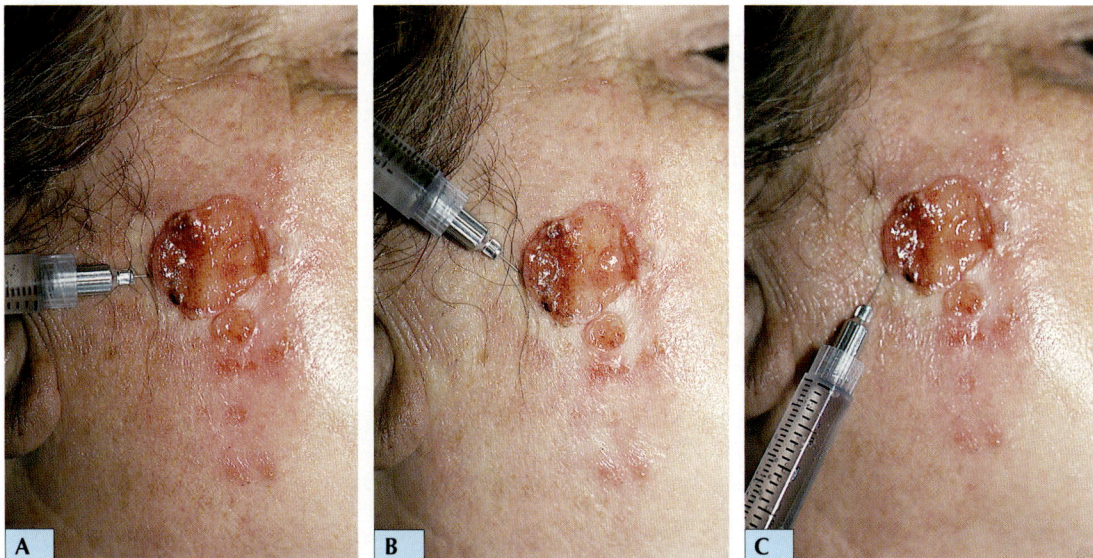

FIGURE 4.12 (A) For a larger lesion a longer needle is used, which is placed to one side of the lesion. The anesthetic is injected while the needle is advanced slowly to its hub. **(B)** The needle is then pulled back but not completely out and is angled inferiorly for injection of the inferior one third of the lesion in the same manner. **(C)** The process is then repeated for the upper one third of the lesion.

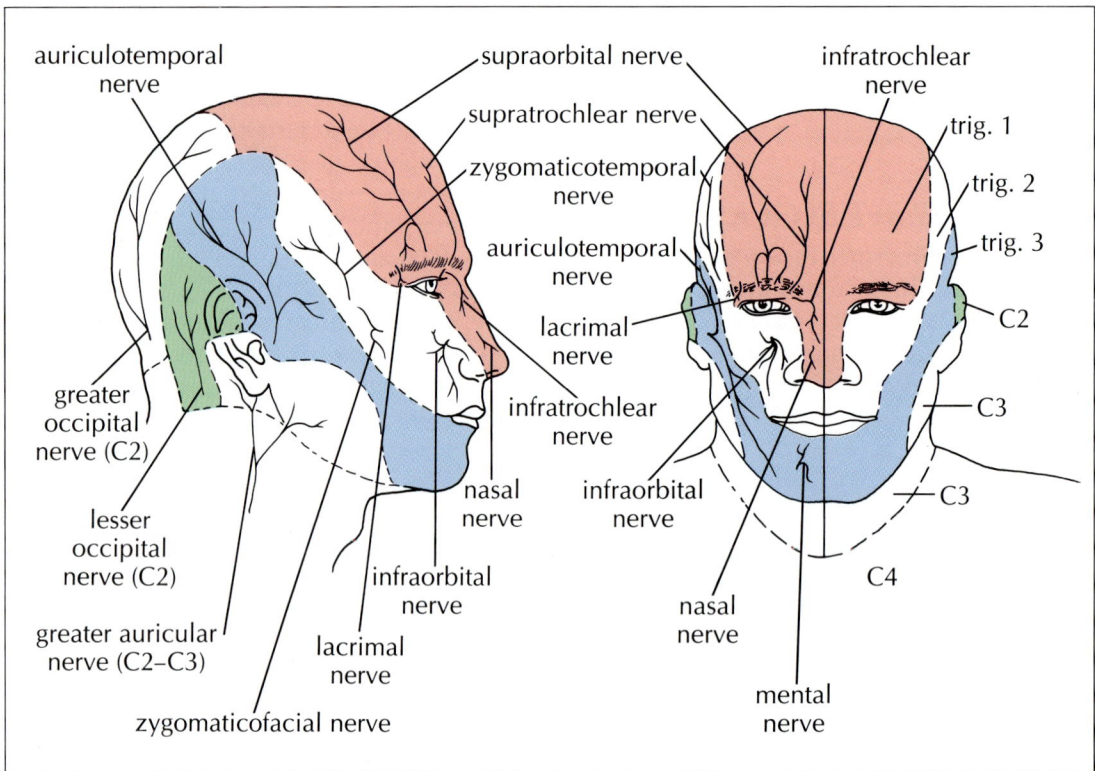

auriculotemporal nerve

supraorbital nerve

infratrochlear nerve

supratrochlear nerve

trig. 1

zygomaticotemporal nerve

trig. 2

auriculotemporal nerve

trig. 3

lacrimal nerve

C2

greater occipital nerve (C2)

infratrochlear nerve

C3

infraorbital nerve

C3

lesser occipital nerve (C2)

nasal nerve

C4

greater auricular nerve (C2–C3)

infraorbital nerve

nasal nerve

lacrimal nerve

mental nerve

zygomaticofacial nerve

FIGURE 4.13 To create nerve blocks, the surgeon must be thoroughly familiar with the anatomy of the area to be anesthetized and with its innervation.

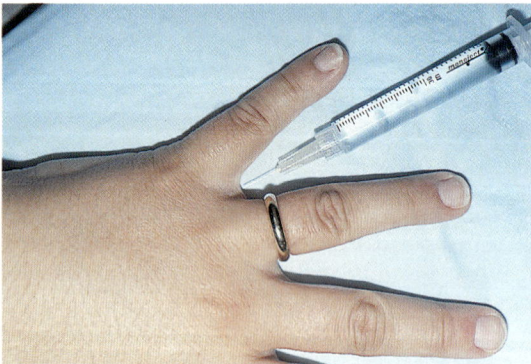

FIGURE 4.14 An alternative to the proximal digital block shown in Chapter 23 is the web-space block. Here, using no epinephrine, 0.5 to 1.0 mL of anesthetic is injected into the web spaces on either side of the finger.

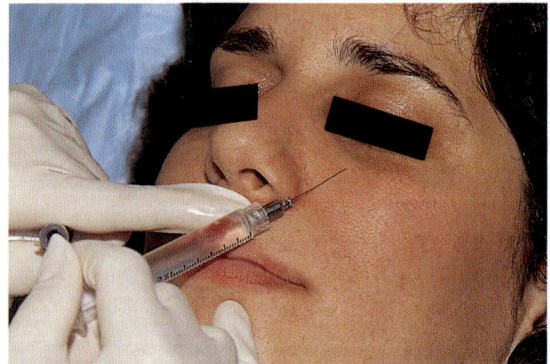

FIGURE 4.15 A long, 1-inch 30-gauge needle is pointed at the infraorbital foramen just below a mid-point in the infraorbital rim. A longer needle is used to enable placement of the anesthetic at a deeper point, nearer the nerve.

erations should be given to nerves in the digits, which also are in confined areas.

The major nerve blocks on the face involve the supraorbital, infraorbital, and mental nerves (Figure 4.13). A digital block is described fully in Chapter 23. The web-space block (Figure 4.14) is a variation thereof. A midface block (Figure 4.15) is described in Chapter 24. Because, with a nerve block, no anesthetic is infiltrated at the surgical site, no hemostatic agent is injected. Some surgeons supplement a distal nerve block with some local infiltration to achieve the effects of the epinephrine as well as of the anesthetic. Because the face is densely innervated, there may be collateral nerves on the face that are not blocked distally. Local infiltration at the site should numb them.

SUMMARY

Local anesthesia revolutionized the horizons of surgery just 100 years ago. Today it is used countless times a day, in all possible medical settings, with a very low incidence of complication. In fact, its use has become somewhat routine. Anesthetics, however, are not innocuous drugs. Their usage should be mastered by the anesthetist–cutaneous surgeon to the extent that any other aspect of the surgical technique is mastered. They are potent drugs, whose side-effects, interactions, and potential toxicity are highlighted in elderly populations. Furthermore, the art of anesthetizing a patient may make the difference between a cooperative and an uncooperative patient both during and after the procedure.

SUGGESTIONS FOR FURTHER READING

Bennett RG. Anesthesia. In: Bennett RG. Fundamentals of Cutaneous Surgery. St Louis, Mo: C V Mosby Co;1988:194-239.

Bezzant JL, Stephen RL, Petelenz TJ, Jacobsen SC. Painless cauterization of spider veins with the use of iontophoretic local anesthesia. J Am Acad Dermatol. 1988;19:869-875.

Fisher DA. Local anesthesia in dermatologic surgery (letter). J Am Acad Dermatol. 1990;22:139-141.

Foster CA, Aston SJ. Propranolol-epinephrine interaction: a potential disaster. Plast Reconstr Surg.1983;72:74-78.

Grekin RC, Auletta MJ. Local anesthesia in dermatologic surgery. J Am Acad Dermatol. 1988;19:599-614.

Reynolds F. Adverse effects of local anesthetics. Br J Anaesth. 1987;59:78-95.

Ritchie JM, Greene NM. Local anesthetics. In: Gilman AG, Goodman LS, Rall TW, Murad F, eds. Goodman and Gilman's the Pharmacological Basis of Therapeutics. 7th ed. New York, NY: Macmillan Publishing Co Inc;1985:302-321.

Stewart JH, Cole GW, Klein JA. Neutralized lidocaine with epinephrine for local anesthesia. J Dermatol Surg Oncol. 1989;15:1081-1083.

Winton, GB. Anesthesia for dermatologic surgery. J Dermatol Surg Oncol. 1988;14:41-54.

chapter 5

THE BIOPSY

Proper biopsy technique is an essential skill for the cutaneous surgeon. The biopsy is used to help diagnose disease, provide histological confirmation of skin cancer, and remove small lesions. The choice of technique is an important factor determining the success of the biopsy. Several techniques may be used, including the shave biopsy, the punch biopsy, the incisional biopsy, the excisional biopsy, and the nail biopsy. The choice depends on the size and location of the tissue being sampled and the suspected diagnosis. The biopsy technique, properly selected and adequately performed, should be efficient, enable histological diagnosis, and leave an acceptable scar (Figure 5.1).

BIOPSY PLANNING AND PREPARATION

In selecting a lesion for biopsy, the surgeon's diagnostic skills are called into play. If there are several lesions to choose from, the one that is relatively new, has the most substance to it, or is the least traumatized should be selected. Lesions irritated by clothing may look the most informative but may yield information only about chronic inflammation. To sample blindly through an area that is suspected of having disease is rarely fruitful. Next, the surgeon should ensure that an adequate amount of tissue is obtained. Care should be taken to avoid removing too little tissue in the interest of speed or with the intention of leaving a small scar. Tissue insufficient for diagnosis results in wasted time, embarrassment, and two scars.

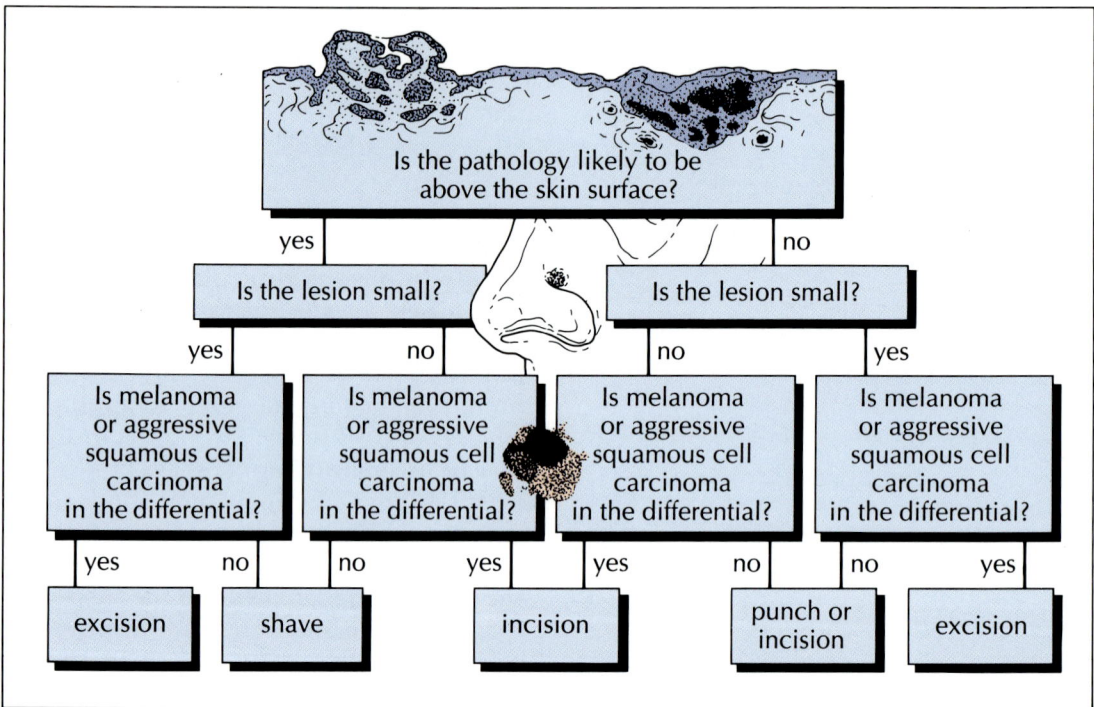

FIGURE 5.1 Algorithm showing decision process for selecting proper biopsy technique.

If only a portion of a lesion is to be sampled, the surgeon should select as he or she would in choosing between multiple lesions. If the lesion is ulcerated, it is usually best to obtain the biopsy from its edge (Figure 5.2A,B). It is always better to remove a nevomelanocytic lesion completely with an excisional biopsy. However, if complete removal is not possible, the area that is the most raised or the darkest should be chosen, which should correspond to the area of deepest invasion and most malignant change (Figure 5.3). If the lesion is a skin cancer, any portion of it will be adequate for biopsy. However, in performing a shave biopsy, the surgeon should take care not to be too shal-

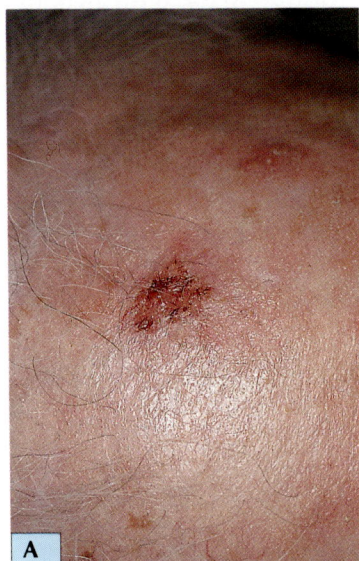

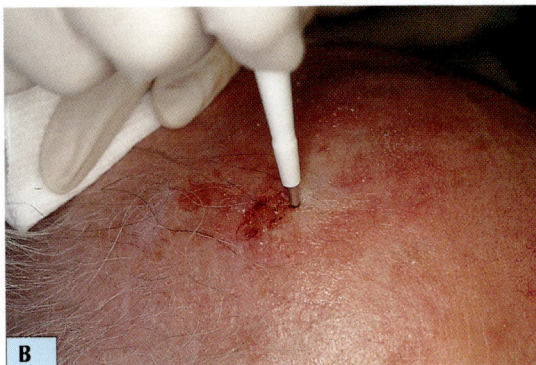

FIGURE 5.2 (A,B) A large, 4-mm punch is used to sample the edge, ulcer, and adjacent normal skin of this lesion.

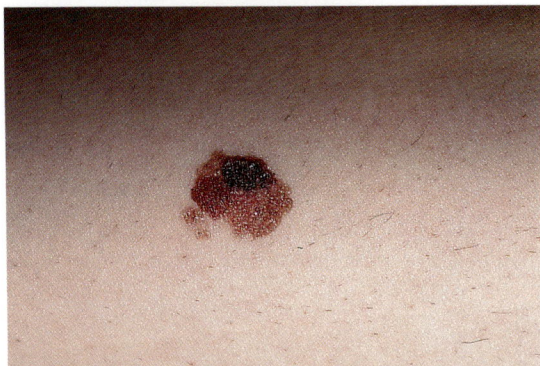

FIGURE 5.3 A large melanocytic lesion on a patient's thigh. An appropriate incisional biopsy should sample the black area at the 12-o'clock position and the adjacent raised dark brown area at the 10-o'clock position to obtain the most accurate histopathology.

low, as inadequate tissue will yield inadequate histological results (Figure 5.4 A,B).

Once the lesion or a portion thereof has been chosen, the surgeon should discuss with the patient the specifics of the procedure, his or her reasons for doing it, and the expected scar. A written consent must be obtained. This is also the time to prepare all instruments and specimen bottles. The bottles should be marked prior to the procedure and they should be kept separate throughout it. This is particularly important when there are multiple biopsy sites. Biopsy specimens should not be placed randomly on trays or counters, as this is the best way to lose them. They should be placed directly in the bottle, or on a specially marked piece of gauze and an assistant should be notified. Next, the surgeon should put on a pair of gloves. Universal precautions must be followed no matter how small the biopsy or how simple the procedure. Next, the skin surface should be prepared. A 2- to 3-minute wipe with alcohol-saturated gauze adequately decreases the number of bacteria on the skin surface. Other cleansers that may be used in addition to, or

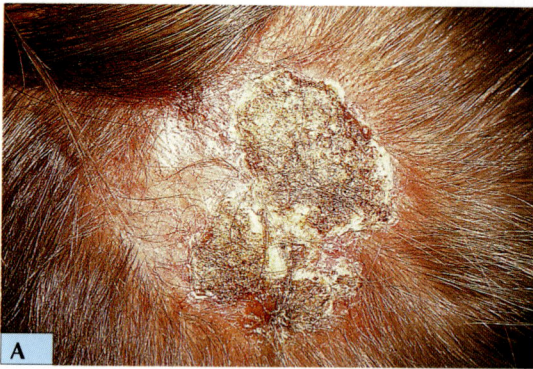

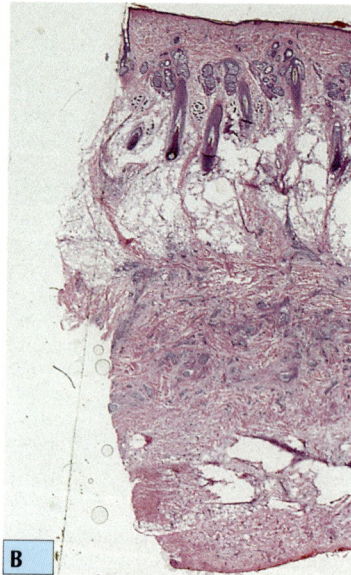

FIGURE 5.4 (A) The large, keratotic crust on this patient's scalp would be inadequately sampled by a shave biopsy. (B) A morpheaform basal cell carcinoma was found underneath normal-appearing epidermis, dermis, and subcutaneous tissue. Only a deep punch biopsy or an incisional biopsy would have yielded the proper diagnosis.

FIGURE 5.5
WAYS TO IDENTIFY A BIOPSY SITE

Leave a portion of the lesion behind

Tattoo the lesion with India ink

Anchor a suture firmly to the site

Draw a detailed body map with the site well marked

Take a Polaroid picture and mark the site on the photo

Show the patient, with mirror in hand, the exact location

in place of, alcohol are povidone-iodine and chlorhexidine. It is also important to mark the area to be sampled with sterile gentian violet or with a sterile skin-marking pen, as the site may be subsequently obscured by the anesthetic as it elevates the surrounding skin or it may be blanched by the epinephrine.

A biopsy is a preliminary study. If a second procedure is anticipated, it is best to re-mark the biopsy site immediately after the initial biopsy is done. This is possible using a variety of techniques (Figure 5.5). The smaller the initial lesion and the more activity on the skin surface in the area of the biopsy, the more critical its identification.

ANESTHESIA

The most common anesthetic is a 1% or 2% solution of lidocaine with epinephrine, injected directly into the skin at the site of the biopsy using a 30-gauge needle. The addition of epinephrine produces hemostasis and prolongs the effects of lidocaine in the area. If epinephrine is not used, the procedure must be performed immediately following the administration of the anesthetic, as the anesthesia is much shorter lived without the vasoconstrictive effects of the epinephrine. When sampling small papules 2 to 4 mm in diameter, a small amount of anesthetic should be used, not more than 0.1 to 0.3 mL. When obtaining samples from the penis or from a digit, no epinephrine should be used. Short-acting, but rapid, anesthesia can also be achieved with liquid nitrogen and is an effective choice for a small snip or shave biopsy, for children, or for someone fearful of needles.

For most biopsies, a single puncture of the needle should be sufficient to administer the necessary amount of anesthetic. An excisional biopsy may require more, in which case subsequent needle punctures should be placed in areas that have already been numbed. If the anesthetic has been correctly placed in the dermis, a small, raised wheal should appear at the site of injection (Figure 5.6). It elevates the skin and should greatly facilitate a snip or shave biopsy. However, the surgeon cannot assume that the area that blanches after the injection corresponds to the total area of anesthesia, and vice versa. Non-white areas may be adequately anesthetized. It is best to check the area with gentle pricks of the needle until the surgeon becomes comfortable with his or her technique.

BIOPSY TECHNIQUES

SHAVE BIOPSY

The shave biopsy is seemingly the simplest of the techniques. It is not the same as a superfi-

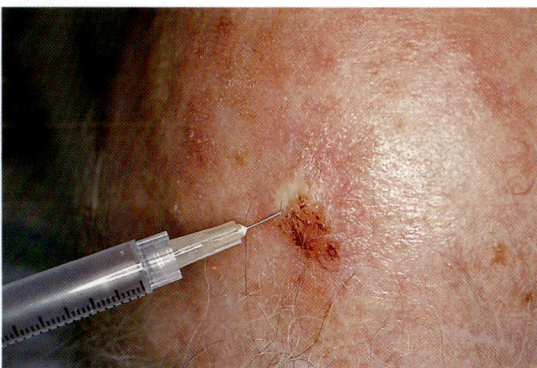

FIGURE 5.6 At the site of intended biopsy, the skin is elevated with a small amount of anesthetic.

cial biopsy, although many treat it as such. Any papular lesion in which the area of pathology is contained within the papule itself and does not lie deep within the under-lying dermis is best served by a shave biopsy. Shave biopsy is also a good choice for any lesion found on a contoured surface such as the nose or the ear. Shave biopsies may not remove a lesion completely if there is a deep component to it, and therefore the possibility of recurrence should be indicated to the patient. Similarly, if the raised papule is mostly eschar, a shave biopsy may fail to obtain tissue for diagnosis. In such a case, it is best to remove the eschar and to perform a deep shave biopsy with better visualization, or to perform a punch biopsy.

As noted earlier, the shave biopsy may be made easier by the creation of a wheal once the anesthetic has been injected. To perform the biopsy, a scalpel with a #15 knife blade is held parallel to the skin surface and is then slid across the base of the lesion (Figure 5.7). One smooth stroke will leave a more even base, although this technique may be difficult for large lesions. Completely encircling the

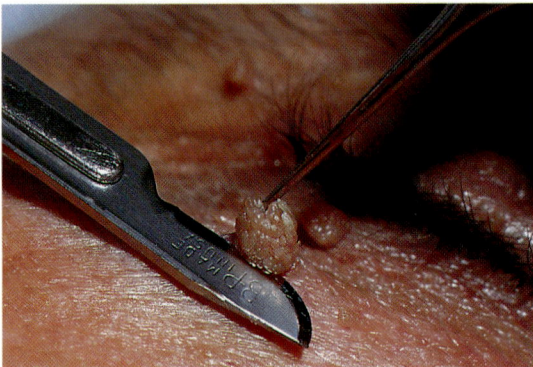

FIGURE 5.7 Putting tension on the lesion by pulling up on it with toothed forceps or by stretching the surrounding skin will aid in obtaining a smooth, single-stroke cut.

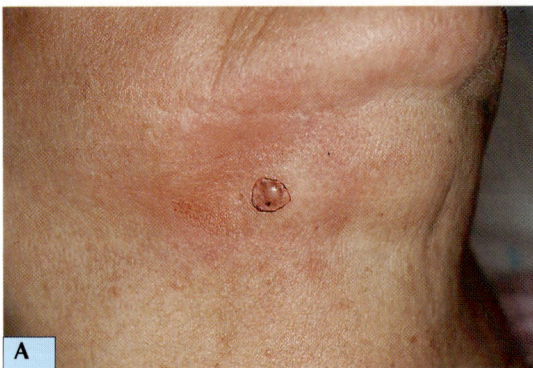

A

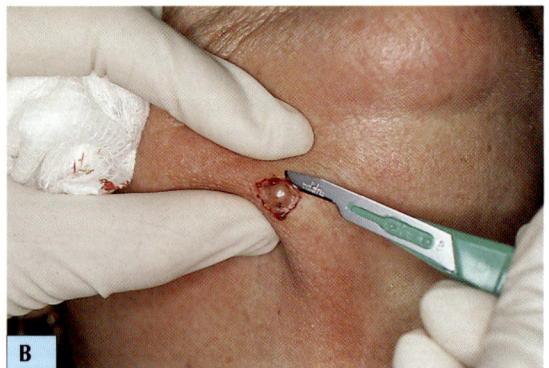

B

FIGURE 5.8 (A) Because it is often difficult to see the entire base of a sessile lesion as it is cut, encircling it provides a guideline that enables the surgeon to remove it completely. The guideline should be deep enough so that the blade falls into it as it moves around the lesion. **(B)** On a concave surface, pinching the skin to give a convex surface facilitates the shave.

area with a superficial incision may provide enough of a guideline to ensure that the entire lesion is removed (Figure 5.8 A,B). This same type of shave technique can also be performed using a wire loop on an electrocautery machine. However, in the latter case, it is important to remember that the pathology at the cutting surface may become distorted, and, therefore, the surgeon must be sure that the suspected pathology is adequately represented throughout the rest of the papule.

If a blade is used, the cutting surface should be angled slightly upward to leave a more even base and to prevent digging of the blade into the dermis, which leaves more of a scar (Figure 5.9). This technique may also be performed using sharp scissors such as fine iris or Gradle scissors (Figure 5.10). The more sessile the lesion, however, the more difficult it is to remove entirely with scissors. Such removal is best reserved for pedunculated lesions.

A shave biopsy that is intended to sample the dermis is called a saucerization, as the cut curves downward in the middle like a saucer. It is accomplished using a #15 knife

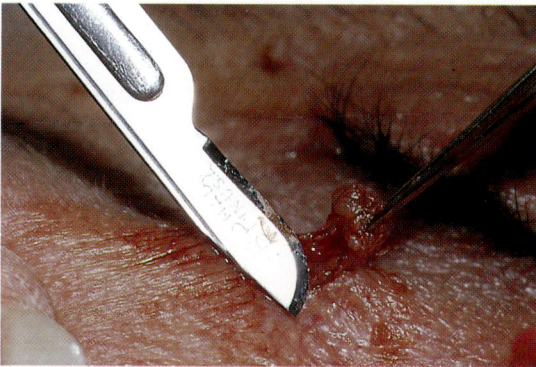

FIGURE 5.9 Upward beveling of the scalpel guards against the natural tendency to advance and cut down into the tissue.

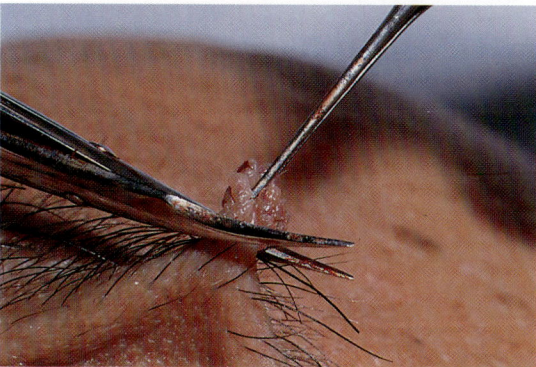

FIGURE 5.10 To obtain the best results, the scissors should be held parallel to the skin surface and at the base of the lesion.

blade or a razor blade bowed in the center (Figure 5.11 A,B). This technique should be used only in specific circumstances, such as when sampling more deeply than a simple shave biopsy, as it will leave more of a scar. Hemostasis with a shave biopsy can be achieved using a topical solution such as ferric subsulfate or aluminum chloride, or with light pinpoint electrodesiccation. A 15% to 35% solution of trichloroacetic acid can also be used, as well as absorbable gelatin/collagen sponges or simple direct pressure.

PUNCH BIOPSY

A punch biopsy, or trephine biopsy, is used to sample a lesion for which dermal or subcutaneous tissue is necessary for the diagnosis.

Unless the histological diagnosis is expected to be evident, as for a basal cell carcinoma, the punch biopsy should be 4 mm in diameter. The area to be sampled is prepped in the same manner as for a shave biopsy.

To perform the punch biopsy, the area to be sampled is drawn tautly between the thumb and the index finger, and the skin is stretched in a direction perpendicular to the skin lines in the area (Figure 5.12). If performed correctly, a cylindrical punch should leave an elliptical hole, which lends itself to closure in a straight line (Figure 5.13). The punch itself should be placed at right angles to the skin surface (Figure 5.14), and rotated and advanced with gentle downward pressure. It is thought by some that unidirectional rotation of the punch is less traumatic to the

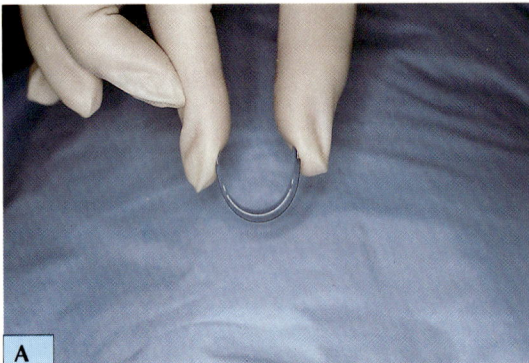

FIGURE 5.11 (A) A razor blade is held in position for cutting. (B) The accompanying schematic shows how the piece of tissue slides right over the blade.

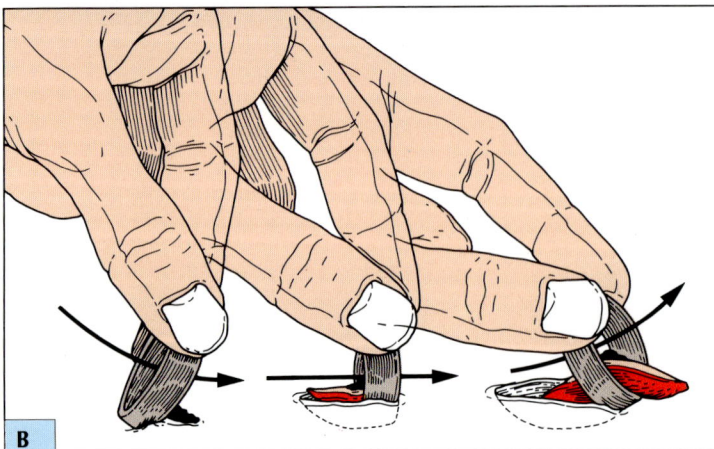

tissue than rotation back and forth. Usually, the punch can be felt popping through to the softer subcutaneous tissue, at which time it can be removed.

Occasionally, the tissue becomes embedded in the punch itself and needs to be extracted (Figure 5.15). Otherwise, the cored out piece of tissue is lifted gently with

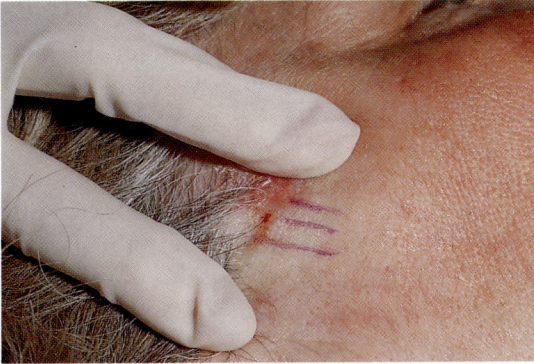

FIGURE 5.12 The dominant skin lines are shown marked with gentian violet and the skin is stretched in a direction perpendicular to them.

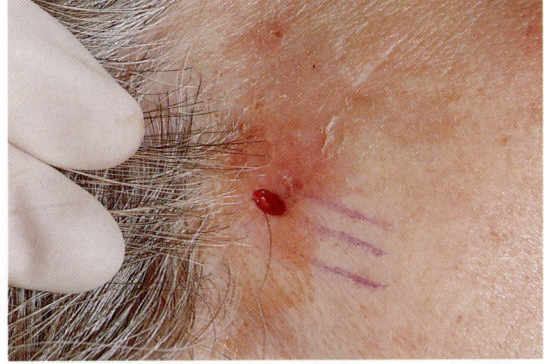

FIGURE 5.13 Once the punch has been done and the skin is released, an elliptical hole should remain.

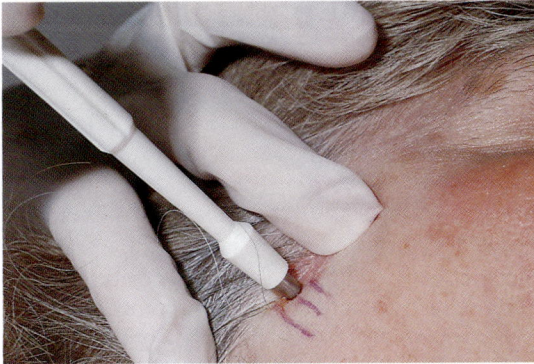

FIGURE 5.14 If the punch is not placed perpendicular to the surface, the closure will be carried out with uneven wound edges, and the defect will not be elliptical.

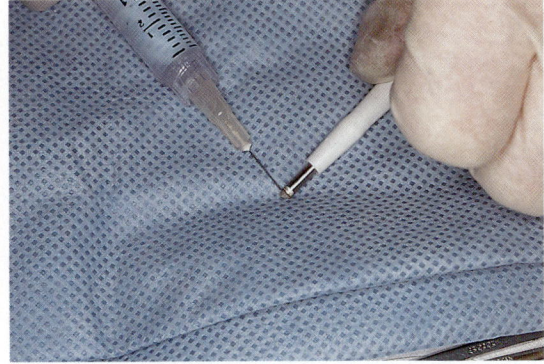

FIGURE 5.15 Small punch biopsies are easily lost. The surgeon should ensure that they are in the trephine itself or still in the defect before anything is wiped from the site. Using the point of a small-gauge needle, the tissue, if lodged in the trephine, can be speared gently and extracted.

toothed forceps or a skin hook and is snipped at its base, which is usually fat (Figure 5.16). To lift extremely small specimens, or to avoid crushing larger ones, the 30-gauge needle that was used to inject the area may be used to elevate the lesion by spearing it and pulling it upward (Figure 5.17). The biopsy site can then be closed using one to three sutures. Suturing may provide adequate hemostasis. However, if suturing is not an option, the defect can be cauterized or filled with an absorbable hemostatic material or pressure can be applied. However, suturing usually provides the best hemostasis and the most acceptable scar (Figure 5.18 A,B).

Biopsies of the scalp should tilt the trephine so that it is parallel to the angle at which the hairs exit. A biopsy there must also penetrate deeply into the subcutaneous tissue to sample the area adequately.

Disposable punches come in various sizes from 1 to 8 mm in diameter. Trephines of 2 to 3 mm can be used to remove small lesions or to obtain biopsies of lesions where the diagnosis can be established easily. A 4- to 6-mm punch is a good sample size for an unknown dermatosis with uniform pathology. A 6- to 8-mm punch obviously gives a larger sample and is faster than an incisional or excisional biopsy of the same size.

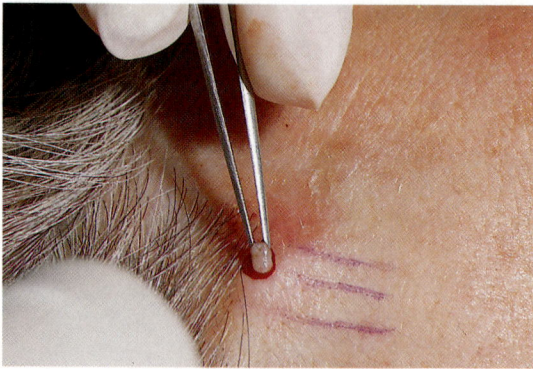

FIGURE 5.16 The cored-out piece of tissue should be snipped at its absolute base to remove it completely, providing the maximum amount of tissue for pathology, and to avoid leaving devitalized fat to necrose in the wound.

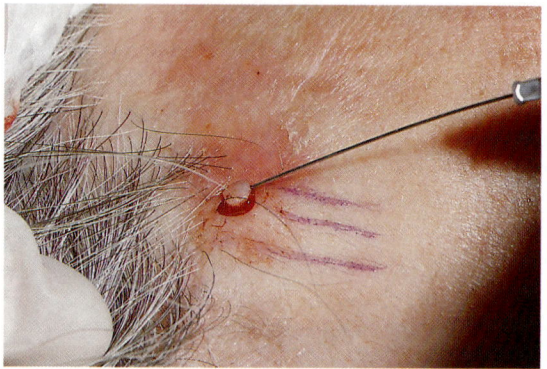

FIGURE 5.17 As it is lifted from the site, a small specimen, or any specimen, should be treated gently. Crush artifacts caused by non-toothed forceps or by mishandling may prevent the pathologist from rendering a diagnosis on an otherwise adequate piece of tissue.

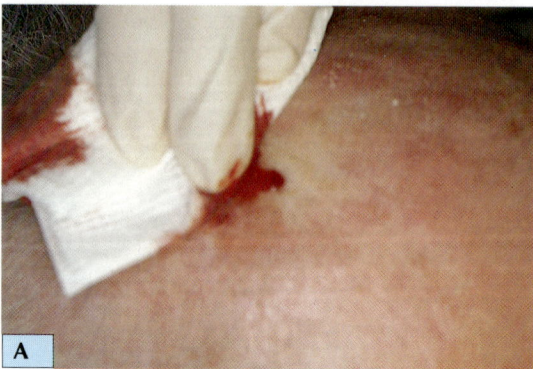

A

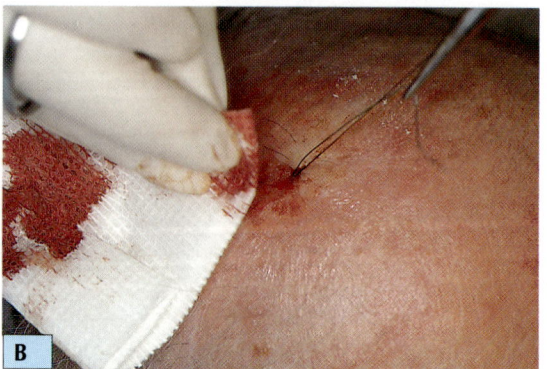

B

FIGURE 5.18 (A) A small punch biopsy on the highly vascular scalp shows rapid bleeding and welling, and requires use of a gauze pad for constant blotting. **(B)** With one suture, the bleeding has stopped completely, and the gauze absorbs no more blood.

However, if such a large sample size is required, a punch may not give enough information about pathology that lies deep in the fat and it may not leave as cosmetically acceptable a scar as one of the excisional sampling techniques. A 6- to 8-mm punch is difficult to close without fairly prominent dog-ears.

INCISIONAL BIOPSY

An incisional, or wedge, biopsy samples a portion of a lesion or an area, but does so more completely than the previously described techniques. It is usually performed when a large portion of a lesion needs to be sampled and/or when the pathology may lie deep within the subcutaneous tissue and an adequately sized specimen needs to be obtained. Examples of this would include a panniculitis, a large melanocytic lesion containing an area that has changed, or a keratoacanthoma that needs to be distinguished from a squamous cell carcinoma. Ulcerated lesions also are often sampled by this technique. In such instances, a single biopsy ideally should sample normal surrounding skin and the edge and base of the lesion. The procedure is that of a simple excision (Figure 5.19).

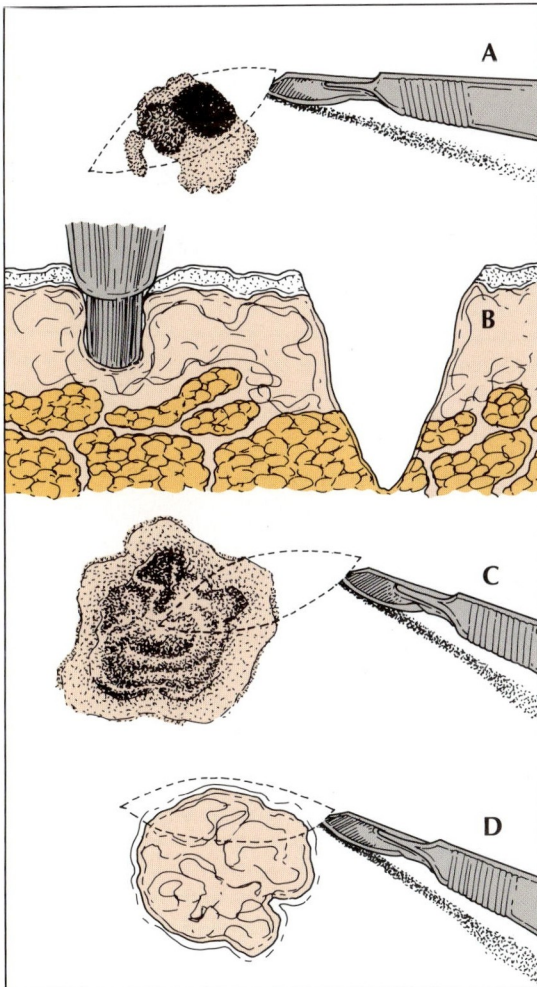

FIGURE 5.19 Schematic drawing showing incisional biopsy technique. (A) To sample part of a large lesion using a scalpel, a classic elliptical incision is made according to the rules of excision for appropriate placement of linear scars. Foremost is removal of the necessary tissue. (B) To sample part of a deep lesion, the cut should extend down to deep fat. A punch biopsy is shown next to the incision demonstrating the depth that it can achieve in sampling deeper tissue. (C) To sample multiple areas of a single lesion such as an ulcer, adequate pathology may be obtained deep in the center, on the border, or in both areas as compared to normal surrounding skin. (D) Distinguishing a keratoacanthoma from a squamous cell carcinoma usually requires a slice through the entire lesion, showing both edges.

EXCISIONAL BIOPSY

An excisional biopsy differs from an incisional biopsy in that it removes the entire lesion instead of just sampling it. It is the preferred technique for a suspicious melanocytic lesion. An excisional biopsy takes margins that are fairly narrow, and it is done to excise the entire lesion and to establish the diagnosis on which to base more definitive surgery. If both the biopsy and the surgery are done at the same time, the procedure is technically not a biopsy, but a true excision. For further discussion of this technique, please refer to Chapter 6, on simple excisions.

NAIL BIOPSY

Biopsies of the nail bed can be done using any of the previously mentioned techniques once the nail plate has been removed. If removal is not possible or if the patient refuses, a double punch biopsy can be performed, utilizing a

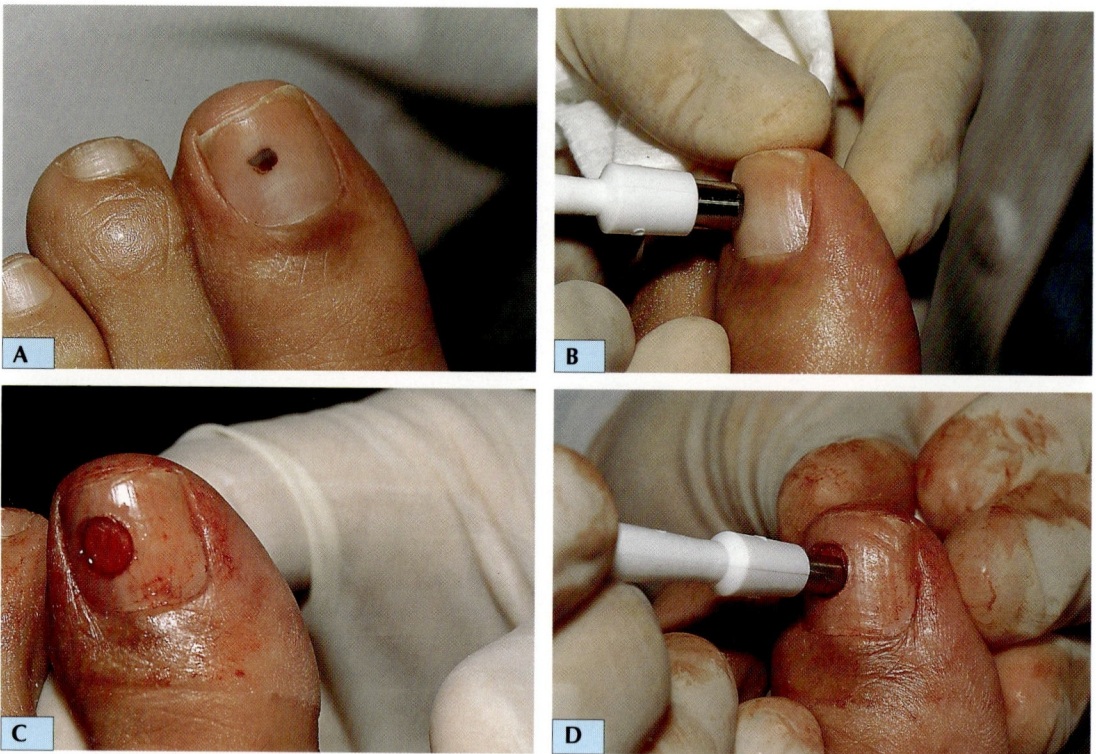

FIGURE 5.20 (**A**) A newly acquired, unchanging pigmented lesion on the big toe requiring biopsy. (**B**) A 6-mm trephine is placed on the overlying nail plate and is rotated and advanced gently. As soon as the firmness of the plate is no longer felt, the trephine is removed. (**C**) The plate is lifted off and snipped at its base. There is an obvious tissue plane between the nail plate and the bed. If this plane is not reached, the trephine should be used again to advance the cut in the nail plate. (**D**) A trephine just slightly smaller than that used for removal of the nail plate is used to obtain a biopsy of the underlying lesion in the nail bed. The nail bed can then be treated as for any other punch biopsy.

larger 4- to 6-mm punch to remove part of the nail plate and a smaller 3- to 4-mm punch to pass through the remaining hole and to obtain tissue from the underlying nail bed (Figure 5.20 A–D). The reader is referred to Chapter 23 for a complete discussion of nail surgery.

Proper biopsy technique is a preliminary to good excisional surgery technique. Apart from adequate surgical skill, the importance of the clinician's judgment is crucial. Both factors, exercised skillfully, will yield consistently good results.

SUGGESTIONS FOR FURTHER READING

Fewkes JL, Sober AJ. How to do a better skin biopsy. Your Patient and Cancer. 1983;3: 67-76.

Robinson JK. Fundamentals of Skin Biopsy. Chicago, Ill: Year Book Medical Publishers Inc; 1986.

Schultz BC, McKinney P. The dermal punch for skin biopsy and small excisions. In: Office Practice of Skin Surgery. Philadelphia, Pa: WB Saunders Co; 1985:51-62.

Winkelmann RK. Skin biopsy. In: Epstein E, Epstein E Jr, eds. Skin Surgery. 6th ed. Philadelphia, Pa: WB Saunders Co; 1987.

chapter 6

BASIC EXCISIONAL TECHNIQUE

Basic excisional technique is fundamental to the practice of cutaneous surgery and relies on principles that must be mastered before more complex excisional techniques can be undertaken. Such basic principles include the proper planning and marking of the excision with regard to its orientation along favorable skin tension lines; appropriate selection of instruments; and proper execution of the excision including stabilization of the surgical site, proper tissue handling, adequate undermining, and sufficient attention to closure.

DEFINING THE AREA OF EXCISION

The simple excision of a cutaneous lesion usually refers to the removal of an elliptical piece of skin. The geometry of the ellipse is critical to the final scar, as is the angle at each end of the ellipse. Establishment of a length-to-width ratio of 3:1 will help the beginning surgeon to obtain an ellipse that has 30° angles at each end. The surgeon will also be aided by the use of a sterile felt-tipped marking pen to trace an outline of the planned excision (Figure 6.1). This should be done before the area is anesthetized or draped, as either may produce distortion of important landmarks. Later, as expertise is gained, the surgeon may successfully execute the ellipse freehand, while also being able to adjust its length and maintain the 30° angles.

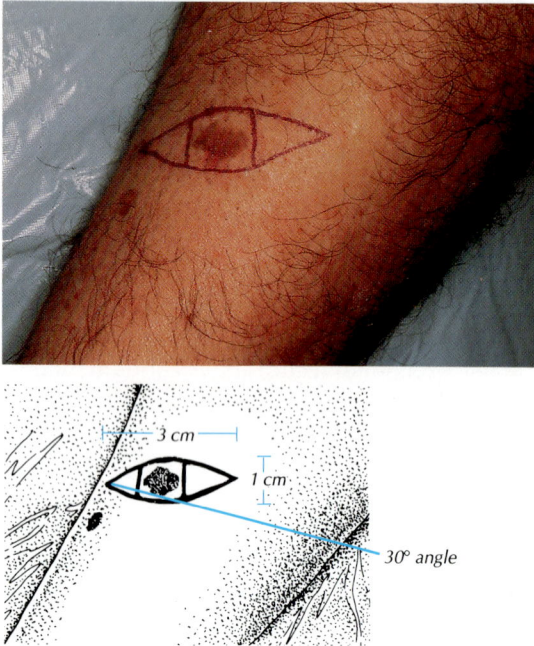

FIGURE 6.1 An elliptical incision can be planned by either measuring the lesion or using a template. For this benign lesion, the margins necessary for its removal are marked. Its width is then measured and the necessary end points are determined using the 3:1 ratio for length to width. The points are then connected to form the elliptically shaped incision, paying particular attention to the 30° angles at each end.

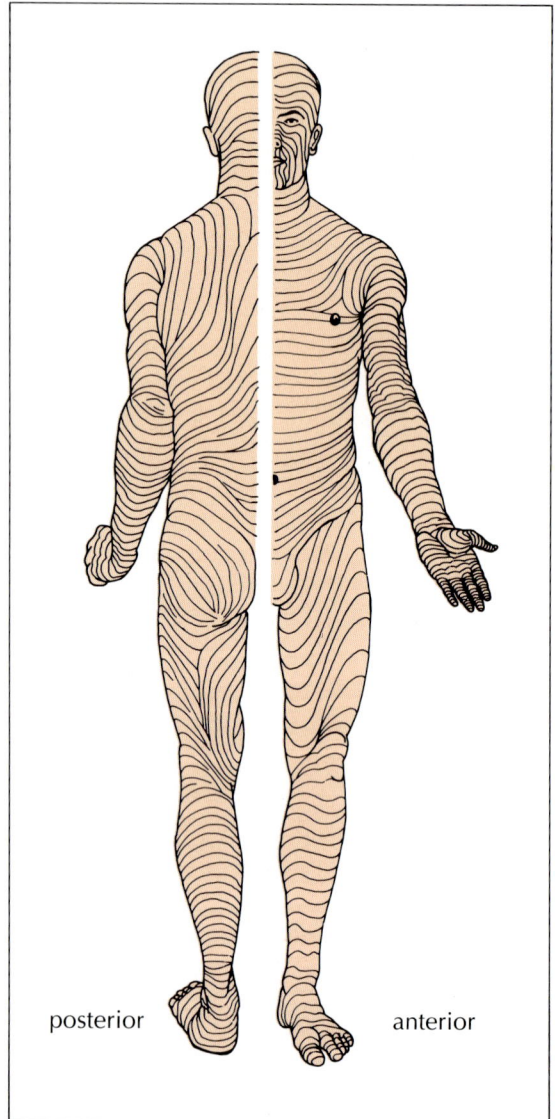

FIGURE 6.2 Schematic diagram showing favorable skin tension lines on the body. Many such charts are available for use when the direction in which to place the suture line is not obvious.

The long axis of the ellipse should lie in an already existing skin crease or in a potential skin tension line. In some individuals, these lines are obvious. In other, especially younger, individuals they may need to be inferred. Relaxed or favorable skin tension lines, the current standard, are lines that usu-ally lie perpendicular to the direction of pull of the underlying muscles (Figure 6.2).

Favorable skin tension lines can also be deduced on an individual basis for each patient. If the lesion is on the face, for example, the surgeon can ask the patient to perform various facial movements that reveal the

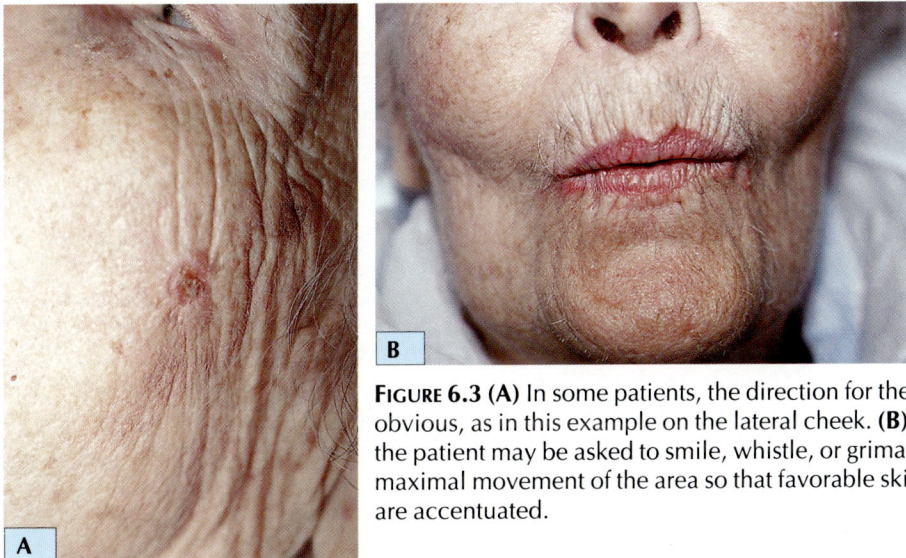

FIGURE 6.3 (A) In some patients, the direction for the ellipse will be obvious, as in this example on the lateral cheek. **(B)** In other cases, the patient may be asked to smile, whistle, or grimace to achieve maximal movement of the area so that favorable skin tension lines are accentuated.

direction of the appropriate lines (Figure 6.3A,B). Similarly, the skin on an extremity may be pinched, which can reveal the area of greatest skin laxity and hence the area that should lie perpendicular to the length of the excision (Figure 6.4A–C).

If the appropriate orientation for an excision cannot be discerned from the methods discussed earlier, a disk excision can be performed in which only the lesion and its margin are excised. The remaining tissues may then be seen to take a shape that follows the direction of maximal skin tension, and the wound is sutured closed appropriately

(Figure 6.5). In the event that there is no obvious direction for closure, as sometimes occurs, the choice for appropriate closure is then in the hands of the surgeon, whose judgment should take into account additional factors determining optimal scar placement. For example, if other scars are found in the area, the new scar should be planned so that it lies parallel to existing scars, thus making it less noticeable. Additionally, the anticipated scar should not cross an aesthetic boundary or extend around a curve, as on the extremities. Ideally, it should run parallel to a favorable skin tension line (Figure 6.6A–C).

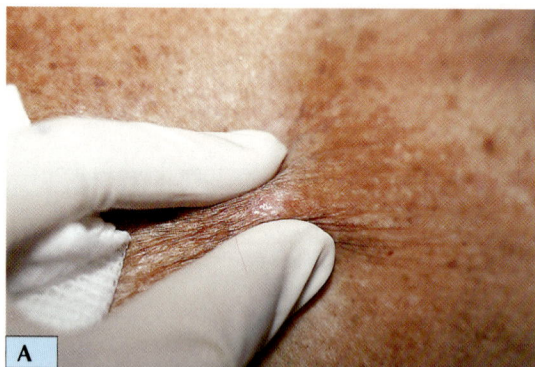

FIGURE 6.4 (A) Pinching of the skin on the upper chest reveals the axis with the greatest amount of skin movement. The incision will be placed perpendicular to this axis. (B) With the patient in a normal sitting position, the skin on his back was relatively smooth. (C) By asking the patient to swing his arm back, the surgeon was able to see the favorable skin tension lines in the area.

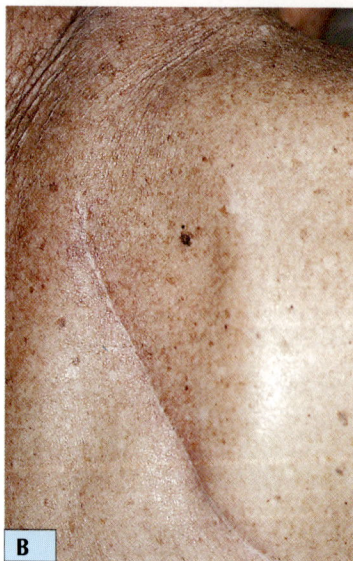

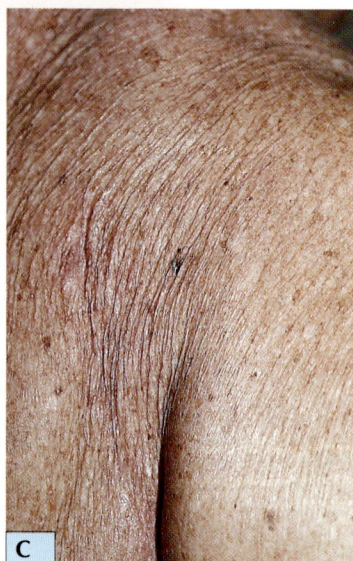

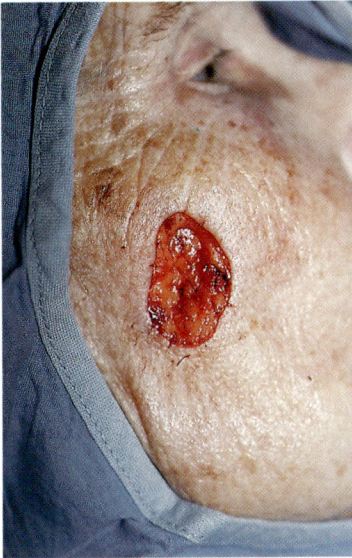

FIGURE 6.5 A large basal cell carcinoma, including appropriate margins, was removed in a circular fashion. Even without undermining, the long axis of the planned closure is evident as the tissue aligns itself along favorable skin tension lines.

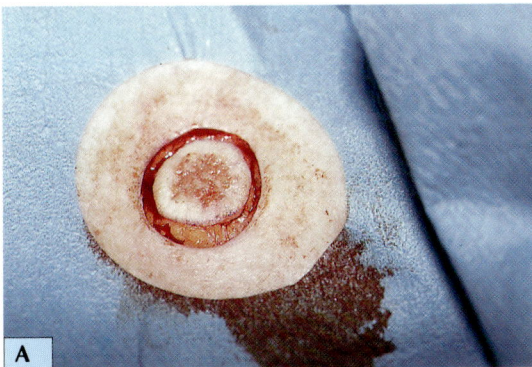

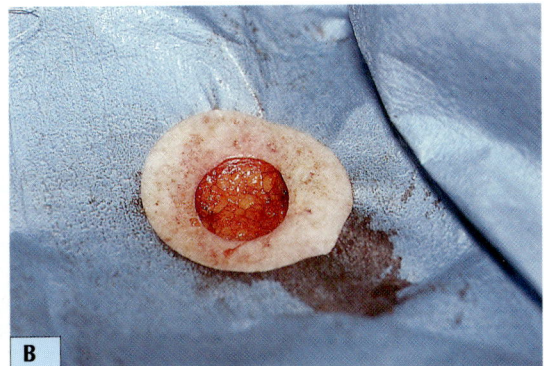

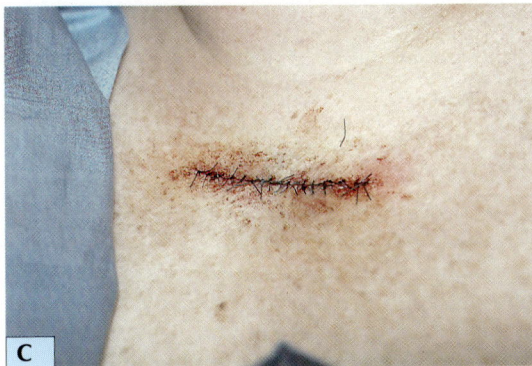

FIGURE 6.6 (A) This lesion of the mid upper chest was removed by disk excision. **(B)** With undermining, no change in the shape of the defect is seen, indicating more or less equal tension in all directions. **(C)** The suture line was placed horizontally in a favorable skin tension line, which was determined by pinching the patient's skin to assess the direction of greatest tissue movement. In addition, there were noticeable horizontal lines on the patient's neck to which the suture line should remain parallel.

SELECTION OF INSTRUMENTS

Once the excision has been planned and delineated, the appropriate tool must be selected. The most commonly used instrument is the #15 blade scalpel, which is made of stainless steel and is very sharp. Disposable scalpels also are available and are useful for shave biopsies. However, they are not as sharp as standard blades and quickly become dull. The Beaver series of blades consists of smaller blades with round handles, which are helpful for working in tight spots such as the pinna, the external auditory meatus, the medial canthus, and the nares (Figure 6.7).

More elaborate cutting instruments also can be found such as the Shaw scalpel, which combines a cutting blade with an electrocoagulation device. This instrument is recommended by some for use in areas that are highly vascular, such as the scalp.

PROPER INSTRUMENT HANDLING

While the choice of blade is important to the success of the excision, the most critical factor is how it is used. With the knife held perpendicular to the skin surface, the tip of the blade is used to begin the incision at one end of the ellipse (Figure 6.8). The knife is then laid

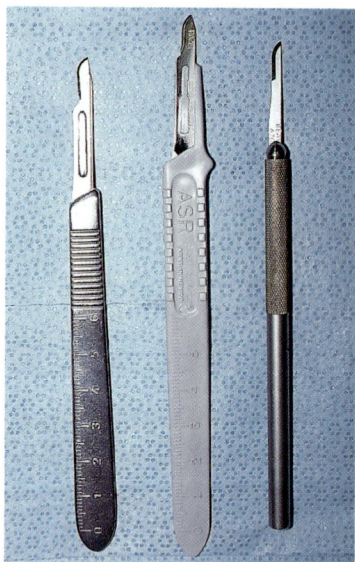

FIGURE 6.7 From left to right, a standard scalpel handle with a #15 knife blade, a disposable handle and blade, and a Beaver handle and blade.

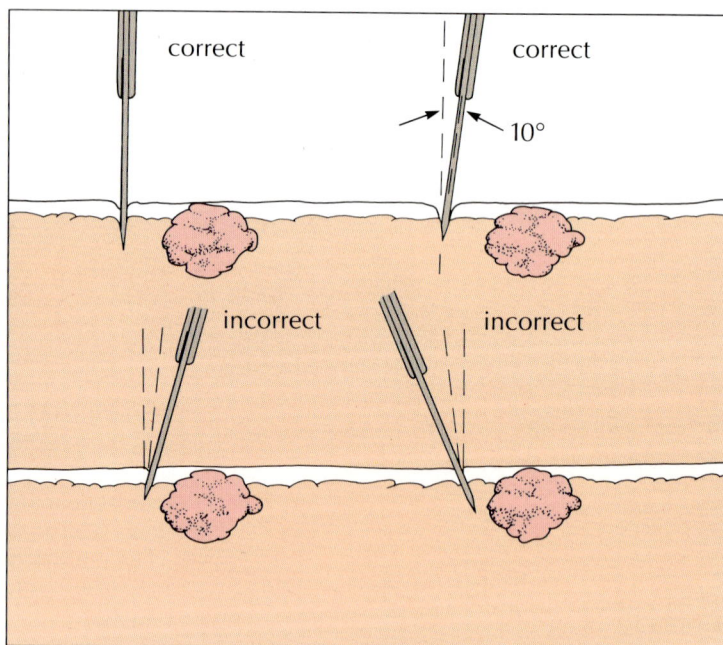

FIGURE 6.8 Schematic diagram showing the correct angle for the scalpel throughout the incision. The scalpel blade should be held perpendicular to the skin surface to achieve as straight a cut as possible, thereby avoiding an overhanging or a beveled edge. Either of these will interfere with wound closure, and also may compromise complete removal of the lesion.

down on its belly while the incision is carried along the remainder of the curve. As the other end of the ellipse is reached, the knife should be brought back onto its tip (Figure 6.9A,B). The scalpel direction is then reversed, so that the surgeon is always cutting toward the center of the excision to avoid cross-hatching (Figure 6.10A,B). In addition, the knife should be handled to cut toward rather than away from the surgeon, to maintain better control.

To stabilize the surface during excision, the skin is stretched tautly. As a result it may fail to lie perfectly flat, for which the surgeon must compensate by adjusting the angle of the scalpel so that he or she is always cutting

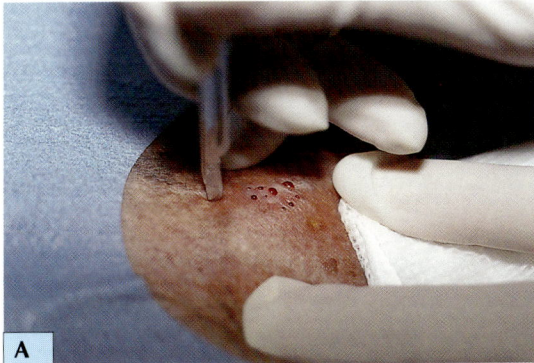

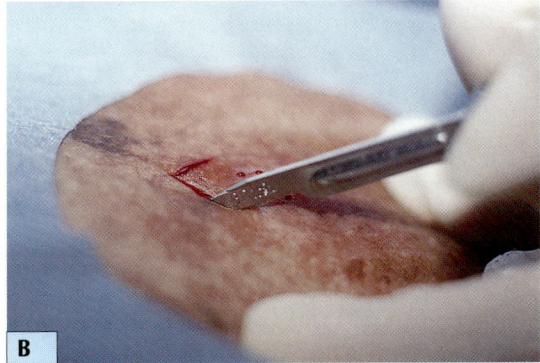

FIGURE 6.9 (A) The incision is begun with the scalpel blade angled on its tip to ensure a sharp point to the ellipse. **(B)** To carry the incision forward to the other end of the ellipse, the belly of the blade is used, with it sharp cutting surface.

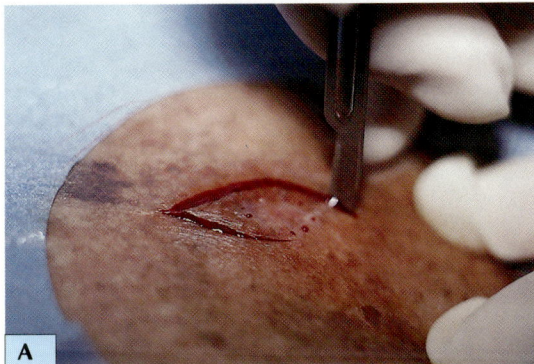

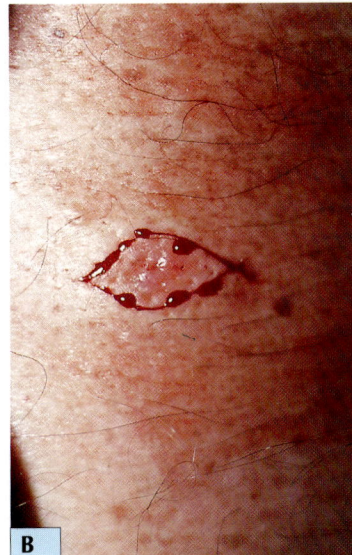

FIGURE 6.10 (A) After creating one angle of the ellipse and incising its upper border, the surgeon creates the second angle by turning the scalpel around and using its fine tip to cut back from the edge toward the center of the ellipse. **(B)** In the absence of proper technique, nicks such as these can result, which may interfere with the final cosmesis of the scar. In this example, the belly of the blade was drawn back too far and overshot the 30° angle, leading to a fish-tail configuration.

with the blade at 90° to the skin surface. One smooth stroke should carry the scalpel blade from one end of the incision to the other. Interruption of this stroke, especially with removal of the blade from the surface, should be avoided as it will result in an uneven cut, with little nicks in it, that may compromise the final cosmetic result.

For most lesions, the incision is taken down to fat. If the incision has been made correctly, the ellipse should be a free-stand-ing island of skin. Toothed forceps are then used to elevate one end of the excised tissue, with a moderate degree of tension applied so that the knife blade can slide easily across the bottom of the cut piece (Figure 6.11A,B). The surgeon should take care to ensure that the knife remains underneath the specimen dur-ing cutting, rather than rising higher into the dermis. The depth of the excision, from one end to the other, should be consistent (Figure 6.12).

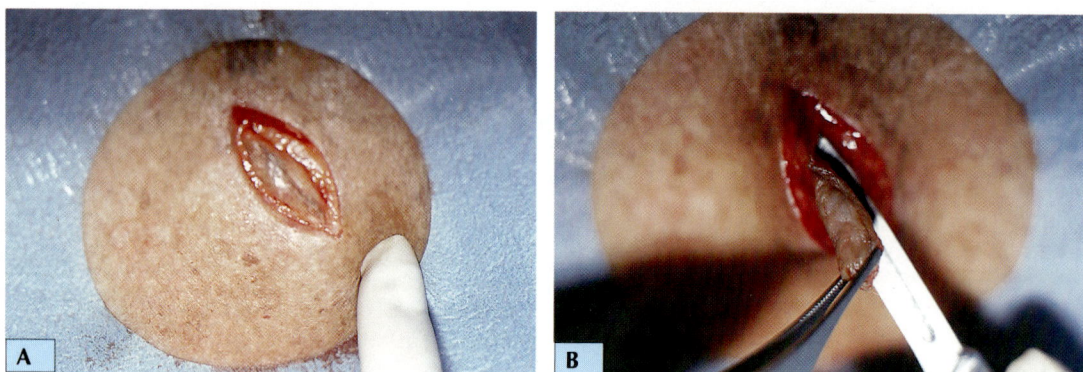

FIGURE 6.11 (A) Note how all attachments to the surrounding dermis have been severed, especially at the tips of this wound. **(B)** With the excised piece of skin elevated, the scalpel is turned parallel to the skin surface, slipped under the piece of tissue, and slid across its remaining attachments to sever it completely, always staying at the same depth in the subcutaneous fat.

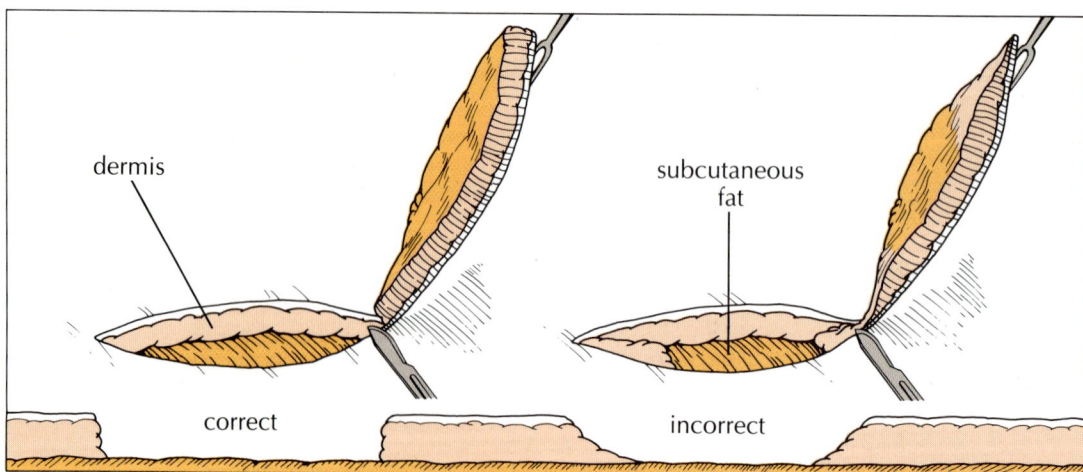

FIGURE 6.12 Schematic diagram showing the proper technique for incising underneath the specimen. It is important that the depth of the incision under the specimen be consistent from one end to the other. A common pitfall is to cut more superficially at either end, thereby increasing the likelihood of dog-ear formation from the excess tissue left behind.

Once the lesion has been excised, the tissue on either side of the wound should be mobilized so that it can be advanced to close the defect. Undermining is performed, the depth of which varies according to anatomic site. On the scalp, undermining occurs in the level deep to the galea aponeurotica, while on most areas of the face undermining is done in the high fat, where there is less of a risk to nerves and vessels. On the nose, the deeper fat is preferred. Undermining on the trunk and extremities occurs in the deep subcutaneous tissue but above the muscle fascia (Figure 6.13A–C). The extent of undermining should be related to the specific needs of the wound closure. To facilitate adequate assessment of these needs, skin hooks or Brown-Adson forceps can be used to approximate

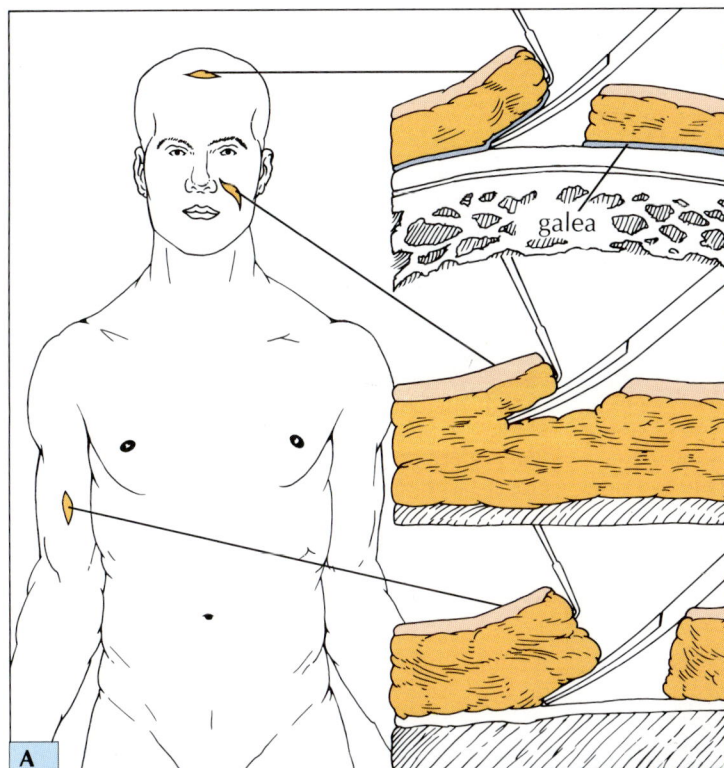

galea

FIGURE 6.13 (A) Schematic diagram showing various levels of undermining that can be done using either a scalpel or scissors. **(B,C)** Blunt-tipped scissors are preferred by most surgeons. They are gently pushed into the wound at the appropriate level and are then opened to push aside the surrounding tissue. This procedure requires a good knowledge of anatomy and a healthy respect for the gentle handling of soft tissue.

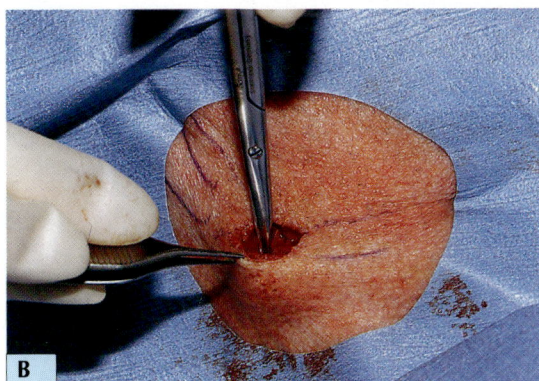

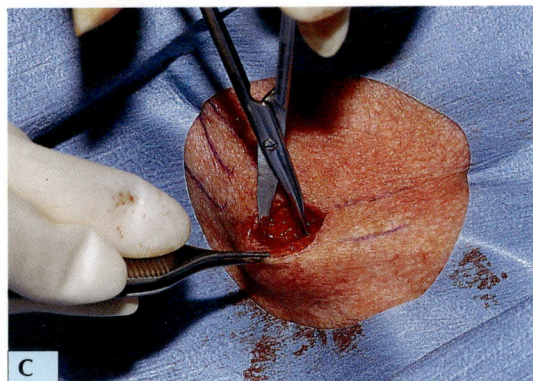

the wound edges. In some cases, no further undermining is necessary beyond that of freeing up the tips of the ellipse to prevent the formation of dog-ears (Figure 6.14A,B).

SUTURING

Once ready for suturing, if the excision has been placed properly with regard to favorable skin tension lines and if proper exci-

sional technique has been utilized along with adequate undermining, the wound should close easily. The use of buried subcutaneous sutures (see Chapter 11) can help to relieve tension on the epidermal sutures used for eversion and coaptation of the wound edges. Careful technique on closure, especially with regard to proper eversion of wound edges, will ensure the most cosmetically acceptable scar (Figure 6.15).

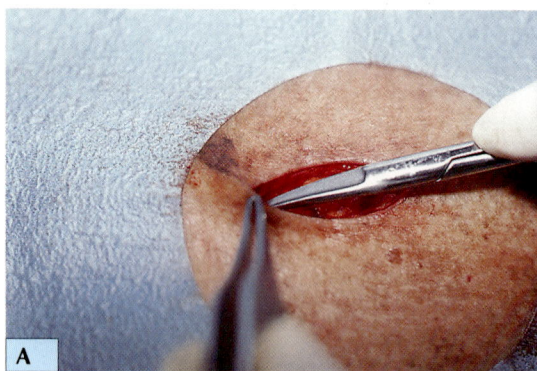

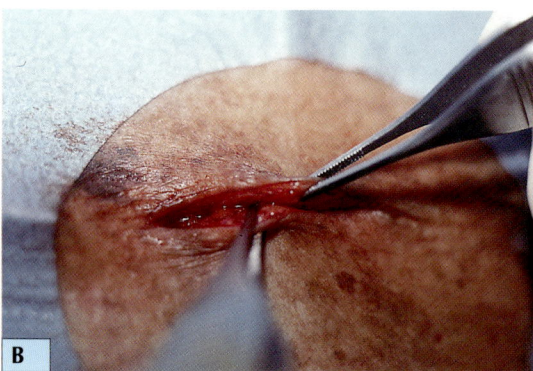

FIGURE 6.14 (A) Undermining at the ends of an elliptical incision should help to decrease the potential for dog-ear formation. **(B)** If the two sides of the wound can easily be approximated, no further undermining is necessary to achieve wound closure with minimum tension.

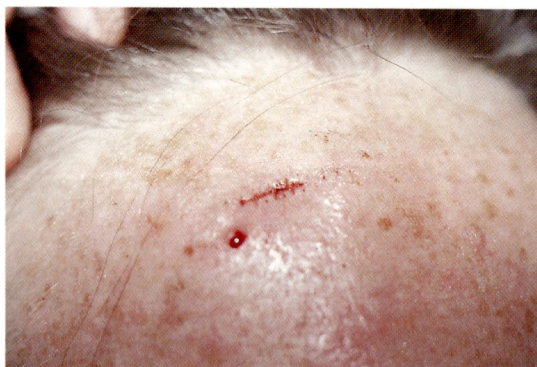

FIGURE 6.15 This wound has been closed without tension, following an elliptical excision made along standard favorable skin tension lines.

SUGGESTIONS FOR FURTHER READING

Bennett RG. Fundamentals of Cutaneous Surgery. St Louis, Mo: C V Mosby Co; 1988.

Stegman SJ, Tromovitch TA, Glogau RG. Basics of Dermatologic Surgery. Chicago, Ill: Year Book Medical Publishers Inc; 1982.

Swanson NA. Atlas of Cutaneous Surgery. Boston, Mass: Little, Brown & Co Inc; 1987.

chapter 7

CURETTAGE

The technique of curettage is used to separate diseased skin or skin lesions from normal skin. Originally adapted from the uterine curet, the dermal curet is accredited to Volkmann in 1870. It is particularly useful for removal of superficial lesions on the cutaneous surface such as seborrheic keratoses, warts, actinic keratoses, superficial basal cell or squamous cell carcinomas, and molluscum contagiosum. When used correctly, it is an effective method of treatment that leaves an acceptable scar.

INSTRUMENTS

Several types of curets are available, which vary in size according to the diameter of the cutting surface. The most commonly used instrument is the Fox curet with its slender handle and 3- or 4-mm diameter. The Piffard curet resembles the Fox curet but its handle is thicker and rounded (Figure 7.1A–C). Disposable curets also are available and are relatively sharp. They have a different "feel" to them, and therefore, require practice before the operator who is accustomed to the Fox or Piffard curet can become proficient in their use. Small curets, 1 to 2 mm in diameter, have been used to ferret out small extensions of a lesion.

TECHNIQUE

The curet should be grasped like a pencil or it should be held with all fingers wrapped around it (Figure 7.2A,B) while the opposite hand draws the patient's skin taut. Then, with a scraping, scooping, or digging motion,

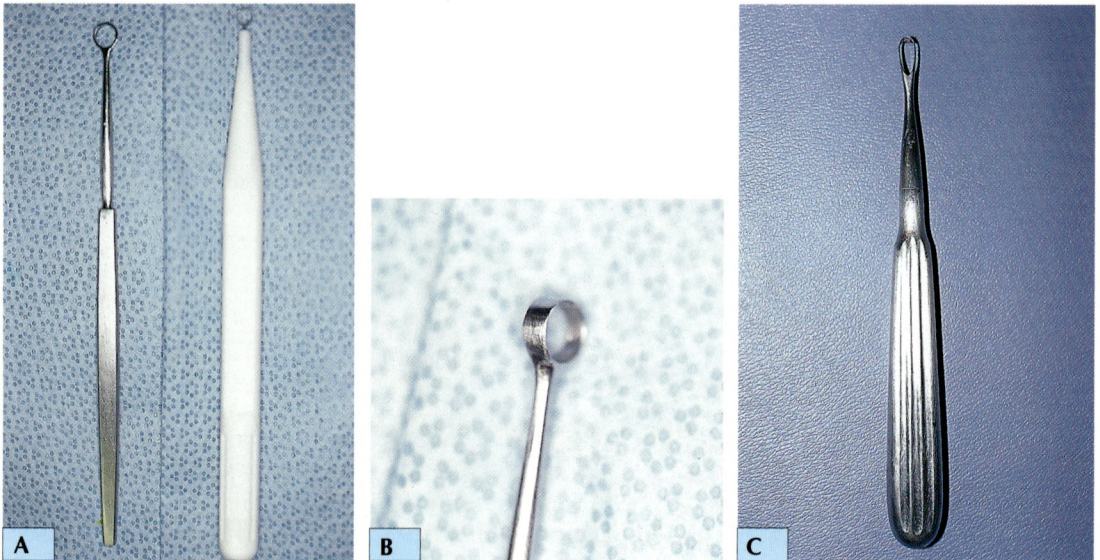

FIGURE 7.1 (A) The Fox curet on the left is the most commonly used instrument. A disposable curet is shown on the right. **(B)** A close-up of the cutting edge on the head of the curet. Only one edge is beveled and sharp; the other edge will not cut. **(C)** A Piffard curet.

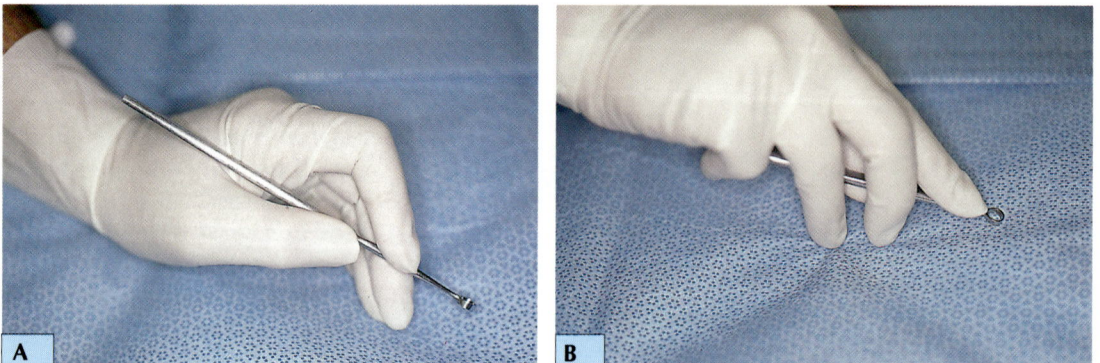

FIGURE 7.2 (A) The curet is held like a pencil with the thumb, index, and middle fingers doing the work. **(B)** The curet also may be held like a peeler, with the entire forearm used to move it back and forth.

the curet is drawn across the lesion in one direction (Figure 7.3). The curet is not meant to be rubbed back and forth across the area. Rather, it should be drawn from the center toward the edge of an imagined circle around the lesion, as if aiming for each of the numbers on a clock face. Alternatively, the curet can be drawn completely across the lesion starting from different points around the edge (Figure 7.4).

In using a curet, the premise is that normal tissue has a different feel to it than lesional tissue, and the more sensitive the operator is to this difference, the more successful he or she will be at removal of the lesion. This type of sensitivity comes with experience. Normal skin is soft and smooth and should not be grated easily by the curet. Lesional skin, by way of contrast, usually has a gritty feel to it. Sometimes the curet may

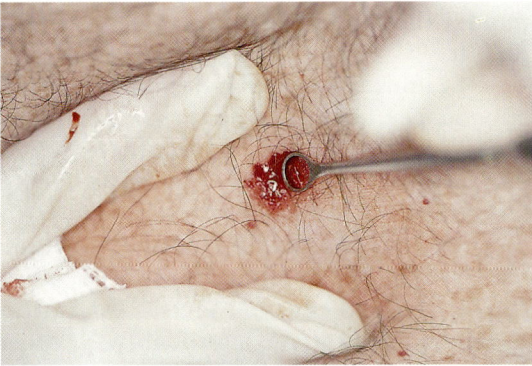

FIGURE 7.3 Two fingers of the opposite hand stabilize the skin as the curet is drawn across the lesion.

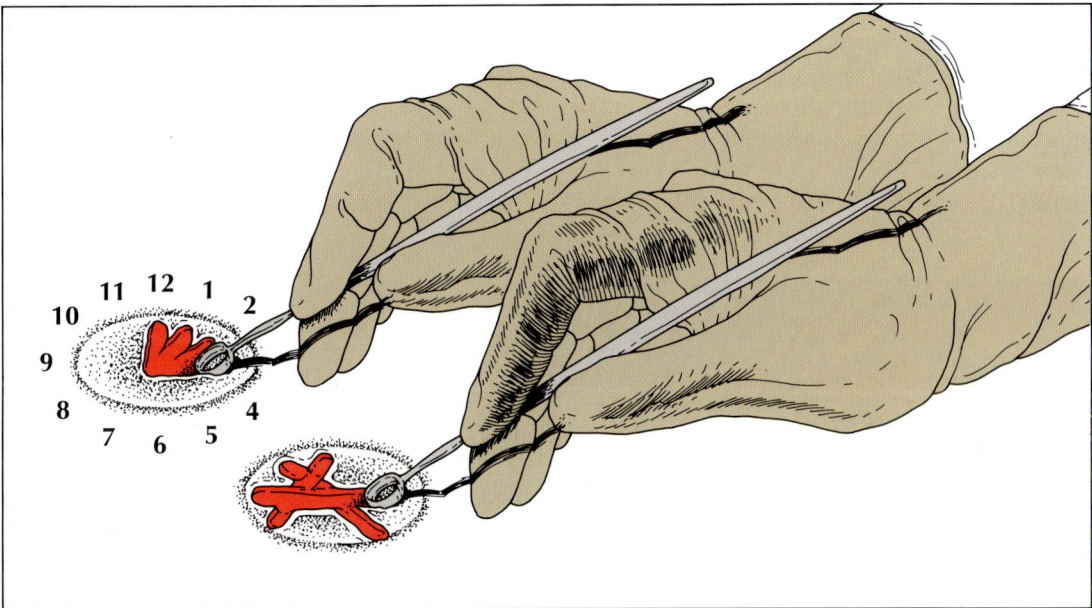

FIGURE 7.4 Schematic diagram showing the direction of the curet as it is drawn across the lesion to ensure that no area is missed.

"fall" into the lesion, finding the tissue friable and easily removed. Once the curet dips down into the skin, the operator must be aware that if the curet is in fat, it can no longer be directed by the "feel" of the lesion. Fat provides a soft, friable background against which the curet is unable to distinguish small lesional extensions. In such a case, another modality for removal of the lesion should be considered. Warts, however, may shell out with a simple digging motion, with the curet placed at the edge of the lesion to scoop it out.

In preparation for the procedure, the site is cleansed with an antiseptic solution such as alcohol or chlorhexidine. While some superficial lesions can be "flicked" off without the need for anesthesia, anesthesia is necessary when electrocautery will be used for hemostasis. While the usual anesthetic is 1% or 2% lidocaine with epinephrine, a light freeze of liquid nitrogen also will suffice. An added advantage of liquid nitrogen is that it hardens the lesion as it freezes it, thus making the lesion easier to scrape off. In addition to electrocautery, hemostasis may be achieved by the use of pressure, Monsel's solution, aluminum chloride, or a gelatin hemostatic sponge. Wound care thereafter consists of daily cleansing with hydrogen peroxide, application of a topical antibac-terial ointment, and a bandaid. Since the resulting defects are superficial, the area should heal rapidly in 2 to 4 weeks.

SELECTION OF LESIONS

In addition to being skilled in the use of the curet, the surgeon must be equally skilled in the selection of lesions for curettage. Lesions that are confined to the epidermis such as warts and keratoses are those most easily "flicked" off with a curet. Curettage should remove the lesion entirely and leave almost no scar.

Lesions that involve dermis or dermal appendages, such as hyperplastic sebaceous glands or syringomas, cannot be removed entirely by curet. They may however be treated by curettage in combination with electrocautery. Light electrocautery is done on the lesion and curettage is used to remove the devitalized tissue. Electrodesiccation followed by curettage is probably the most commonly performed dermatologic procedure. In cases where curettage is performed first and electrodesiccation second, the procedure is not correctly referred to as electrodesiccation and curettage. The former can be used simply for hemostatic purposes or to provide a larger rim of destruction following curettage, as in the case of warts or

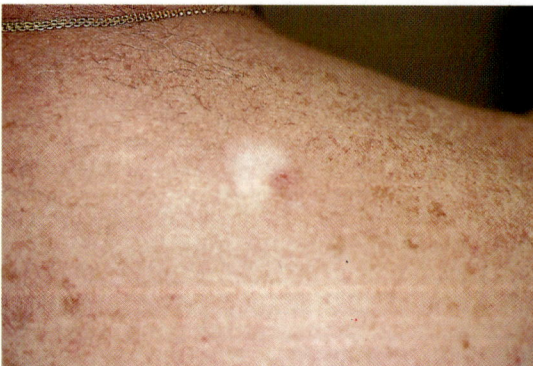

FIGURE 7.5 Because minimal electrocautery was used, the scar left from previous curettage is flat and white even in an area notorious for hypertrophic scarring (the cape area). Notice also the recurrence of a superficial basal cell carcinoma at the 4-o'clock position. Recurrences occur most commonly at the border, which is the most difficult area to clear. The junction of normal and diseased skin is subtle. Therefore, the curet in this location must be used with great sensitivity and should be drawn out at least 2 mm beyond the "feel" of the lesion.

superficial skin cancers. However, electrodesiccation with extension of destruction into dermis may result in a hypertrophic, contracted, or hypopigmented scar. Therefore, for cosmetic purposes, it is best to use the electrocautery lightly and to alert the patient to the possibility of scarring. In the best of outcomes, the scar is flat, smooth, and slightly hypopigmented (Figure 7.5).

Curettage followed by electrodesiccation is also the most commonly used treatment for basal cell carcinoma. In such a case, electrodesiccation is used to provide further destruction. Whether it is necessary is of considerable debate in the literature. Recommendations for treatment range from curettage × 1, curettage × 2, or curettage × 3 with or without electrodesiccation. Recurrence rates range from less than 3% to 26%. Discrepancies in recurrence rates may reflect the operator's expertise in using the curet or the appropriateness of the lesion chosen for treatment.

Lesions on the torso and extremities lend themselves best to curettage because the skin in the area can be stretched easily to provide a firm base against which to work (Figure 7.6A–D). The more difficult areas for curettage are the abdomen and the face, on which it is more difficult to get a firm base

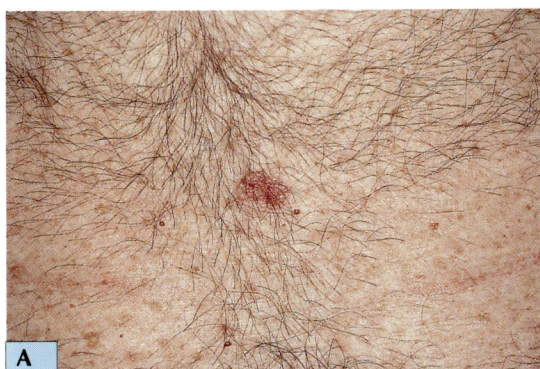

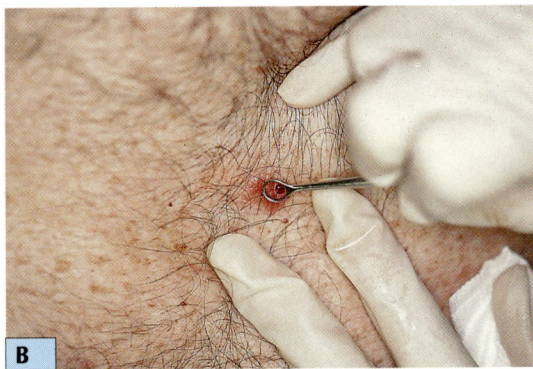

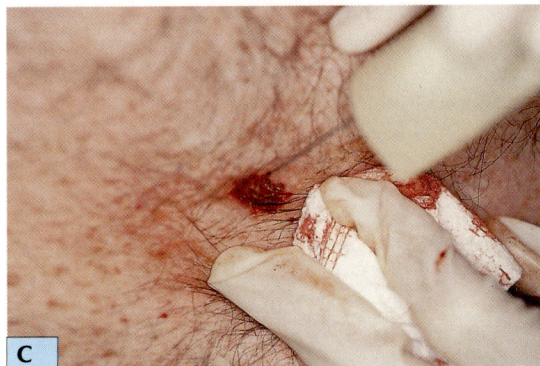

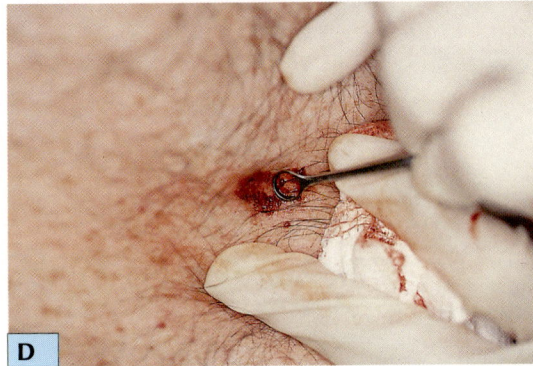

FIGURE 7.6 (A) A superficial basal cell carcinoma on the midchest. (B) The lesion is curetted with the surrounding skin under tension provided by the fingers of the free hand and the pinkie of the hand with the curet. This position also serves to stabilize the operating hand. With the curet held like a pencil, the first three fingers of the hand draw it across the lesion. The involved skin is easily curetted and the epidermis comes off. (C) Light electrodesiccation is done especially around the border as that is the area most likely to contain residual tumor. (D) The charred portion is then curetted again. The gritty feel should now be gone from areas adequately treated and the operator can focus better on any remaining abnormal tissue. The entire procedure is repeated three times.

except perhaps for the forehead and lateral cheeks. In addition, the hypopigmented disk that remains on the face following treatment does not take makeup well and therefore is more noticeable than an excisional scar.

Lesions that are recurrent and contain scar tissue will deceive the curet. Fibrous tissue, whether it be scar or a morpheaform basal cell carcinoma, also will affect the feel of the curet. Such lesions therefore should be removed by other means. The curet, however, may be used to provide an acceptable biopsy of the area for diagnosis. If the resulting diagnosis is beyond question, the definitive procedure can be done immediately follow-

ing curettage (Figure 7.7A–C). If the procedure must be delayed, the tumor site is well preserved, the patient has no need to return for suture removal, and the feel of the tumor may have helped the physician decide upon the best method for removal.

Thus the curet is a multipurpose instrument that can be used for biopsy, removal, or definition before removal of many cutaneous lesions. Furthermore, it is simple and cost effective. However, the technique is mastered and refined only through experience, which must include use of the curet as well as patient follow-up to evaluate success, scar formation, and patient satisfaction.

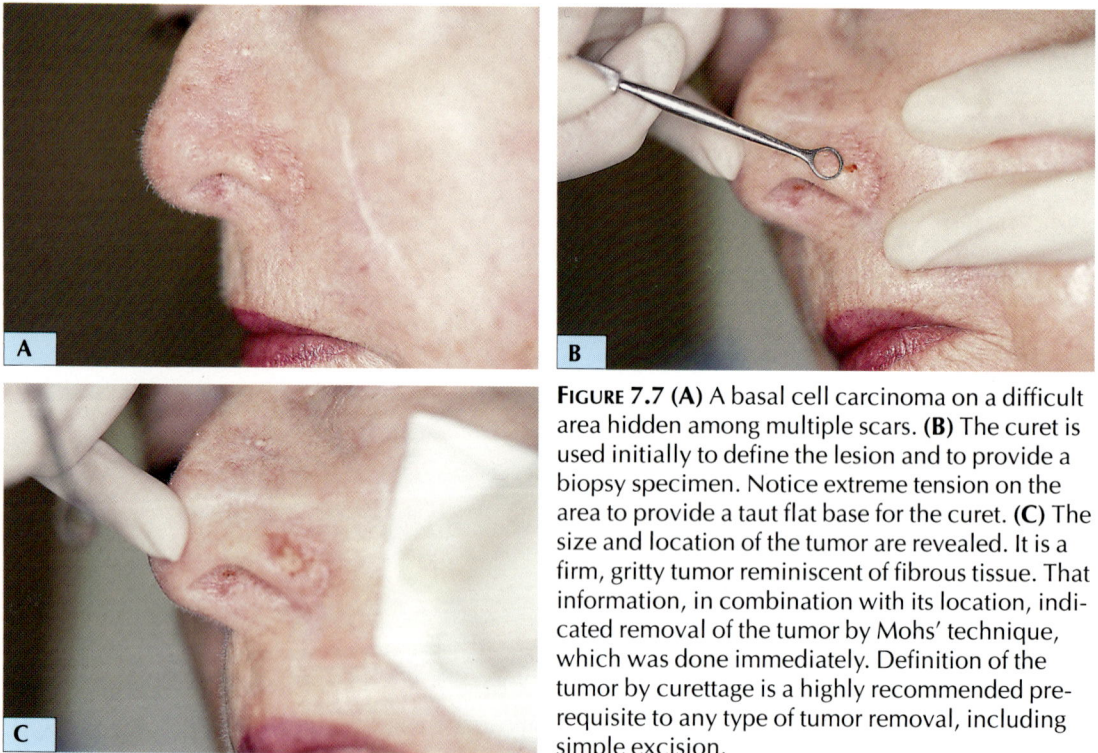

FIGURE 7.7 (A) A basal cell carcinoma on a difficult area hidden among multiple scars. **(B)** The curet is used initially to define the lesion and to provide a biopsy specimen. Notice extreme tension on the area to provide a taut flat base for the curet. **(C)** The size and location of the tumor are revealed. It is a firm, gritty tumor reminiscent of fibrous tissue. That information, in combination with its location, indicated removal of the tumor by Mohs' technique, which was done immediately. Definition of the tumor by curettage is a highly recommended prerequisite to any type of tumor removal, including simple excision.

SUGGESTIONS FOR FURTHER READING

Adam JE. The technique of curettage surgery. J Am Acad Dermatol. 1986;15:697-702.

Bennett RG. Curettage. In: Bennett RG. Fundamentals of Cutaneous Surgery. St Louis, Mo: C V Mosby Co;1988:532-552.

Cott RE, Wood MG, Johnson BL. Use of curettage and shave excision in office practice. J Am Acad Dermatol. 1987;16:1243-1251.

Dubin N, Kopf AW. Multivariate risk score for recurrence of cutaneous basal cell carcinoma. Arch Dermatol. 1983;119:373-377.

Kopf AW, Bart RS, Schrager D, et al. Curettage–electrodesiccation treatment of basal cell carcinomas. Arch Dermatol. 1977;113:439-443.

Krull EA. Surgical gems: the little curet. J Dermatol Surg Oncol. 1978;4:656-657.

Spiller WF, Spiller RF. Treatment of basal cell epithelioma by curettage and electrodesiccation. J Am Acad Dermatol. 1984;11:808-814.

Wheeland RG, Bailin PL, Ratz JL, Roenigk RK. Carbon dioxide laser vaporization and curettage in the treatment of large or multiple superficial basal cell carcinomas. J Dermatol Surg Oncol. 1987;13:119-125.

chapter 8

CRYOSURGERY

The era of cryosurgery began at the turn of the century, when several European scientists successfully liquefied mixtures of oxygen and carbon monoxide and of nitrogen and oxygen. The result was liquid air, which was used by physicians to freeze off small benign lesions. In 1907, carbon dioxide snow was introduced as an additional cryogen, and skin cancers were added as another indication for cryosurgery. It was not until 50 years later that the now most popular refrigerant, liquid nitrogen, was introduced by HV Allington. Its use stimulated the creation of better delivery systems and the more efficient use of cryogens, thereby greatly expanding the field of cryosurgery. Research and development in fields such as cryophysics, cryobiology, and cryogenetics was able to begin in earnest.

Freezing of tissue, which occurs at around 0°C, produces necrosis. At −50°C, maximum damage is done to cells. The necrosis occurs as a direct result of ice formation both inside and outside of the cell. If ice forms intracellularly, more destruction is done and the cell has less chance of survival. Therefore, to increase the effectiveness of cryosurgery, rapid freezing is indicated, which precipitates the formation of ice intracellularly. Slow freezing precipitates ice formation extracellularly. The amount of time it takes for the frozen tissue to lose all evidence of freezing is called the total thaw time, or, the rewarming time. The slower the thaw time, the more damage done to the cells. Multiple repetitions of freeze–thaw cycles are even more lethal to cells. Thus, for maximal killing of cells as in skin cancers, freezing should be rapid, achieve temperatures of −40°C to −60°C, and thaw slowly. For benign lesions, lighter and shorter freezes are indicated, which thaw rapidly.

Cells are differentially sensitive to cryosurgery, with rapidly growing cells, nerve cells, and melanocytes being those most sensitive. Because melanocytes are frequently destroyed, cryosurgical scars are usually hypopigmented, especially after treat-

ments involving longer application of the cryogen, as is used for skin cancers. Where cosmetic considerations are especially important, this side effect must be communicated clearly to the patient before he or she undergoes treatment. Care should also be taken in freezing areas in which there are superficial nerves, as at the elbow or on the digits. Patients should be forewarned of the possibility of temporary anesthesia following treatment. Sensation almost always returns although it may take up to 18 months to do so. As this phenomenon is not dose related, even very short freeze times may affect sensation.

Lesions reportedly treated with success by cryosurgery include angiomas and venous lakes, dermatofibromas, granuloma faciale, keloids either before or just after the injection of steroids, actinic keratoses, leukoplakia,

FIGURE 8.1
MINIMUM TEMPERATURES OF COMMONLY USED CRYOGENS

CRYOGENIC AGENT	MINIMUM TEMPERATURE
carbon dioxide	−79°C
nitrous oxide	−90°C
fluorocarbons	
Freon 114	−33°C
Freon 12	−60°C
Freon 22	−70°C
Freon 13	−90°C
liquid nitrogen	−196°C

seborrheic keratoses, lentigines, mucoceles, prurigo nodularis, sebaceous hyperplasia, trichiasis, warts, certain deep fungal infections, molluscum contagiosum, benign and malignant lesions of the oral mucosa, and skin cancers. While several modalities exist to treat each of these lesions, the choice of cryosurgery versus other treatment modalities depends on a variety of factors including the expertise of the operator, the availability of the cryogen and delivery system, specific characteristics of the lesion including its location and diagnosis, the age of the patient, the desired cosmetic result, the color of the skin surrounding the site, the patient's level of tolerance, and whether the patient is able to comply with wound care, sometimes prolonged, either through self-care or through care provided by another.

TOOLS

CRYOGENIC AGENTS

Cryogens used to freeze tissue include carbon dioxide, nitrous oxide, fluorocarbons and liquid nitrogen. Carbon dioxide is used in stick form or as a snow or slush, the latter being a mixture containing acetone or alcohol. Fluorocarbons are often used as hardening sprays during dermabrasion. Because of their minimum temperatures (Figure 8.1), they should be used only in the treatment of superficial lesions. Liquid nitrogen is the preferred cryogen with a minimum temperature of −196°C. It is inexpensive, readily available, and can be stored conveniently in an insulated container and refilled regularly as needed or as it evaporates (Figure 8.2A–C).

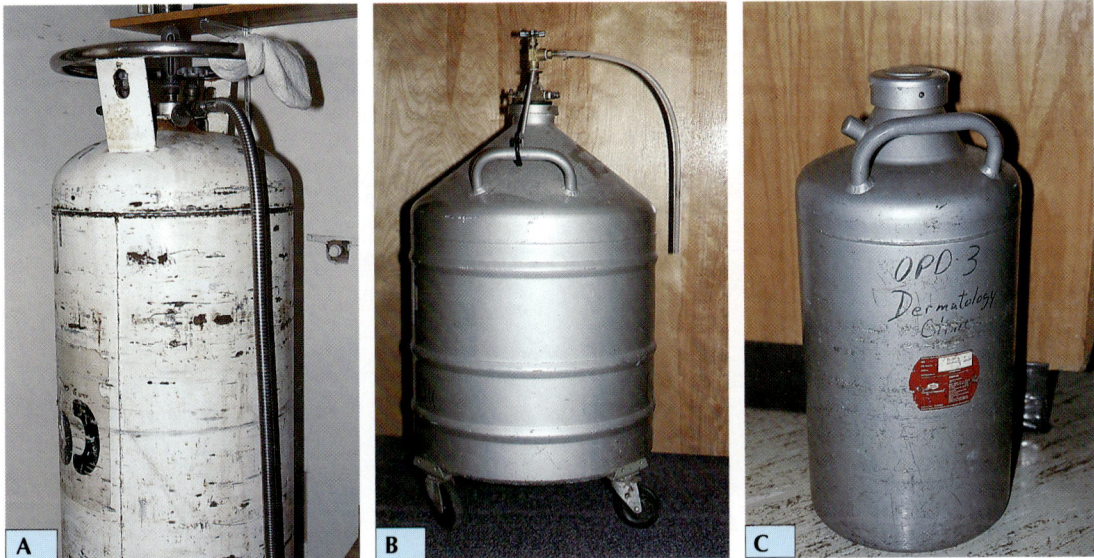

FIGURE 8.2 Tanks of various sizes are available for the storage of liquid nitrogen. (A) The largest such tank (160 L) is delivered full at whatever interval of time it takes to empty one. In a large, busy, hospital clinic, it is refilled every 2 weeks. (B) The more common, medium-sized container (50 to 80 L) is portable and has to be taken to a larger receptacle for more frequent filling. (C) The smaller container (10 to 20 L), which is easily carried, can be taken to a satellite clinic for use over a short period of time.

CRYOSURGICAL INSTRUMENTS

Most dermatologists use a cotton-tipped applicator dipped in a styrofoam cup of liquid nitrogen to freeze the majority of small lesions. A modern version of this swab, called the Frigipoint, has a larger absorbent member, which, when placed within the housing, allows treatment of several lesions in succession without the need for replenishment of the cryogen.

In the 1960s, Irving Cooper developed a cryoprobe unit to deliver liquid nitrogen to sites in the brain and to monitor tissue temperature at the site of destruction. The principles of his instrumentation ushered in modern day cryosurgical practices and formed the basis for later delivery systems.

The cryoprobe is a cold object that acts as a heat sink by drawing heat to itself from the warmer tissues. In 1964, Setrag Zacarian made a cryoprobe using copper disks that were cooled in liquid nitrogen, which were then placed on the lesion. Modern cryo-probes are sometimes attached to the cryogen container, which constantly circulates the cryogen through them to maintain a low temperature during application.

When uniform freezing of the tissue is done, the physical laws that govern the formation of the ice ball allow the clinician to estimate the depth of the freeze by measuring its lateral extent. The two measurements should be equal, so that if a 5-mm rim of normal tissue is frozen around a lesion, a 5-mm deep freeze should be achieved when using a cryoprobe or a restricted spray. The advantage of probes is that there is no spray to affect surrounding structures. Similarly, there is no precipitation of cryogen, as occurs during long freezes, which may run off and freeze normal tissue adjacent to the site or distant to it. Probes also are necessary for endoscopic and neurosurgical use. Another advantage is that they can be pressed down onto the skin surface to produce deeper freezes (Figure 8.3A,B).

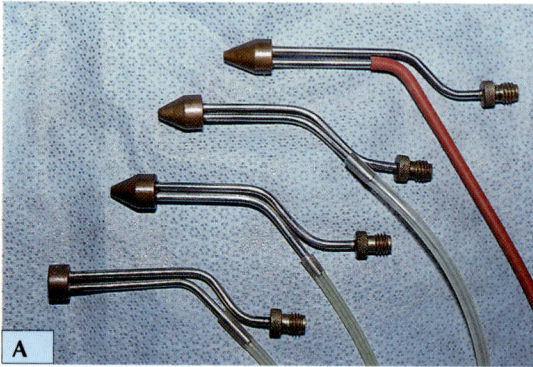

FIGURE 8.3(A) Cryoprobes of various sizes and shapes are shown. The size and shape of the probe selected should fit the size and shape of the lesion.(B) The probe is attached to a hand-held unit. Liquid nitrogen flows to the probe and as it evaporates is vented through the attached tubing. The tubing should be directed away from the patient.

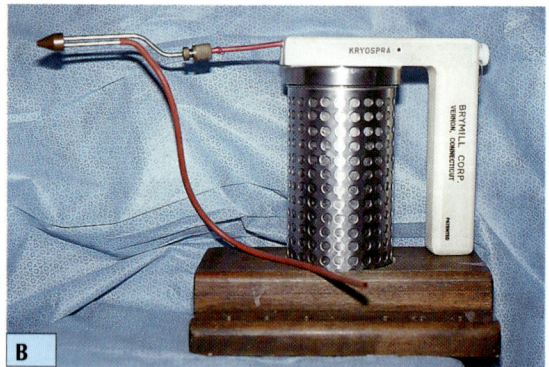

The disadvantage of the probe is that, at its interface with the cutaneous surface, uneven contact may result in uneven freezing of the area, from such factors as dry skin, surface irregularities, or movement of the probe. However, application of petroleum jelly between the skin and the instrument may counteract this problem.

In 1965, Douglas Torre introduced a spray unit for delivery of liquid nitrogen that became the forerunner of our modern hand-held units. The spray allows direct application of the cryogen to the site at its coldest or minimum temperature. By contrast, a probe introduced between the cryogen and the target site elevates the minimum temperature available. Furthermore, with the spray there are no interface problems. It can be moved back and forth freely to give a wider field of any shape, although the freeze itself will be more shallow than that achievable with a probe (Figure 8.4). Neoprene cones can be used with the open spray to direct it and make it more concentrated. More rapid freezing is therefore possible, with subsequently longer thaw times (Figure 8.5). Tips of various sizes also are available to attach to the spray unit, thereby enabling the surgeon to

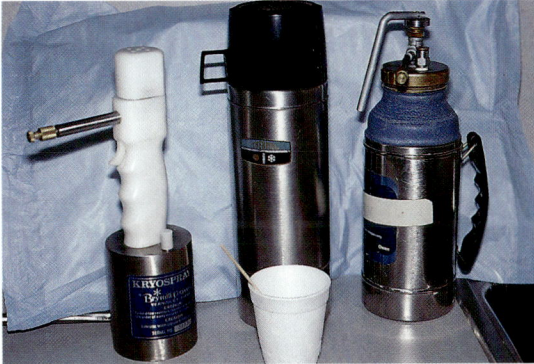

FIGURE 8.4 Various containers are used in cryosurgery. On the left is a hand-held spray unit, with a small receptacle and a thin handle with a trigger mechanism for delivery. It is fairly lightweight. On the right is a larger, heavier model that delivers a spray when the L-shaped bar is pressed toward the container. The thermos in the center is used to transport and hold small amounts of cryogen and to act as a reservoir for its use in styrofoam cups.

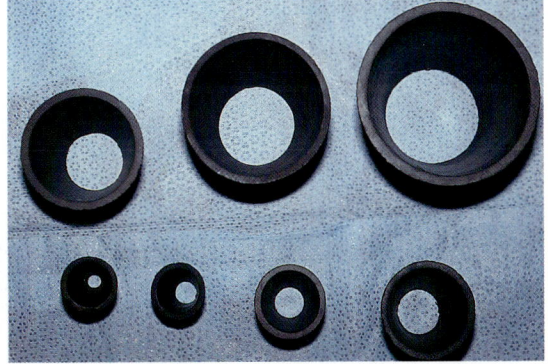

FIGURE 8.5 Neoprene cones of various sizes, ranging from an aperture of 5 mm to 37 mm, can be placed on the skin surface with the cryogen sprayed through them onto the skin. When the cone is used in the treatment of tumors, its size should correspond to the size of the lesion. For example, to produce a 5-mm rim of frozen tissue around a lesion for margin control, the frozen area should extend about 3 to 4 mm beyond the edge of the cone, to allow for the 2- to 3-mm thickness of its rim.

change the caliber and/or direction of the spray (Figure 8.6A–C).

Thermocouples (see page 8.9) are recommended for those who are new at cryosurgery and for those who plan to treat skin cancers, especially large or deep ones. By monitoring temperature at the depth of a lesion, they ensure adequate freezing. Adequate freezing of a lesion also can be determined by measuring changes in electrical impedance in the area, a method that was introduced by PJ LePivert in the late 1970s.

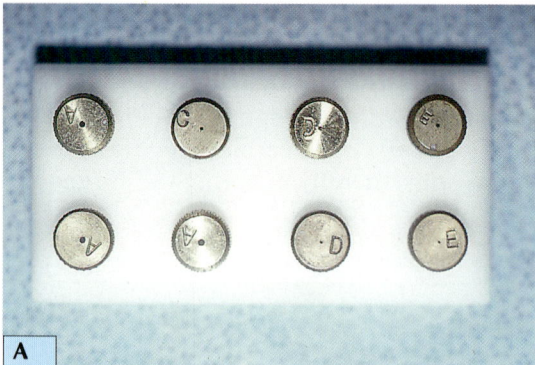

A

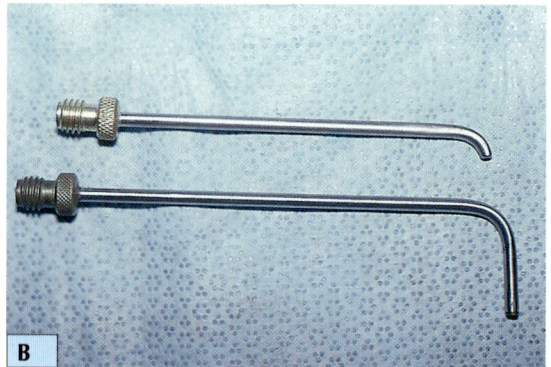

B

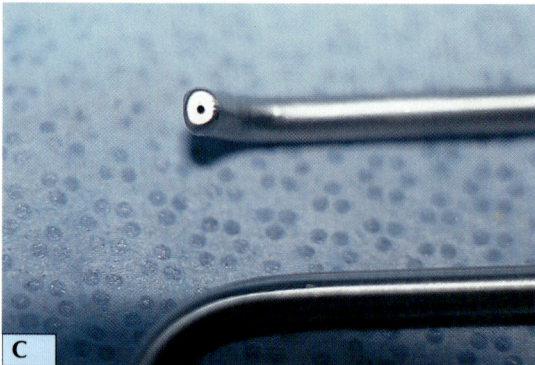

C

FIGURE 8.6(A) Tips of different sizes are available for the spray unit. Larger sized "A" holes are used to treat larger tumors while tinier "E" holes are used to deliver a more precise spray.(B,C) Curved tips with small apertures can be used to spray around curves, as in the nares or on the ear.

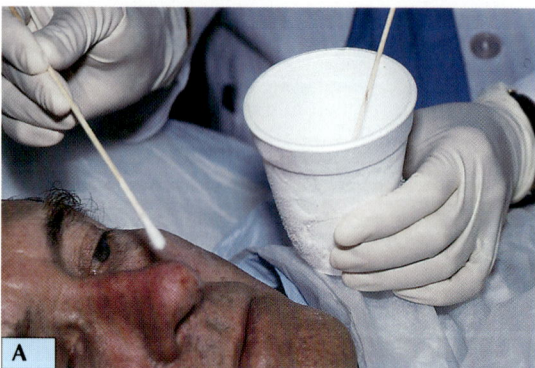

A

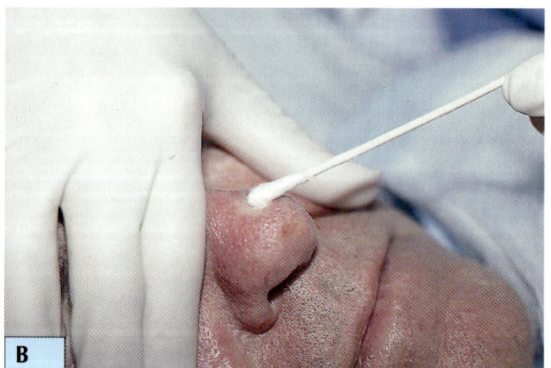

B

FIGURE 8.7(A) With one cotton-tipped applicator in the cup, the other is used to freeze a small actinic keratosis on the nose.(B) By rapidly changing the applicators, a sustained freeze can be maintained even when small swabs are used. During freezing, especially when using a spray, the patient's eyes and mucous membranes should be protected from the spray and from any precipitate.

TREATMENT OF BENIGN LESIONS

DIRECT APPLICATION METHOD

A cotton-tipped applicator is the most commonly used instrument for the removal of cutaneous lesions by cryosurgery. Liquid nitrogen is placed in an insulated container, such as a styrofoam cup, to protect the operator's hand from the cold liquid. A small or large swab, depending on the size of the lesion, is placed in the container. It is recommended that two swabs be used, rather than one, as one swab can be left in the cup to reabsorb the liquid while the other is being used to treat the lesion (Figure 8.7A,B). By alternating swabs in this manner, a lightly frozen lesion will not have time to thaw between applications.

The size of the swab chosen should correspond to the size of the lesion. Larger swabs may be used, which absorb more liquid. They are rolled out at their tip to provide a finer delivery point (Figure 8.8). A 10-second freeze, during which the entire lesion is kept frozen or white, should be adequate for the treatment of superficial lesions. A small rim of normal skin should also be included in the freeze. A total thaw time of 20 to 45 seconds is recommended. This method works well in the treatment of actinic keratoses, lentigines, seborrheic keratoses, and warts.

With modern methods available for the delivery of liquid nitrogen, the direct application method should be reserved for superficial, small lesions for which little destruction is necessary and an optimal cosmetic outcome is desired. Because of the risk of hypopigmentation, it is often better to underfreeze rather than to overfreeze the lesion. The surgeon should explain to the patient beforehand the possibility that a second treatment

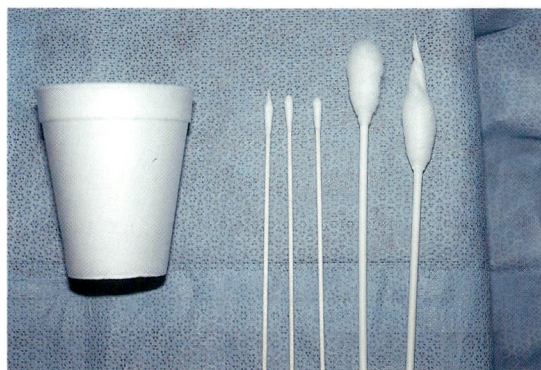

FIGURE 8.8 Any cotton-tipped applicator can be adapted to the size of the lesion.

may be necessary. The site, the individual, and the freeze all can be determining factors in the variable response of any one lesion to a simple, 10-second freeze. Only through experience can the surgeon learn to predict each patient's response to treatment.

SPRAY TECHNIQUE

The spray technique administers a constant flow of liquid nitrogen to the lesion allowing for a very rapid freeze. Three patterns of application have been described: (1) an ever-enlarging circular spray; (2) spraying of the entire lesion from side to side as if making strokes back and forth with a paint brush; and (3) freezing of a central point on the lesion, from which expansion of the ice ball will cover the lesion evenly, along with a perimeter of normal skin. However, most

lesions can be frozen with little movement of the spray unit (Figure 8.9A,B).

TREATMENT OF SKIN CANCERS

Cryosurgery is one of the most frequently used modality for the treatment of skin cancers in the outpatient setting. Success rates up to 97% have been reported. Such encouraging results relate directly to the educated choice of lesions for treatment and to the expertise of the operator. However, most studies report an 85% to 95% success rate. Cryosurgery is recommended for primary lesions, superficial lesions, and nodular tumors (Figure 8.10A–C). It is not recommended for the treatment of poorly defined lesions, morpheaform tumors, and deeply invasive lesions.

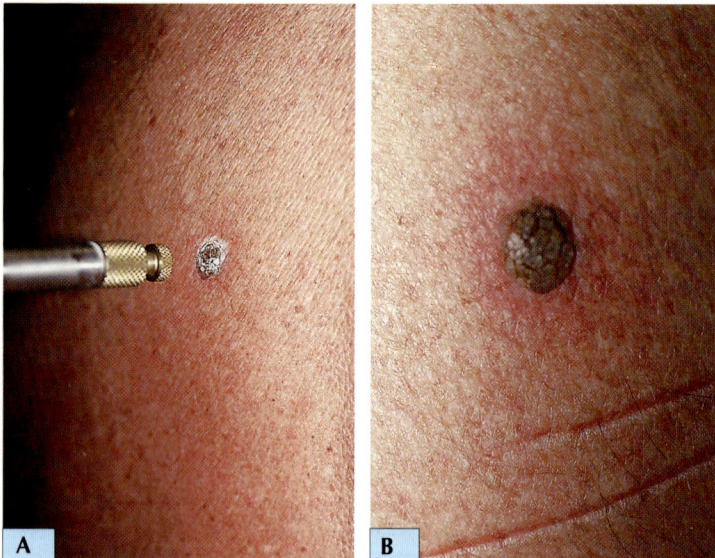

Figure 8.9(A) With the tip of the unit held 5 to 10 mm away from the surface, a seborrheic keratosis on the back is frozen until white, including a small rim of normal skin. It took 20 seconds for the area to thaw.**(B)** Note the immediate rim of erythema around the lesion.

For the initiate to the use of cryosurgery for tumors, thermocouples are recommended to monitor the temperatures achieved at the depth of the lesion (Figure 8.11). Temperatures between –40°C and –60°C are desirable. Depending on factors such as the delivery system used, the size of the spray, whether a neoprene cone is used, and the

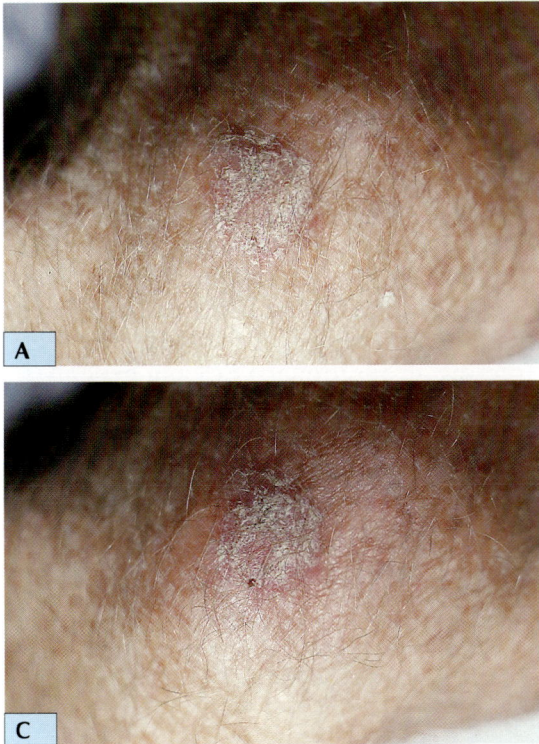

FIGURE 8.10(A) A primary actinic keratosis with a small focus of squamous cell carcinoma in situ is seen on the dorsum of the hand.(B) Using the open spray technique, the entire lesion is frozen, along with a 3-mm rim of normal skin. The total freeze time for the area was 40 seconds, with a total thaw time of 1.5 minutes.(C) Erythema is immediately evident. Pain was minimal, and the patient was warned about the possibility of a temporary loss of sensation.

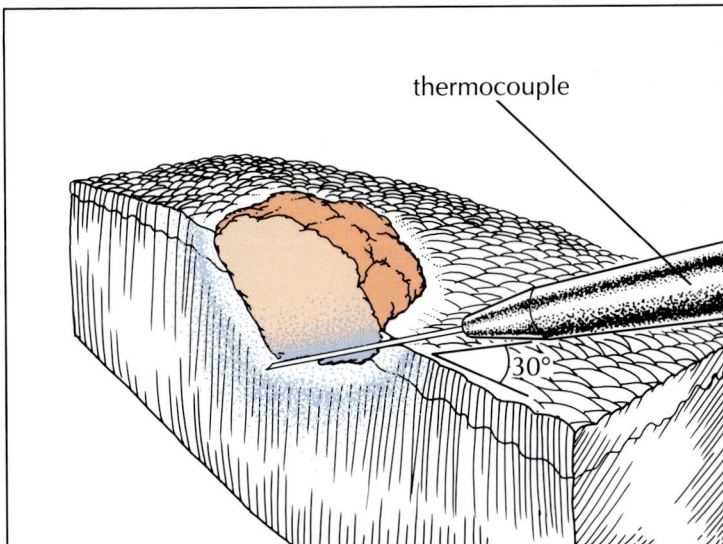

FIGURE 8.11 Schematic drawing showing how the thermocouple may be placed below the lesion to monitor temperature.

location of the tumor near large vessels or bone, adequate freezing times for particular lesions will vary. The thermocouples can help to familiarize the operator with adequate freeze times for different situations, and can then be dispensed with for routine cases. Experts in the field, however, do recommend the use of thermocouples all of the time for tumors of the scalp, ala nasi, nasolabial fold, preauricular skin, and medial canthus. These locations account for many of the recurrences seen after treatment with cryosurgery, perhaps reflecting inadequate treatment at the deepest part of the lesion.

Since intense freezing is uncomfortable, and since the thaw cycle may cause burning and throbbing, the lesion first may be anesthetized using plain lidocaine. Epinephrine is not used as it may extend the area of destruction by enhancing ischemia. Anesthesia is a must if thermocouples are to be used. For lesions near the eye, plastic shields may be used to protect the eye from the spray. Eyelid

tumors should be treated by experts, where caution must be exercised to avoid notching of the lid margin or the development of ectropion. Other areas of concern are the lip margin, where a contracted cryosurgical scar may cause distortion, and in hair-bearing sites, where treatment may result in alopecia (Figure 8.12).

For freezing of a superficial tumor that is not deeper than 3 mm, an open spray, a neoprene cone, or a cryoprobe may be used. As all of these systems are effective, the choice of technique usually depends on the operator and the expertise that he or she has developed with each system. Some surgeons curet the lesion first for better definition of its margins. The cryogen is then applied evenly, freezing an additional 3 to 5 mm beyond the tumor for margin control. The area should be frozen as rapidly as possible to cause lethal destruction to the tumor cells.

Several methods are available by which the adequacy of freezing may be judged. One

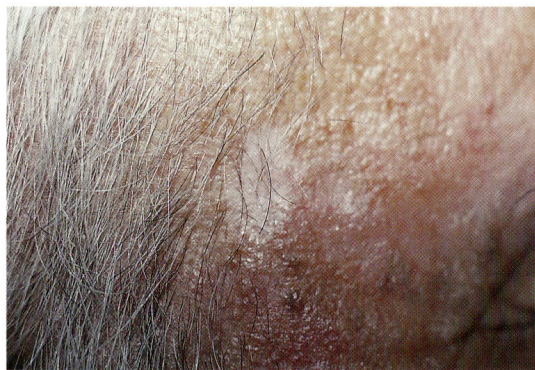

FIGURE 8.12 The classic hypopigmented flat scar created by a short freeze cycle did not cause alopecia, which is more likely to occur with longer freezes.

such method is the halo thaw time, which refers to the time it takes for the 3- to 5-mm margin of noncancerous tissue to lose all evidence of freezing (Figure 8.13A–D). Total thaw time also may be used, which applies the same phenomenon as halo thaw time but does so to the entire frozen area. Another method is the total time that it takes to freeze the area. It is important that each surgeon establish a consistent method of evaluating all treated lesions and that he or she adhere to that method to enable assessment of its effectiveness in his or her hands in terms of cure rate and cosmetic outcome.

If halo thaw time is used, 60 seconds is recommended for adequate freezing. Total thaw time can be 1.5 to 5 minutes. Total freeze time should be 60 to 90 seconds. Total freeze time also may be counted as 30 seconds from the time at which the advancing frost line has reached the tumor margin. These measurements will vary depending on the site, type of lesion, and expertise of the operator. If a thermocouple is used, freezing is stopped for all superficial lesions when the thermocouple reaches –25°C to –30°C.

One freeze–thaw cycle is considered adequate by some for superficial lesions such

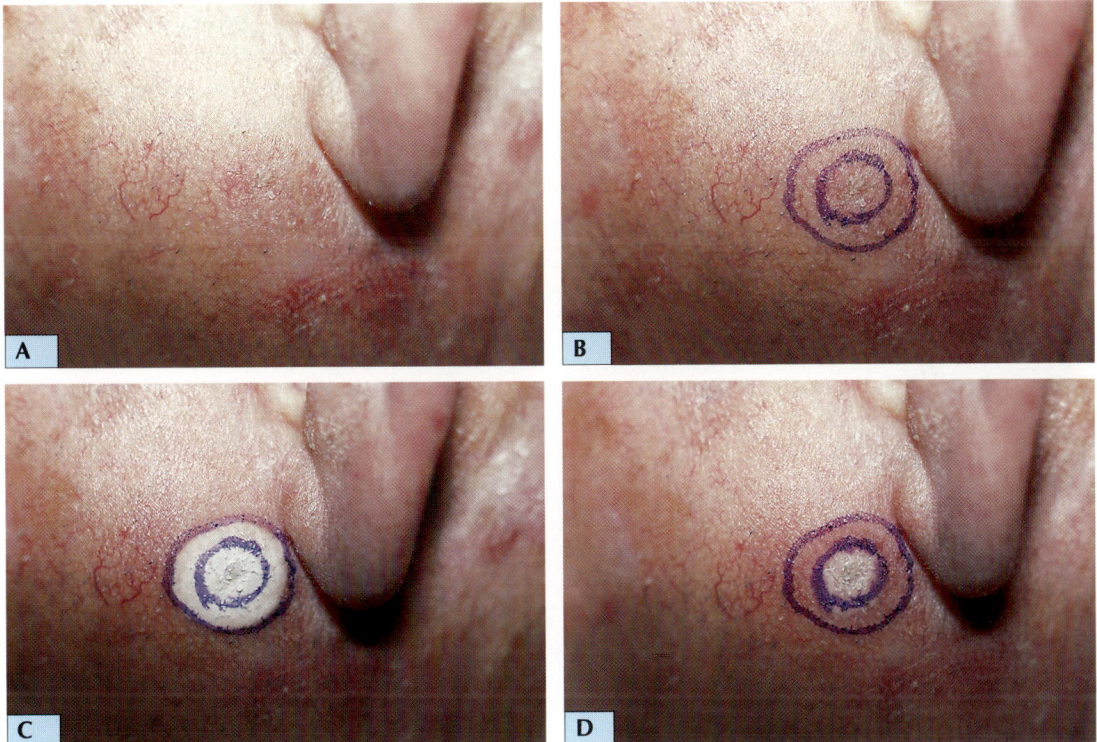

FIGURE 8.13(A) A small superficial basal cell carcinoma located preauricularly.(B) The lesion is marked and a 3-mm margin of normal tissue is drawn around it.(C) The total freeze time is 60 seconds.(D) The halo thaw time, in this case 60 seconds, is when the lesion remains white but the margin has returned to normal.

as superficial basal cell carcinomas and superficial squamous cell carcinomas. All other lesions require two cycles. The second cycle obviously will have a faster freeze time than the first, because some of the tissues, vessels, and cells remain affected from the first freeze.

For deeper lesions, a cryoprobe is useful since it can be placed on the skin, pressed down on it, or even pressed into the lesion to achieve a deeper freeze. For lesions close to underlying bone, freezing can extend to the bone or it can last until the lesion has become fixed to it. Small tumors rarely invade bone and either method gives an adequate deep margin for treatment.

COMPLICATIONS

Cryosurgery is contraindicated in patients with cryoglobulinemia, cold sensitivity, and cryofibrinogenemia. It should be considered with caution in patients with autoimmune diseases and pyoderma gangrenosa. Lesions on the lower extremities frequently are superficial and therefore lend themselves well to this technique. Leg lesions, however, especially in the elderly, heal slowly. Therefore patients undergoing cryosurgery on the lower leg should be prepared for the possibility of prolonged wound healing, up to as much as 6 months (Figure 8.14). Lesions overlying cartilage may be frozen without harm to the cartilage unless the tumor has already invaded it. Such invasion, however, may be difficult to assess clinically.

If performed correctly and in carefully selected patients, cryosurgery has few complications. Most patients experience edema and erythema in the area of treatment, which may begin immediately after freezing (Figure 8.15A,B). These side effects may be marked with longer and larger freezes. In the periorbital area, edema actually may swell the eyelids shut. To prevent this potential complication, some clinicians advocate the use of systemic steroids to decrease inflammation.

While most patients complain of some

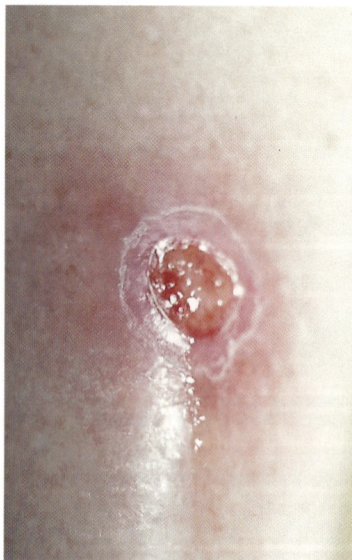

FIGURE 8.14 A cryosurgical wound 4 weeks after treatment of a superficial basal cell carcinoma on the lower posterior leg. The wound healed completely in 3 months.

discomfort during and after treatment, it is easily controlled with a mild analgesic. With freezes done on the forehead, scalp, or temple, patients may complain of a post-therapy headache. Patients should be forewarned of this possibility, and if analgesic therapy is initiated soon after treatment, the headache usually remains mild to moderate.

Infection following cryosurgery is un-usual. A more frequent complication is that of hypopigmentation, which is more marked in lesions treated by longer freezes. The lighter the individual's skin and the less mottled the surrounding skin, the less noticeable the scar (Figure 8.16). For cosmetic reasons, the possibility of a hypopigmented scar should be evaluated before cryosurgery is selected and factors in its choice should be explained to

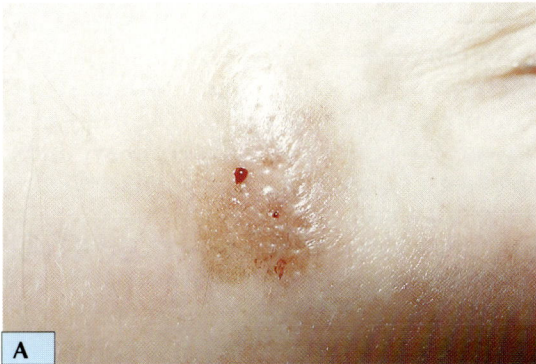

A

FIGURE 8.15(A) A portion of a large lentigo is frozen for 20 seconds, with immediate swelling and redness seen in the area. The remaining half was frozen 6 weeks later, to minimize the patient's discomfort and morbidity following treatment.**(B)** After 5 years there is no recurrence, although the area remains slightly hyperpigmented. This was camouflaged easily by makeup.

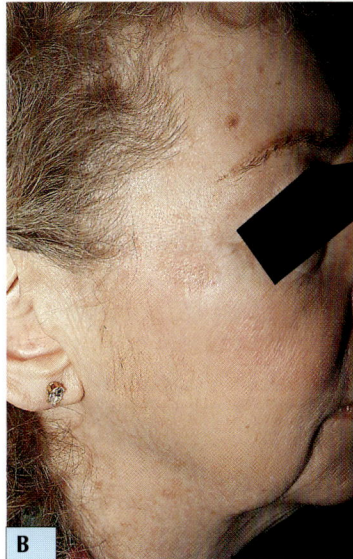

B

FIGURE 8.16 A cryosurgical scar on the cheek of a fair-skinned individual with surrounding lentigines, telangiectasia, and sebaceous hyperplasia. Note that the scar is fairly prominent.

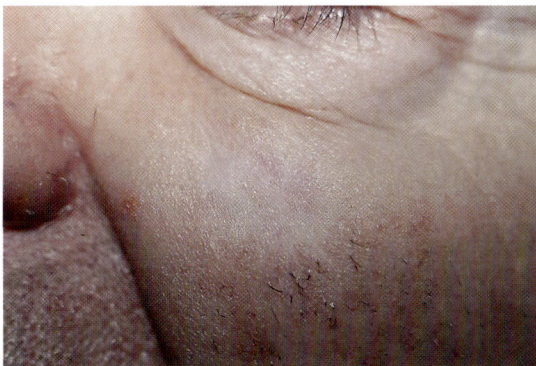

the patient. The patient is unlikely to be satisfied with a large, white shiny round facial scar that is not camouflaged easily by make-up (Figure 8.17).

Hypertrophic scars are seen much less frequently with cryosurgery than they are with electrodesiccation and curettage. If such scars occur with cryosurgery, most are likely to involute spontaneously in less than 1 year. To avoid the possibility of hypertrophic scar formation, curettage followed by cryosurgery is often recommended over electrodesiccation for the treatment of many skin tumors. Superficial nerves also may be affected by the application of the cryogen, as noted previously. Fortunately, sensation almost always returns, although sometimes after more than 1 year.

WOUND CARE

The destruction caused by liquid nitrogen becomes evident immediately after treatment. Initially, swelling and erythema occur, which may vesiculate or develop into a thin eschar depending on the extent of the freeze. In the patient who has undergone a light freeze and who is not particularly sensitive to treatment, the eschar will take 1 to 2 weeks to disappear completely. The site will then likely remain erythematous for several more weeks, as fading occurs gradually. Deeper freezes will produce more evidence of tissue necrosis and may take up to 4 weeks to heal,

after which time the skin becomes erythematous and eventually hypopigmented.

Routine wound care consists of daily cleansing of the area with hydrogen peroxide, and application of a topical antibacterial ointment to speed wound healing, maximize cosmetic outcome, and prevent infection. During the first few days, the wound may be very exudative and require frequent changes of an absorptive, gauze dressing. Sometimes drying treatments are necessary, such as saline soaks or treatment with Domeboro solution for several days. Following treatment of a skin cancer, most wounds heal completely in 4 to 6 weeks. The healing of lower extremity wounds, scalp wounds, extremely large lesions, or wounds involving bone may take longer. Some have recommended the use of topical steroids during wound healing to decrease the inflammatory response to treatment.

SUMMARY

Cryosurgery is an easy and inexpensive way to treat many cutaneous lesions. It can be performed quickly in the physician's office, with little equipment. Most patients tolerate treatment well, even if multiple lesions are involved. Because anesthesia is not always needed, patients in whom anesthesia is contraindicated can be treated by cryosurgery. Furthermore, there are relatively few complications.

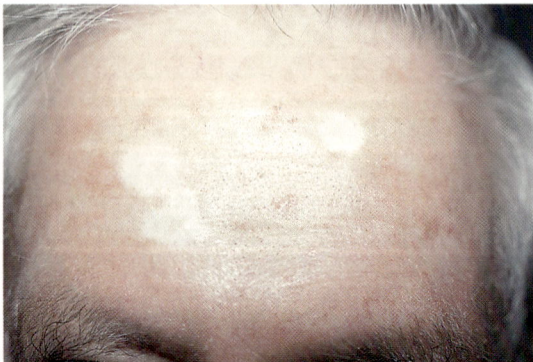

FIGURE 8.17 Many small lesions have been treated on this patient, leaving multiple small white blotches that give an overall unacceptable cosmetic result.

Cryosurgery, however, is not for all lesions. Its limitations must be recognized so that it can be applied appropriately. For example, in the treatment of skin cancers, cryosurgery does not provide margin control. The cryosurgeon uses clinical judgment in deciding where to treat. If adequate margins of a skin cancer are not taken, recurrence is possible. Furthermore, since the depth of a tumor can be unpredictable, it would seem unwise to use cryosurgery in areas of embryonic fusion planes, such as on the midface or the ears, where the depth of the tumor is difficult to assess.

Recurrences following cryosurgery have been seen many years after treatment, with as few as 86% of recurrences seen in the first 3 years. Thus, treatment areas must be followed for many years. Residual tumor may occur at the deep margin as well as the lateral borders, and therefore scars need to be palpated, with biopsies obtained of any suspicious finding. With these precautions in mind, and with appropriate selection and application of the technique, cryosurgery is a modality that greatly expands the outpatient treatment capabilities for many cutaneous lesions.

SUGGESTIONS FOR FURTHER READING

Gage AA. Probe Cryosurgery. In: Epstein E, Epstein E Jr, eds. Skin Surgery. Philadelphia, Pa: WB Saunders Co; 1987:465-479.

Karakashian GV, Sweren RJ. Frigipoint: a new cryosurgical instrument. J Dermatol Surg Oncol. 1989;15:514-517.

Kuflik EG, Webb W. Effects of systemic corticosteroids on post-cryosurgical edema and other manifestations of the inflammatory response. J Dermatol Surg Oncol. 1985;11:464-468.

Lubritz RR. Superficial cryosurgery. In: Epstein E, Epstein E Jr, eds. Skin Surgery. Philadelphia, Pa: WB Saunders Co; 1987:448-456.

Lubritz RR. Cryosurgical spray patterns. J Dermatol Surg Oncol. 1978;4:138-139.

Zacarian SA. Cryosurgery of Malignant Tumors of the Skin. In: Epstein E, Epstein E Jr, eds. Skin Surgery. Philadelphia, Pa: WB Saunders Co; 1987:457-464.

Zacarian SA. Cryosurgery for Skin Cancer and Cutaneous Disorders. St Louis, Mo: C V Mosby Co; 1985.

chapter 9

ELECTROSURGERY

Electrosurgery is a procedure by which tissue is removed or destroyed by the use of electrical energy. This energy, in the form of high-frequency alternating current, is converted to heat within the treated tissues as a result of resistance to its passage.

Over the years, devices for electrosurgical treatment have become increasingly sophisticated. A variety of electrical outputs, each with a characteristic waveform and use, can be generated by a single apparatus. Clinical application of the appropriate output results in selective incision, excision, ablation, or coagulation of tissue.

To optimize the use of an electrosurgical device, the clinician should have some understanding of how such equipment functions. The circuitries of all electrosurgical instruments share certain design features necessary for production of suitable electrical outputs for electrosurgery. Standard household current first passes through a transformer, which alters the voltage, providing the levels and characteristics required for the instrument's various circuit functions. The current next travels through an oscillating circuit, which increases its frequency. Finally, it is delivered to the treatment electrode.

Electrosurgical oscillating circuits may employ a spark gap, a thermionic vacuum tube, or solid-state transistors to increase electrical frequency. The generated outputs and their resultant capabilities will vary depending on the method by which they are produced. Some electrosurgical units, such as the Birtcher Hyfrecator, the Sybron Coagulator, the Burton Electricator, and the Cameron–Miller Technicator, are limited in function to electrodesiccation and, in some models, electrocoagulation. Other popular units, including the Ellman Surgitron, Sybron Bantam Bovie, Sybron Bovie Specialist, Valleylab Surgistat, Birtcher Blentome, and several models manufactured by Cameron–Miller, Aspen Laboratories, and Elmed also provide bipolar cutting currents.

ELECTROSURGICAL OUTPUTS

Each variety of electrosurgical current produces its own unique wavy pattern of current flow, or waveform. The waveforms thus produced can be visualized on the screen of

FIGURE 9.1
APPLICATIONS OF DIFFERENT WAVEFORMS IN ELECTROSURGERY

MODALITY	WAVEFORM	
Electrodesiccation	*Markedly damped*	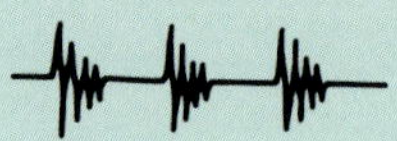
Electrofulguration	*Markedly damped*	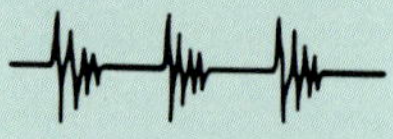
Electrocoagulation	*Moderately damped*	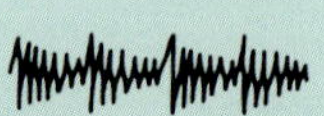
Electrosection with coagulation	*Slightly damped*	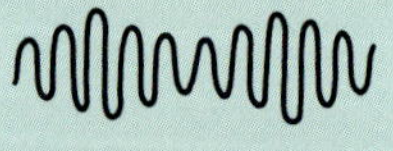
Pure electrosection	*Undamped*	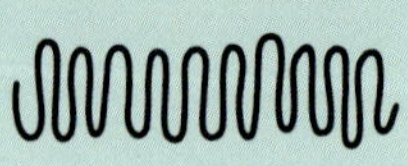

an oscilloscope or traced on an oscillograph. They may be either damped or undamped, depending on the type of oscillating circuit used. In general, damped waveforms provide electrodesiccation and electrofulguration, whereas the application of undamped currents results in electrocoagulation and cutting currents. The spark gap generator produces a damped wave, consisting of bursts of energy in which successive wave amplitudes gradually return to zero. This is caused by the resistance presented by the gap. As the voltage is lowered, damping decreases and the resultant wave trains occur closer together.

Use of a thermionic tube results in a more uniform output. The valve tube circuit is able to neutralize the internal resistance responsible for the damping effect seen in the spark gap circuit, and the amplitude of output therefore remains unchanged. Depending on the circuitry used, the output can be moderately damped (partially rectified) or slightly damped (fully rectified). A filtered, fully rectified output is essentially continuous and uniform, similar to an undamped wave. The different types of waveforms are used for different electrosurgical procedures (Figure 9.1).

CLINICAL APPLICATIONS OF ELECTROSURGERY

The simplest way to think of electrosurgical applications in the clinical setting is to consider the three major capabilities of electrosurgery units. These include superficial tissue destruction (electrodesiccation), deep tissue destruction (electrocoagulation), and cutting (electrosection). Destruction or excision of skin lesions by electrosurgery should be accomplished with the smallest possible amount of damage to normal tissues. Whether electrosurgery, cryosurgery, or CO_2 laser surgery is used, the greater the penetration of the destructive modality into the skin, the greater the likelihood that unacceptable scarring will result. Because the destructive effects of electrocoagulation extend more deeply than those of electrodesiccation, the clinician must consider the histological characteristics of the lesion to be treated in selecting the appropriate current.

ELECTRODESICCATION

For very superficial lesions, such as those involving only the epidermis, electrosurgical destruction by electrodesiccation can be achieved with little if any scarring. The markedly damped, high-voltage current generated by spark gap electrosurgical units causes superficial tissue damage by dehydration of the treatment site (from the Latin *desiccare*, to dry up). The current is delivered in a monoterminal (concentrative) fashion. If the electrode is held at a slight distance from the tissue, a spark is formed between the electrode and the tissue. This technique, termed electrofulguration (from the Latin *fulgur*, lightning), achieves only very superficial destruction because the surface carbonization it produces insulates the underlying tissues from electrosurgical damage.

Electrodesiccation is the method of choice when the most superficial type of tissue destruction is desired. For example, it is ideal for treatment of epidermal lesions such as seborrheic or actinic keratoses, achrochordons, plane warts, or small epidermal nevi (Figure 9.2A,B). Hemostasis of mild capillary bleeding can also be achieved by use of this type of current. A standard technique for treating keratoses by this method is to move the electrode slowly across the surface of the lesion (for small lesions) or to insert it directly into the lesion (for larger lesions), while applying current at a low power setting. After a few seconds the lesion bubbles as the epidermis separates from the underlying dermis. It can then be easily removed with a curette or simply by rubbing a piece of gauze across the treatment site. The clinical endpoint in treating epidermal lesions is punctate bleeding, which is controlled with pressure, by spot electrocoagulation, or by topical hemostatic agents such as aluminum chloride (Figure 9.3A–D). More profuse bleeding indicates probable damage to the

dermis, with a greater likelihood of subsequent scarring. Extremely small superficial lesions can be treated by electrofulguration, which causes the least amount of damage to adjacent tissues.

We ordinarily use a local anesthetic (1% lidocaine), except for treatment of very small lesions that usually require no anesthesia. Before the procedure, the lesion and the surrounding skin should be cleansed with an agent such as Hibiclens or povidone iodine. Because there is the potential for alcohol to be ignited during electrosurgery, it should be avoided as a skin cleanser (or allowed to evaporate thoroughly). Standard postoperative wound management, incorporating semi-occlusive dressings, is followed. Patients should be warned of the possibility of delayed bleeding and should be reassured that it can be controlled by 20 to 30 minutes

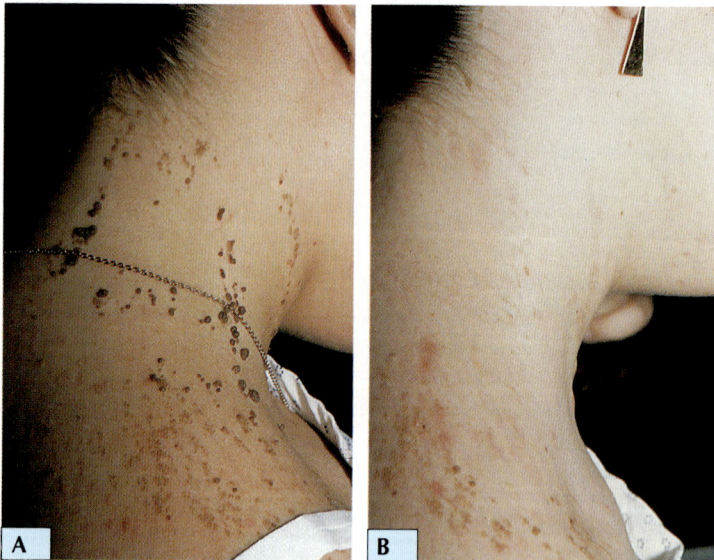

FIGURE 9.2 (A) Epidermal nevi on the neck of a teenage girl before electrosurgical treatment. **(B)** Same patient after three treatments using electrodesiccation. Each lesion is touched lightly with the electrode until charring occurs. Note some residual erythema subsequent to the last treatment, 1 month earlier.

of constant direct pressure over the wound. They should also be told that scarring may occur but that this is usually minimal.

ELECTROCOAGULATION

In electrocoagulation (from the Latin *coagulare*, to curdle), a moderately damped current is applied in a biterminal manner. (Both concentrative and dispersive electrodes are used.) This current is of higher amperage and lower voltage than that utilized for electrodesiccation. Because this type of current penetrates more deeply, it has the potential for greater tissue destruction.

Electrocoagulation is particularly useful for deep tissue destruction and surgical hemostasis. It is our preferred modality for treating small and uncomplicated primary basal cell and squamous cell carcinomas, as well as other lesions such as trichoepithelioma, which extend into the dermis. The electrode is brought into direct contact with the tissue to be treated and is moved slowly across the lesion, which eventually becomes charred. A curette is then used to remove the

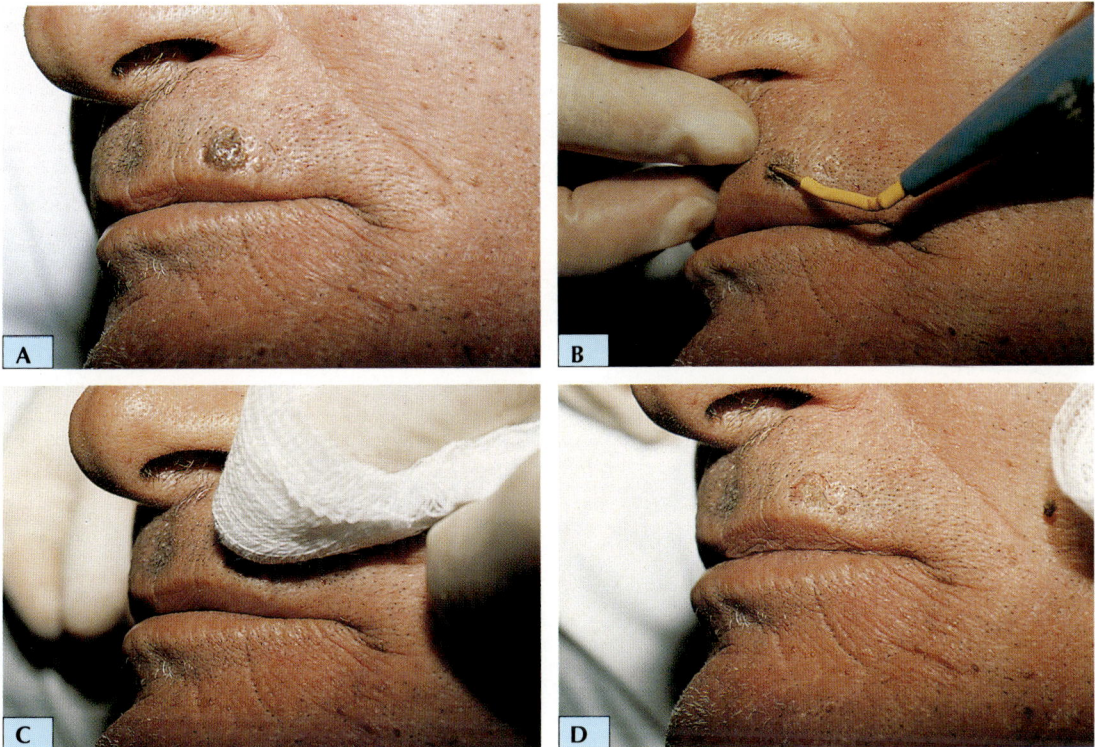

FIGURE 9.3 (A) A seborrheic keratosis on the upper lip. This is a histologically superficial lesion. Electrosurgical destruction should employ a current that provides the most superficial type of tissue damage. (B) Under local anesthesia, the lesion is treated by electrodesiccation. Delivery of current is stopped when the lesion begins to "bubble." (C) In lieu of a curette, a gauze pad is useful for removing charred tissue after desiccation of superficial lesions. (D) There is minimal bleeding, indicating that damage does not penetrate deeply into the dermis.

charred tissue. For treatment of skin cancers we repeat this procedure two more times in an attempt to remove any small tumor extensions. During the last curettage a small curette is often used to remove the final tiny "roots" of the tumor. Scarring must be expected with this procedure, as with any other tissue-destroying therapy, and must therefore be discussed with the patient when therapeutic alternatives are considered. Electrocoagulation is also effective for treatment of superficial telangiectases (Figure

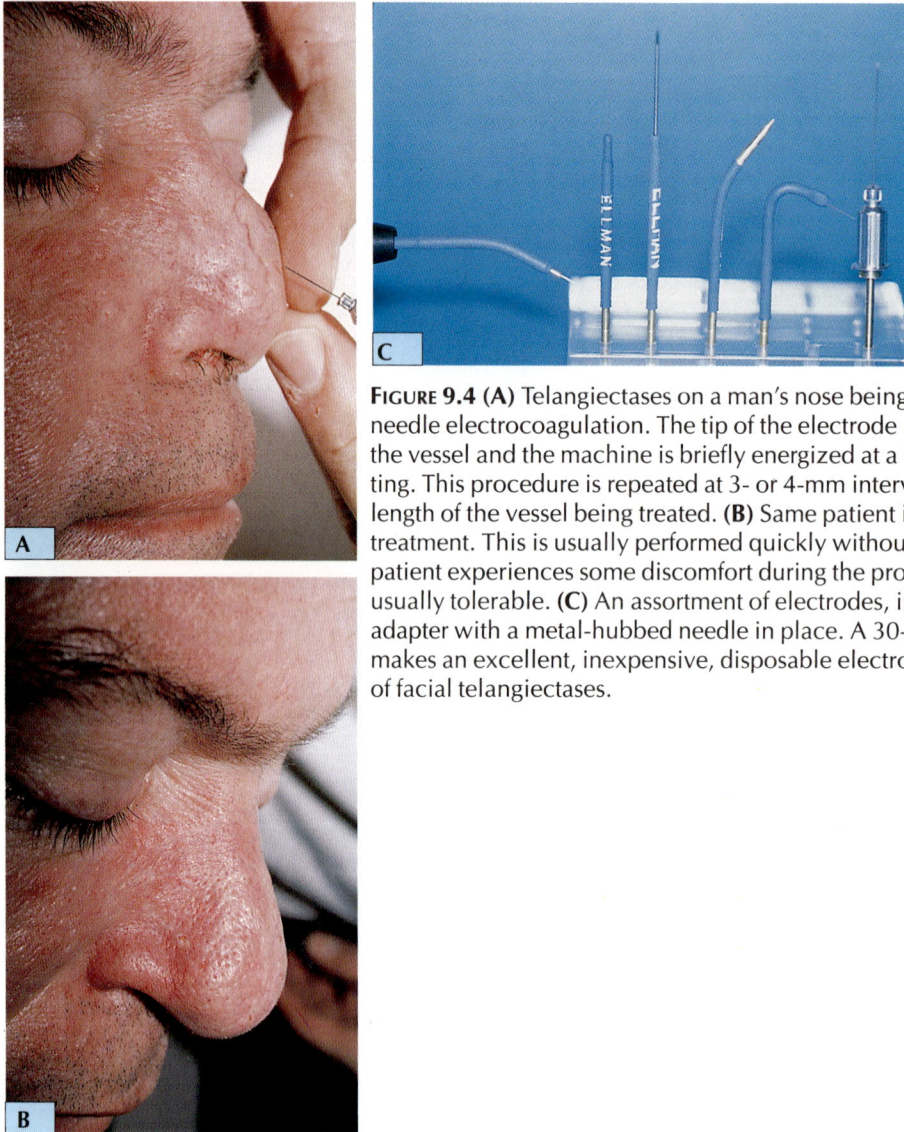

FIGURE 9.4 (A) Telangiectases on a man's nose being treated by fine-needle electrocoagulation. The tip of the electrode is placed inside the vessel and the machine is briefly energized at a low power setting. This procedure is repeated at 3- or 4-mm intervals along the length of the vessel being treated. **(B)** Same patient immediately after treatment. This is usually performed quickly without anesthesia. The patient experiences some discomfort during the procedure, but it is usually tolerable. **(C)** An assortment of electrodes, including a hub adapter with a metal-hubbed needle in place. A 30-gauge needle makes an excellent, inexpensive, disposable electrode for treatment of facial telangiectases.

9.4A–C), unwanted hair (electro-epilation), and ingrown toenails (electrosurgical *matricectomy*) (Figure 9.5A–D).

Hemostasis using electrocoagulation can be achieved by either monopolar or bipolar means. Because the electrosurgical energy may be transmitted for several millimeters along the vessel wall, it is important to use the minimum effective exposure time and power setting to prevent delayed bleeding from damaged vessels. We often use monopolar electrocoagulation, in which the electrode is touched directly to the bleeding vessel. Coagulation can also be achieved by touching

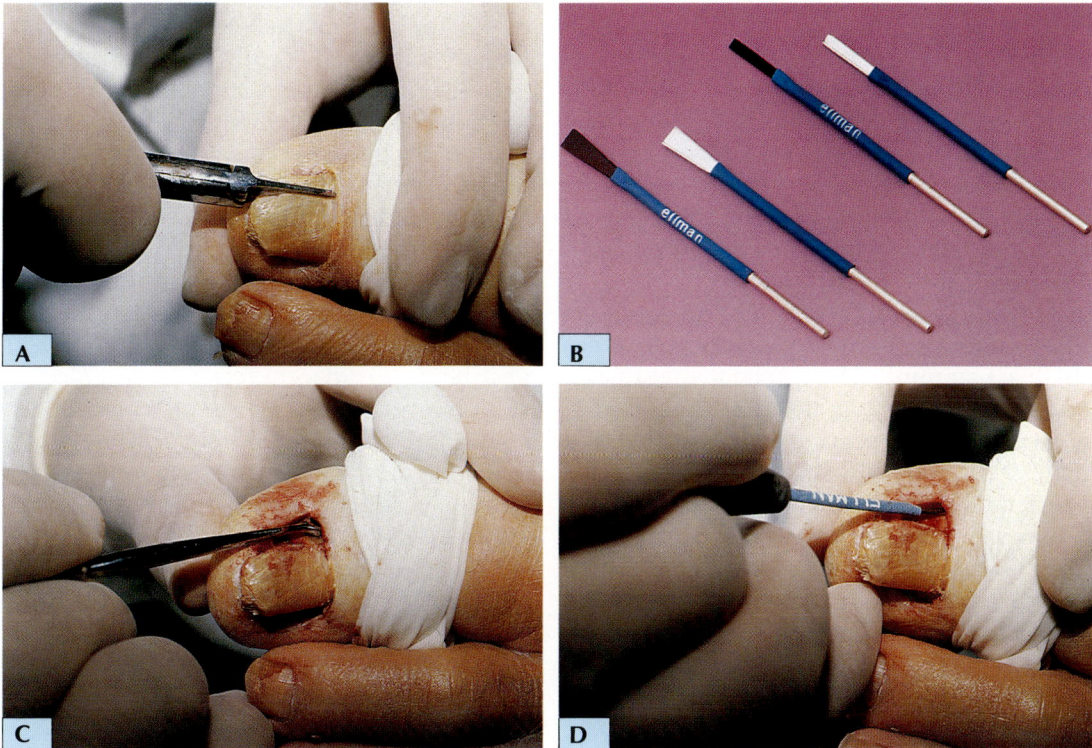

FIGURE 9.5 (A) An ingrown toenail requiring matricectomy. (B) Matricectomy electrodes. (C) After digital block anesthesia and removal of the offending portion of nail plate, the corresponding matrix is curetted with a small (2- to 3-mm) dermal curette. (D) The matricectomy electrode is then inserted into the space overlying the matrix with the teflon-coated portion facing upward. This prevents damage to the undersurface of the proximal nail fold. With no downward pressure, the underlying matrix is destroyed with a short burst (5 seconds) of electrocoagulation current. (Combined electrosection/electrocoagulation current has also been reported effective.) This is repeated a second time. Postoperative healing is generally complete in about 4 weeks. During healing, patients soak the involved foot twice daily in epsom salt solution, and apply an antibiotic ointment and a dry dressing. Pain, discharge, infection, or bleeding rarely complicate this procedure.

the electrode to a hemostat that has been clamped on the severed vessel. In bipolar electrocoagulation, a bipolar forceps is used to provide more directed pinpoint hemostasis (Figure 9.6). Electrocoagulating current delivered in this manner causes less adjacent tissue damage but requires a dry operative field to be effective.

ELECTROSECTION (CUTTING)

Electrosection involves the biterminal application of a slightly damped current. The current, of low voltage and high amperage, causes minimal lateral heat spread and tissue damage, and has the additional advantage of simultaneously achieving hemostasis and cutting.

"Pure" cutting can be obtained using a true undamped tube current, which provides the least amount of lateral heat spread and causes vaporization of tissue without hemostasis. When electrosection is performed using a filtered, fully rectified current, subsequent spot electrocoagulation can be achieved by changing to the electrocoagulation current.

Electrosection can be used to perform rapid and effortless electrosurgical excisions or incisions. Virtually no manual pressure by the operator is required. Electrodes configured as loops, triangles, or diamonds can be used for quick removal of skin tags, papillomas, nevi, and other exophytic lesions (Figure 9.7A–D). A straight, narrow electrode is most often used to incise the skin and is applied to the tissue in brisk, continuous paintbrush-like strokes. The difference between electrosection and scalpel excision is immediately apparent to the first-time user of electrosection. At the appropriate power setting the electrode passes smoothly through the tissue like a "hot knife through butter." If perceptible sparking occurs during incision, the power setting is too high; if the electrode "drags," the power setting is too low.

Slightly damped currents cause some charring at the margins of the excised tissue. This can be minimized by developing a smooth, rapid hand motion for performance of electrosection. In addition, vacuum tube units tend to provide outputs that are less destructive to adjacent tissues when electrosection is performed. However, when a specimen suitable for histopathological analysis is required, the filtered current should be used because it does not create significant electrosurgical artifact. We recommend that the initiate to electrosection develop technical skills and concepts by practicing on beefsteak before utilizing these techniques in the clinical arena.

The major advantage of electrosection over scalpel surgery is that hemostasis is

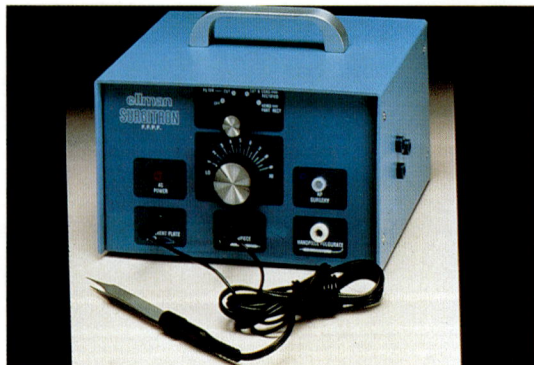

FIGURE 9.6 Bipolar forceps attached to an electrosurgical apparatus. These are useful for providing pinpoint electrocoagulation in hemostasis.

achieved immediately as the incision is made. However, larger blood vessels (more than 2 mm in diameter) require additional spot electrocoagulation at the completion of the excision. A drawback is that vaporization of the tissue generates a smoke plume, which can be unpleasant for both the patient and the operator and may contain potentially infectious viral particles (see page 9.12). Consequently, effective smoke evacuation equipment should be available during such procedures (Figure 9.8).

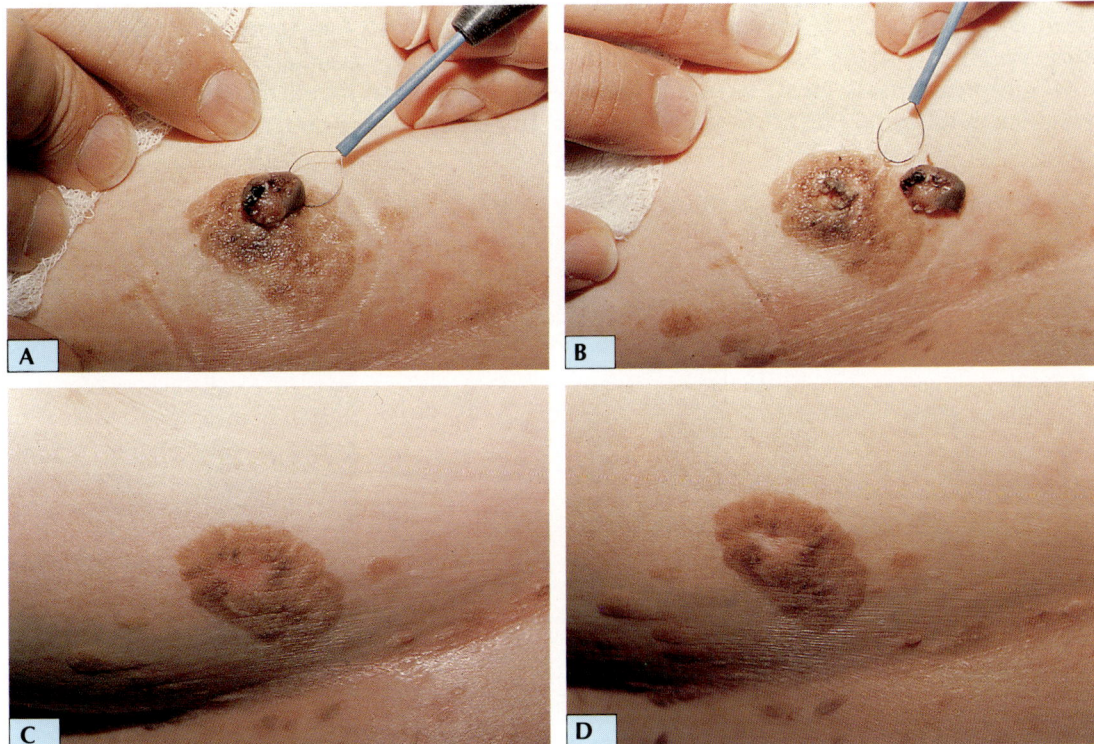

FIGURE 9.7 (A) A loop electrode is used to remove the exophytic portion of a seborrheic keratosis by electrosection. (B) Lesion removed without bleeding owing to the inherent coagulating feature of the current. (C) Operating site 5 weeks after surgery shows only a small amount of erythema. (D) Post-operative photograph taken at 6 months. The erythema has subsided and no scar is visible owing to the superficial nature of the tissue injury.

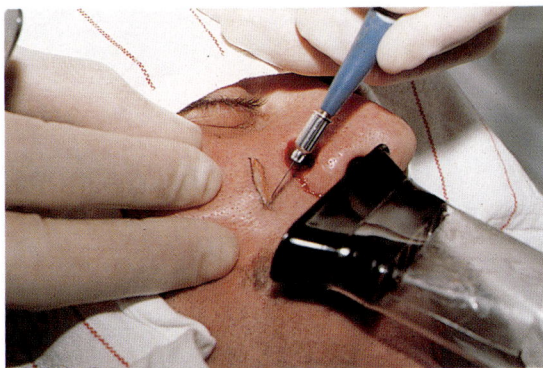

FIGURE 9.8 A smoke evacuator is used to remove the smoke plume generated by electrosection during preparation of a rhombic skin flap. To be effective in removing viral particles, the suction must be placed at a distance no greater than 2 cm from the operative site.

Electrosection is extremely useful for achieving relatively bloodless excision of large, bulky lesions, such as acne keloidalis nuchae and rhinophyma (Figure 9.9A–C), in which the surgical defect is allowed to heal by second intention. Electrosurgical excision followed by primary closure can also be undertaken with no impairment of wound healing, as compared to conventional scalpel surgery. This modality has been used, without complications, to create skin flaps with excellent outcomes (Figure 9.10A–C).

POTENTIAL HAZARDS OF ELECTROSURGERY

ELECTROSURGERY AND CARDIAC PACEMAKERS

Fixed-rate (asynchronous) pacemakers stimulate the heart at a regular rate, independent of the intrinsic heart rate. They are resistant to external electromagnetic interference such as that caused by electrosurgery. However, in recent years fixed-rate pacemakers have

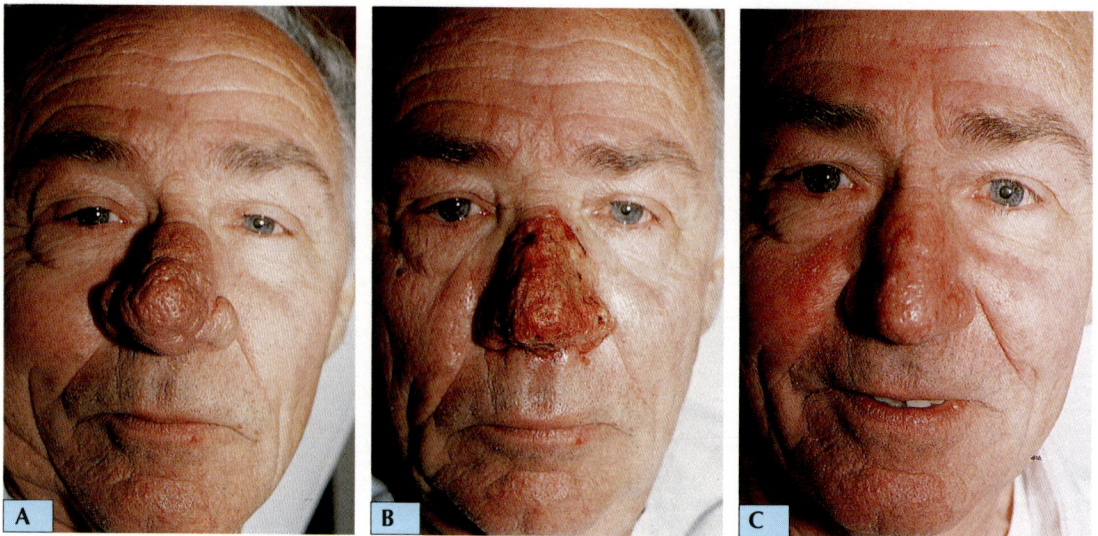

FIGURE 9.9 (A) Moderately severe rhinophyma in a middle-aged man. (B) Immediately after electrosurgical planing of excess sebaceous material. Care is taken to perform subtotal removal, as very aggressive therapy can lead to significant scarring and possible deformity caused by scar contracture. (C) Four weeks later, healing with good cosmetic outcome is noted. During healing, the wound is kept moist with an antibiotic ointment and semi-occlusive dressings.

largely been replaced by noncompetitive demand (synchronous) pacemakers, which use a sensor to detect the heart's spontaneous rhythm. Triggered electrical impulses are sent to the heart when the spontaneous rhythm is slower than the pre-set pacemaker rate. The most commonly used ventricular-inhibited pacemaker is suppressed when impulses from normal ventricular activity are received. If no ventricular activity is detected after a pre-set interval, it fires at a fixed rate. Since this type of pacemaker is completely inhibited by sensed interference, asystole could occur if a patient has no spontaneous rhythm and electrical interference is prolonged. Because safety factors are built into modern units, including improved shielding and rejection circuits, magnetic and radio-frequency fields rarely cause clinical problems. Nevertheless, electrosurgery is best avoided in particularly unstable cardiac patients and for treatment of skin lesions overlying a pacemaker.

FIRE

There is a risk of fire or explosion if electrosurgical procedures are conducted in the presence of alcohol, oxygen, or bowel gases (methane). Care should be taken to be certain that the operative site is free of alcohol residue. Oxygen is usually not a problem except in the operating room setting. Bowel gases are highly inflammable! Use care in the perianal region.

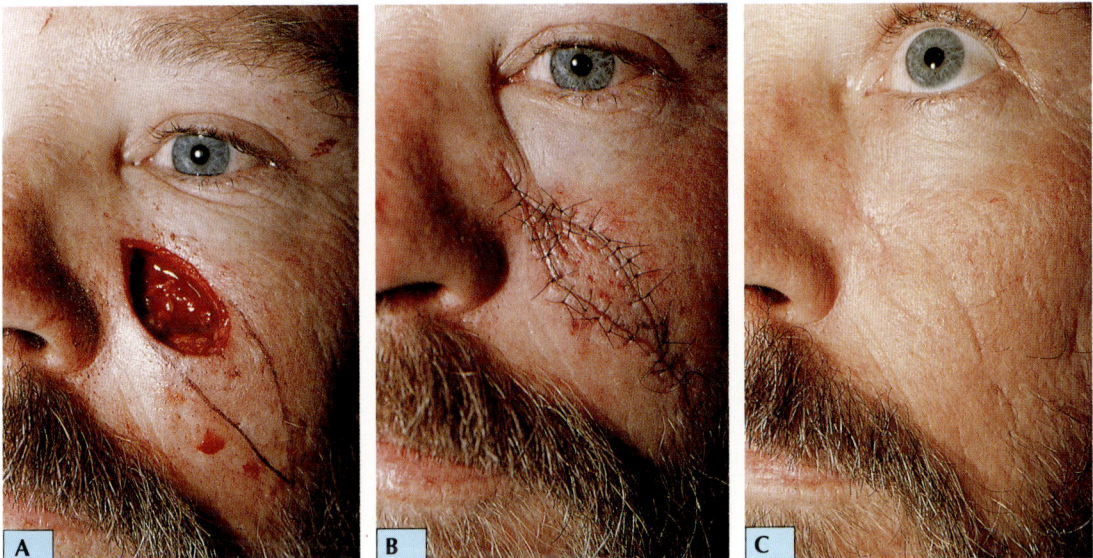

FIGURE 9.10 (A) Postoperative defect after removal of a large basal cell carcinoma. An island pedicle flap is planned. (B) After creation of the flap using electrosection instead of a scalpel, interrupted nylon sutures are placed. No complications were noted and healing took place as would be expected after scalpel surgery. (C) Five-month follow-up shows satisfactory cosmetic outcome. The flap margins were dermabraded at approximately 2 months post surgery to improve the outcome.

MICROORGANISM TRANSMISSION

The potential exists for transmission of microorganisms either via electrode or via smoke plume inhalation. Neither possibility has been investigated in sufficient depth to yield conclusive results. Practitioners should minimize the risk of possible electrode transmission by considering the use of disposable or sterilized electrodes. Adapters are available that allow disposable metal hypodermic needles to be used as electrodes.

With electrosection and extensive electrocoagulation, as with CO_2 laser surgery, a smoke plume is generated. Intact viral particles have been recovered from smoke plumes from both procedures. A smoke evacuator, with the intake held not less than 2 cm from the operative site, is indicated for intensive electrosurgical procedures in which a smoke plume is generated, particularly those involving lesions of viral origin.

SUGGESTIONS FOR FURTHER READING

Bennett RG: Electrosurgery. In Bennett RG: Fundamentals of Cutaneous Surgery. Philadelphia, WB Saunders, 1987, pp. 553–590.

Blankenship ML: Physical modalities. Electrosurgery, electrocautery, and electrolysis. Int J Dermatol 1979;18:443–452.

Boughton RS, et al: Electrosurgical fundamentals. J Am Acad Dermatol, 1987; 16:862–867.

Crumay HM: Alternating current: electrosurgery. In Goldschmidt H, ed. Physical Modalities in Dermatologic Therapy. New York, Springer-Verlag, 1978, pp. 203–227.

Jackson R: Basic principles of electrosurgery: A review. Can J Surg, 1970; 13:354–361.

Pollack SV, Grekin RC: Electrosurgery and electroepilation. In Roenigk HR Jr, Roenigk RK, eds. Dermatologic Surgery: Principles and Practice. New York, Marcel Dekker, 1989, pp. 187–203

Popkin GL: Electrosurgery. In Epstein E, Epstein E Jr, eds. Skin Surgery. Philadelphia, W.B. Saunders Co., 1987, pp. 164–183.

Sebben JE: Electrosurgery and cardiac pacemakers. J Am Acad Dermatol, 1983; 9:457–463.

Sebben JE: The hazards of electrosurgery. J Am Acad Dermatol, 1987;16:869–872.

chapter 10

HEMOSTASIS

Wound hemostasis is essential for the avoidance of complications from bleeding that may not be stopped adequately by normal activation of the clotting cascade. The failure to activate normal clotting mechanisms may be due to abnormal clotting parameters, to severing of medium- and large-sized vessels during surgery, to delayed bleeding due to reversal of the vasoconstrictive effect of epinephrine as it wears off, or to disruption of a fragile clot by increased blood pressure and pulse when the patient becomes ambulatory.

The first such cause should be detected by the surgeon when the patient's medical history is taken. The surgeon should always ask the patient if he or she has any history of bleeding problems. Specific questions should be directed toward problems with previous surgical procedures and with medications such as aspirin, nonsteroidal anti-inflammatory drugs, and anticoagulants. To avoid bleeding problems from these medications, the patient is asked to discontinue taking them 5 to 7 days prior to surgery but only

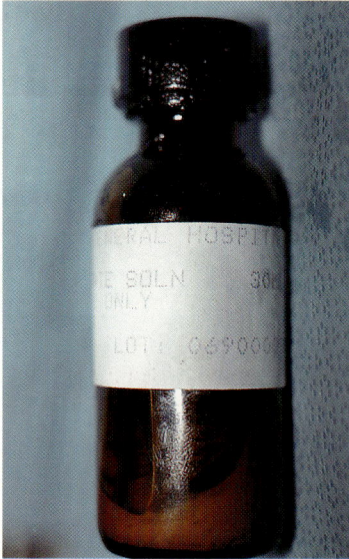

FIGURE 10.1 Ferric subsulfate (Monsel's solution) in a dark glass bottle with precipitate at the bottom. Because the precipitate may be responsible for the tattooing reported with this agent, when the cotton swab is placed in the bottle it should be kept away from its edges. To prevent sticking of the bottle cap due to the precipitate, the cap can be covered with vaseline. The bottle then becomes very slippery and thereafter should be handled with care.

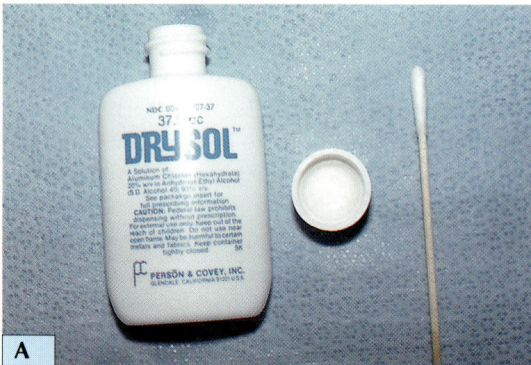

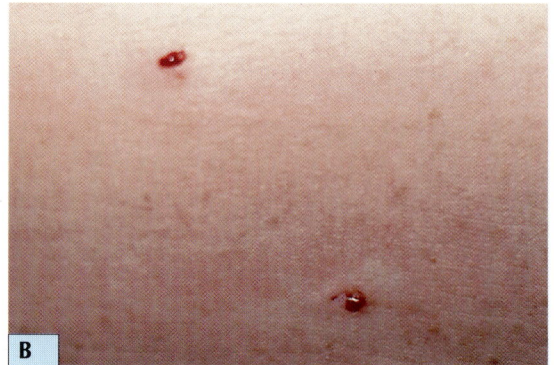

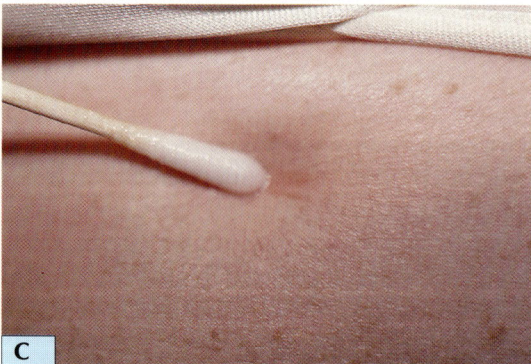

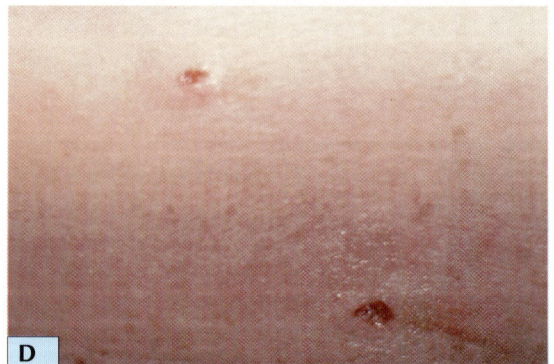

FIGURE 10.2 (A) For the application of aluminum chloride hexahydrate (Drysol), the wound should be as dry as possible. **(B)** Two small shave biopsy sites with welling up of blood in each one. **(C)** One cotton swab can be run over the wound to dry it, quickly followed by another containing aluminum chloride. If no anesthetic has been used for the procedure, the patient should be forewarned that the aluminum chloride may sting. **(D)** Hemostasis is achieved.

after checking with their internist. While some surgeons routinely order clotting studies for all outpatient procedures, for the majority of routine procedures, such studies are probably unnecessary.

With regard to the second cause of bleeding, large vessels usually need to be tied off. Cauterization of such vessels cannot be expected to be sufficient. Delayed bleeding, the third cause, can be controlled during surgery by adequate hemostasis, tying off of large vessels, and application of an adequate pressure bandage. The last cause, dislodgment of a clot, can be managed to some extent by postoperative instructions to the patient. Such instructions may include restrictions as to certain activities, avoidance of bending forward (for surgery in the head and neck region), and restrictions regarding the intake of analgesics with anticoagulant activity, such as aspirin and certain nonsteroidal anti-inflammatory drugs.

HEMOSTATIC AGENTS

TOPICAL STYPTICS

Monsel's solution, or ferric subsulfate, is a good hemostatic agent for use in very superficial wounds. Usually it is applied with a cotton swab that has been dipped into the solution, which is then rolled across the wound. Because of reports of tattooing, Monsel's solution is not recommended for use in areas where the dermis has been exposed. An additional problem with Monsel's solution is that it precipitates out onto the bottle, making the bottle cap difficult to reopen. Because precipitate also accumulates at the bottom of the bottle, care should be taken to ensure that the precipitate does not get onto the cotton swab for application onto the skin (Figure 10.1).

Aluminum chloride hexahydrate (eg, Drysol) in general is not as good a styptic as Monsel's solution, although for superficial wounds it works equally well. A clear liquid that can be stored in a plastic bottle, it has not been associated with tattooing. It is applied in a similar fashion to that of Monsel's (Figure 10.2A–D).

Silver nitrate sticks, although less effective than either Monsel's solution or aluminum chloride, are convenient to use, easy to store, and quick acting. When a bleeder is touched lightly by the stick, the area rapidly turns silver (Figure 10.3A,B). Because application of the stick is slightly painful and causes a burning sensation, the patient should be so warned.

Certain styptics may be too irritating or too caustic to use in areas such as the perior-

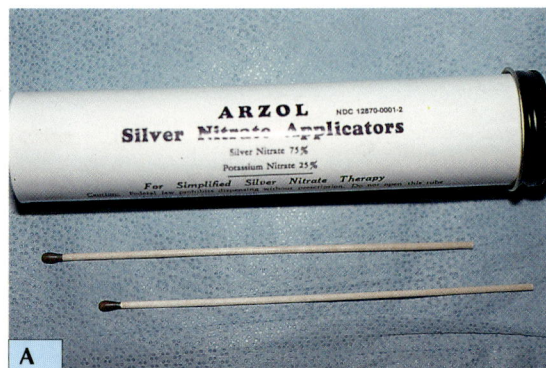

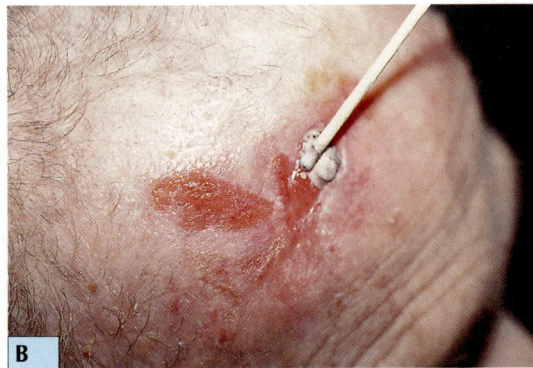

FIGURE 10.3 (A) Silver nitrate applicators are supplied in tubes containing 100 sticks. (B) Note how both the stick and the wound turn silver when the applicator touches a bleeder. Silver nitrate sticks also can be used for the superficial destruction of hypergranulation tissue to allow advancement of epithelium. Thus, the potential for tissue destruction should be kept in mind when these convenient sticks are chosen for superficial hemostasis.

bital region. In such locations, simple pressure may be sufficient to stop the bleeding. Note that the application of pressure should be continuous. Although the temptation is great to apply pressure for a minute or two and then to "peek" to see if the bleeding has stopped, it is best to apply pressure continuously for 10 minutes, without interruption (Figure 10.4A,B). Furthermore, when removing a pressure dressing from the skin surface, the surgeon should be careful to avoid dislodgment of any clots. Successful removal of the dressing is facilitated by the use of a relatively nonadherent material against the wound surface.

SPONGES AND OTHER HEMOSTATIC MATERIALS

Sponges are useful for hemostasis and absorption of blood in wounds that are not superficial or which continue to ooze after other modalities have been tried. A sponge that absorbs the blood, applies pressure, and

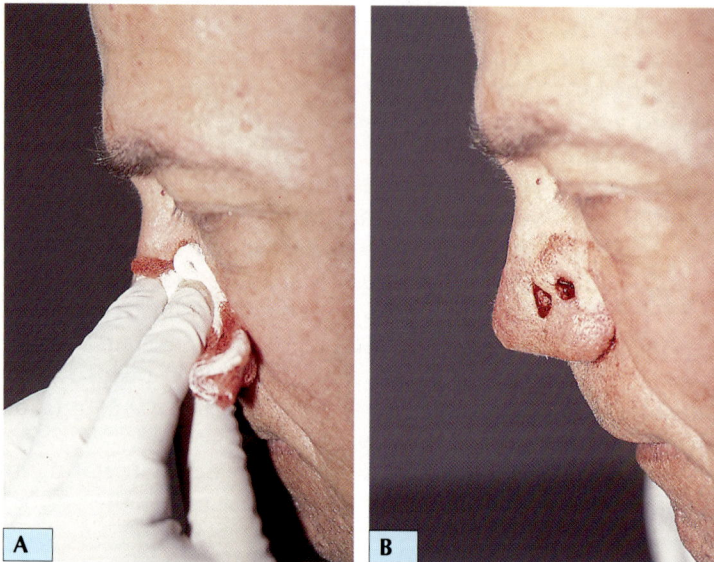

FIGURE 10.4 (A) This wound was oozing blood. Cauterization of the bleeders was ineffective as the defect was too small to visualize them adequately. Random cautery would place too much devitalized tissue in the wound. (B) Pressure was applied to the wound for 10 minutes, with excellent results obtained.

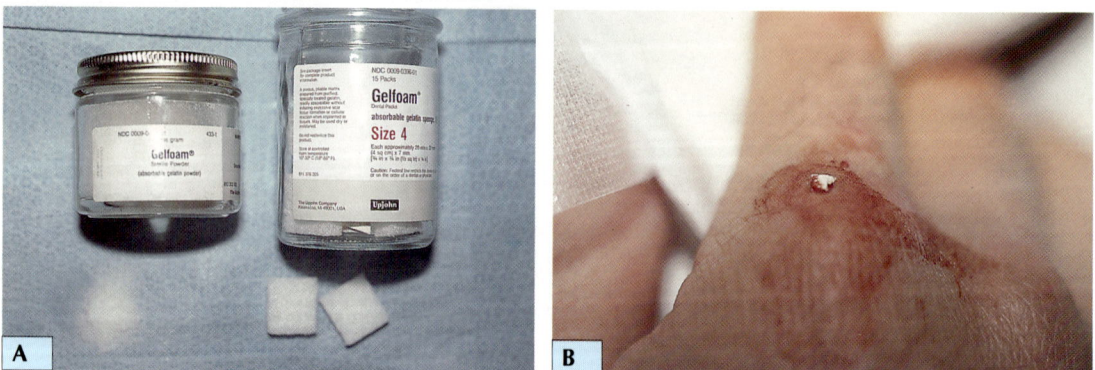

FIGURE 10.5 (A) Gelfoam is packaged in powder form or as a sponge. Gelfoam should not be compressed totally into a wound or it will soon become saturated and lose its strength. (B) Here it is used for hemostasis at a biopsy site. Note how it fills the site and extends above it.

later dissolves is a useful tool. Two helpful products are Gelfoam, a porous gelatin matrix that comes in powder form or in square styrofoamlike sponges (Figure 10.5A,B), and Helistat, an absorbable collagen-based sponge (Figure 10.6A–C). Other hemostatic materials include Oxycel (oxidized cellulose), Avitene (microfibrillar collagen), and topical thrombin. These substances can be pressed into the wound to which they will conform, with a pressure dressing placed over them. Gelfoam, which is highly absorbent, completely dissolves within 4 to 6 weeks. During that time, however, it can act as a foreign body in the wound and thus increase the possibility of infection. Therefore, it should not be buried deeply in wounds.

ELECTROCAUTERY

Electrocautery (discussed at length in Chapter 9) is the hemostatic agent used most commonly for surgery. It is used with the intent of achieving hemostasis by causing the least possible amount of tissue destruction. Thus, the lowest possible power setting should be used. The exact location of the bleeding should be identified, with the current ap-

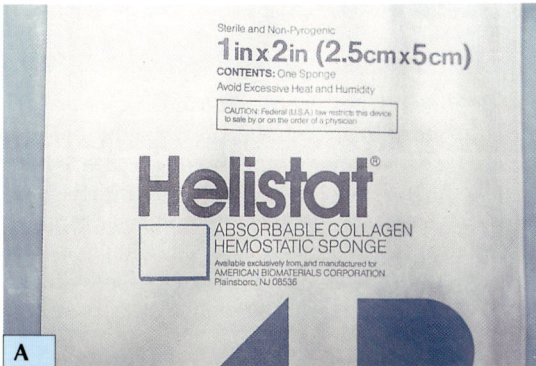

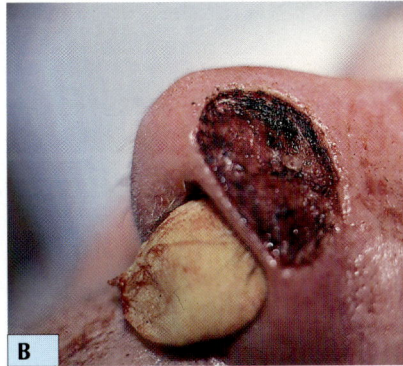

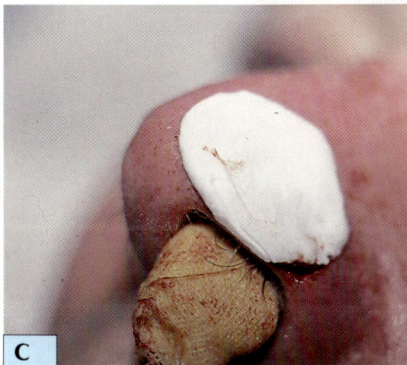

FIGURE 10.6 (A) Helistat sponges are supplied in individual packages. The collagen probably causes aggregation of platelets and precipitates the clotting cascade. (B) This superficial wound has been left to heal by second intention according to the patient's request following removal of a basal cell carcinoma. (C) After Helistat has been placed on the wound, the patient is instructed to perform routine wound care around the insert. The sponge, which will be completely absorbed, has not been found to enhance bacterial growth in vitro.

plied directly to it (Figure 10.7). For hemostasis, a smaller tip is recommended as a larger tip will cause more tissue destruction (Figure 10.8). As an alternative, jeweler's forceps may be used to grasp the bleeder, with current delivered to the lower one third of the forceps (Figure 10.9A,B). If the procedure needs to be done in a sterile fashion, the equipment, including the electrocautery machine, needs to be handled as such. Dispos-

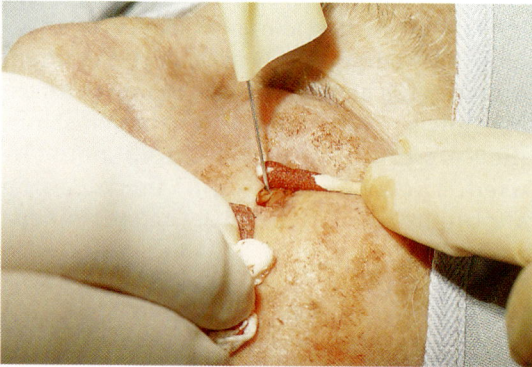

FIGURE 10.7 An effective means of identifying a bleeder is to roll a cotton swab across the area while applying pressure. Since this technique compresses a small amount of tissue at one time, the vessel will start to bleed as soon as the swab rolls off of it and precise cauterization can be done leaving a very small eschar.

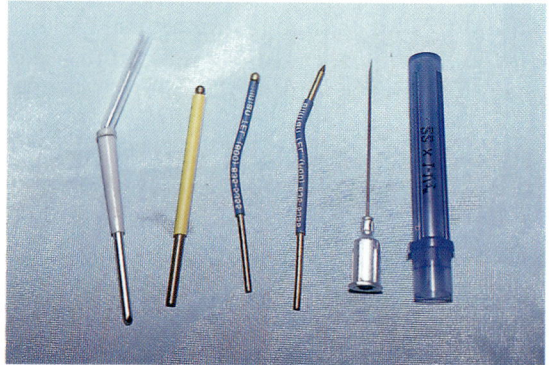

FIGURE 10.8 Tips of various sizes and shapes usually are supplied with an electrocautery machine. They should be disposable or they should be able to be sterilized. The larger the tip, the more tissue destruction occurs. The 25-gauge, large-bore needle attached to an adapter on the far right, and the needle with a slightly thickened point next to it, provide pinpoint hemostasis without piercing the tissue.

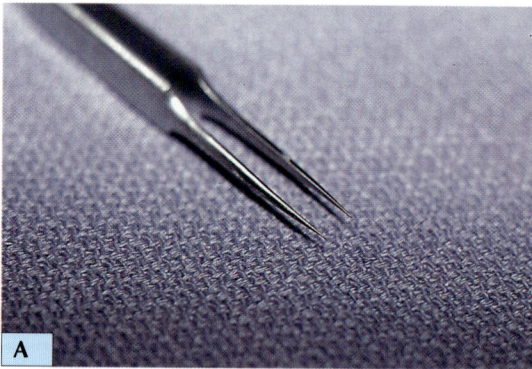

A

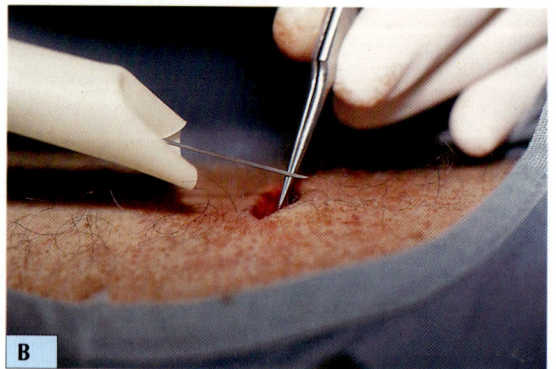

B

FIGURE 10.9 (A) Jeweler's forceps, which taper to a very fine point, can be used to grasp small vessels. **(B)** They can also be held against the area that is bleeding and used like an electrical conductor, without the need for grasping. Note that the cautery tip is touching the proximal one third of the instrument.

able handles for the electrocautery machine are available, but expensive. An alternative to their use is a sterile Penrose drain slipped over the cautery handle (Figure 10.10; see also Figure 10.9B).

A common mistake made by those new to electrocautery is to char an area of bleeding repeatedly, thereby creating a large area of necrotic tissue and greatly increasing the chances of infection (Figure 10.11). If identification of the source of bleeding proves difficult, the tissue can be stretched and pulled until visualization is possible. A suction machine also may be helpful for large defects, for defects located in difficult areas such as at the medial canthus, or for areas of rapid bleeding. Bleeding also can be controlled by the application of pressure at the edge of a wound (on the forehead, for example) to enable the bleeder to be identified. Because of its destructive action upon tissue, electrocautery should not be used at epidermal wound edges, if a primary closure is intended.

OTHER TECHNIQUES

Hemostasis of larger vessels is best obtained by tying of the vessel with a loop of absorbable suture, such as chromic gut. The loop is made around the vessel, including a bit of surrounding tissue, and is then tightened. Alternatively, a "figure-of-8" suture can be used. The tail of the suture should be cut short so that a minimal amount of foreign material remains in the wound (Figure 10.12).

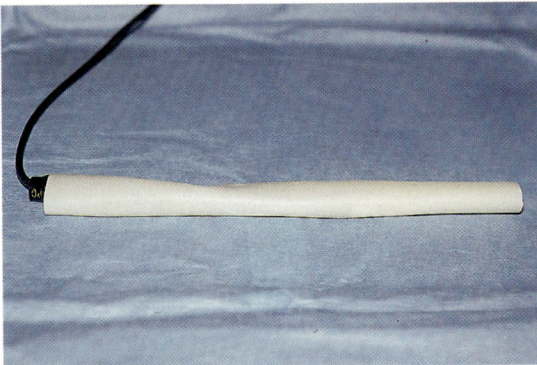

FIGURE 10.10 A sterile Penrose drain is placed over the cautery handle and serves the same purpose as would an expensive disposable handle.

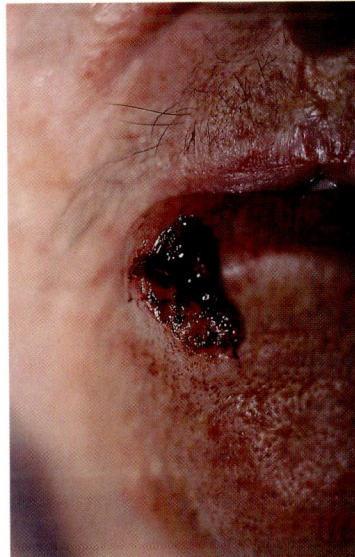

FIGURE 10.11 Excessive hemostasis was obtained at this wound on the lower lip, leading to a blackening of the entire base of the excision site.

Other devices that aid in the stoppage of bleeding are the Shaw scalpel and the laser. These devices may be helpful in areas that are highly vascular as they provide some degree of hemostasis during removal of the lesion.

The degree of hemostasis that should be undertaken in any wound varies with the surgeon and with the particular circumstances of the case. Certainly, no active bleeding should remain. However, it is not neces-sary that the defect be bone dry. Once the defect has been closed, a cotton swab can be rolled across the suture line with gentle pressure applied to the tissues to express any remaining blood. In the event that there is active bleeding that is not stopped easily by pressure, the wound should be reopened and adequate hemostasis obtained (Figure 10.13). Rarely is a drain necessary to evacuate a possible accumulation. The drain itself can in-

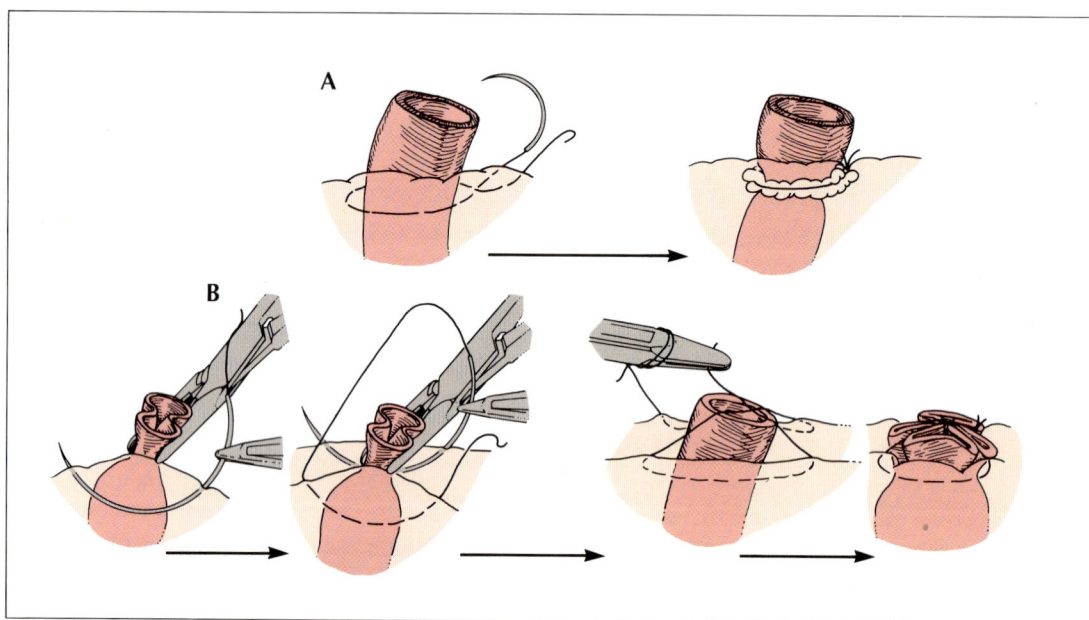

FIGURE 10.12 Schematic drawing to illustrate hemostatic suturing. **(A)** A simple vessel tie. **(B)** A "figure-of-8" suture.

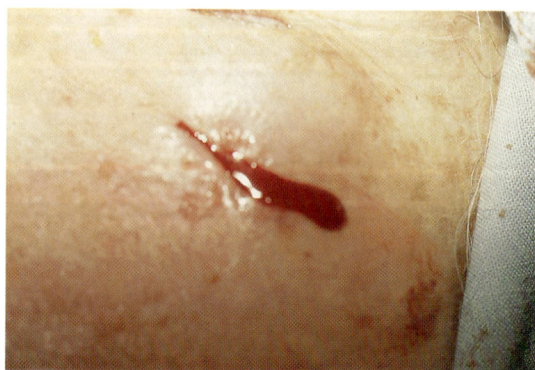

FIGURE 10.13 This closed wound shows active bleeding, beyond that which can be controlled by pressure. Therefore, the wound should be reopened, adequate hemostasis obtained, and the wound re-sutured.

crease the risk of infection by providing a route through which bacteria can enter the wound.

Finally, a pressure dressing should be placed on the wound. The majority of such dressings are left in place for approximately 48 hours, although sometimes they are best left on until suture removal. Because of the possibility of postoperative bleeding, surgical patients should always be given a number that they can call in case of an emergency. Before being seen, the patient with postoperative bleeding should first attempt to control the bleeding by the *continual* application of pressure to the area for 20 minutes while lying down, without removal of the original dressing.

If sustained direct pressure proves inef-fective, the patient should return to the office for evaluation. Sometimes bleeding ceases by the time the patient arrives, as indeed most such episodes stop on their own. If bleeding continues, however, the surgical site may need to be taken down. A frequent cause of persistent postoperative bleeding is inade-quate hemostasis of a large vessel, which has been cauterized instead of tied off. Another source of bleeding may be inadequate instruc-tions given to the patient regarding postoper-ative restrictions. Even with these important considerations in mind, if hemostasis is obtained carefully using good surgical tech-nique, postoperative bleeding should be a rare complication of most cutaneous surgical procedures.

SUGGESTIONS FOR FURTHER READING

Hicks PD, Stromberg BV. Hemostasis in plas-tic surgical patients. Clin Plast Surg. 1985;12:17-23.

Larson PO. Topical hemostatic agents for der-matologic surgery. J Dermatol Surg Oncol. 1988;14:623-632.

Stegman SJ, Tromovitch TA, Glogau RG. Hemostasis. In: Basics of Dermatologic Surgery. Chicago, Ill: Year Book Medical Publishers Inc; 1982: 32-35.

chapter 11

SUTURING TECHNIQUES

The idea of suturing flesh wounds is found in ancient Greek and Indian medical texts. Evidence of suturing goes back even further, to its use by the ancient Egyptians on mummies. However, suturing was not a prominent feature of early wound care, perhaps because of infection. Sutures act as foreign bodies in a wound and may prevent the drainage of serosanguinous fluids. Pooling of fluid deep in the wound may result, which then acts as a nidus for bacterial growth.

The ancients knew that wounds could heal naturally with relatively few complications. They often used various kinds of adhesives to hold wounds together or to close them partially. When sutures were placed, it was to improve the ultimate cosmetic outcome without increasing the risk of infection or other complication. Even today, when suturing cannot be undertaken without an increase in such risks, alternatives to full clo-sure must be sought. Sutures can be used for partial wound closure, to approximate wound edges, to decrease wound-healing time, to orient wound healing in a certain direction, or to minimize distortion in an area (Figure 11.1A–C). Basic suturing techniques and examples of their use are the subject of this chapter.

SIMPLE INTERRUPTED EPIDERMAL SUTURE

The simple interrupted epidermal suture is the basic suture upon which other, more advanced, suturing techniques are based. It must be mastered before other such tech-niques are attempted. The sutures are attach-ed or swaged on to the needle, which should

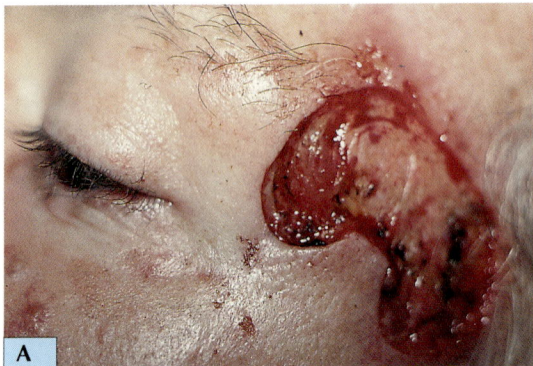

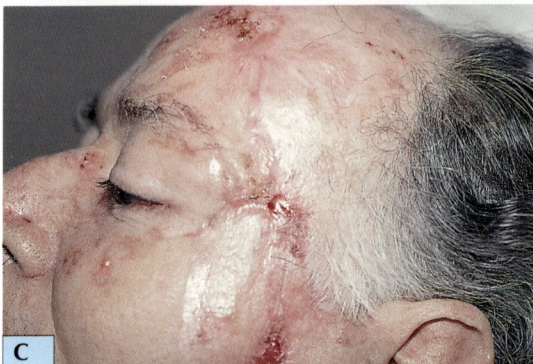

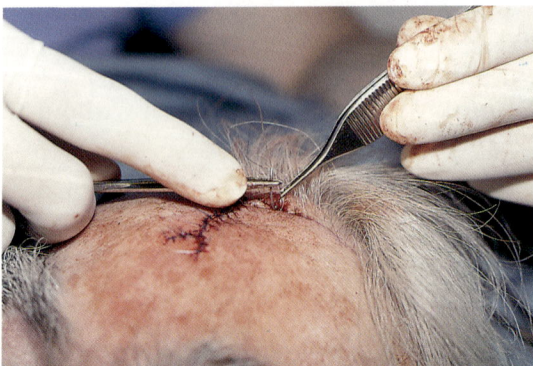

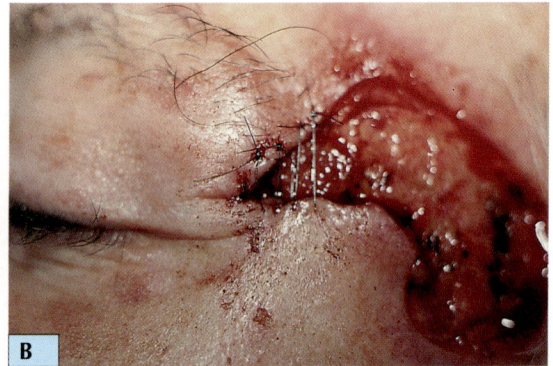

FIGURE 11.1 (A) This wound just lateral to the left eye is the result of removal of a squamous cell car-cinoma by Mohs' technique. **(B)** Guiding sutures have been placed to decrease the tendency for wound contraction, causing the upper lid to retract upward. **(C)** The fully healed scar is horizontal, causing no retraction of the lateral lid margins.

FIGURE 11.2 With the needle in position to begin suturing, the needle holder is held as shown, with placement of fingers in the holes of the instrument avoided and with its tip stabilized by the index fin-ger. This facilitates manipulation of the needle holder as it rolls between the fingers and follows the curvature of the needle for correct suture place-ment. Toothed forceps or a skin hook may be used for better placement of the skin edge to meet the needle at 90°.

be grasped by a needle holder one half to three fourths of the way back from its point (Figure 11.2). The curvature of the needle is essential for proper suture placement in the tissue. If the needle becomes bent during placement, it usually indicates that the surgeon is using too much force to direct the needle into an unnaturally straight line.

Instead, as soon as the needle is placed on the skin it should be directed by the needle holder through a 90° turn that carries the suture through the tissue and everts the wound edges (Figure 11.3A,B). This is most easily accomplished in locations where the epidermis and dermis are thick, as on the back. By contrast, on the face and extremities,

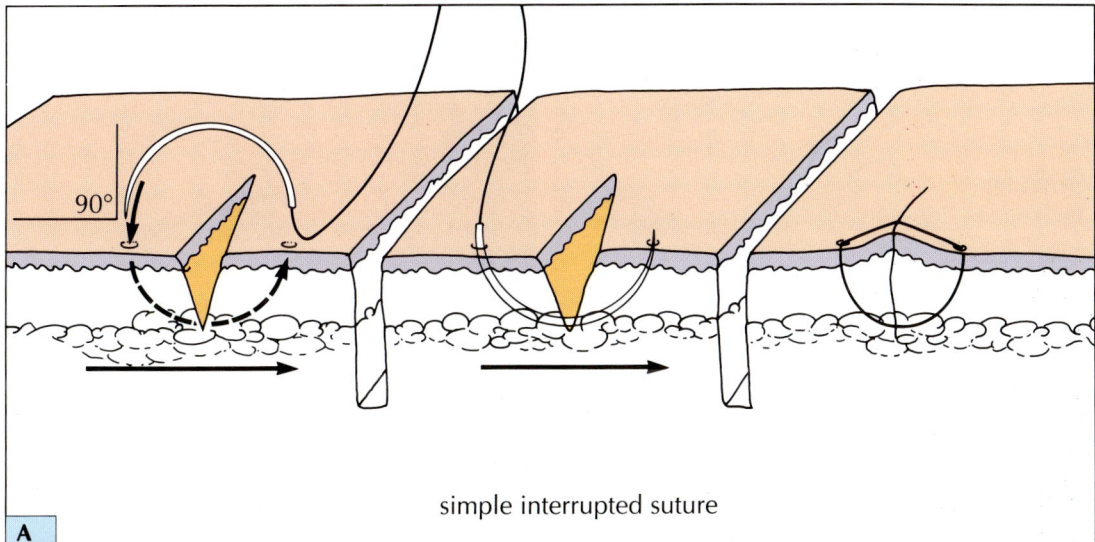

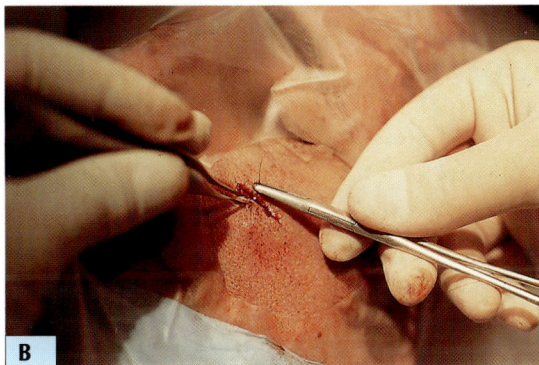

simple interrupted suture

A

B

Figure 11.3 (A) Schematic diagram showing the basic technique for simple interrupted sutures. The needle enters at a 90° angle and picks up dermis and some fat depending on the level of undermining. It then enters the other side of the wound at 90° and, using the curvature of the needle, exits the epidermis. The final exit point of the needle should be at the same distance from the cut edge of the wound as was its initial entry point. **(B)** When the needle exits, it can be grasped by forceps or by the needle holder. To avoid crushing of the finely honed point, the needle should always be grasped behind the point.

especially in older patients, the epidermis is very thin and has little support from the dermis. In such areas, eversion of the edges of the wound may be more difficult (Figure 11.4A,B). Eversion of wound edges is important as it allows wound healing to occur evenly with regard to the skin surface. If healing occurs below the surface, a slight trough will occur along the suture line, which will detract from the final cosmetic result.

Three throws are necessary to position and secure the suture (Figure 11.5A–C). The first throw should merely approximate the wound edges, the second should tighten and seat the knot, and the third should tie the

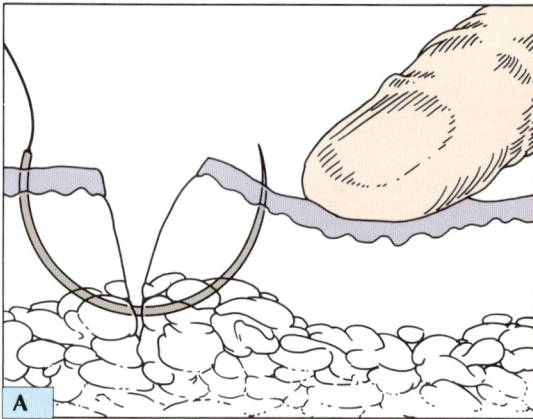

FIGURE 11.4 (A) Another method of everting wound edges is to pull the overhanging epidermis back before insertion of the needle, using either the needle tip or pressure applied to the area by the finger.

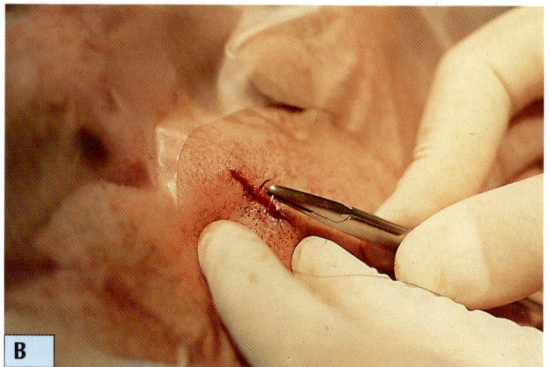

(B) This technique is most useful in areas where the epidermis is thin, such as on the face. Note the tip of the needle entering the skin at 90°.

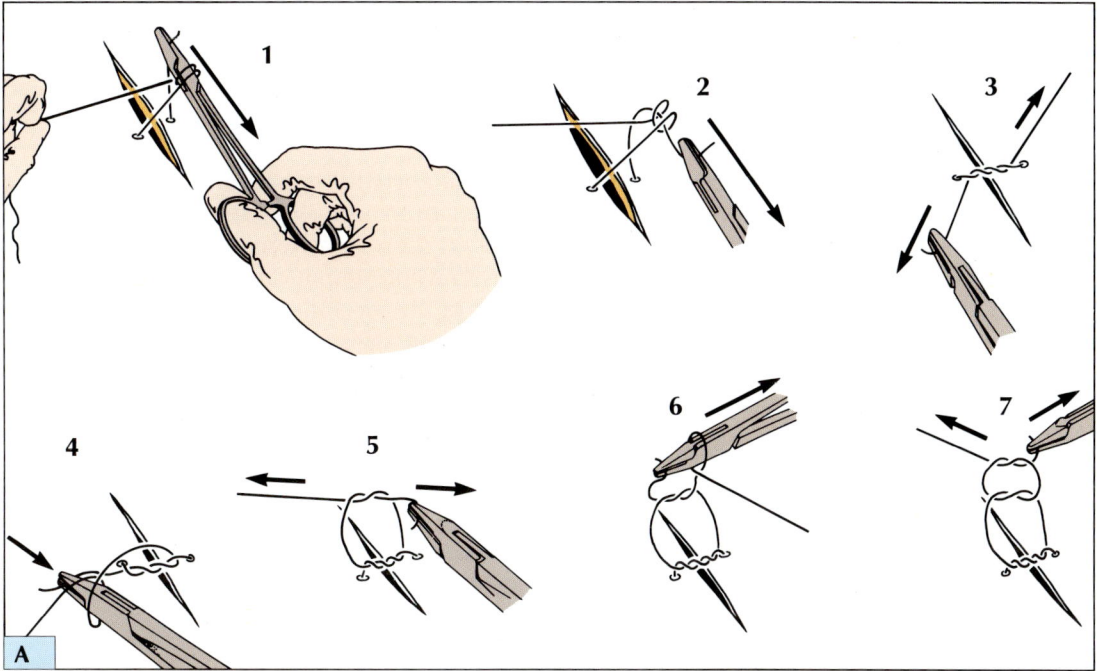

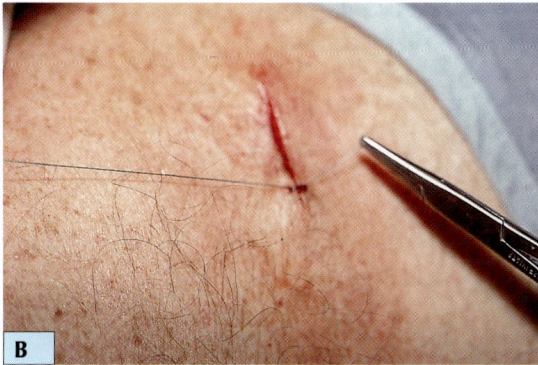

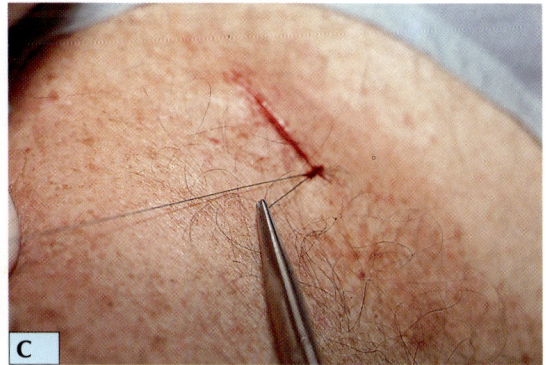

FIGURE 11.5 (A) An instrument tie is used to provide a square knot, which is done by wrapping the long end of the suture twice around the needle holder and then grasping the short end and pulling it through. The suture is then wrapped around the needle holder once, going in the opposite direction. For the third tie, the suture is wrapped around the needle holder once in the original direction. **(B,C)** To secure the first tie if it slips, tension should be kept on the tie, with one hand being brought over to the other to cinch the knot and allow the other two ties to be made without knot slippage.

knot firmly. With monofilament or coated sutures, more throws can be added to ensure that the knot is secure. However, the surgeon should take care to avoid the tying of sutures too tightly, as the surrounding skin will become ischemic and risk necrosis and poor cosmetic outcome (Figure 11.6).

It is not necessary that sutures be placed at points equidistant throughout the suture line. The closer together they are, the less tension there is on each individual stitch; for this reason, sutures are often placed closer together in the center of a wound becoming more widely spaced toward its ends. Knots should be placed to one side of the wound so that they do not interfere with the wound healing process, and the tails of the cut sutures should not be sticking into the wound.

The initial epidermal suture may be placed anywhere along the suture line, especially if there is no tension on the wound. If tension is present, it can be reduced for placement of the centrally located sutures by starting at the sides and working toward the center of the wound. The surgeon may also start at the ends when working in cosmetically sensitive areas, to minimize the forma-

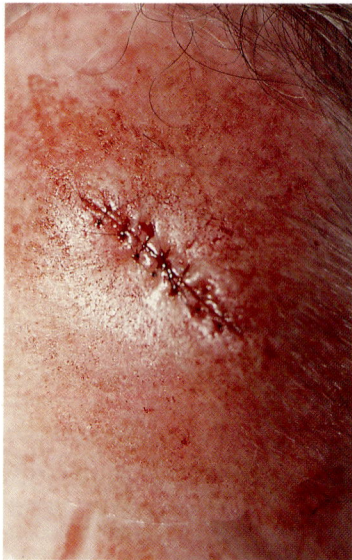

FIGURE 11.6 The five sutures along the suture line from its midpoint to the right side of the photograph have been tied too tightly. The adjacent skin is white and there are small mounds of tissue between each stitch. These may fail to resolve totally during healing, allowing small crusts to form along the suture line that may disrupt the cosmetic outcome. Note the improved technique in the two sutures at the left upper pole of the suture line, with looser stitches placed more closely together.

tion of dog-ears and to push any excess tissue toward the center where it may be less noticeable in the final result.

VERTICAL MATTRESS SUTURE

The vertical mattress suture is another technique that can be used to evert wound edges. It can also be used to close dead space (gaps in the tissue below the skin surface) and to decrease tension on wound edges, which oth- erwise may lead to dehiscence, widening of the scar, and/or hypertrophic and keloidal scar formation. However, because this tech- nique leaves four suture holes instead of two, it should be used only when these indica- tions exist and there are no other options. In some cases, one centrally placed vertical mat- tress suture may be used to direct wound edges, to close dead space, or to absorb ten- sion, following which wound closure can be completed using simple interrupted sutures (Figure 11.7).

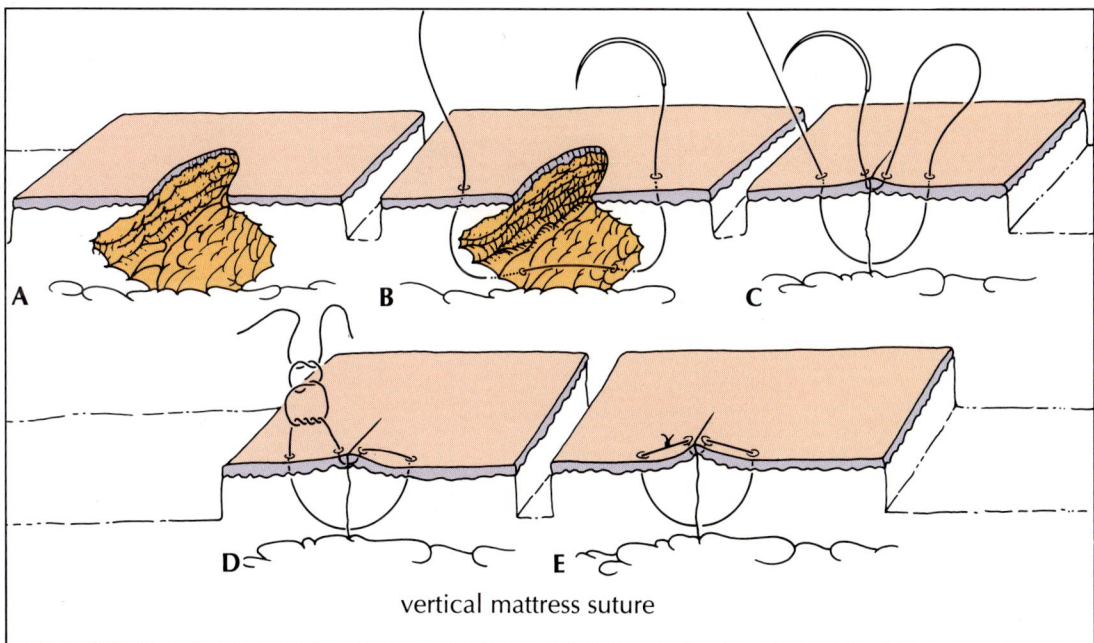

vertical mattress suture

FIGURE 11.7 A classic example of the vertical mat- tress suture is its use in closing a wound following removal of a cyst. **(A)** There is a large dead space and usually overhanging epidermal edges due to the thinned epidermis that was stretched over the cyst. **(B,C)** A wide interrupted suture is placed first to close the dead space, after which the needle is reinserted on the same side but closer to the wound edge, to evert the epidermis. The stitch is complet- ed on the opposite side, in the epidermis. **(D,E)** The knot lies entirely on the skin surface. If the knot is tied too tightly and/or pressed into the skin surface by tension, it may leave a scar.

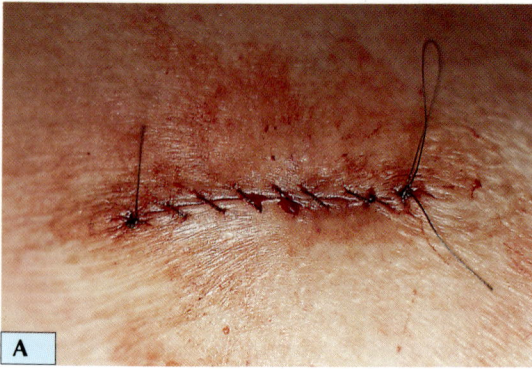

FIGURE 11.8 (A) A running suture technique is useful for the closure of long wounds. The first knot is a simple interrupted suture tie. **(B)** The running locked suture is thought by some to secure the running suture and to decrease the possibility of dehiscence. However, it also has the potential for increasing suture marks on the skin and ischemia along wound edges. The final knot is tied onto the last running suture, as shown here.

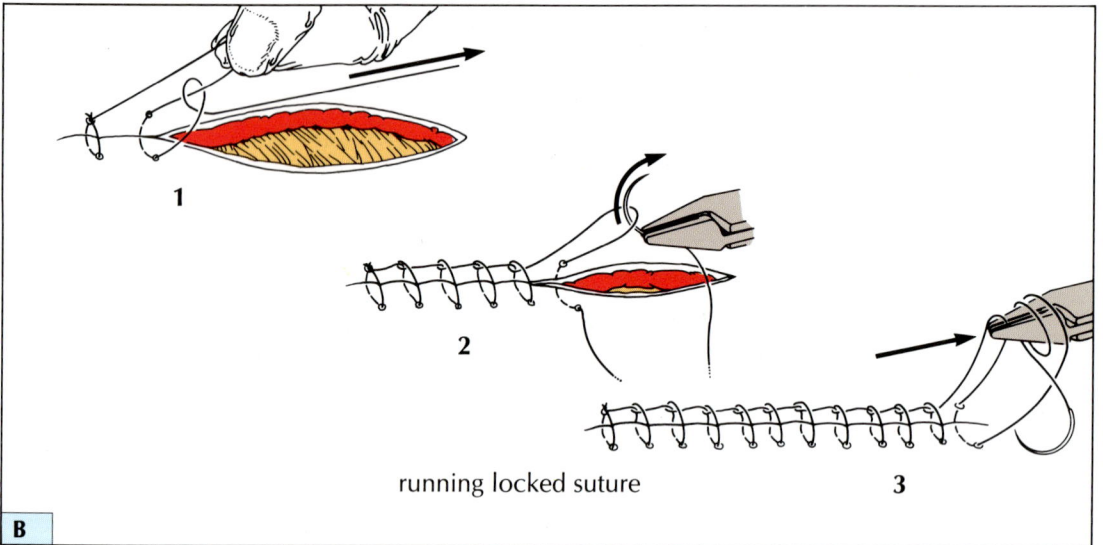

1

2

running locked suture   3

RUNNING SUTURE

The running suture (Figure 11.8A) is a continuous simple interrupted suture. Because it is faster to perform, it is often used for the closure of long wounds. However, it is not recommended for wounds whose sides are of unequal length and need to be adjusted or for the eversion of wound edges. It is also not indicated if there is tension on the wound, since if one area experiences dehiscence, there is risk to the entire suture line. This suture can also be "locked," which is accomplished by looping each stitch under the previous stitch (Figure 11.8B).

HORIZONTAL MATTRESS SUTURE

The horizontal mattress suture is based on the same principles as the vertical mattress suture, although the reentering stitch is placed adjacent to the first stitch on the same side of the wound, at a point equidistant to the wound edge. It is usually used to secure large flaps (Figure 11.9). Because this suture is used primarily to decrease tension, it is likely to leave telltale marks on the epidermis by the two lines of suture tying on the skin surface. Therefore, it should be considered for early removal. The occurrence of such marks

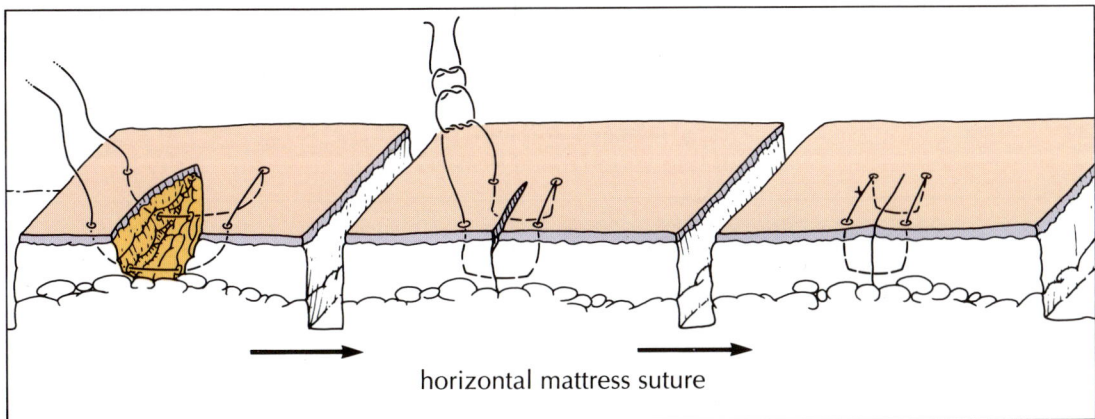

horizontal mattress suture

FIGURE 11.9 The horizontal mattress suture can pull together a wider expanse of tissue and spread the tension over a larger distance.

may be minimized by the use of a half-buried horizontal mattress suture or a bolster (Figure 11.10A–C).

RUNNING SUBCUTICULAR SUTURE

The running subcuticular suture removes almost all suturing from the epidermis and with it the possibility of any suture tracks in the final scar. However, it does not evert wound edges and cannot finesse a closure by approximating the epidermal edges perfectly. Therefore, it should be used when there is no tension on the wound edges or when it is expected or desired that the sutures remain in place for a prolonged period of time (Figure 11.11A,B). A monofilament suture such as Prolene is recommended, as it causes little tissue reaction and is easily pulled through

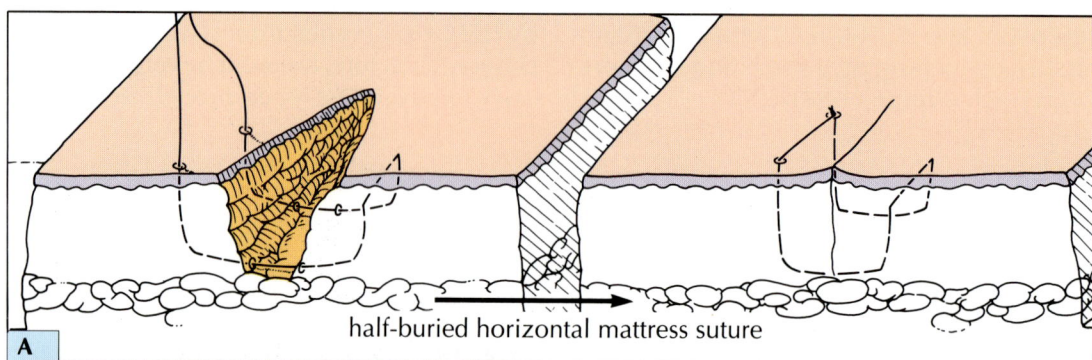

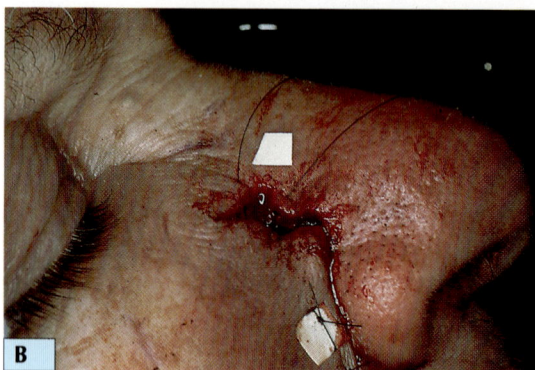

half-buried horizontal mattress suture

FIGURE 11.10 (A) Schematic drawing of a half-buried horizontal mattress suture. The buried side must be secured firmly in dermis to support the tension that is usually placed on this suture. **(B)** To decrease the possibility of the suture cutting into the skin, a bolster is sometimes used, which can be cut from the sterile insert in the suture package and slipped under the suture. **(C)** These same principles may be used to create half-buried vertical mattress sutures.

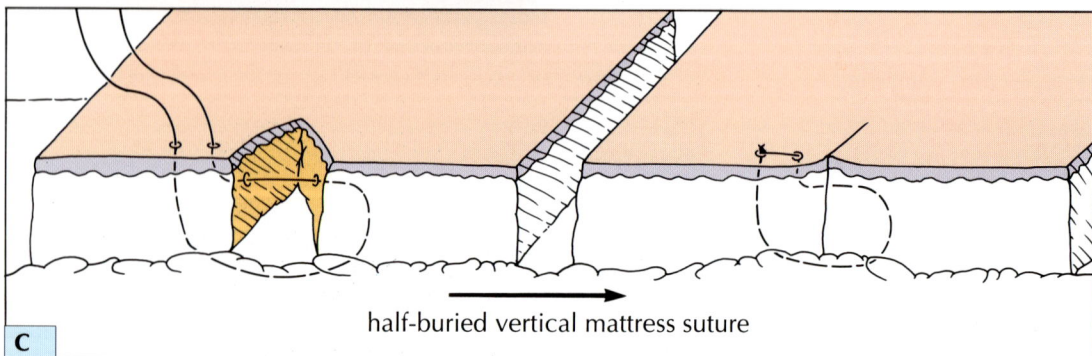

half-buried vertical mattress suture

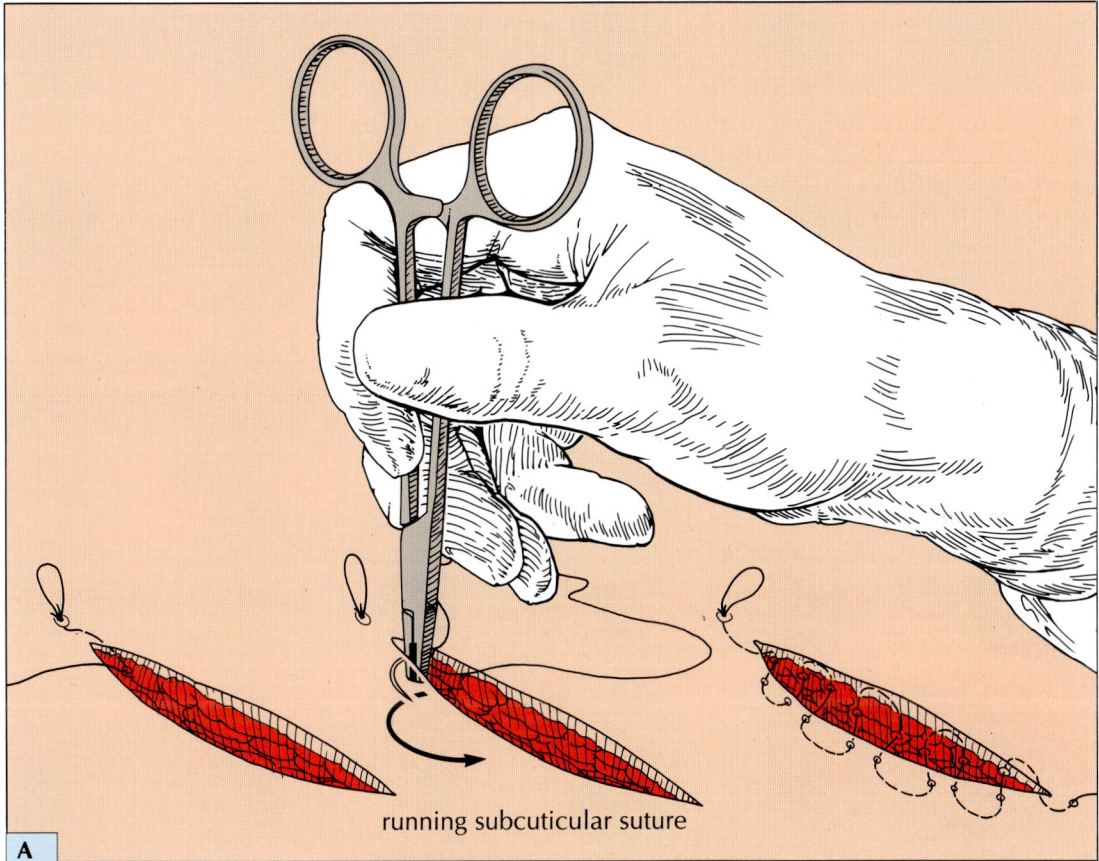

running subcuticular suture

A

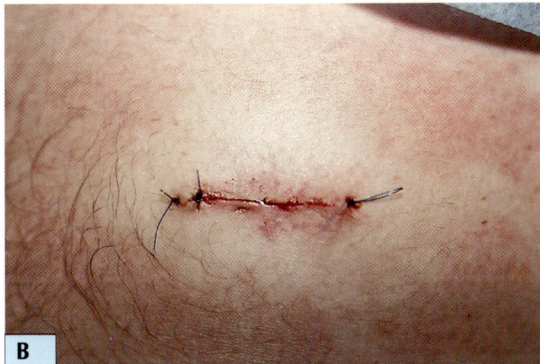

B

FIGURE 11.11 (A) The running subcuticular suture may be started at one pole or to the side of the wound. The needle enters the epidermis normally, but exits the wound just below the epidermis. Then, with the needle placed parallel to the skin surface, it enters and exits each side of the wound at the same level. To prevent gaping, each entry point of the needle should be placed slightly behind the exiting stitch on the other side. Any gaping along the suture line may be closed by small interrupted sutures or with Steri-Strips. The final exit is the reverse of the start of the suture with regard to level and placement of the needle at the pole or to the side of the wound. **(B)** A clinical example of a completed running subcuticular suture.

the wound at the time of suture removal (Figure 11.12). For long closures, it is best that the sutures come through the epidermis and over the suture line and that they reenter on the opposite side to continue the stitch every 2 to 3 cm to facilitate removal. This suture, which is an epidermal closure stitch, should not be confused with a buried subcutaneous suture.

CORNER SUTURE

An important stitch to know, the corner suture combines the epidermal suture with the buried horizontal suture. It is used to effect closures in cases where there are more than two epidermal edges to oppose, such as for an M-plasty, Burow's triangles, an A to T closure, and others (Figure 11.13). Most cor-

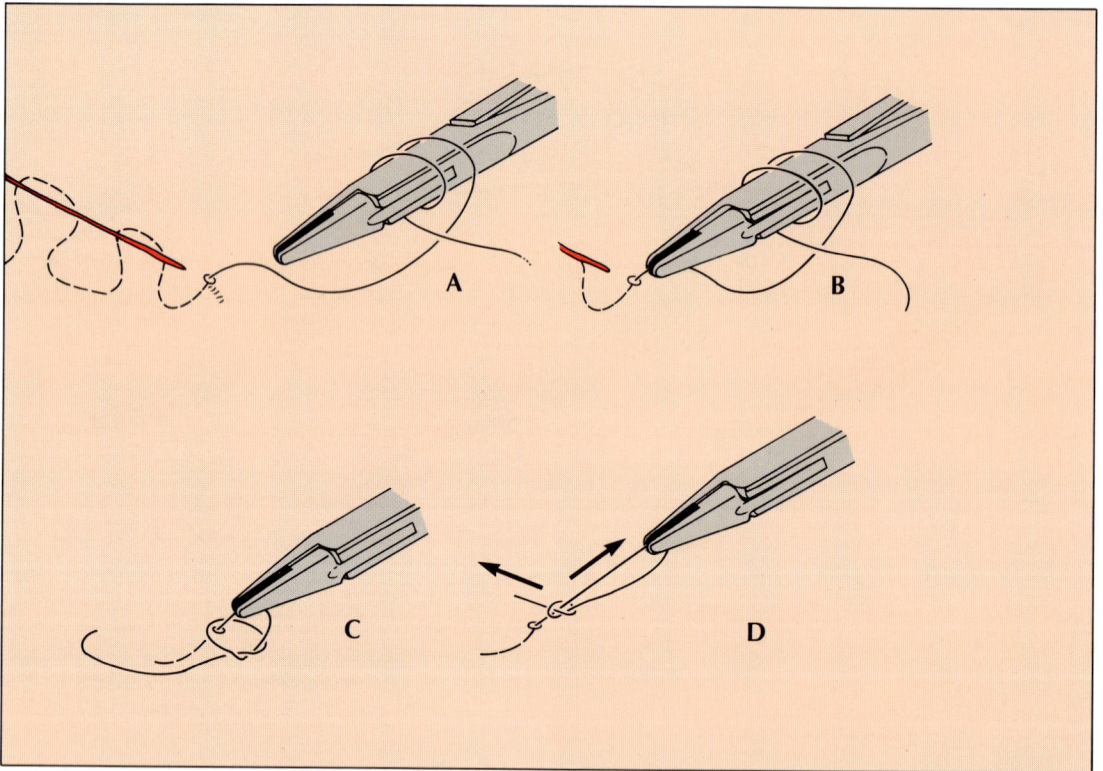

FIGURE 11.12 The tie for a running subcuticular suture is the same as that for a regular instrument tie except that the long and short ends of the suture are the same strand. **(A,B)** The suture is wrapped around the needle holder, which grabs it at the skin surface. **(C)** The knot should be slid down the suture *without* tightening it around the needle holder. **(D)** Once the knot reaches the skin surface, both sides are pulled to tighten it. The resultant loop should be large enough to prevent slippage of the knot. This maneuver is then repeated six to ten times to secure the knot.

ner sutures are used to pull the piece of tissue into the defect and therefore should be placed slightly ahead of the flap tip. If the suture is to be tied directly over a fragile flap tip, care should be taken to ensure that the suture is not tied too tightly as necrosis of the tip may result.

BURIED SUBCUTANEOUS SUTURE

The buried subcutaneous suture is a tension-reducing suture that is also meant to close dead space. The sutures are placed in the fat and dermis. Absorbable suture material usu-

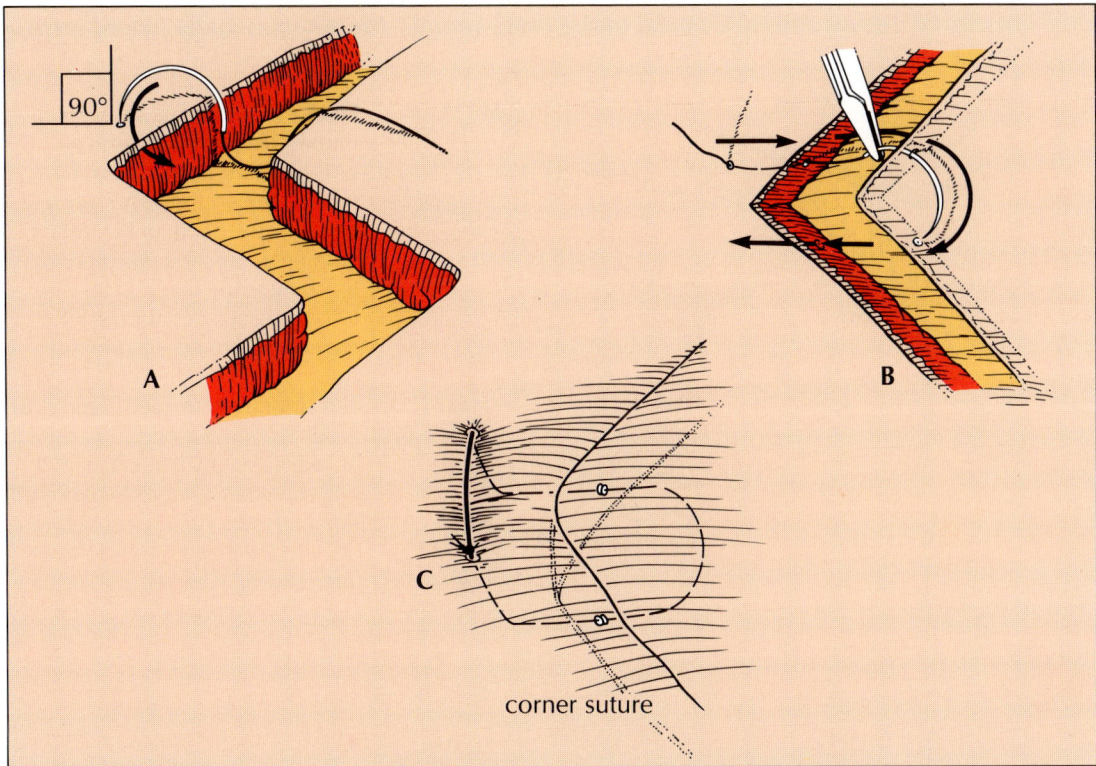

FIGURE 11.13 Schematic diagram showing a corner suture. (A) It begins as an epidermal suture. (B) The needle is then turned horizontally to enter the tip of the other piece of tissue in dermis and exit its other side, remaining at the same dermal level and distance from the tip as at the entering side. (C) The stitch then finishes as an epidermal suture. Note how the epidermal portion of the suture is placed so that its tied portion does not overlie the tip and pulls it forward into the defect.

ally is used, although nonreactive, clear permanent suture also can be buried if long-term tension reduction is sought.

    Variations include the standard vertical suture, the horizontal, or pursestring, suture, and the running horizontal subcutaneous suture (Figure 11.14A–C). The sutures should be placed deep enough to prevent spitting or extrusion through the epidermis. To avoid this, only three throws should be used to tie

each suture. In very deep wounds, two layers may be needed to close the dead space adequately. Since closure of a deep wound often makes it difficult to place additional buried sutures, all of the necessary sutures can be placed without tying (held by a clamp, if necessary) and then can be tied once the last buried suture has been placed (Figure 11.15). Deep sutures are placed and tied like epidermal sutures. More superficially placed buried

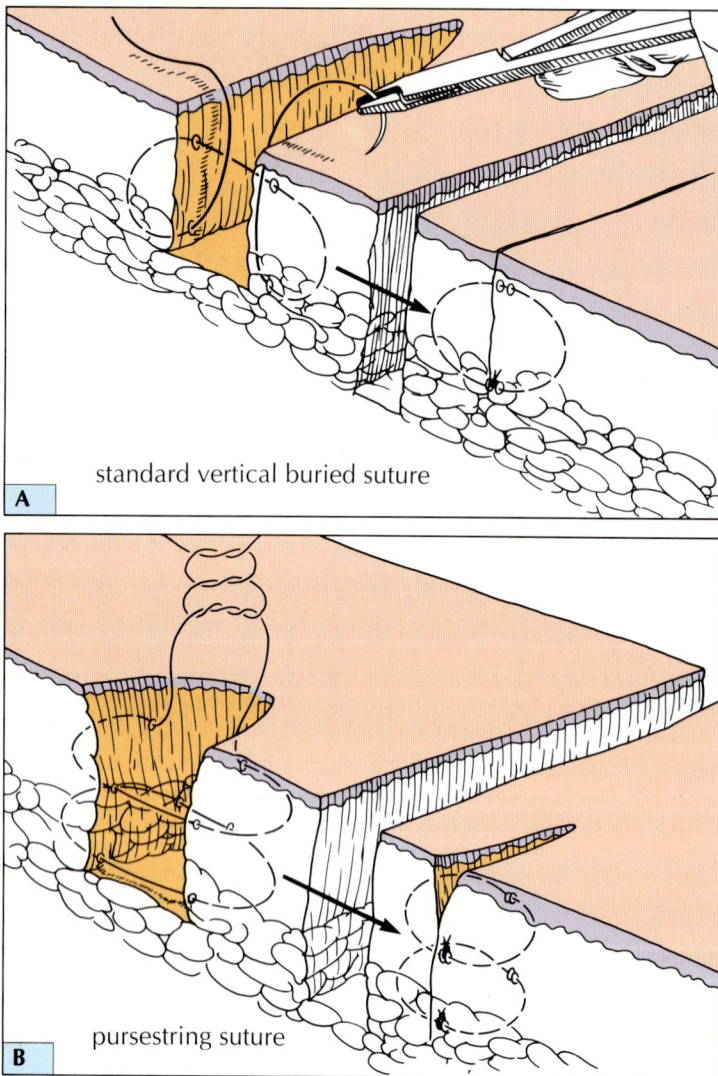

standard vertical buried suture

A

pursestring suture

B

FIGURE 11.14 Buried suture techniques. **(A)** Standard vertical buried suture, with knot placement at the bottom. The suture is begun at the depth of the defect, coming up into the dermis and finishing at the depth. If the suture is to be buried deeply, the knot may be placed on top and the suture placed in the same fashion as a simple interrupted suture. **(B)** A pursestring buried suture may be placed at any level of skin. It pulls together a wider expanse of skin and is useful in closing the dead space that remains following removal of a cyst.

(continued on next page)

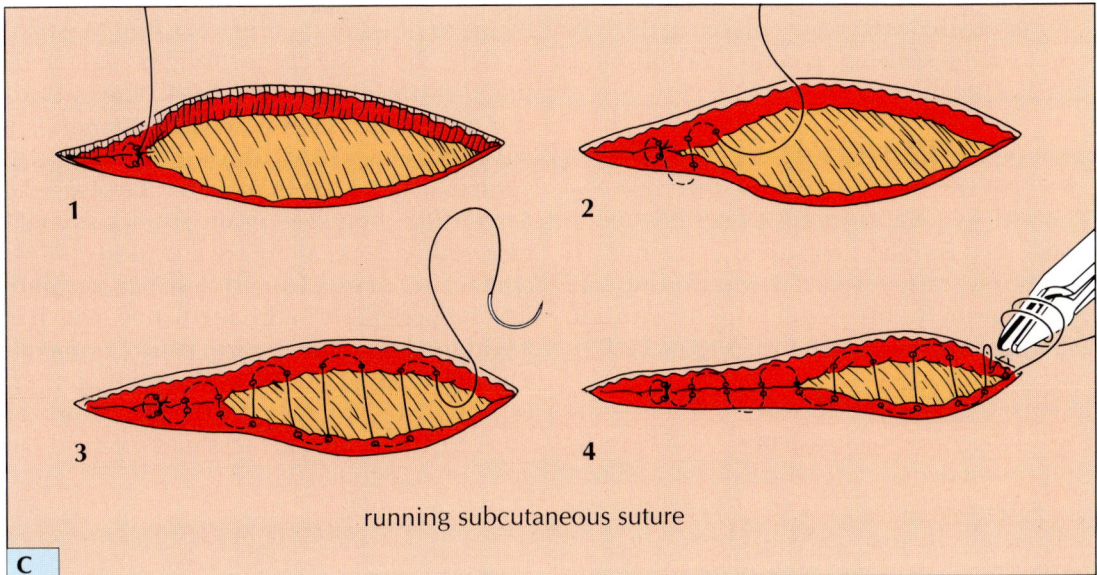

running subcutaneous suture

C

(C) The running subcutaneous suture is often used to close wounds without tension after a deeper layer of sutures has been placed. It removes any tension from the epidermal sutures and may lead to an improved cosmetic result.

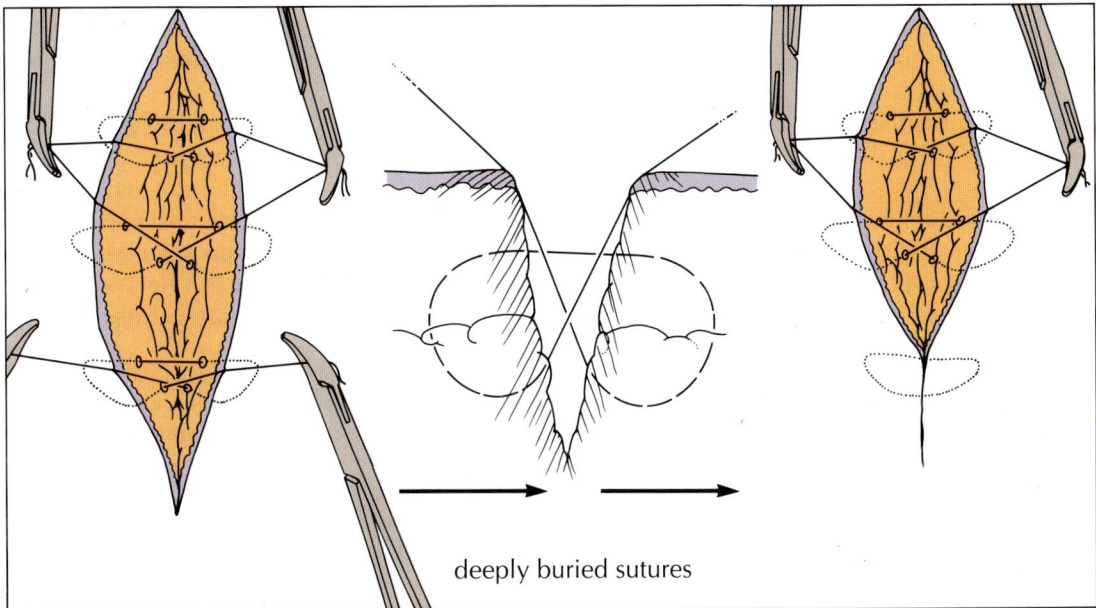

deeply buried sutures

FIGURE 11.15 Schematic drawing showing deeply buried sutures held by a clamp until all buried sutures have been placed. Each suture is then tied.

sutures are tied with knots placed at the bottom to avoid spitting, wound disruption, or bulging (Figure 11.16).

SELF-REMOVAL SUTURE

The self-removal suture is a useful stitch to know, as it enables the patient to remove his or her own stitches easily should there be good reason for the patient not to return to the surgeon for suture removal (Figure 11.17).

SUTURE REMOVAL

Sutures on the face are usually removed at 5 to 7 days following surgery. Eyelid sutures and sutures in areas lacking tension may be removed at 3 days. For areas where there are dense appendageal structures that may rapidly re-epithelize and lead to railroad tracking scars, such as on a very sebaceous nose, suture removal at 3 to 5 days is recommended. Neck and extremity sutures are retained for 7 to 10 days, while sutures in areas of greater tension and thicker skin should be retained for up to 14 days. Sutures in the torso should be removed after 10 to 14 days.

Individual judgment must be exercised in each case. Patients can always be asked to return for a wound check, at which time some of the sutures can be removed and Steri-Strips applied in their place, using Mastisol to help them adhere for longer than their usual duration of 3 to 7 days. The patient can then return later to have the remaining sutures removed. Running subcuticular sutures may be left in place for 3 to 4 weeks to allow the wound to regain as much strength as possible. Since there are only two epidermal suture marks from this stitch, they are usually preferable to the alternative, which is a widened scar due to early suture removal. Suture removal can be avoided altogether, especially on children, by the use of tape or Steri-Strips, which are less painful for them and not as frightening.

COMPLICATIONS

Causes of wound dehiscence or suture failure include poorly secured knots, excessive tension on the wound, infection, and trauma to the suture line. Slippage of sutures can be avoided by the use of proper suturing technique, proper choice of suture material, and proper suture cutting. Excessive tension can be reduced by orientation of incisions along appropriate skin tension lines, adequate undermining, adequate hemostasis to prevent hematoma formation, and the use of a sufficient number of sutures. Infection and trauma to the suture line can be avoided by attention to proper surgical technique, ade-

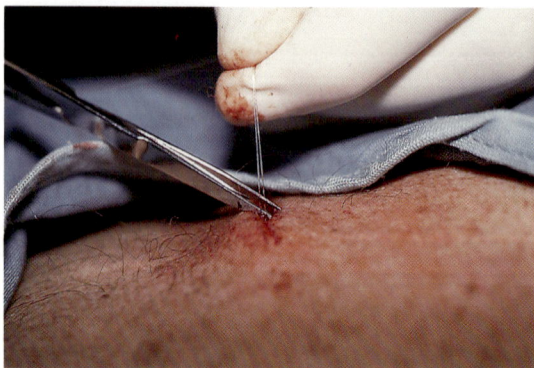

FIGURE 11.16 To cut suture, the scissors are slid down the suture to the knot and turned at a 45° angle. The suture is then snipped. Only scissors specifically intended for cutting sutures should be used. Fine tissue-cutting scissors will rapidly become dull if used for this purpose.

quate hemostasis, and effective communication between patient and physician regarding appropriate postoperative restrictions.

In situations where suturing may be difficult, the likelihood of complications can be assessed before suturing is undertaken, with healing by second intention offered as an appropriate alternative (see Chapter 13). In this regard, it is important to remember that not all wounds need to be sutured.

Buried sutures can also spit or extrude through the epidermis, usually presenting as small pustules or holes directly on the suture line. Often occurring weeks after surgery,

they usually cause the patient some concern. Once the pustule has been incised, the dissolving suture usually can be expressed easily. The wound closes and no discernible mark should remain on the suture line.

The suturing techniques described throughout this chapter can be combined for any single closure. They are essential to achieving the highest quality result with the least visible or troublesome scar. Indeed proper choice of suturing technique and competence in its mastery are vital indicators of the final cosmetic result.

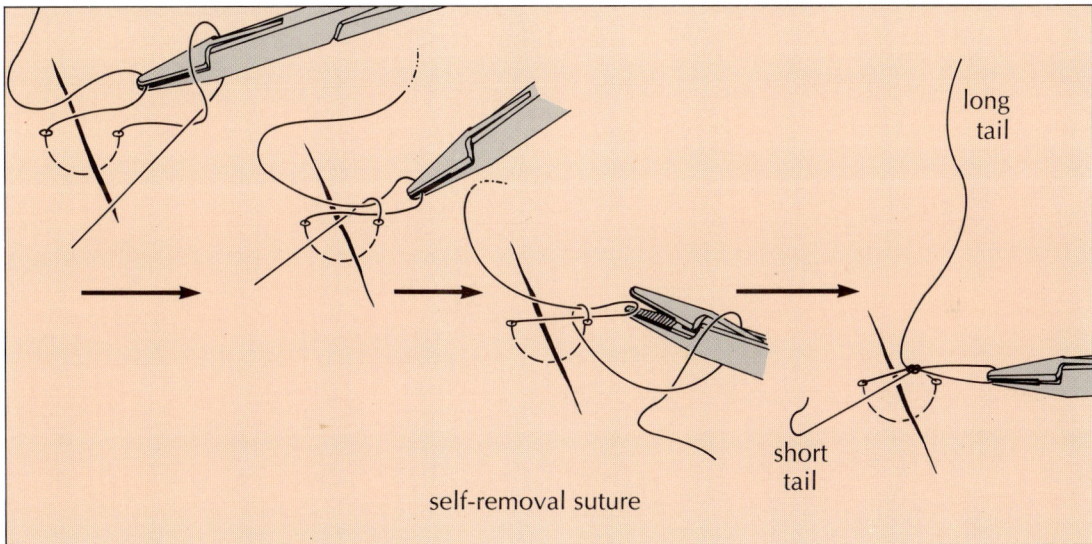

FIGURE 11.17 Self-removal suture. This stitch is tied on itself, with its long end being left for the patient to pull out. In this case, a monofilament suture is preferred.

SUGGESTIONS FOR FURTHER READING

Stegman SJ, Tromovitch TA, Glogau RG. Basics of Dermatologic Surgery. Chicago, Ill: Year Book Medical Publishers Inc; 1982.

Stegman SJ. Fifteen ways to close surgical wounds. J Dermatol Surg Oncol. 1975;1:25-31.

Swanson NA. Atlas of Cutaneous Surgery. Boston, Mass: Little, Brown & Co Inc; 1987.

chapter 12

DRESSINGS

Bandages are described in the oldest complete medical text, the Smith Papyrus. They consisted of an adhesive (usually a resin) and an antibacterial (sometimes honey or copper powder) and were secured in place using strips of linen or silk, and later, gauze. The wounds were cleansed first with alcohol or beer and with various potions. If the dressing was to be placed over a bleeding wound, pressure was emphasized. Although little else could be done for the wounded patient, the ancients realized the importance of bandaging and understood its basic principles: to protect, to cover or to hide, to absorb, to promote healing, to decrease infection, and to decrease pain.

Modern research on wound healing shows that wounds heal faster when they are kept moist and not allowed to dry out. Therefore, most wounds are now covered. The most simple wound coverage is a band-aid with a central piece of nonadherent material. The bandaid can breathe, get wet, and be replaced if it falls off. It can be used with or without placement of a topical antibiotic ointment on the wound. However, bandaids provide no pressure on the wound and the adhesive backing often is irritating to the skin. Even so, they have become something of a prototype for the layered, postsurgical wound coverings that combine a nonadherent layer against the wound, a slightly absorbent layer on top of that, and an outer layer to hold the inner dressings in place.

COVERAGE FOLLOWING SIMPLE EXCISION

Many different approaches to wound coverage exist, including the idea of no coverage at all. However, most cutaneous surgeons adhere to the principle of keeping a wound covered with an antibacterial ointment and some variation of a bandage. Since the bandage is

an integral part of each surgical procedure, bandages are discussed throughout this volume as they relate to the specific surgical procedure at hand. The basic principles of wound coverage are discussed at length in Chapter 13 in the context of wound healing by second intention. The present chapter describes only the most basic dressing for wound coverage, the principles of which can be applied to the coverage of any wound.

The dressing for a simple excision begins with hydrogen peroxide, which is used to clean the wound. It is then wiped off (Figure 12.1A,B). The suture line is then covered with an antibacterial ointment (Figure 12.1C) and the wound is surrounded by the liquid adhesive, Mastisol (Figure 12.1D). Tincture of benzoin also can be used but is more difficult to work with. Then, using paper tape, an "inner layer" of dressing is glued onto the suture line (Figure 12.1E,F). Paper tape is less irritating to the skin than

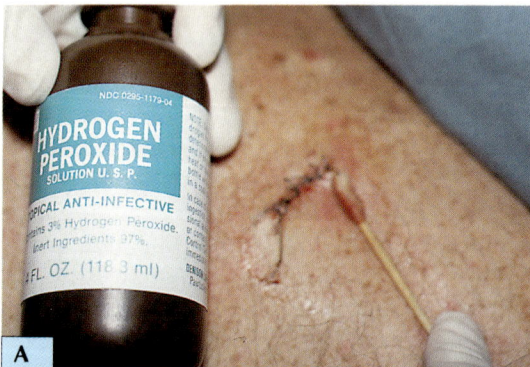

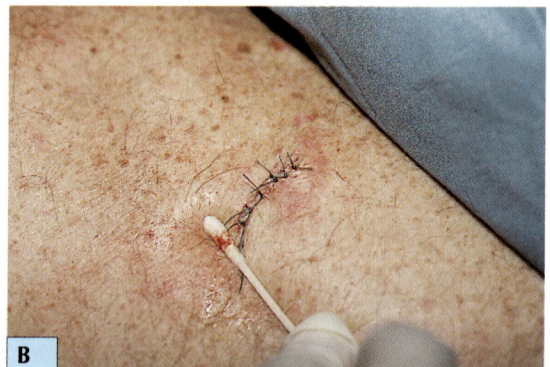

FIGURE 12.1 Basic dressing regimen following simple excision and suturing of a basal cell carcinoma on the middle of the back. **(A)** Hydrogen peroxide is applied to the wound using a cotton-tipped applicator. **(B)** It is then wiped off along with any residual blood. **(C)** Bacitracin ointment is applied to clean the wound surface, keeping it only on the suture line. **(D)** Mastisol is applied around the

wound using two cotton-tipped applicators to give a wider stroke to the application. **(E)** Flesh-colored paper tape is cut to the size of the suture line and is reinforced by placement of two to three pieces of tape on top of one another. **(F)** The paper tape is applied to the suture line with Mastisol acting as the adhesive. **(G)** Pressure is applied using a dental roll. **(H)** This is secured in place using more tape.

some of the more adhesive varieties of tape. It is also supplied in white or flesh-color, the latter of which creates a more cosmetically acceptable bandage. In most cases, this inner layer should remain in place until the sutures are removed. On top of this layer an "outer layer" is applied, which forms the pressure bandage (Figure 12.1G,H). The area of applied pressure should be confined to the suture line and the surrounding undermined area. Multiple layers of gauze folded over itself, dental rolls, or cotton balls all can be

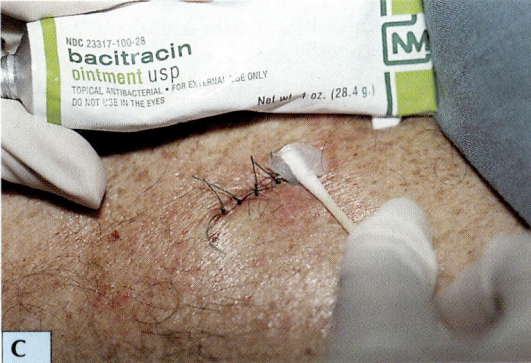

C

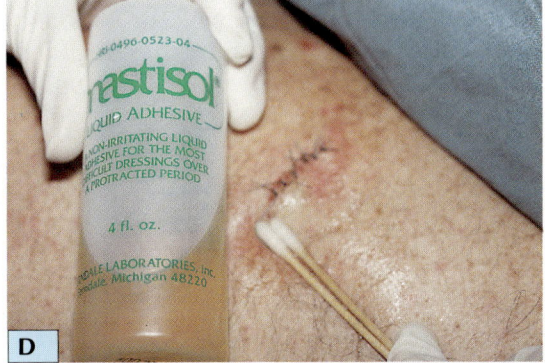

D

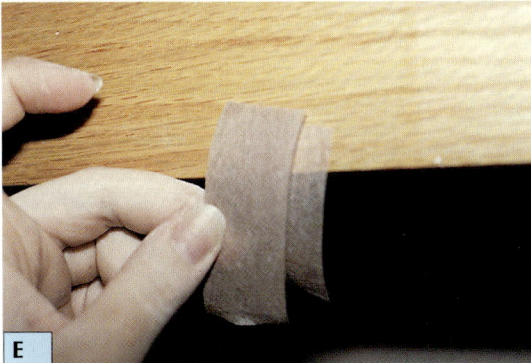

E

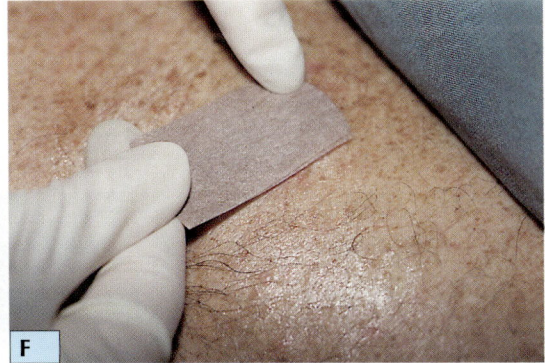

F

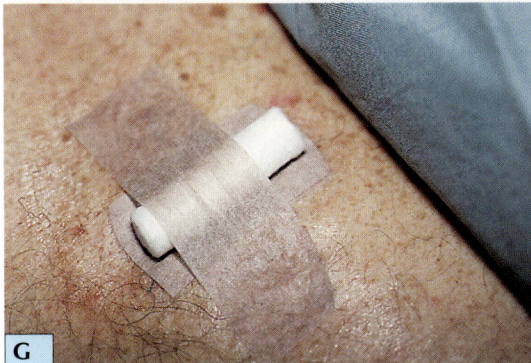

G

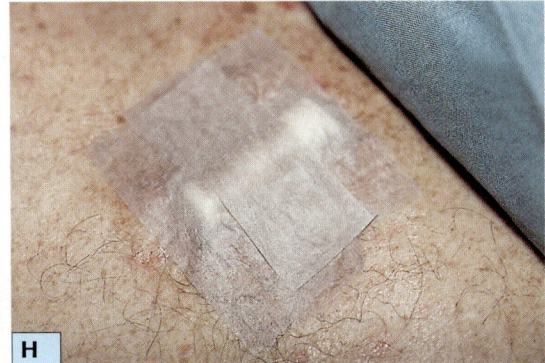

H

used to provide pressure. Whichever of these materials is used, it should be molded so that it fits over the wound as well as the contour of the body part to be covered (Figure 12.2A–D).

Patients are instructed to remove the outer bandage after 48 hours. If the wound is on the face, the entire bandage should be left in place until suture removal. The bandage should also be kept dry. If the dressing falls off, the wound may be covered with a simple bandaid so that the sutures are not irritated.

Some practitioners advocate daily care of sutured wounds, consisting of hydrogen peroxide for cleansing and drying, application of an antibacterial ointment, and coverage with a bandaid or nonadherent layer such as Telfa and tape to hold it in place. Others advocate the use of soap and water for gentle cleansing of the wound several times daily. Advocates of the latter approach claim low infection rates equal to those of the more complicated wound care regimen, with equally good cosmetic results.

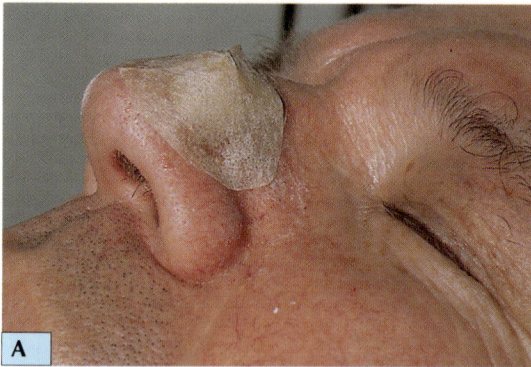

FIGURE 12.2 Examples of bandages on various parts of the body: (A) the nose, (B) the neck, (C) the back of the ear, and (D) the shin.

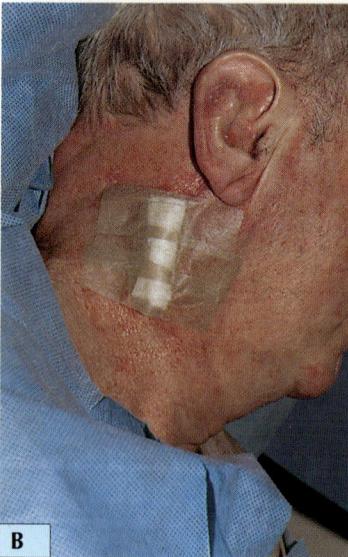

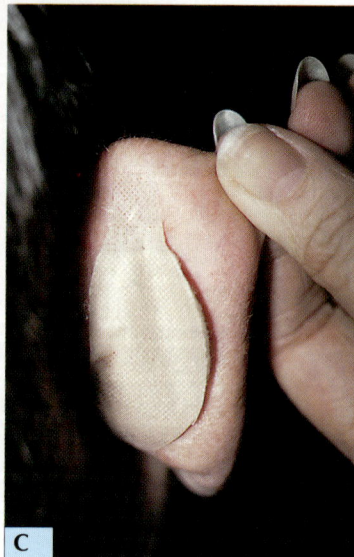

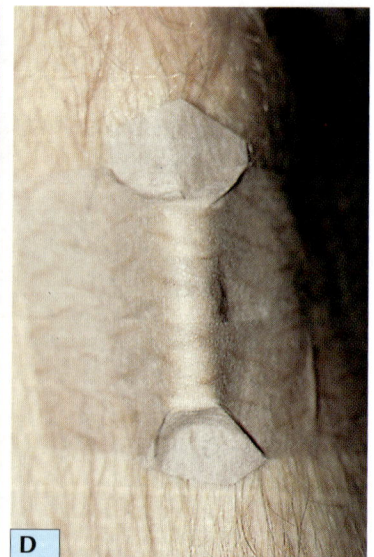

Most scalp wounds are dressed with a head roll, as it is virtually impossible to secure a bandage in a hairy area. Furthermore, given the potential amount of bleeding associated with scalp wounds, a good pressure dressing is essential. Patients who have been forewarned of this need are better able to accept it, and also have the opportunity to bring a hat or scarf to the office to camouflage the bandage at the conclusion of the procedure. Once the head roll is removed, the wound should be cleansed two times daily with soap and water, following which an antibacterial ointment is applied. Hydrogen peroxide should not be used in hair as it will bleach it, causing understandable distress to the unsuspecting patient.

Despite the endless variety of wound care materials manufactured, many such products are not available on a local basis. Therefore, if dressing changes are to be a part of a patient's wound care regimen, the surgeon can best serve the patient's needs by knowing what is available in local pharmacies at reasonable cost and by using these materials to create the best possible bandage according to the principles set forth in this chapter.

SYNTHETICS

Synthetic wound coverings are discussed elsewhere in this Atlas at somewhat greater length (see Chapter 13). The prototypical synthetic dressing is Op-Site, which is a polyurethane film. This dressing is semipermeable (permeable to water vapor and gases but not to water), transparent (permitting inspection of the wound site), and adherent only at its edges (allowing for easier application). Because the dressing is non-absorbent, when it is used with an exudative wound, large amounts of serosanguinous fluid may pool underneath it. To express the fluid, a small incision can be made in the Op-site, with the fluid drained through it. Op-site also conforms to the surface to which it has been applied. Op-site probably does not increase the risk of infection. Other polyurethane films include Bioclusive, Tegaderm, and Polyskin. The most popular uses for these dressings are to cover donor sites for split-thickness skin grafts and for coverage of ulcers.

SUMMARY

The fashioning of adequate bandages takes time and experience. As a general rule, a few standard products should be used and the dressing's primary purpose should always be kept in mind. Patients are often concerned about the size and appearance of the bandage and therefore it is desirable to attempt to make the bandage look as presentable as possible. First and foremost, however, the bandage must serve its primary purpose, be it pressure, coverage, stability, or protection of the wound.

SUGGESTIONS FOR FURTHER READING

Bennett RG. Fundamentals of Cutaneous Surgery. St Louis, Mo: C V Mosby Co; 1988.

Zitelli JA. Wound healing and wound dressings. In: Roenigk RK, Roenigk HH Jr, eds. Dermatologic Surgery. Principles and Practice. New York, NY: Marcel Dekker Inc;1989:97-135.

chapter 13

HEALING BY SECOND INTENTION

Surgical wounds of the skin are allowed to heal by second intention for a variety of reasons. Certain procedures, notably electrosurgery, cryosurgery, and CO_2 laser surgery, often result in the creation of relatively superficial defects that are not well suited for primary closure or repair but do well with second intention healing. For saucerized wounds in certain anatomic regions, particularly in areas of concavity, the outcome seen with natural wound healing is often superior to that seen with complicated reconstruction. Finally, occasional excisional procedures are complicated by wound infection or hematoma, which results in wound dehiscence and necessitates that the open wound be allowed to "heal by granulation." Every cutaneous surgeon, therefore, has reason to be familiar with the principles of healing by second intention.

THE WOUND HEALING PROCESS

To manage wounds effectively, the clinician must have some familiarity with the wound healing process. For ease of understanding, this process can be divided into four components, namely, the inflammatory response, epithelization, fibroplasia, and neoangiogenesis. Despite their presentation here as discrete compartmentalized entities, these components are, in fact, clinically inseparable and occur concurrently during wound repair.

THE INFLAMMATORY RESPONSE

When a wound is created, a large number of chemical substances, including various growth factors, are generated. Some of these substances are chemotactic for inflammatory cells (neutrophils and monocytes) while others increase local vascular permeability. A stranding network of fibrin forms in the wound space and is important later for cellular ingress and collagen deposition (Figure 13.1A).

Neutrophils and macrophages, in numbers proportionate to their presence in peripheral blood, appear in the wound within the first few hours of injury. Polymor-

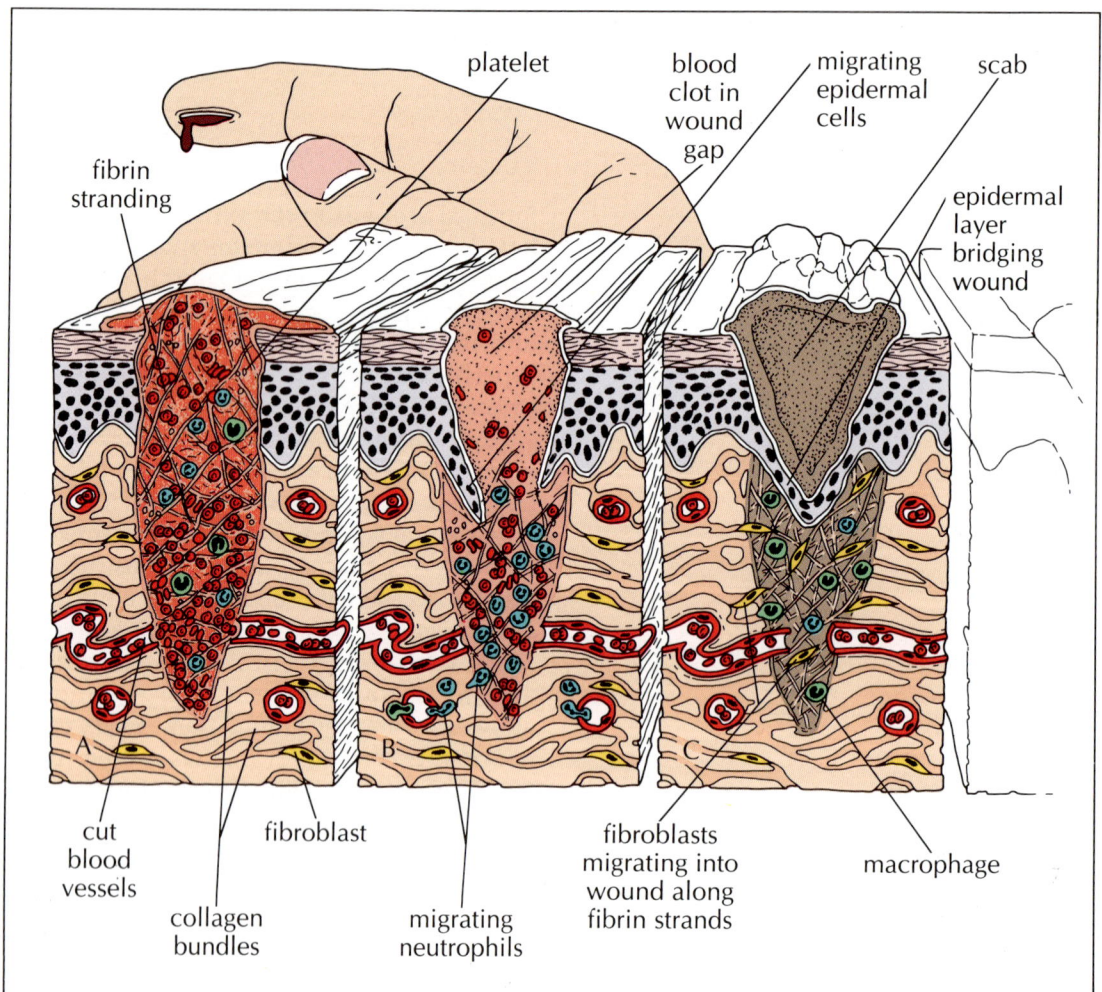

FIGURE 13.1(A) Laceration, day 1 (at the time of wounding). Blood constituents, including cells and soluble factors, enter the wound space. Platelet aggregation and blood coagulation proceed rapidly. A stranding network of fibrin forms within the blood clot and becomes cross-linked with fibronectin. **(B)** Laceration, day 2. Numerous polymorphonuclear leukocytes have migrated to the wound to phagocytose bacteria and wound debris. The surface epidermis exhibits mitotic activity, and peripheral epithelial cells, guided by the fibrin

(continued on next page)

phonuclear leukocytes initially predominate and remove contaminating bacteria and wound debris for a period of 3 to 4 days (Figure 13.1B). They are then replaced largely by tissue macrophages, which are derived from circulating monocytes that enter the wound. These cells phagocytose any remaining microorganisms, scavenge tissue debris, and release multiple biologically active substances, including chemotactic and growth factors, vasoactive mediators, and enzymes.

Some of these substances play a role in subsequent fibroblast activation (Figure 13.1C).

EPITHELIZATION

Within 24 hours of injury, proliferating epidermal cells at the wound margins give rise to migrating cells that move across the wound from all directions (see Figure 13.1B). Once inwardly migrating epidermal cells come into contact with one another at the

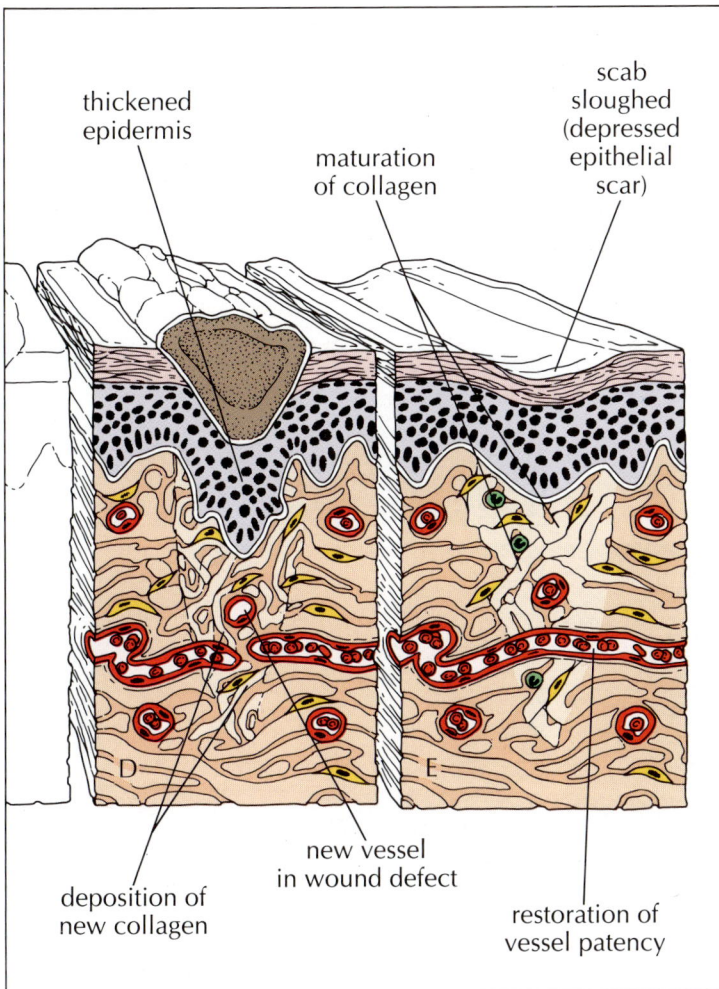

thickened epidermis

maturation of collagen

scab sloughed (depressed epithelial scar)

deposition of new collagen

new vessel in wound defect

restoration of vessel patency

network, begin to migrate across the wound, within the blood clot. **(C)** Laceration, day 3. The short-lived neutrophils have been replaced by macrophages. Among the many activities of these cells are the elaboration and release of chemotactic and growth factors for endothelial cells and fibroblasts, both of which exhibit increased migration into the wound. Granulation tissue components are being secreted by fibroblasts. **(D)** Laceration, day 5. Collagen fibers are being deposited haphazardly on the framework of fibronectin. These fibers will be reoriented in the future by the process of collagen remodeling. The epidermal cells, having already covered the wound surface, have ceased migrating and are now dividing to increase epidermal thickness. **(E)** Laceration, day 10. The eschar has sloughed and normal epidermal stratification is reappearing. Some new collagen is being secreted and wound strength is increasing. Severed blood vessels have undergone repair. The processes of wound maturation and wound remodeling will improve final wound contour and add strength to the scar.

center of the wound surface, migration ceases ("contact inhibition") and the epidermis begins to thicken (see Figure 13.1C).

To maintain viability during their transit, migrating epithelial cells seek a moist environment. They must tunnel beneath dehydrated surface tissues and do so by releasing collagenases, proteases, and plasminogen activators.

FIBROPLASIA

Under the influence of various chemoattractants, fibroblasts migrate into the wound along the fibronectin-coated fibrin lattice (see Figure 13.1C). Proliferation of these cells is stimulated by various growth factors, thrombin, and certain lymphokines. Fibronectin appears to act as the template for collagen deposition.

Early granulation tissue, which contains a great deal of type III collagen, fibronectin, and hyaluronic acid, is conducive to cell migration and proliferation (Figure 13.1D). With maturity, scars gain increased resilience and tensile strength. Type I collagen, dermatan sulfate, and sulfated proteoglycans become the major scar constituents (Figure 13.1E).

As water and mucopolysaccharides are lost from early scar tissue, the collagen fibrils become compressed, allowing closer approxi-

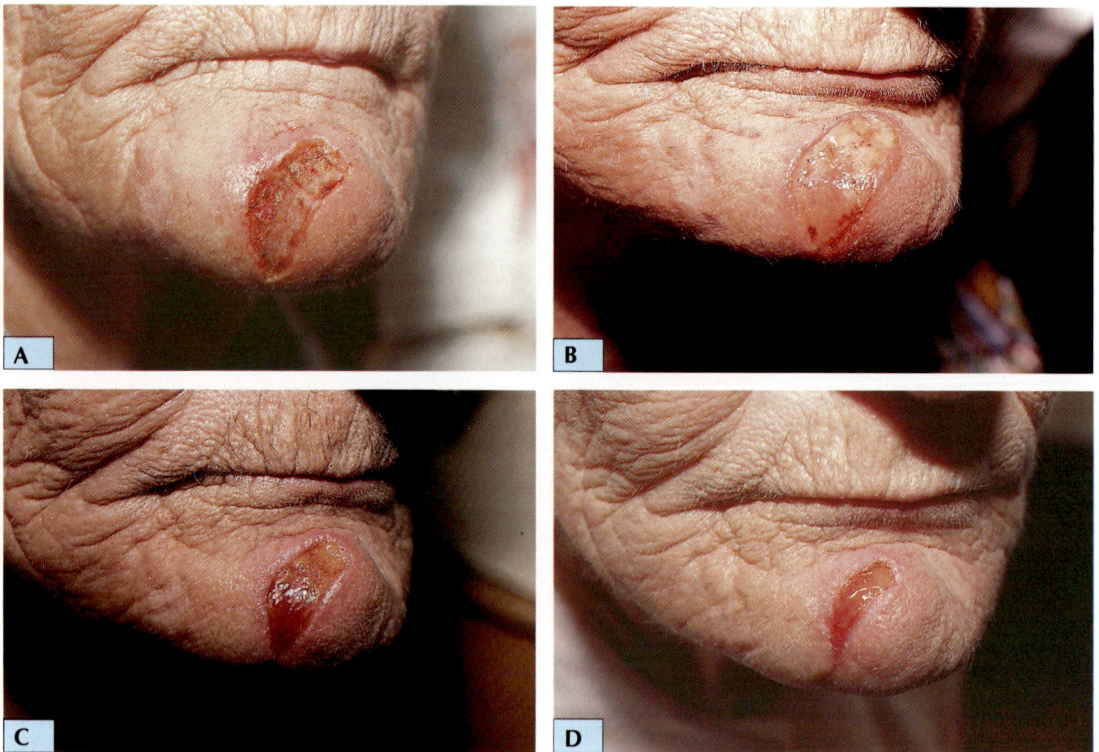

FIGURE 13.2 Healing of a full-thickness wound. **(A)** A full-thickness wound on the chin of an elderly woman following skin cancer surgery. **(B)** At 1 week following surgery, there is no appreciable decrease in surface area. A pseudomembranous exudate at the wound surface is a normal finding despite the use of semi-occlusive wound dressings. **(C)** At 2 weeks, some wound contraction is evident. Note also the "halo of erythema" that frequently is seen during this stage of wound healing. **(D)** At 3

mation of cross-linking sites. This, in turn, permits intermolecular and intramolecular covalent bond formation, both of which are essential for connective tissue strength. As the covalent bonds become more numerous, collagen fibrils become completely insoluble. This process is referred to as "collagen maturation."

Another late event in fibroplasia is the process of "collagen remodeling." Due to the haphazard arrangement and fragile nature of the newly deposited collagen fibrils, many are destined to serve little toward imparting ultimate tensile strength to healing wounds (see Figure 13.1D). During "remodeling," many such fibrils are digested and removed while new fibrils continue to be produced.

WOUND CONTRACTION

The surface area of a wound allowed to heal by second intention usually diminishes during the first few weeks of healing. Following wound contraction, any remaining exposed surface area will epithelize by epidermal cell migration (Figure 13.2A–H).

The forces responsible for wound contraction reside in myofibroblasts within the granulation tissue that fills the healing wound. These cells align themselves along the radial axis of the defect. The force of wound contraction, generated by actin bundles within the myofibroblasts, is transmitted to the sides of the wound by cell-cell and cell-stroma links.

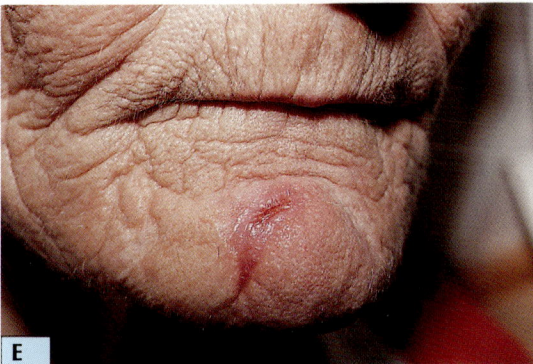

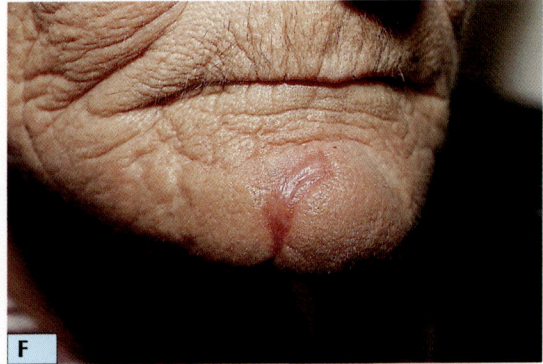

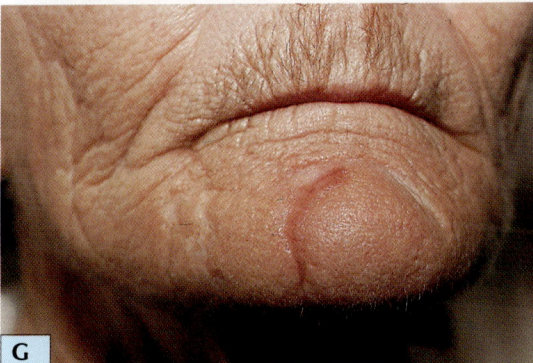

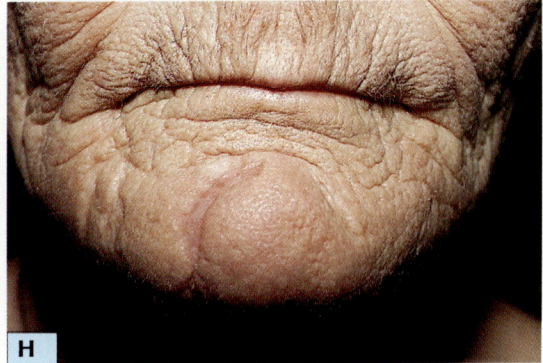

weeks, appreciable diminution in surface area can be seen. **(E)** At 4 weeks, the remainder of the wound surface has almost entirely re-epithelized. No further surface area reduction has occurred. **(F)** The wound is completely resurfaced at 5 weeks.

(G) At 3 months, the scar is slightly narrower and less erythematous than before. **(H)** The erythema has subsided by 1 year and the scar has softened, thinned, and become less obvious.

In anatomic areas of cutaneous laxity, wound contraction may be significant (Figure 13.3A,B). On the face, where the skin is attached to structures such as the eyelid, nose, or lip, wound contraction may result in distortion, causing ectropion, retraction of the alae nasi, or eclabium. When wound contraction occurs over a joint, a flexion contracture may result. Wound contraction ceases when the countervailing force in surrounding skin begins to exceed the force of contraction (Figure 13.4A,B). The mobility of the skin surrounding a wound therefore determines how much contraction will occur.

In general, round wounds do not contract as quickly or as completely as do rectangular, elongate, or stellate defects of equal surface area. In this regard, Zitelli has suggested that the expected healing time of a wound is proportionate to the diameter of the largest circle that can be contained within its margins.

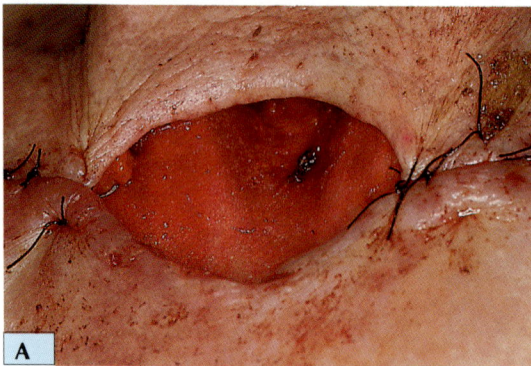

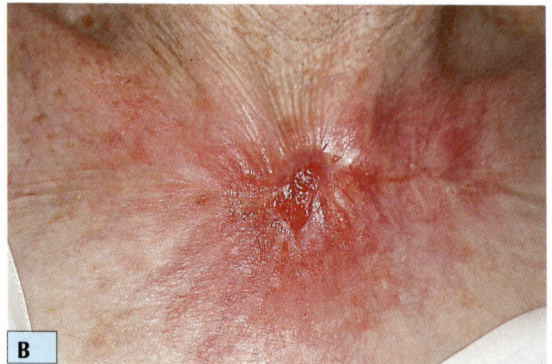

FIGURE 13.3 Contraction of a large surgical defect at the presternal region of an elderly woman. **(A)** Skin approximation was undertaken at the ends of the wound, but the mid-portion of the defect could not be approximated and was left to "granulate in." **(B)** Six weeks later, significant wound contraction has occurred. The remainder of the defect went on to heal completely by epithelization.

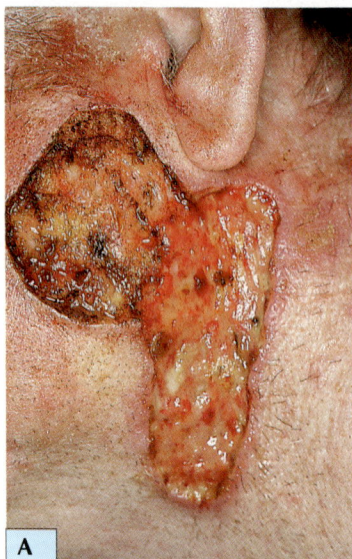

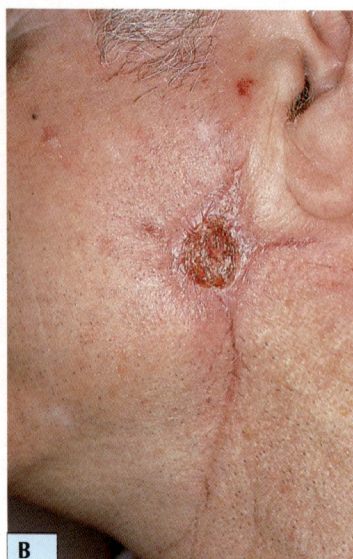

FIGURE 13.4 Healing of a large, surgical defect at the mandibular area in a middle-aged man. **(A)** The wound contained both circular and linear components. It was allowed to heal by second intention with daily wound dressings applied by the patient. **(B)** Seven weeks later, the linear portion of the wound had healed with a narrow scar, while the circular portion (with obviously greater counteracting skin tension) was incompletely healed. The remainder of the surface area went on to heal by epithelization.

NEOANGIOGENESIS

New blood vessel formation, or "neoangiogenesis," occurs in healing wounds to support the metabolic requirements of the wound healing process and to deliver the necessary substrate materials. It is likely that tissue hypoxia in wounded tissue stimulates macrophages to release various chemical mediators, including macrophage-derived angiogenesis factor.

The initial event in neoangiogenesis is migration into the wound of endothelial cells lining adjacent venules. These cells link up to form new arcades of capillaries, following which lumina appear in the center of the cords and blood flow begins. As healing proceeds and new blood vessel formation follows, increased oxygen tensions in the healing site eventually serve to curtail the secretion of angiogenesis factors, with subsequent regression of the neovasculature. Thus, the wound is transformed from capillary-rich, highly cellular tissue into a comparatively avascular, cell-free scar composed of dense collagen bundles. In clinical terms, a red, raised scar becomes a uniformly hypopigmented (porcelain white) flat scar.

FACTORS AFFECTING WOUND HEALING

Many local and systemic factors have the potential to affect wound healing adversely (Figures 13.5 and 13.6). In practice, those that appear to be the most detrimental to normal healing are edema, impaired microvasculature, and infection. Edema is primarily a problem of the lower extremity. Wounds in this location normally require 6 to 12 weeks to heal by second intention as compared to the 4 to 6 weeks usually required for facial wounds of a comparable size. If edema is present, healing time can be prolonged. Normal healing time can be restored by the institution of supportive measures for edema reduction, such as support hose or elasticized bandage wraps.

Impaired microvasculature is also of limited concern, as most cutaneous surgical procedures are performed on the richly vascularized head and neck. With the exception of wounds located on the lower extremity, microvascular patency is rarely a problem. When a paucity of local blood vessels exists, as in areas of chronic radiodermatitis, signifi-

FIGURE 13.5
LOCAL FACTORS ADVERSELY AFFECTING WOUND HEALING

Surgical Technique
- *traumatic tissue handling*
- *tightly tied sutures*
- *excessive tension*
- *inadequate hemostasis*
- *destructive method of wounding*

Hematoma Formation

Infection
- *bacterial*
- *yeast*

Hypothermia

Edema

Foreign Body Reaction

Desiccation

Tissue Ischemia
- *prior radiotherapy*
- *microvascular disease*
- *physical*

Topical Medications
- *topical corticosteroids*

cant fibrosis, or prior major surgical intervention, healing can be significantly delayed due to compromised neoangiogenesis.

Regarding infection, while most open wounds quickly become colonized with resident bacteria, clinical infection is rare. When infection does occur, healing is delayed. In fact, delayed healing may be the only sign that infection is present since during the early weeks of healing a certain degree of inflammation, exudation, and slight local tenderness is expected. During this period, it is not uncommon for patients to call the surgeon to report that they have "an infection" in the wound. What they are usually seeing is the halo of erythema that accompanies the normal inflammation and new blood vessel ingrowth seen with wound healing (see Figure 13.2C). Nonetheless, when significant pain, redness, swelling, and malodorous exudate appear in a granulating wound, bacterial infection should be suspected and systemic antibiotics promptly administered following a swab for culture and sensitivity. In superficial wounds, such as those following dermabrasion or chemical peeling, delayed healing in association with extreme erythema, pustulation, and burning discomfort should alert the surgeon to the possibility of yeast infection.

FOREIGN BODY REACTION

Over the years, a number of cutaneous surgeons have noted occasional hyperproliferation of granulation tissue ("proud flesh"), particularly in wounds located in hair-bearing regions (Figure 13.7A–C). A heaped-up, gel-like mass of vascular, beefy red tissue appears in the wound, often overhanging it. Occasionally, it resembles a pyogenic granuloma. This finding is usually the result of embedded hair or other foreign body. Removal of the excess granulation tissue seems to aid in subsequent healing, particularly when the excess tissue overhangs the wound edge. An attempt should also be made to remove the inciting foreign body. Often this requires trimming of the local hair.

FIGURE 13.6
SYSTEMIC FACTORS ADVERSELY AFFECTING WOUND HEALING

Deficiency States
- *malnutrition*
- *vitamin deficiency*

Disease States
- *hereditary (Ehlers-Danlos syndrome)*
- *metabolic (diabetes, chronic renal failure)*
- *vascular (vasculitis, hypertension)*
- *immunologic (deficiency states)*
- *other (malignancy, cirrhosis)*

Systemic Medications
- *glucocorticosteroids*
- *anticoagulants*
- *salicylates*
- *antineoplastic agents*

Impaired Oxygenation
- *cardiopulmonary disorders*

Aging

MANAGEMENT OF GRANULATING OPEN WOUNDS

The role of the clinician in managing the healing of open wounds is to support the natural healing process and to avoid situations that impair it. By providing an optimally sustaining environment for the wound and by ensuring that it remains free of infection, the clinician can fulfill his or her "secondary" function in second intention healing.

WOUND DRESSINGS

It is well established that wounds left open to the air take longer to heal. Desiccation of the wound slows epithelization by forcing the migrating epithelial cells to travel beneath the surface eschar to seek a sustaining "water table." By keeping the wound moist and preventing dehydration, occlusive or semi-occlusive dressings can enhance epitheliza-

tion by 30% to 45%. Such dressings also decrease pain in granulating wounds.

Currently there are seven distinct dressing types available, and composites thereof:

(1) Non-adhesive perforated plastic films with absorptive backing (eg, Telfa);

(2) Non-adhesive impregnated dressings that require a secondary wrap (Vaseline gauze);

(3) Adhesive polyurethane films (eg, Op-Site);

(4) Hydrogels containing a high percentage of water in a cross-linked polymer lattice (eg, Vigilon);

(5) Hydrocolloids containing hydrophilic colloidal particles (gumlike materials) formulated in an adhesive mass (eg, Duoderm);

(6) Non-adhesive sponge-like foams (eg, Synthaderm); and

(7) Alginate fibers high in calcium and sodium content (eg, Kaltostat).

The polyurethane films tend to be most

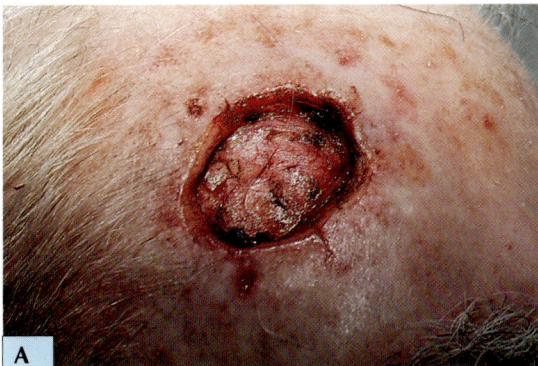

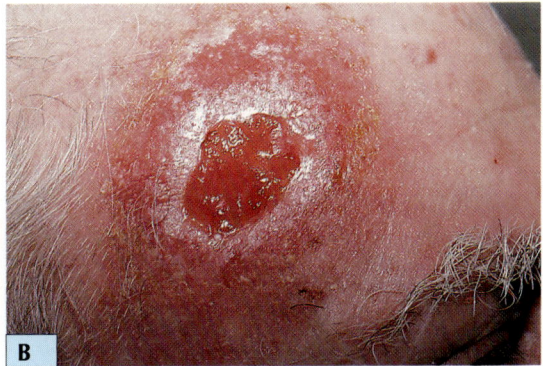

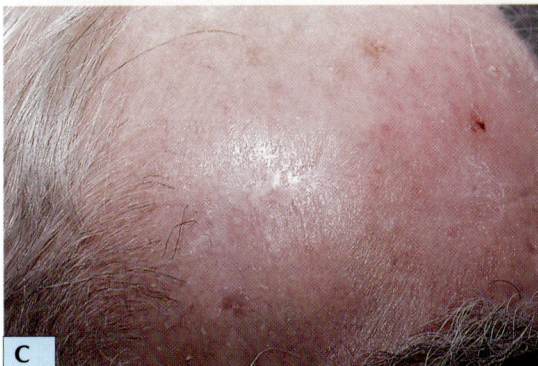

FIGURE 13.7 (A) A full-thickness defect following Mohs' micrographic surgery for a large squamous cell carcinoma on the brow of an elderly man. (B) Six weeks later, a mass of gelatinous granulation tissue is present, which is found to overhang the edge of the wound. The "proud flesh" was removed by gentle curettage, following which hemostasis was achieved. The wound healed without further complication during the following few weeks. (C) Three years later, the cosmetic outcome is quite acceptable.

valuable in the coverage of superficial wounds, while the other types listed have shown utility in the treatment of both superficial and deep wounds.

WOUND CARE

Most clinicians now recognize the benefit of using wound dressings, usually polyurethane films (Figure 13.8), in the treatment of split-thickness skin graft donor sites. They also use a variety of wound dressings routinely for the treatment of deep defects, such as those following saucerization of large skin cancers. In the postoperative management of dermabrasion, some clinicians have noted enhanced epithelization when semi-occlusive dressings such as Vigilon (Figure 13.9) are applied daily until the wound is healed.

To cover common superficial wounds, however, such as those following dermabrasion or electrosurgery, many, and possibly most, clinicians do not insist upon wound dressings beyond the immediate postoperative period. They do, however, frequently instruct patients to apply an ointment (or a vegetable-oil-based cream) to the operative site several times a day. This ointment, which provides an interface with the air, minimizes surface dehydration and eschar formation and could reasonably be thought of as a rudimentary semi-occlusive "dressing" that promotes healing.

Many cutaneous surgeons employ a padded, perforated plastic film dressing (Telfa) held in place with flesh-colored microporous paper tape (Micropore) for many of their wound care needs. Since the dressing is "custom made" for each wound, it can be used for large, small, superficial, and deep wounds. A typical wound care regimen performed by the patient, patient's friend, or family member at each dressing change is shown in Figure 13.10A–F. Patients are instructed to wear the dressing 24 hours a day. Epithelization is usually complete in approximately 4 weeks for superficial lesions and in 4 to 6 weeks for full-thickness skin wounds.

PREDICTING OUTCOMES

Young scars remain active for quite some time after the wound surface has healed. New blood vessels, which cause scars to be red, regress over a period of 3 months or more. Likewise, collagen maturation and collagen remodeling can continue up to 1 year. For this reason, it is only after 6 to 12 months that the

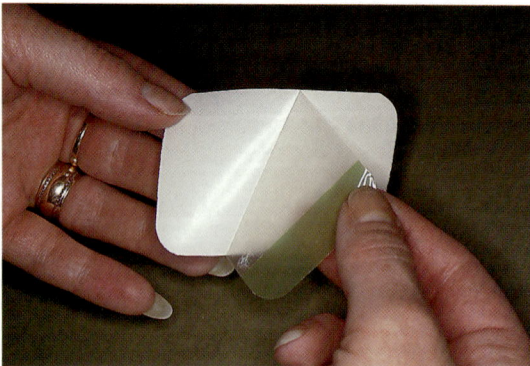

FIGURE 13.8 Op-Site is one of the adhesive polyurethane occlusive film dressings used frequently in the management of split-thickness skin graft donor sites.

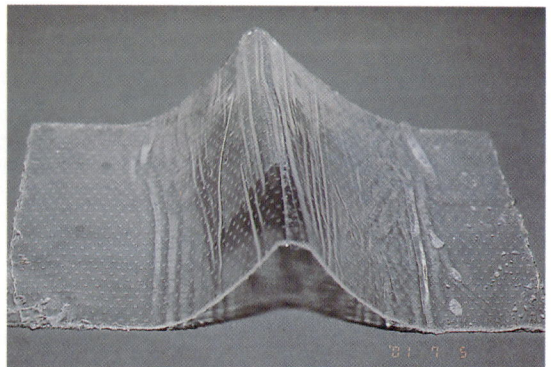

FIGURE 13.9 Vigilon, a hydrogel dressing, is used by many clinicians in the management of dermabrasion sites and other superficial wounds. In addition to providing a semi-occlusive environment, this and similar dressings are capable of absorbing significant amounts of exudate.

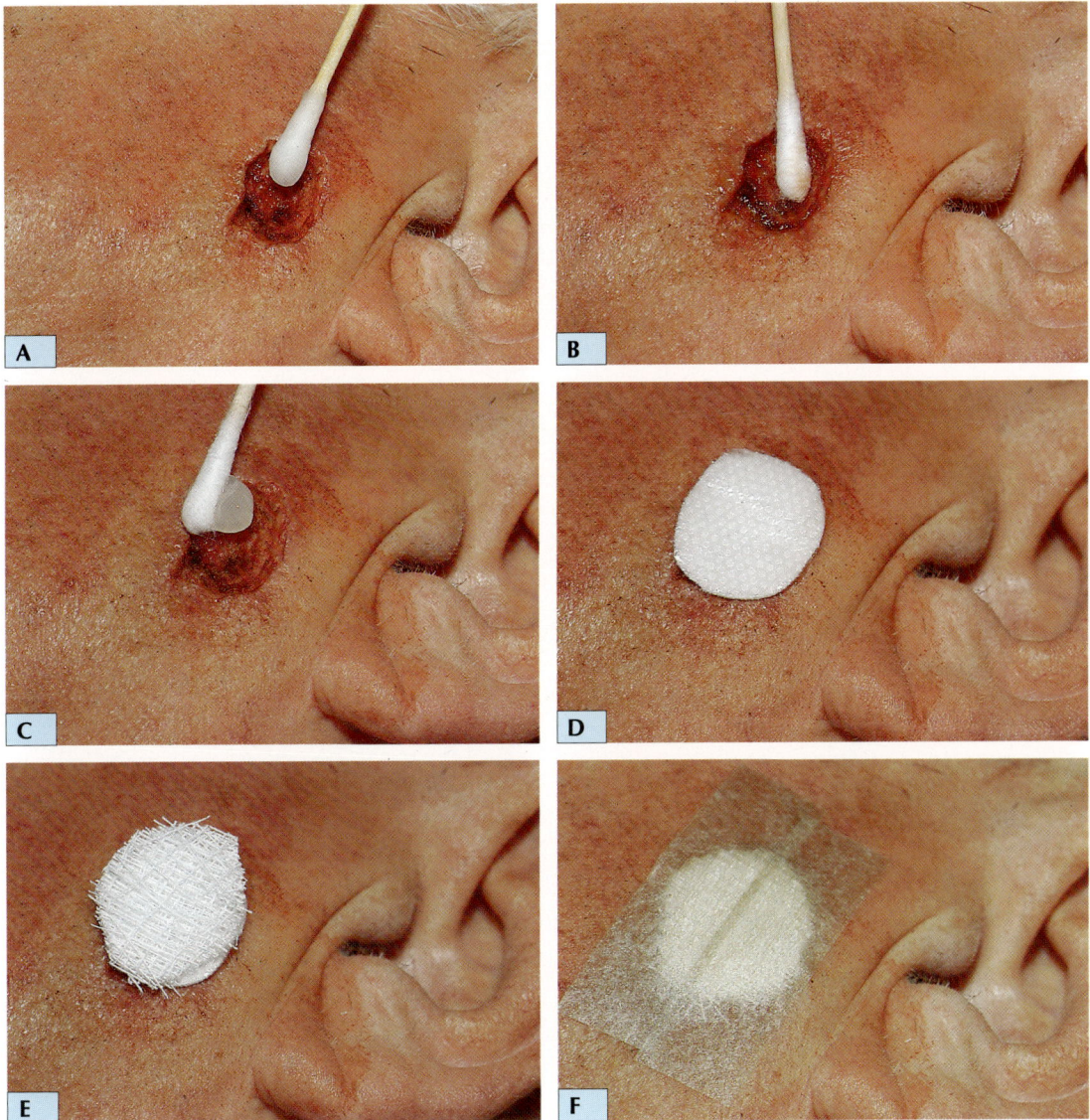

FIGURE 13.10 A common wound-care regimen for full-thickness skin defects. The dressing is changed twice daily until drainage subsides and once daily thereafter. **(A)** The wound surface is cleansed gently with a clean, cotton-tipped applicator dipped in 3% hydrogen peroxide or other cleansing solution. **(B)** Another clean, cotton-tipped applicator is used for gentle removal of any residual cleanser from the wound bed. **(C)** A thin layer of antibiotic ointment is applied to the wound surface. **(D)** A piece of Telfa dressing, cut slightly larger than the wound, is applied to the wound surface. **(E)** For heavy drainage, an absorptive layer of gauze, cut to size, is placed over the Telfa. This layer is omitted when the drainage subsides. **(F)** One or more strips of Micropore tape are used to hold the Telfa and gauze layers in place.

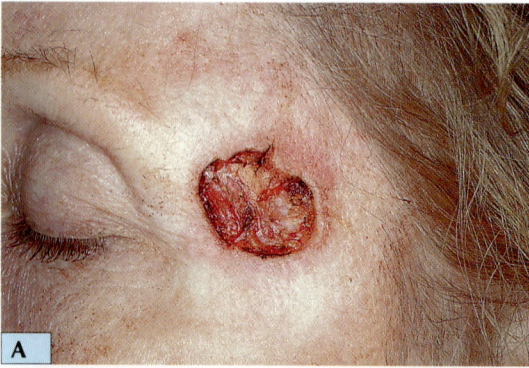

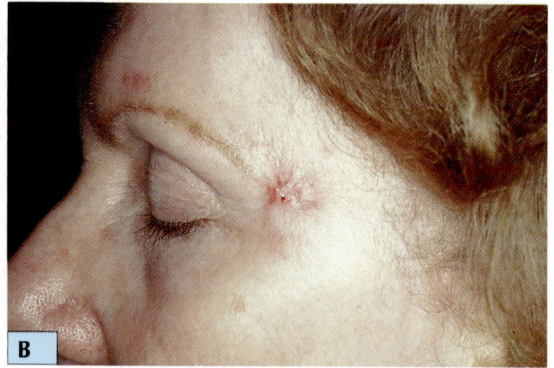

FIGURE 13.11 Healing of a full-thickness wound at the temple of a middle-aged woman. **(A)** Defect following Mohs' micrographic surgery for basal cell carcinoma. **(B)** Appearance of the operative site 2 months after surgery. The scar is red and lumpy. **(C)** One year later, after removal of makeup, the scar is seen to be completely flat and hypopigmented.

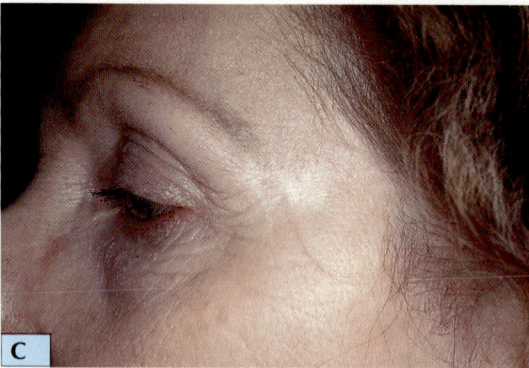

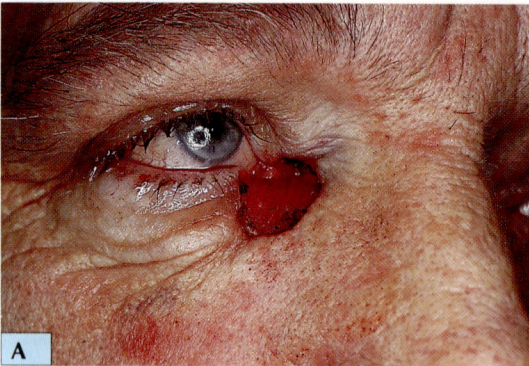

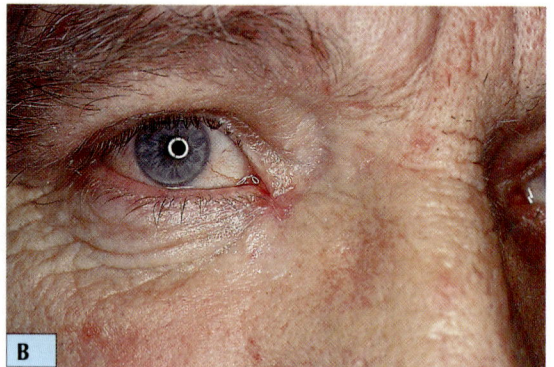

FIGURE 13.12 (A) A full-thickness defect at the inner canthus following treatment of a skin malignancy in a middle-aged man. **(B)** After 5 weeks, the defect has healed by second intention, with minimal distortion.

final cosmetic outcome of second intention healing can be assessed. Initially, the epithelized wound is lumpy, red, and firm. Within 3 months the erythema usually resolves, and over the next 3 to 9 months the wound flattens and softens (Figure 13.11A–C).

Outcomes for full-thickness wound healing vary with wound size, depth, and location as well as patient age and skin color.

Wounds located in concave areas (medial canthus, nasal alar crease, nasolabial fold, temple, postauricular sulcus, auricular concha) heal with excellent cosmetic results (Figures 13.12A,B and 13.13A,B) while those situated on convex surfaces (malar cheeks, nasal tip, vermilion border) usually yield obvious scars (Figure 13.14A,B). The latter are best managed, when possible, by a reconstructive pro-

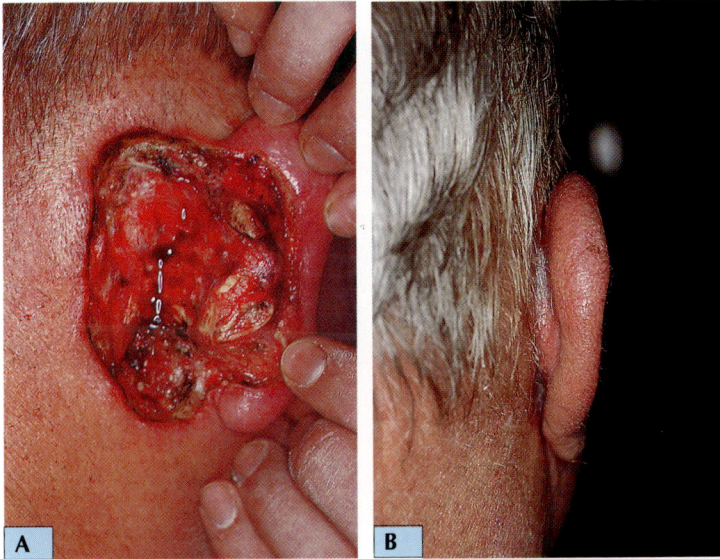

FIGURE 13.13 (A) This large, full-thickness defect at the postauricular sulcus resulted from treatment of an aggressive skin malignancy in an elderly man. **(B)** The wound was allowed to heal by second intention and 6 weeks later had closed with minimal distortion. No sutures were used in this case.

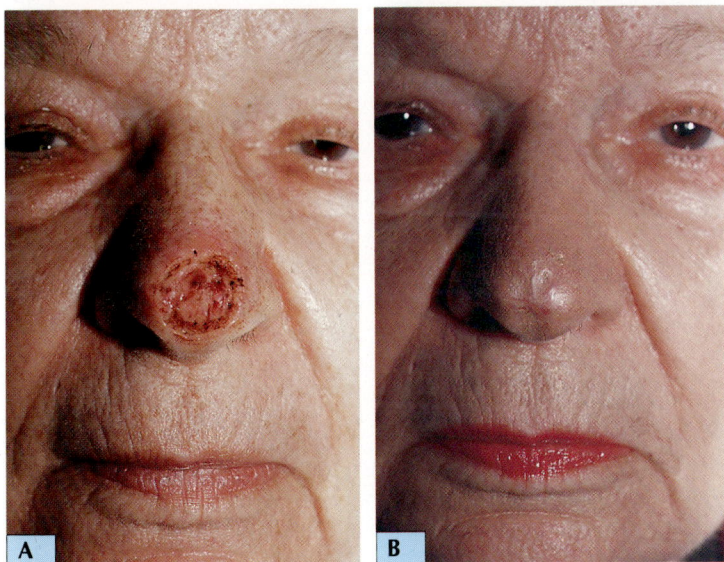

FIGURE 13.14 (A) A full-thickness defect at the nasal tip of an elderly woman following skin cancer removal. **(B)** The appearance of the scar following second intention healing is adequate at 5 months.

cedure. An intermediate outcome (Figure 13.15A,B) is seen with full-thickness wounds present on flat skin surfaces (forehead, sides of nose, periorbital region).

Wounds that expose bone or cartilage are also amenable to second intention healing, and the same principles of moist wound healing apply. Although cosmetic outcomes are generally satisfactory to excellent depend-ing on location, healing times are usually prolonged (Figure 13.16A–C). This is because granulation tissue must migrate into the wound from the periphery. In the case of large areas of exposed skull, the outer table of bone may necrose and shed, often exposing a granulation tissue base. Based on the collective experience of Mohs' surgeons who have seen this phenomenon many times, and

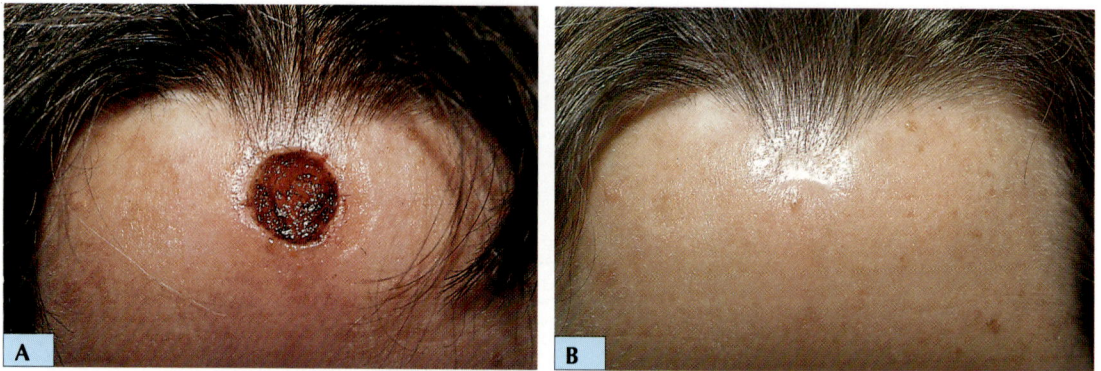

FIGURE 13.15 (A) A relatively large, full-thickness defect at the forehead of a middle-aged woman follow-ing skin cancer surgery. **(B)** The result, 9 months later following second intention healing, is satisfactory.

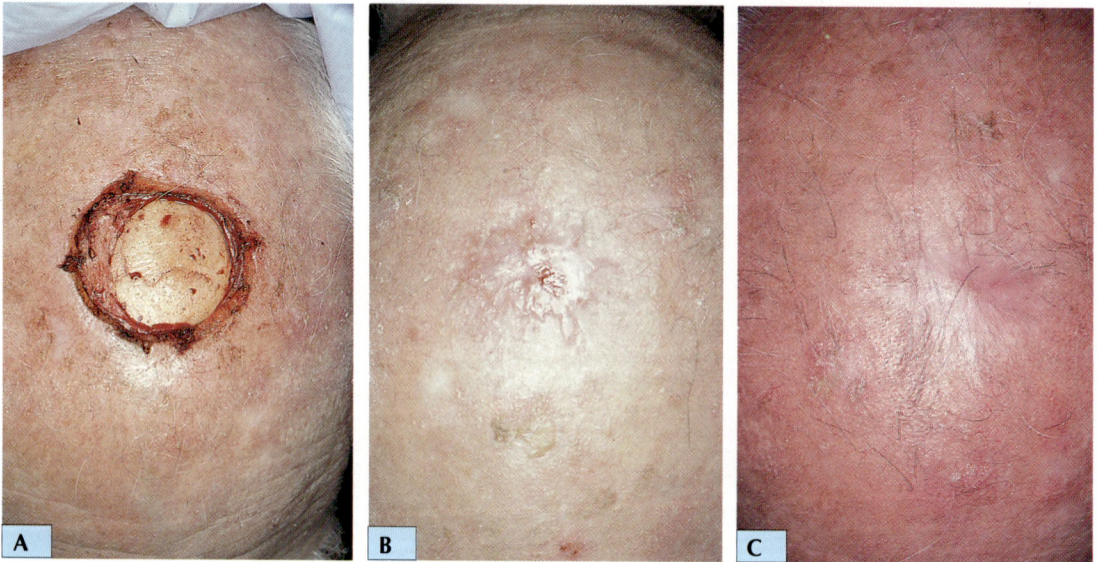

FIGURE 13.16 (A) This wound, which includes removal of periosteum, resulted from Mohs' micrographic surgery in an elderly man. **(B)** The wound healed with a somewhat thickened scar in approxi-mately 12 weeks. **(C)** Twelve weeks later, wound remodeling has occurred with excellent cosmetic outcome. The final result rivals that which could be expected with reconstructive surgery.

contrary to classical surgical teaching, osteomyelitis is a rare event in such situations. Nonetheless, preservation of periosteum or perichondrium should be undertaken whenever possible since these structures can contribute to the formation of granulation tissue.

When cartilage is exposed, a simple, but uniformly effective, maneuver can be undertaken to facilitate rapid healing (Figure 13.17A–D). Small plugs of full-thickness cartilage are removed using a 2-mm dermal punch, with care taken to expose but not to penetrate the underlying skin or mucosa. Multiple punch excisions of cartilage are performed, leaving cartilage bridges of 3 mm or more between them to serve as supportive scaffolding. As healing proceeds, buds of granulation tissue will arrive rapidly at the wound base through these fenestrations.

Older patients tend to heal with softer, less obvious scarring. This is especially true

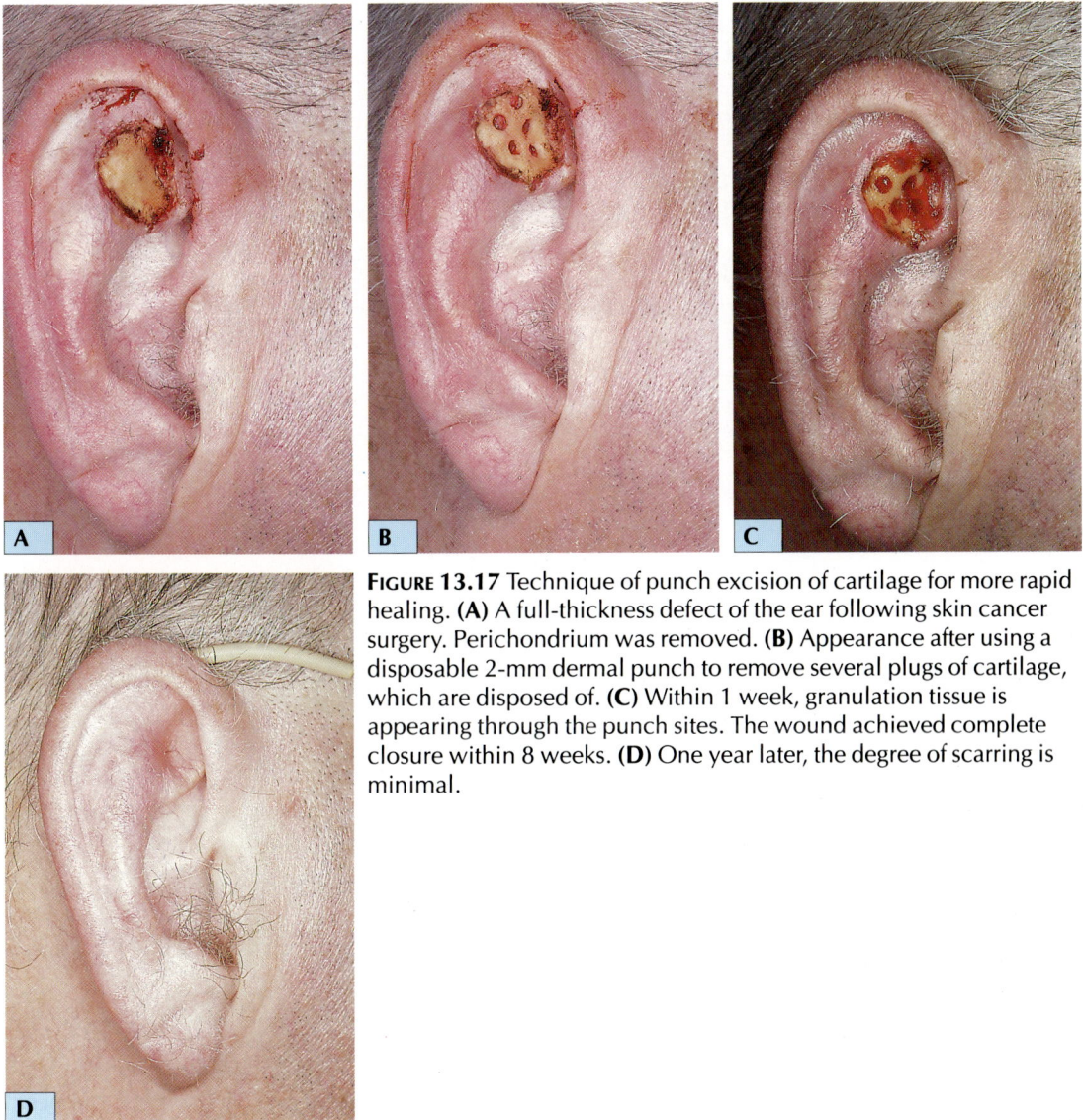

FIGURE 13.17 Technique of punch excision of cartilage for more rapid healing. (A) A full-thickness defect of the ear following skin cancer surgery. Perichondrium was removed. (B) Appearance after using a disposable 2-mm dermal punch to remove several plugs of cartilage, which are disposed of. (C) Within 1 week, granulation tissue is appearing through the punch sites. The wound achieved complete closure within 8 weeks. (D) One year later, the degree of scarring is minimal.

in individuals who have sustained a modicum of actinic skin damage resulting in a mottled skin coloration. Since all full-thickness scars exhibit the porcelain white coloration mentioned earlier, scarring tends to be less obvious in fair-skinned individuals.

The utility of second intention wound healing in a variety of clinical situations makes it an important modality with which to become familiar. As increasingly sophisticated wound dressings and topical medicaments appear and our knowledge of biologic mediators involved with wound healing increases, we may find ourselves taking a more active role in determining outcomes in second intention healing.

SUGGESTIONS FOR FURTHER READING

Clark RA. Cutaneous tissue repair: basic biologic considerations. I. J Am Acad Dermatol. 1985;13:701-725.

Eaglstein WH, ed. Clin Dermatol. 1984;2:1-153, 1984.

Falanga V. Occlusive wound dressings. Why, when, which? Arch Dermatol. 1988;124:872-877.

Goslen JB. Wound healing for the dermatologic surgeon. J Dermatol Surg Oncol. 1988;14:959-972.

Pollack SV. Wound healing 1985: an update. J Dermatol Surg Oncol. 1985;11:296-300.

Reed BR, Clark RA. Cutaneous tissue repair: practical implications of current knowledge. II. J Am Acad Dermatol. 1985;13:919-941.

Zitelli JA. Wound healing and wound dressings. In: Roenigk RK, Roenigk HH Jr, eds. Dermatologic Surgery. Principles and Practice. New York, NY: Marcel Dekker Inc; 1989.

chapter 14

COMPLICATIONS

Complications are events that occur unexpectedly. In surgery, most are avoidable by adherence to good surgical practice; others are unavoidable. In this regard, all surgical patients must sign an informed consent form that delineates, within reason, all of the most likely complications related to the procedure at hand (see Chapter 1). Most such documents are fairly nonspecific and list such general complications as loss of function, bleeding, and pain. To this list the surgeon should add specific information regarding the procedure for which the patient is signing. The form should be reviewed carefully by the patient, who can then ask specific questions. This interactive process tends to make the patient feel more comfortable with the planned procedure as well as with the surgeon. There is no doubt that careful and compassionate communication between patient and physician will be comforting to the patient, who in the event of an unforeseen or disturbing complication may be less likely to lodge a formal complaint and more likely to work with the surgeon to correct it.

Good surgical practice relates not only to the technical competence of the surgeon but also to his or her detailed attention to all aspects of surgery. After the informed consent has been signed and before the procedure, the surgeon must obtain from the patient a detailed medical history. Potential problems can be avoided if the surgeon knows the patient's past and present medical problems, regular medications, allergies, and home situation. The latter may help the surgeon to determine the level of wound care available to the patient, the patient's need for assistance, and the general support that the patient can anticipate at home.

Throughout this Atlas, specific surgical complications are discussed within the context of each chapter as they relate to a specific surgical technique. In the present chapter, general complications are discussed.

TISSUE HANDLING

Gentle handling of tissue in general, and of wound edges in particular, can decrease the chances of complication due to pinching, crushing, and tearing. Forceps crush and pinch. Specimens sent to the laboratory for histological evaluation may be insufficient for evaluation, especially with regard to their margins, if their edges have been crushed with forceps. Toothed forceps should be used at all times for tissue handling. To elevate wound edges, a skin hook is the least traumatic instrument. Sutures also can crush and pinch tissue if they are tied too tightly. If ischemia results, the wound edge may necrose and interrupt a smooth suture line (Figure 14.1). Elderly skin is particularly fragile, and therefore may tear if just a moderate amount of force is applied to it in pulling.

WOUND DEHISCENCE

Adequate surgical planning, including careful preoperative planning, is necessary to prevent wound dehiscence. Such planning begins with the patient interview. Postoperative restrictions should be carefully explained to the patient, who should be able to comply with them. This means that the patient must agree to take time off from work, avoid exercise and sports activities, and be available for timely suture removal to the extent that the particular procedure requires it. In addition, the excision should be planned so that it is properly oriented with regard to favorable skin tension lines.

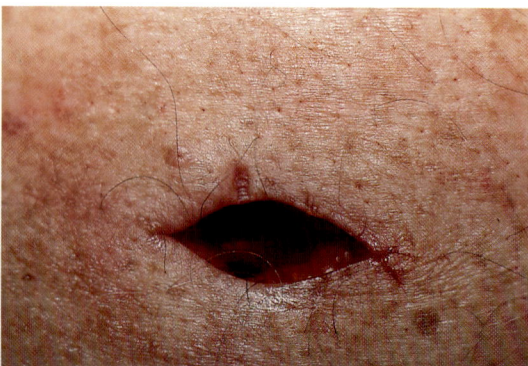

FIGURE 14.1 The edges of this wound have been crushed by tightly closing smooth forceps. An indentation from the forceps can be seen at the 11-o'clock position and can be expected to persist and mar the final suture line.

The appropriate suture material and suturing technique must be chosen. In addition, proper suture tying technique must be practiced. A gaping wound can be the result of sutures that have slipped. Monofilament sutures as well as teflon-coated sutures may need extra instrument ties to increase knot security (Figure 14.2A,B). Buried sutures will hold wounds together and should be placed at any location where there will be tension on the wound. To minimize added tension, patients should restrict movement of the area following surgery. Even so, some wounds do end up being closed under greater tension than expected or do not close at all. In such cases, instead of risking wound dehiscence and the problems that go with it, partial closure of the wound should be considered or no closure at all. Undoubtedly, the patient will understand and appreciate the surgeon's vigilance throughout the procedure and his or her carefulness in dealing with an unexpected occurrence.

If wound dehiscence is clean, the wound can be resutured. However, if the reasons for the wound's spread are not eliminated, there is little reason to re-close it. In a common example, a wound may be found to be ragged because the stitches have pulled through it and therefore further placement of sutures cannot be tolerated. In such a case, routine wound care is given. The physician should then discuss with the patient in a reasonable and straightforward manner the factors responsible for the dehiscence, the scar that will probably result, and the measures that might be undertaken to correct any unacceptable scar.

HEMATOMA FORMATION

Careful history taking, meticulous surgical technique, and adequate hemostasis all should contribute to a minimal amount of postoperative bleeding. However, if such bleeding should occur, which cannot be

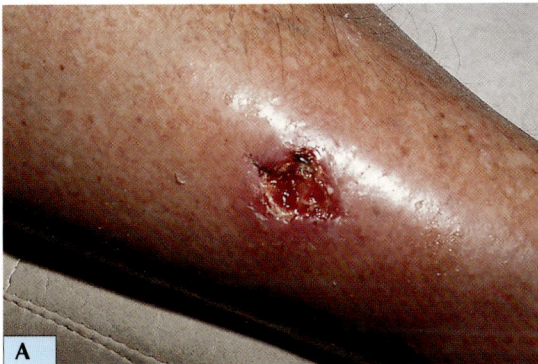

FIGURE 14.2 (A) Wound dehiscence has occurred due to tension that pulled the sutures through the wound edges. The sutures can still be seen as green pieces of thread in the wound. (B) The wound was left to heal by second intention, which is complete at 6 weeks.

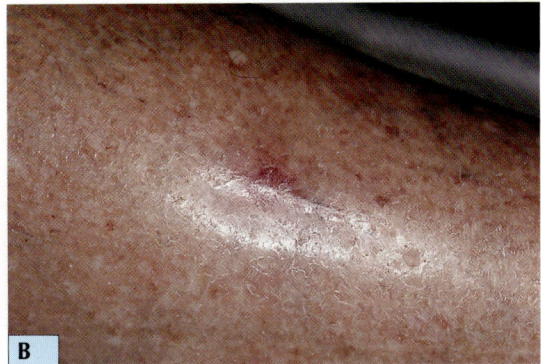

stopped by the sustained application of direct pressure, the wound must be taken down and the bleeder identified and eliminated.

Hematoma formation should be avoided deep in the wound as it may disrupt wound closure and cause dehiscence or infection. If circumstances allow it, the hematoma should be evacuated by removal of some of the sutures to make an opening (Figure 14.3). If active bleeding is still present, its source must be identified and eliminated. In most cases, however, no such source can be found.

Drains are not recommended as the wound is already at risk for infection and a drain can provide a route for the entry of microbes as much as it provides an exit for blood. The patient should be placed on antibiotics and the wound left open to drain. An adequate pressure dressing should be applied, which is left in place for 48 hours. The patient should then be seen frequently to assess reaccumulation.

INFECTION

Infection is a rare complication of outpatient surgery. However, it may occur due to an inadvertent break in antiseptic technique, inoculation of the wound following surgery, or increased risk from hematoma formation or wound dehiscence. The patient should be instructed to look out for increased soreness, redness, or swelling around the operative site, and to report any such findings without delay (Figure 14.4).

For certain types of excisions, including large excisions, those with a good deal of tissue manipulation, undermining, or increased tension on closure, or excisions in certain areas of the body where infection would be particularly serious, such as the fingers, toes, and penis, antibiotics are prescribed at the time of surgery. Antibiotics should also be prescribed for patients with poor hygiene or for those who show questionable compliance

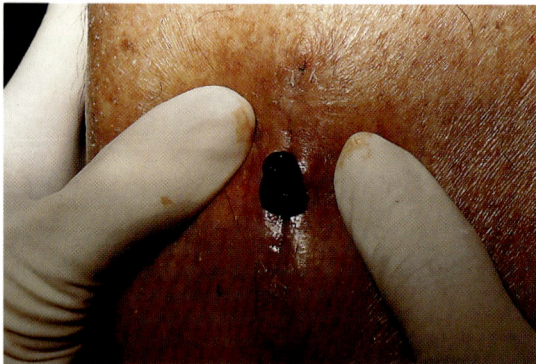

FIGURE 14.3 Following patient complaints of tenderness and redness of the wound, this organized clot was expressed after the sutures were removed. The wound was then cleansed, pressure bandages were applied, and antibiotics were prescribed. For wounds that are infected, it is recommended that sutures be removed to prevent them from eliciting a foreign body response.

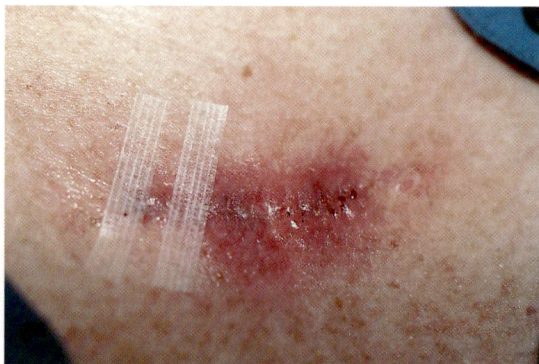

FIGURE 14.4 Swelling, tenderness, and erythema denoted infection even though there was no expressible pus in this wound. Following suture removal, the wound was covered with Steri-Strips and antibiotics were prescribed.

with postoperative instructions. As with any break in operating room technique, a postoperative infection must be taken seriously and its source or explanation found and corrected. For a more detailed discussion of antiseptic technique in cutaneous surgery, the reader is referred to Chapter 3 of this Atlas.

NERVE DAMAGE

Through an adequate knowledge of anatomy, nerve damage can be somewhat anticipated and explained to the patient *in advance* of surgery. Two possibilities must be explained. The first is the possibility of temporary nerve dysfunction, which almost always occurs with infiltration of the anesthetic at the oper-

ative site, especially if it is close to a large nerve. The patient should be forewarned of this likelihood and of its consequences. For example, if the eyelid does not close, the patient should be instructed to close it manually so that the cornea does not dry out. The patient should also be apprised that nerve function will return to baseline as the anesthetic wears off (Figure 14.5A,B). The second possibility is that of permanent dysfunction, which may result from severing of a major motor nerve. In fact, nerves may dysfunction without actually being cut or handled. For example, Bell's palsy has been known to occur from surgery in the lateral cheek area that did not involve nerves, infection, or swelling (Figure 14.6). The patient should

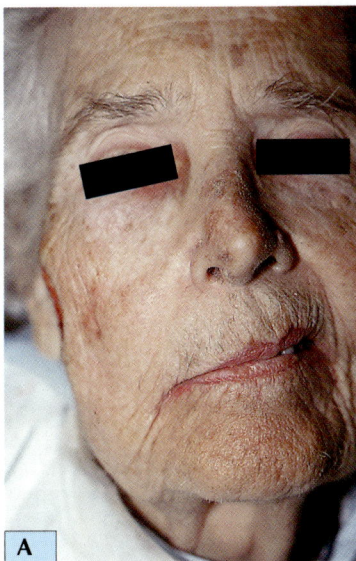

FIGURE 14.5 (A) Hemifacial paralysis was induced by infiltration of the anesthetic. The patient was forewarned regarding drooling and the intake of hot liquids and

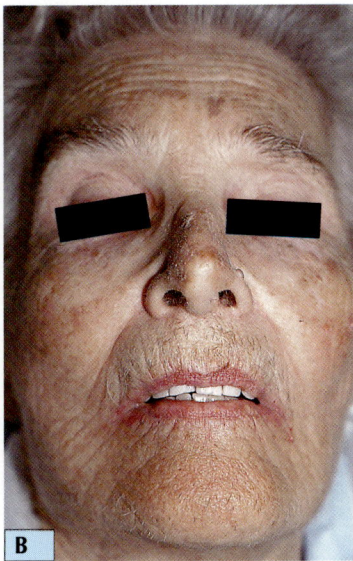

she was assured that the loss would be temporary. **(B)** By the time the patient left the office, most of the function had returned.

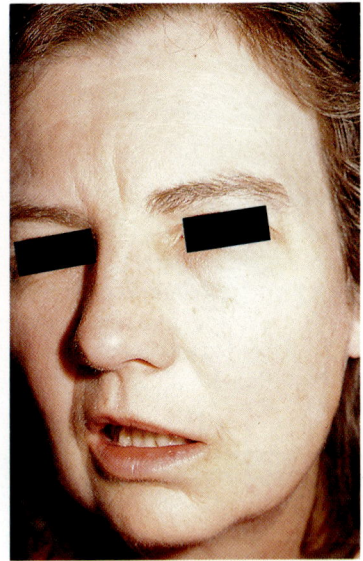

FIGURE 14.6 Bell's palsy after excision of a superficial skin cancer. Nerve dysfunction lasted more than 6 months. Careful evaluation by an otolaryngologist neurologist reassured the patient that although the nerve was not functioning it was electrically healthy and had not been severed.

also be apprised that the sensation at or around the surgical site may not return to normal for 1 year or longer. Patients are usually able to tolerate this well as long as they have been adequately informed in advance.

Lastly, whenever possible, photographs should be taken to document preoperative and postoperative function, especially in situations where nerve damage is anticipated. This is especially true for those patients who present at the time of surgery with nerve dysfunction due to other causes.

PAIN

Pain is usually minimal following most outpatient procedures and therefore analgesics are not routinely prescribed. However, the surgeon's assessment of the patient's tolerance of postoperative discomfort should be ongoing. Analgesics may cover up discomfort due to complications such as infection or hematoma. Therefore, patients should be told to notify their surgeon if they experience any severe discomfort. Even so, surgery in certain

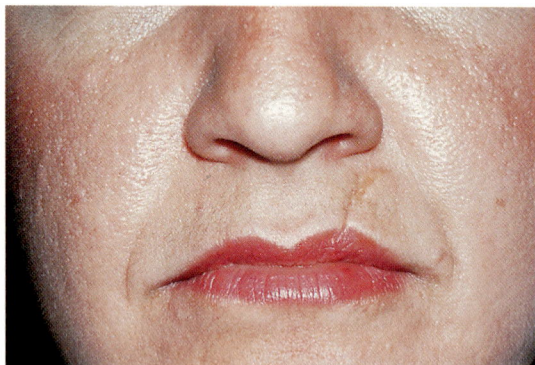

FIGURE 14.7 This patient's vermilion border had not been aligned properly before the repair. The surgeon working in this area must pay particular attention to the border and sew it together. The patient had not been forewarned adequately of the possibility of this complication and therefore was quite upset.

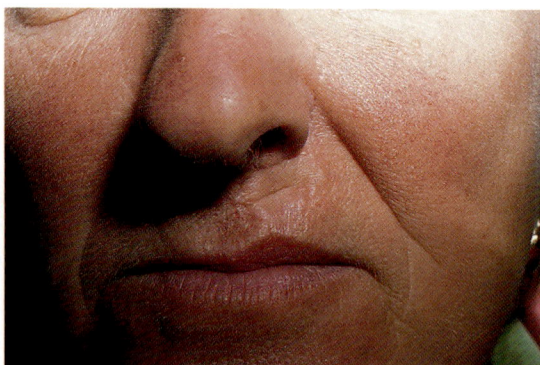

FIGURE 14.8 Wound contraction, following placement of a temporary graft at the site of removal of a large morpheaform basal cell carcinoma. While the patient had been forewarned of the possibility of some contraction, because of the thinness of her lips the problem was more noticeable than expected.

FIGURE 14.9 This young patient was more concerned with the hypertrophic scars resulting from three small punch biopsies than she was with the congenital hemangioma.

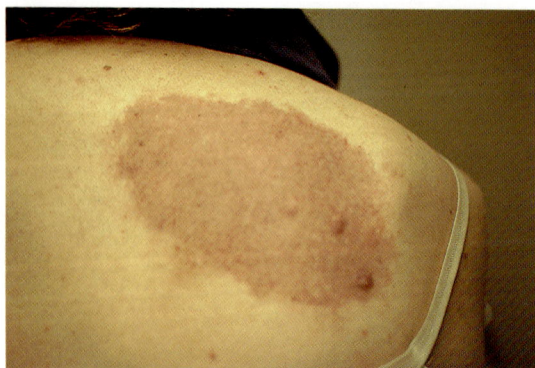

anatomic areas does require special consideration regarding discomfort. Surgery on the forehead and scalp, for example, usually results in headaches. We recommend that patients begin taking acetaminophen every 3 to 4 hours following surgery and continue to do so for the first 24 hours to prevent the headache from developing. Surgery on the fingers or toes also can be quite painful and therefore analgesics are often prescribed at the time of the procedure.

UNSATISFACTORY COSMESIS

An unsatisfactory cosmetic result may exist in the eyes of the patient or the surgeon. The patient should be encouraged to discuss how he or she feels about such a result and exactly what about it is troublesome. Sometimes the patient's concerns will differ markedly from those of the surgeon, and it is important that the surgeon be aware of these differences as correction of the surgeon's concerns will not necessarily help the patient.

In certain instances, a scar that is unexpectedly troublesome may result from a previously explained complication (Figures 14.7 and 14.8). In the cape area, including the upper back, chest, and shoulders, hypertrophic scarring almost always occurs (Figure 14.9). Therefore, special attention should be given to reducing wound tension as much as possible during surgery and the patient should be forewarned about the potential outcome.

Preoperative, intraoperative, and postoperative complications undoubtedly will occur at one time or another in the routine practice of cutaneous surgical procedures. If the patient feels that the surgeon is on his or her side throughout the procedure and through any eventual complications, the patient will be more cooperative and understanding of the ultimate outcome should it fall short of his or her expectations.

SUGGESTIONS FOR FURTHER READING

Amonette RA, Thomas RM. Emergencies in skin surgery. In: Roenigk RK, Roenigk HH Jr, eds. Dermatologic Surgery. Principles and Practice. New York, NY: Marcel Dekker Inc;1989:71-84.

Salasche SJ. Acute surgical complications: cause, prevention, and treatment. J Am Acad Dermatol. 1986;15:1163-1185.

SECTION THREE

INTERMEDIATE TECHNIQUES

chapter 15

FACIAL SCAR REVISION

Patients with traumatic and surgical scars of the face often seek advice for scar improvement. The surgeon must evaluate the scar to determine which revision technique can be applied to the reconstruction as scars vary in terms of their location, their surface contour, the amount of scar tissue and fibrosis present, and the degree of hypertrophic response to trauma. Psychological considerations of the patient also are factored into the management plan, as facial scars by nature are difficult to conceal and therefore are of greater concern to the patient than are scars located in other anatomic areas. While this chapter deals primarily with facial scar revision, the principles and techniques presented here are equally applicable to other regions of the body.

Scars in the facial region that are wider than 1 to 2 mm may be improved by conventional revision techniques such as simple scar excision and re-closure, along with geometric broken-line techniques. Physical characteristics of unfavorable scars include trapdoor deformities, poor orientation of the scar to favorable skin tension lines (FSTLs), hypertrophic scar formation, keloids (discussed in Chapter 22), and significant discrepancy in the height of the scar margins. These physical characteristics result from a variety of factors including the patient's individual response to soft-tissue trauma, the anatomic location of the scar in terms of cutaneous thickness, the orientation of the scar to lymphatic drainage, and the degree of attention given to primary closure of the wound including proper suture

selection, careful suturing technique, and appropriate tissue debridement.

FSTLs are best described as natural contour lines that are produced by and run perpendicular to the direction of pull of the facial muscles and in some patients may be more or less noticeable than in others. These natural contour lines may be identified by accurately noting the orientation and direction of muscle contraction beneath the skin of the surgical area. The pattern of the FSTL should be noted by the surgeon and utilized in the design of an elective incision, which should be placed parallel to it (Figure 15.1). If not

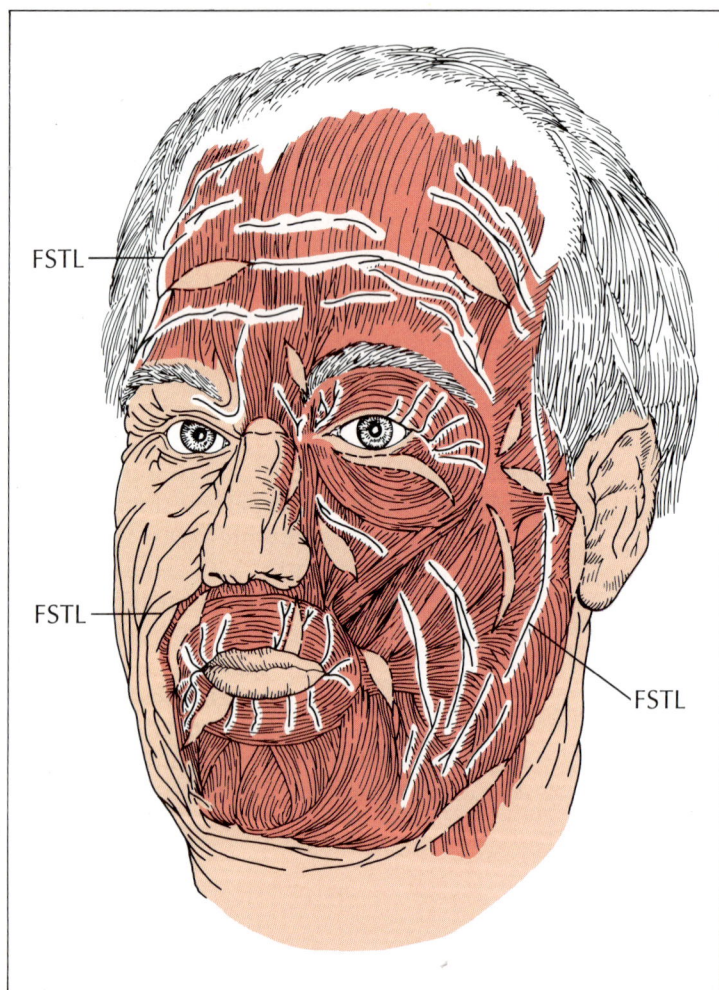

FIGURE 15.1 Schematic diagram showing favorable skin tension lines (FSTLs) on the face, which lie perpendicular to the direction of action of the facial muscles. Elective incisions should be designed so that the long axis of the incision runs parallel to the FSTL. Incisions not properly oriented will have a tendency to widen over time due to the action of the facial muscles.

oriented properly, both elective incisions and traumatic scars tend to widen with time, making scar camouflage difficult. Subcutaneous and cutaneous suturing techniques also are major factors in long-term scar results.

PREOPERATIVE PLANNING

Preoperative planning is especially important for the successful surgical correction of facial scars. Initial preoperative planning begins with a thorough analysis of the patient's scar in terms of location, secondary functional defects, the pattern of facial muscle movement, and the age and surface anatomy of the patient. In addition the surgeon should consider the length and width of the scar, the thickness of the surrounding skin, and the functional requirements of the soft tissue and muscle involved. Thorough planning prior to surgery is aided by accurate photographic documentation obtained at the initial visit. In addition to the physical findings thereby provided, the surgeon can employ such documentation to educate the patient as to the likely long-term result.

The timing of scar revision also is important and depends on a number of factors including the rate at which wound maturation occurs, the presence or absence of foreign bodies within the scar, the condition of the surrounding skin, the presence or absence of primary or secondary soft-tissue infection, and the amount of trapped edema produced by the scar. As a general rule, it is best to delay scar revision for a period of 6 to 12 months. However, in certain situations such as impending osteomyelitis of exposed facial bone, functional disability caused by the scar, and progressive contracture of the scar causing

distortion of facial landmarks, earlier intervention may be warranted.

As with other cutaneous surgical procedures, preoperative instructions to the patient include the careful avoidance of aspirin and aspirin-containing medications and the avoidance of alcohol for at least 3 weeks prior to the procedure. A complete history and physical examination also are necessary, with a careful review of current medications. These precautions serve to minimize the risk of prolonged soft-tissue bleeding and/or hematoma formation. In addition, scar revisions that involve the perioral or perinasal regions are particularly susceptible to local tissue necrosis in patients who smoke in the perioperative period.

The method of anesthesia selected is dependent on the location, depth, and length of the scar, its proximity to vital facial anatomic structures (eg, the facial nerve), and the general psychological makeup of the patient. As part of the patient's preoperative education, the surgeon should also review any accessory techniques that may be necessary after the initial revision technique has been performed, in particular, the potential use of dermabrasion and/or scar camouflage. Patient education also should firmly establish the concept that successful scar revision is a long-term process.

REVISION TECHNIQUES

SIMPLE ELLIPTICAL EXCISION

Scars that are wide but properly oriented to FSTLs can be improved by simple elliptical excision of the scar. The skin is undermined using sharp and blunt soft-tissue techniques that employ a #15 knife blade, skin hooks, and sharp soft-tissue scissors. Adequate undermining requires 2 to 3 cm of cutaneous elevation in all directions to minimize tension on closure. The closure is maintained with absorbable subcutaneous suture (either 3-0 or 4-0 PDS or Vicryl) and 5-0 or 6-0 polypropylene externally. This technique works well for a large percentage of simple, small, well-oriented scars. Its usefulness is limited, however, for large, complex, or poorly oriented scars.

Z-PLASTY

The Z-plasty is a time-honored technique used for the management of scars oriented perpendicularly to FSTLs or scars that are characterized by webbing or contracture across the scar. It is best to design the central limb of the Z-plasty as the scar excision and utilize its lateral limbs as extensions from the scar. The angle of the lateral limbs in relation to the central limb may vary to suit the specific clinical problem at hand. As a general rule,

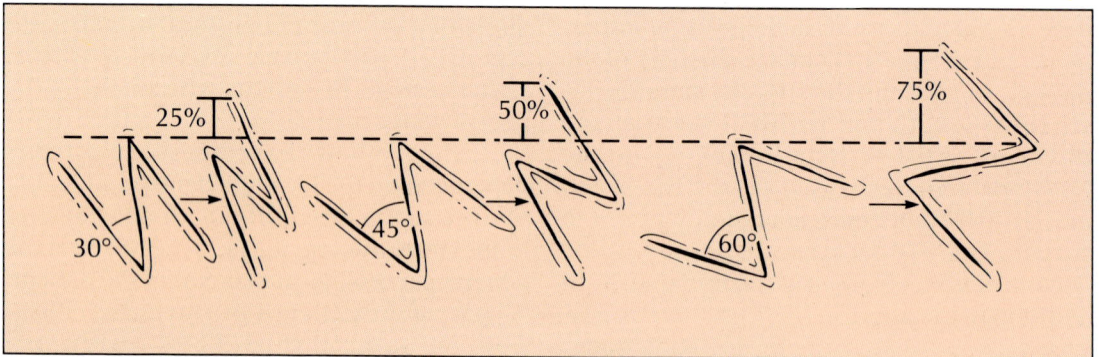

FIGURE 15.2 The design of a Z-plasty can vary depending on the need for increased length. Increased length may be particularly helpful for the revision of scar webbing.

utilization of wider angles at the junction between the two lateral limbs and the central limb of the Z-plasty results in increased length and a wider distribution of tension across the scar (Figure 15.2).

Although the use of Z-plasty will result in a longer scar, if the Z-plasty is well designed it can be used to change the orientation of and correct contracted, webbed scars. Longer scars are best reconstructed using multiple Z-plasties rather than one large Z-plasty (Figure 15.3A–D). Successful closure requires the use of a two-layer technique in a tension-free soft-tissue environment.

W-PLASTY

W-plasty is a technique utilized for scar camouflage. It produces an irregular scar pattern without the addition of length. It is particularly well suited for the correction of curvilinear defects. The pattern is that of a series of

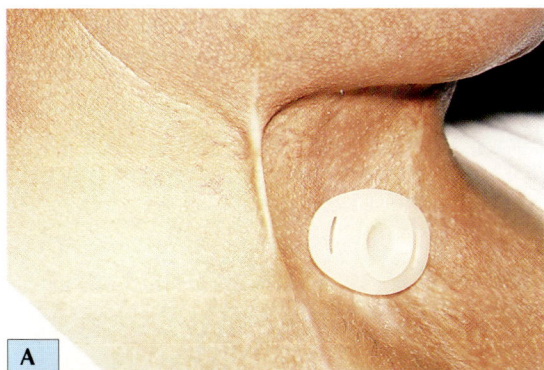

FIGURE 15.3 (A) Patient with a contracted, webbed cervical band and a complaint of decreased range of cervical motion. (B) Multiple Z-plasties are planned to reduce tension, correct the webbing, and increase mobility. (C) The immediate postoperative result. (D) The result at 6 months.

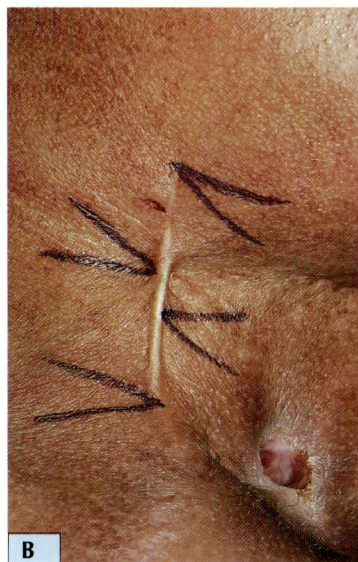

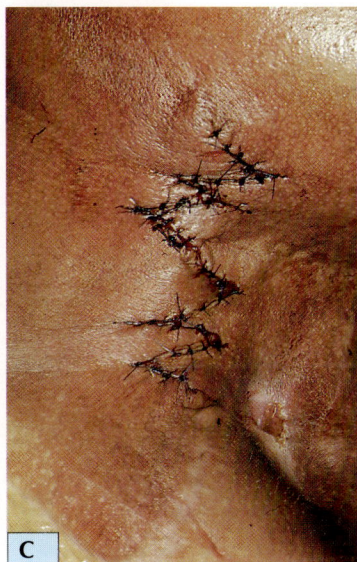

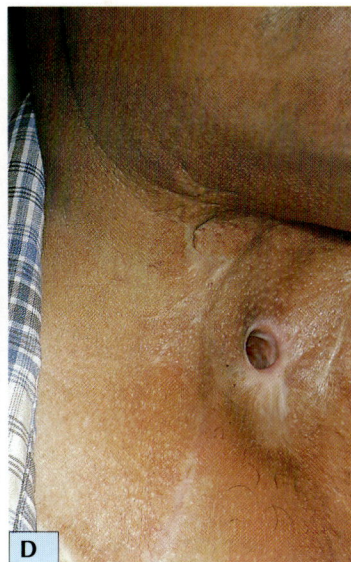

triangles with no linear segment being greater than 5 mm (Figure 15.4). The wound edges are carefully tailored using a #11 knife blade, followed by wide subcutaneous undermining (2 to 3 cm) in all directions using a #15 knife blade, skin hooks, and sharp soft-tissue scissors. The wound edges are then advanced and stabilized using a two-layer closure technique (Figure 15.5A–E).

W-plasty is also particularly useful for the correction of persistent trap-door deformity, which results in uneven wound margins across the scar. To achieve correction of this deformity, W-plasty techniques are used in combination with appropriate resection of soft tissue and scar across wound margins. Trap-door revision should be carefully monitored for recurrence of edema and scar tissue, so that intralesional injections of triamcinolone acetonide can be implemented should recurrence be noted.

GEOMETRIC BROKEN-LINE CLOSURE

The geometric broken-line closure is a modification of the W-plasty technique in which irregular geometric lines are used in a random pattern such that scar camouflage is maximized. It is based on the principle that

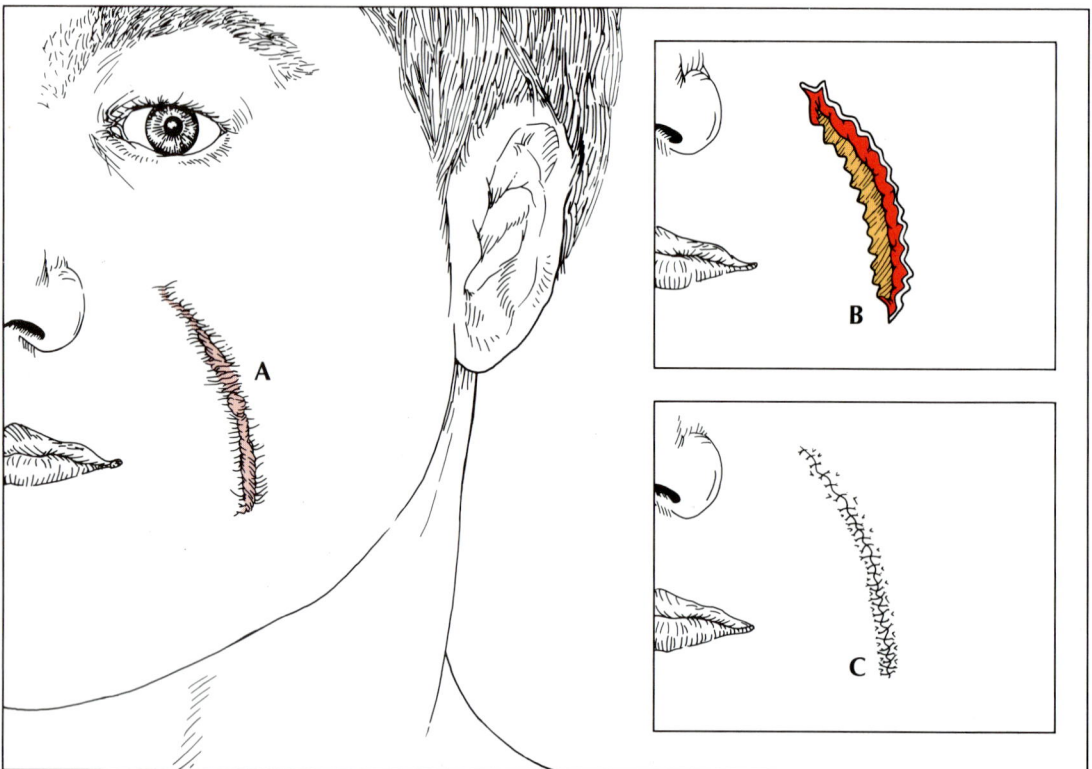

FIGURE 15.4 (A–C) Schematic diagram illustrating running W-plasty.

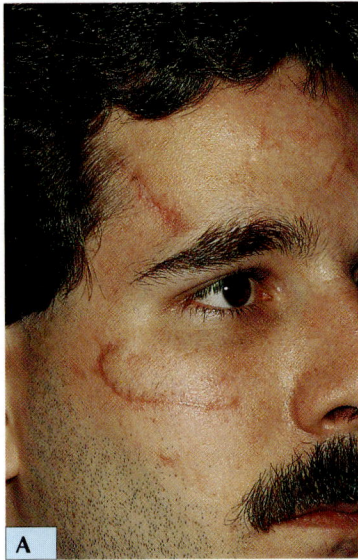

FIGURE 15.5 (A) This 25-year-old man was seen 6 months following a motor vehicle accident in which he sustained multiple facial lacerations including a right curvilinear cheek scar. **(B)** A W-plasty design is utilized for correction of the scar. **(C)** Cutaneous closure is established using 4-0 PDS in the subcutaneous layer and 6-0 nylon externally. **(D)** The wound edges are reinforced and tension is minimized by the prolonged use of Steri-Strips. **(E)** Postoperative result at 4 months.

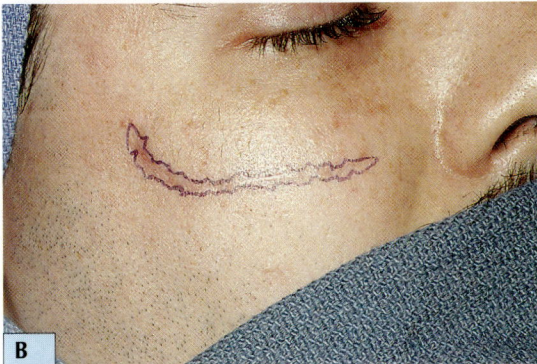

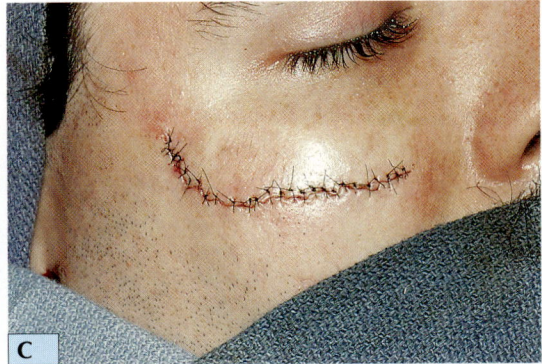

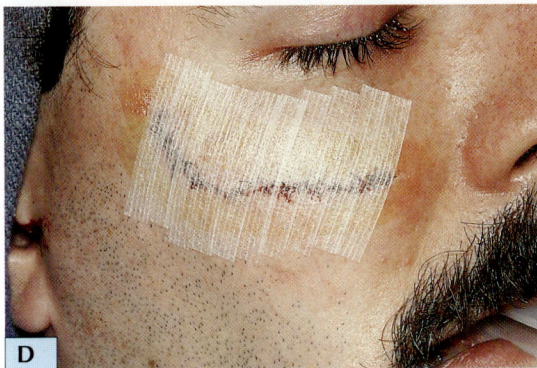

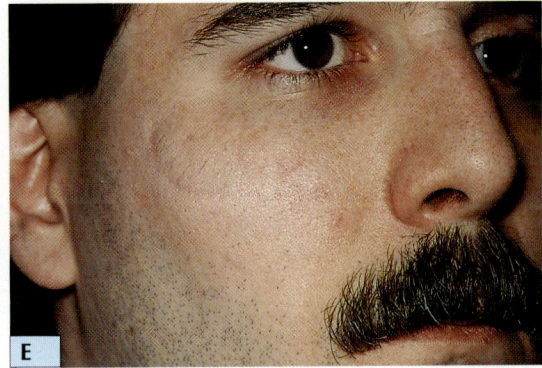

the pattern of the revised scar is more difficult to recognize than is the unbroken pattern of the original scar. The appropriate pattern for the revised scar should be carefully established, such that the length of any of its linear segments does not exceed 5 mm. The technique used for geometric broken-line closure is the same as that described for W-plasty. The method is dependent on careful design, adequate soft-tissue undermining, and accurate subcutaneous and epithelial approximation of the sharp angles of the geometric design (Figure 15.6A–G). Precise closure relies on accurate approximation of the corners, which is best achieved by use of the corner suture (see Figure 11.13).

DERMABRASION

Dermabrasion is a useful adjunct for the successful refinement of results once initial scar revision techniques have been utilized (see Figure 15.6F,G). The technique is helpful for improving minor color mismatches and cuta-

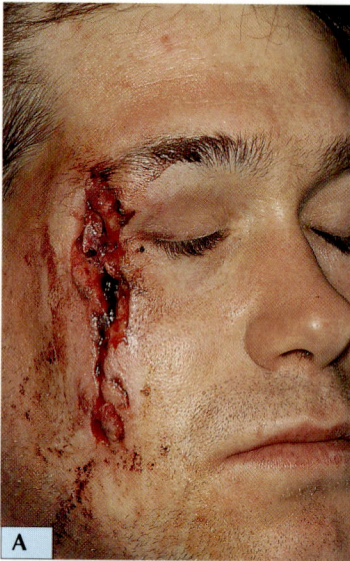

FIGURE 15.6 (A) Patient with complex facial laceration following chain-saw injury. (B,C) After debridement and primary closure the laceration was allowed to mature for 6 months, after which time a geometric broken-line revision was performed.

(continued on next page)

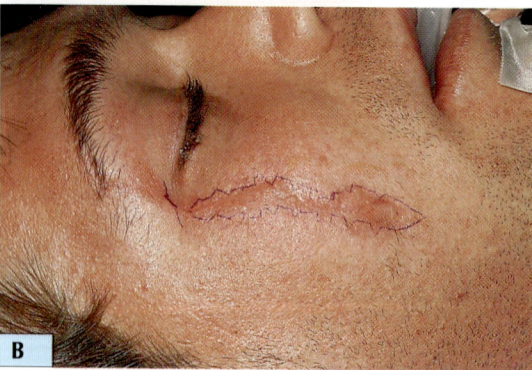

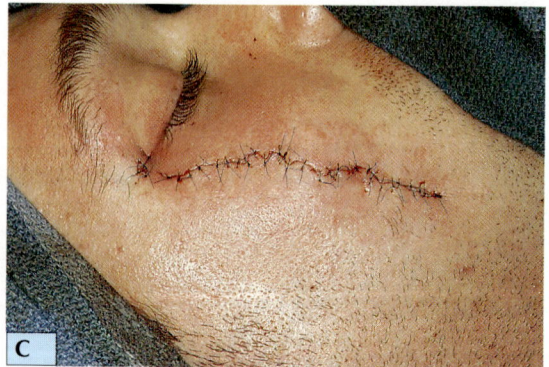

neous irregularities. The scar should be well healed before dermabrasion is performed, with a customary delay of 6 to 12 months. However, in selected cases in which scar maturation is complete in less than 6 months, earlier dermabrasion can be considered. Either a wire brush or diamond fraise can be used, with the wire brush producing a deeper more uniform abrasion. The former, however, must be used with care to prevent irregular gouges in the skin. The diamond fraise, by contrast, is safer to use for more superficial scars.

Preoperative evaluation of the scar and of characteristics of the surrounding skin will help to identify appropriate candidates for this technique. Darker skinned individuals are more likely to experience hypopigmentation of the abraded area, which may persist after dermabrasion. Additionally, dermabrasion is most effective when it is used to modify scars that are raised as opposed to those that are depressed. A more detailed description of dermabrasion can be found in Chapter 26 of this Atlas.

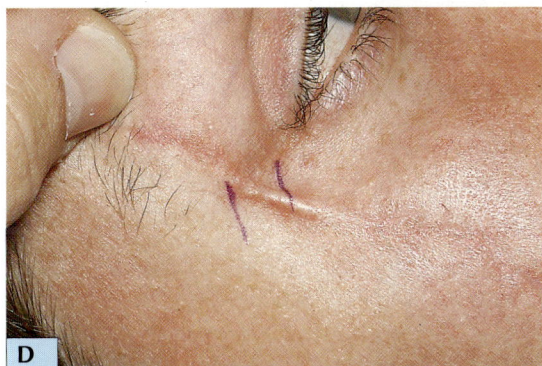

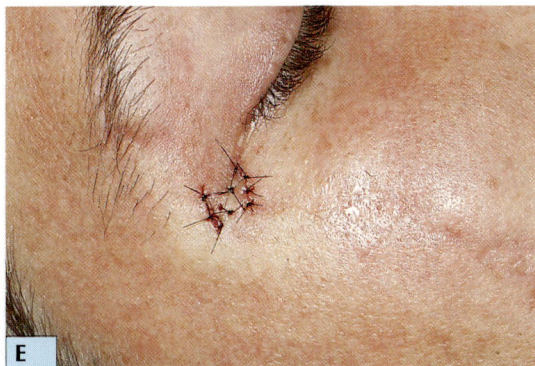

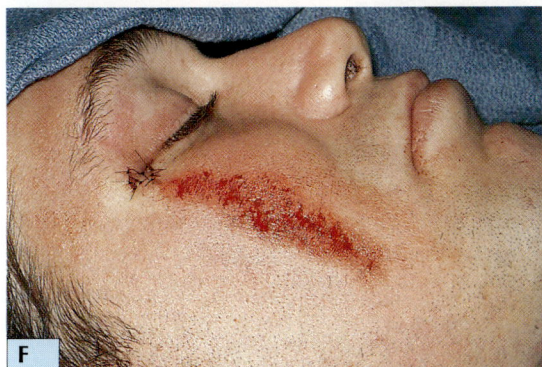

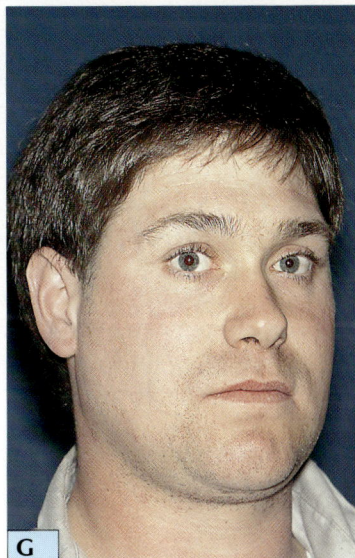

(D,E) Three months later, a Z-plasty of the lateral canthal web was performed to eliminate secondary contracture of the scar. (F) In addition to the Z-plasty, wire brush dermabrasion was performed. (G) The result at 6 months.

MAKEUP TECHNIQUES

Makeup techniques also have been utilized with success in the treatment of facial scars. They are helpful for scar camouflage in the immediate postoperative period of scar revision as well as for long-term support for scars that lie in a prominent area of the face. Expert medical makeup artists can provide the patient with appropriate education as to the techniques available to reduce the visibility of facial scars during the period of scar maturation (Figure 15.7A,B).

In summary, successful revision of a facial scar requires thorough preoperative planning and analysis, experience on the part of the surgeon with a wide variety of techniques, and adequate preoperative education of the patient as to the goals of surgery and the time needed to achieve the final result.

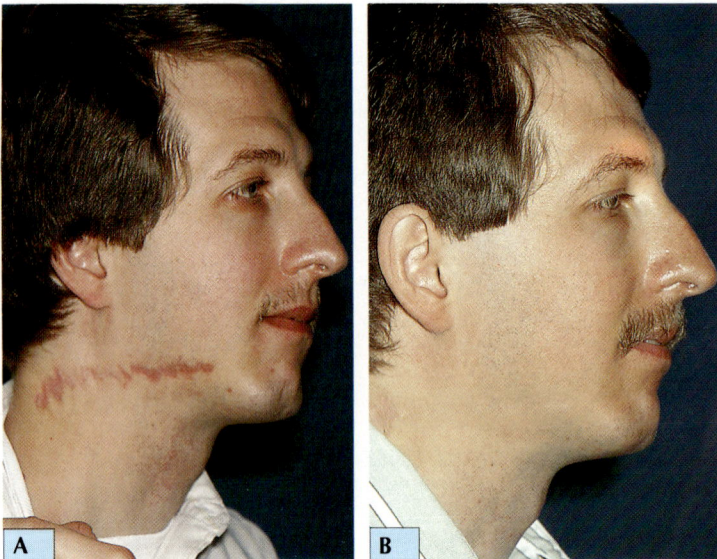

FIGURE 15.7 (A) Patient 2 weeks after geometric broken-line closure of a cervical scar. (B) Makeup techniques have been utilized for temporary coverage.

SUGGESTIONS FOR FURTHER READING

Bernstein L. Z-plasty in head and neck surgery. Arch Otolaryngol. 1969;89:574-584.

Borges AF. Elective Incisions and Scar Revisions. Boston, Mass: Little, Brown & Co Inc; 1973.

Gunter JP. Camouflaging scars in the head and neck area. J Otolaryngol. 1978;7(1): 75-87.

Thomas JR, Holt GR, eds. Facial Scars. Incision, Revision, and Camouflage. St Louis, Mo: C V Mosby Co; 1989.

Webster RC, Smith RC. Scar revision and camouflaging. Otolaryngol Clin North Am. Symposium on Plastic Surgery of the Face. 1982;15(1): 55-68.

Zoltan J. Atlas of Skin Repair. New York, NY: S. Karger. 1984.

chapter 16

COMPLEX EXCISIONS

For many types of cutaneous lesions requiring removal, a simple elliptical excision will suffice in which the lesion and its surrounding skin are removed (see Chapter 6). However, in certain situations where even the best-designed ellipse will not produce an acceptable result, additional techniques exist that enable the surgeon to achieve adequate removal of the lesion while also producing a cosmetically acceptable scar. Some of these techniques, namely dog-ear correction, repair of wound edges of unequal length, and M-plasty, are the subject of this chapter.

DOG-EAR CORRECTION

Dog-ears are the most commonly occurring problem with imperfect elliptical closures. Characterized by puckering at either or both ends of the ellipse, they are the result of an elliptical incision where the angle at the edge of the ellipse is greater than 30°, where the site of the excision is a curved surface such as the arm, forehead, or nose, where the sides of the ellipse are of different lengths, or where a lesion is removed in a circular fashion. As some of these factors are uncontrollable, knowledge of dog-ear repair is critical for even the cutaneous surgeon who plans to do nothing more than simple elliptical excisions.

A dog-ear usually takes the form of a standing pyramid or triangle of tissue (Figure 16.1). To locate the midpoint of the excess tissue, which will determine the direction of the repair, toothed forceps or a skin hook is used

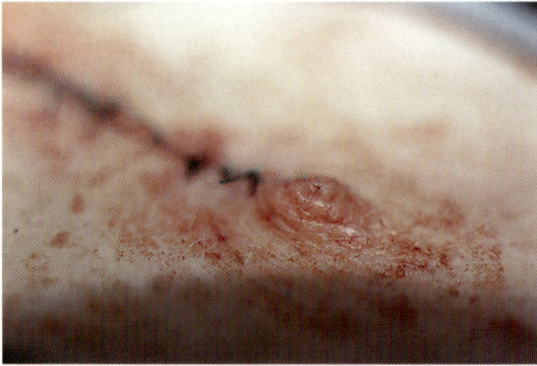

FIGURE 16.1 After removal of a lesion in a circular fashion, followed by central closure, a pucker or pyramid of tissue remains at one pole of the excision. This is commonly referred to as a dog-ear.

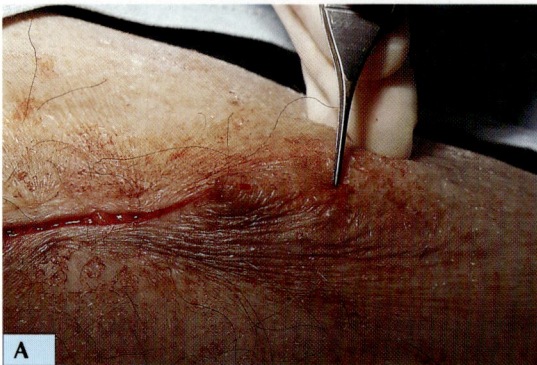

FIGURE 16.2 (A) Forceps are placed at the midpoint of the dog-ear, which is located at a point at the base of the pyramid away from the excision, where equal amounts of tissue lie on either side of an imaginary line drawn from this point to the near end of the excision. (B) If the dog-ear is only at one end of the closure, its repair may consist of a straight extension of the original elliptical incision or it may be slightly angled, as in a "hockey stick" repair.

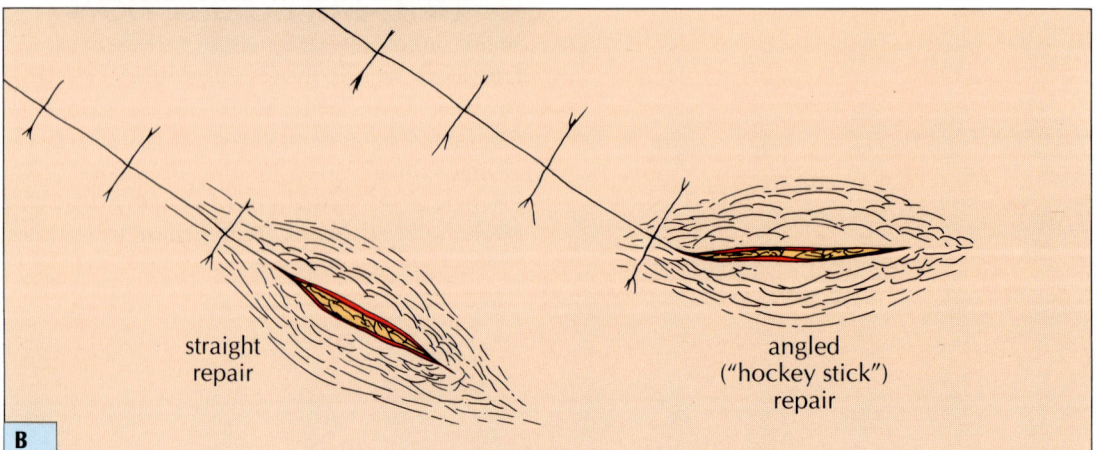

straight repair

angled ("hockey stick") repair

(Figure 16.2A,B). Once the direction of the repair has been established, the pyramid of tissue is then elevated using the skin hook or forceps and it is incised at one side of its base, beginning at the edge closest to the wound and extending distally to the edge farthest from the wound (Figure 16.3A,B). This maneuver should release a triangular piece of tissue, which is stretched out and excised by cutting across its base (Figure 16.3C). Alter-

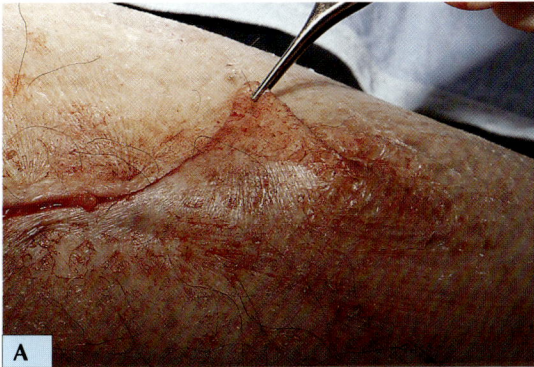

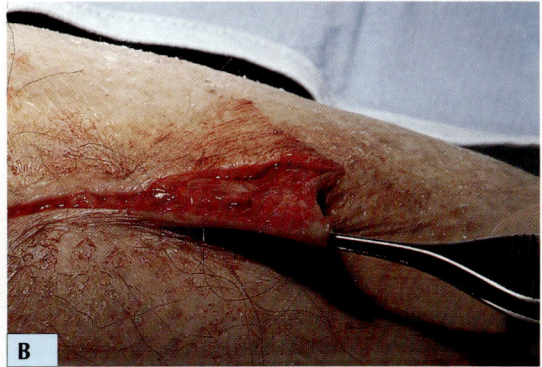

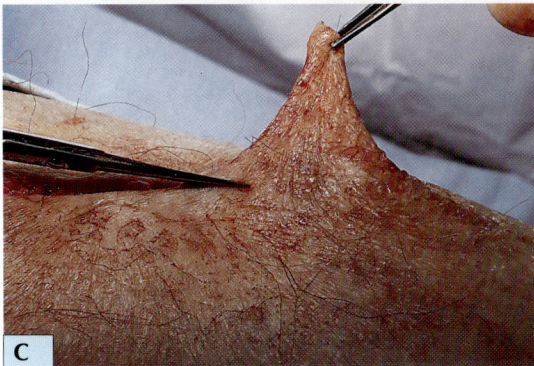

FIGURE 16.3 (A,B) The pyramid is lifted up and one side of it is cut with fine tissue scissors, such as iris or gradle scissors. (C) The resulting triangular piece of tissue is then pulled over and cut at its base. The surgeon should take care to ensure that the skin is always cut at an angle of 90° to the surface, despite the angle at which the piece of tissue is held, by keeping the cutting surface of the scissors or blade perpendicular to the skin.

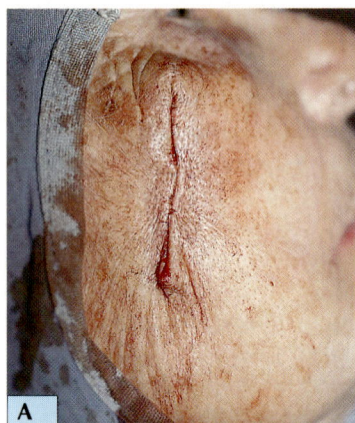

FIGURE 16.4 (A) A dog-ear is evident inferiorly following closure of this large defect with buried sutures. **(B–E)** To correct the dog-ear, it is first bisected to form two triangles. Each triangle is then incised at its base in the manner described earlier. **(F)** The resultant wound looks like an ellipse with a 30° angle at its tip that will be a straight extension of the original excision line.

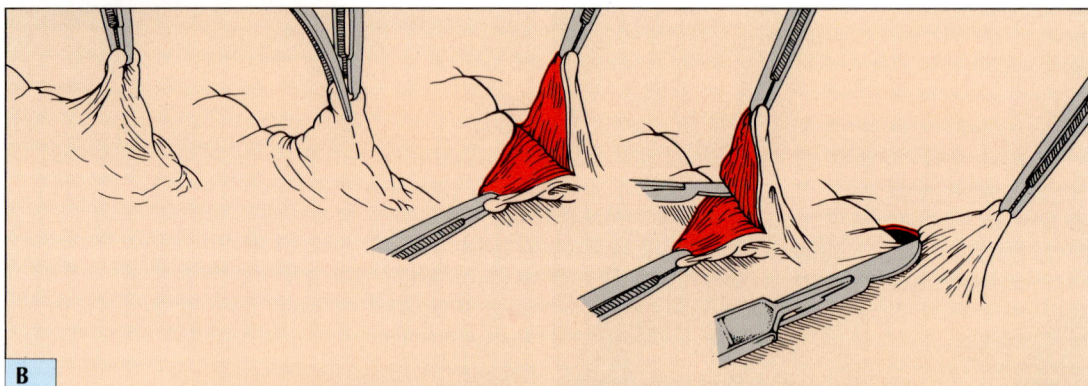

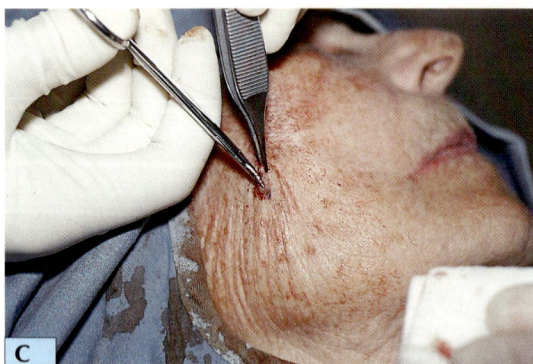

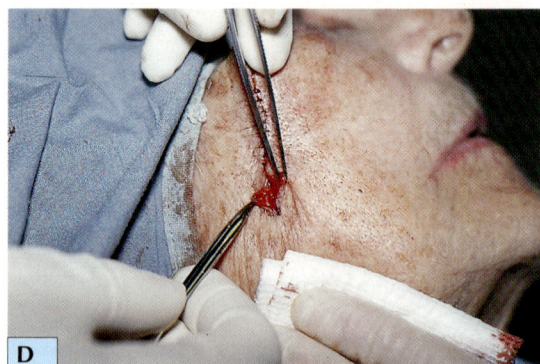

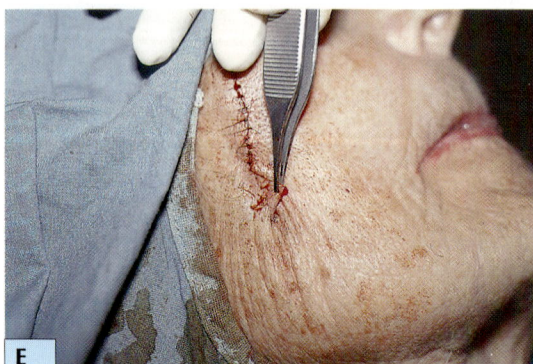

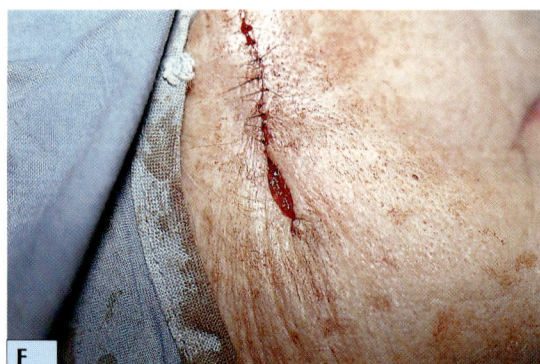

natively, some surgeons prefer to bisect the dog-ear into two triangles and then carry out the procedure on both triangles, which are first pulled toward one side and then toward the other (Figure 16.4A–F). To compensate for excess tissue that is located slightly off center to the midline, or to achieve proper alignment with regard to expression lines in the area, the repair may be placed at an angle (Figure 16.5). Although fine tissue scissors provide better control in making these incisions, a scalpel may be used and indeed may be necessary when the tissue is thick and bulky.

REPAIR OF WOUND EDGES OF UNEQUAL LENGTH

Wound edges of unequal length may occur following the removal of a lesion by elliptical incision. Whether they are intentional, as in the case of an incisional line that is curved as in the nasolabial fold, or unintentional, as occurs during the early stages of learning excisional surgery when elliptical incisions are imperfectly drawn, various techniques can be used for their repair. A useful technique for closure of the defect is the principle of halves (Figure 16.6), which can be applied

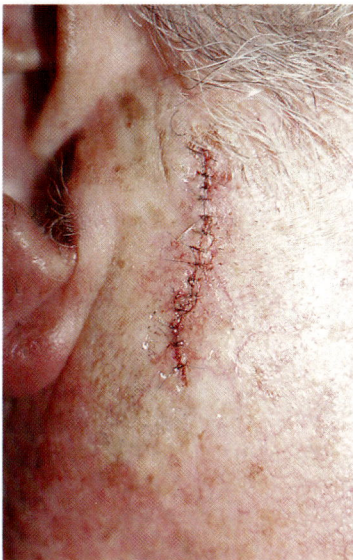

FIGURE 16.5 The side-to-side closure of a large defect following removal of a basal cell carcinoma by Mohs' technique created a dog-ear inferiorly. Correction was made at an angle to create a "hockey-stick" repair, since the excess tissue was more bulky medially than laterally.

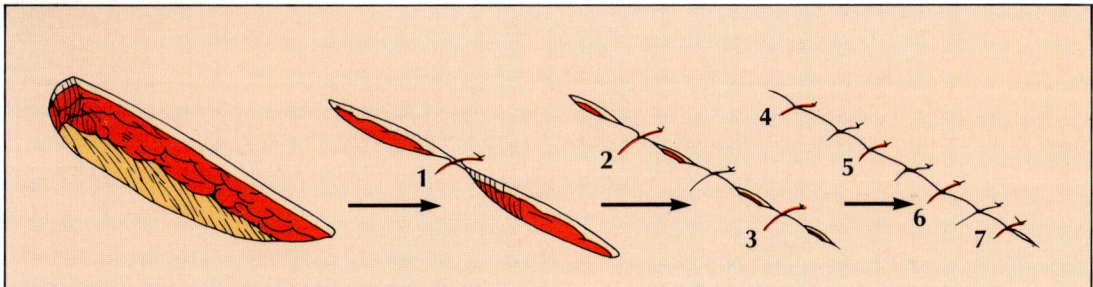

FIGURE 16.6 Schematic diagram illustrates the principle of halves for the repair of wound edges of unequal length.

even to small discrepancies between the two sides (Figure 16.7A,B). Alternatively, a small dog-ear correction may be used, which can be placed anywhere along the longer side of the incision, depending on the location of excess tissue or of natural skin lines (Figure 16.8).

M-PLASTY

A useful technique for the planning of excisions is the M-plasty, which is used most commonly to shorten an excisional line or scar or to direct it along a natural expression

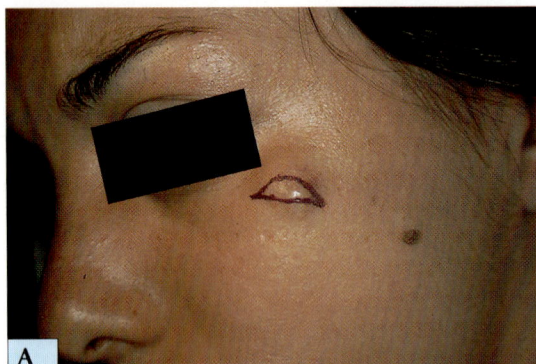

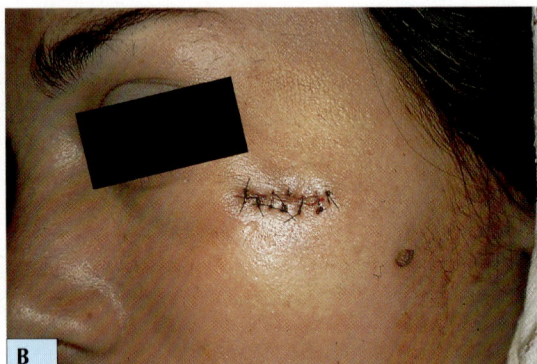

FIGURE 16.7 (A) To contour this excision to the curvature of natural skin lines, the ellipse has been drawn so that it is more curved superiorly. (B) Using the principle of halves, the incision line was halved with each placement of the sutures such that no dog-ear corrections were necessary and the sutured wound lies perfectly flat.

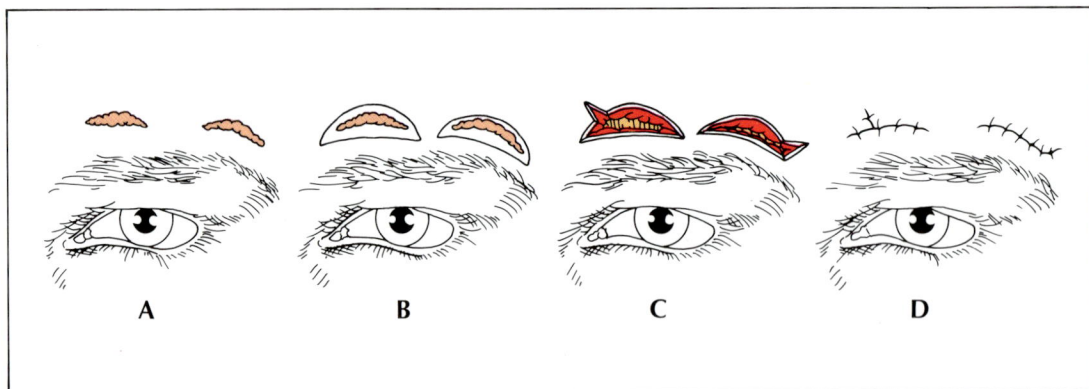

FIGURE 16.8 (A,B) Schematic diagram showing the repair of an excision having two unequal sides due to the shape and location of the lesion being removed. (C,D) A dog-ear correction is performed to shorten the longer side at a point where the resulting suture line falls into a natural skin crease.

line. Classic locations for M-plasty are the lateral canthus and the corner of the mouth, and it may be performed at one or both ends of the incision (Figure 16.9). It can be planned for use at the time of the excision or it can be used following excision to correct a dog-ear. It is probably easier to do the latter.

When an M-plasty is used to correct a dog-ear, a line is cut back to the middle of the free edge of the pyramid of tissue from a point midway along its side. The incision is then repeated on the other side of the pyramid. The V-shaped piece of tissue that results is then drawn into the defect using a corner suture that is placed slightly ahead of the tip (Figure 16.10A–D).

The corrective techniques described in this chapter can be used to solve almost any problem encountered in the attempt to create a smooth line following excision of a cutaneous lesion. However, for lesions that cannot be treated adequately by these techniques in combination with those described in Chapter 6, the use of skin flaps may be indicated. Skin flaps are described in Chapter 20 and represent an additional level of complexity for the surgical removal of cutaneous lesions.

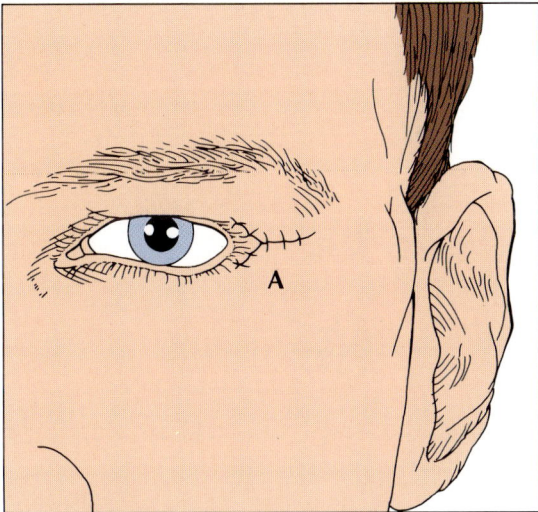

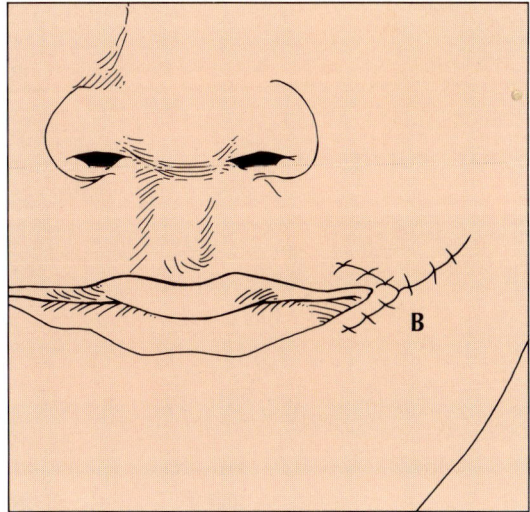

FIGURE 16.9 Schematic diagram showing the classic locations for M-plasty: (**A**) lateral canthus; (**B**) corner of mouth.

SUGGESTIONS FOR FURTHER READING

Dzubow LM. The dynamics of dog-ear formation and correction. J Dermatol Surg Oncol. 1985;11:722-728.

Swanson NA. Atlas of Cutaneous Surgery. Boston, Mass: Little, Brown & Co Inc; 1987.
Webster RC, Davison TM. M-plasty techniques. J Dermatol Surg. 1976;2:393-396.
Zitelli JA. TIPS for a better ellipse. J Am Acad Dermatol. 1990;22:101-103.

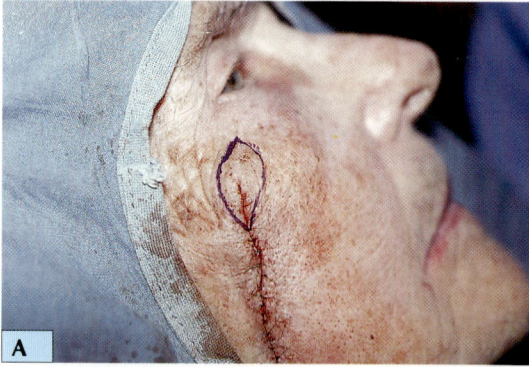

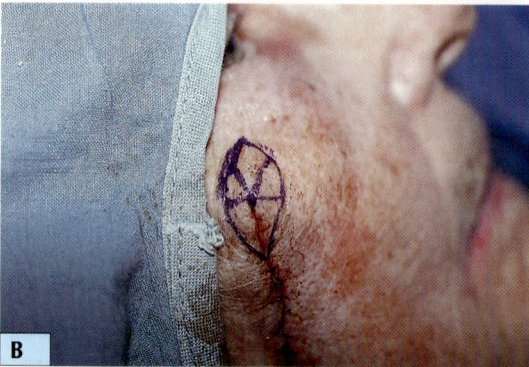

FIGURE 16.10 (A) The dog-ear is outlined. (B) An M-plasty is designed to shorten the dog-ear and to place it in natural skin creases. A line drawn at the edge of the incision transects the ellipse. From a point midway between this line and the far tip, another line is drawn, creating a 30° angle with the outer line, back to the end of the incision. (C) The lines are then cut and the M appears. (D) The wound is then sutured closed using 5-0 chromic gut for buried sutures and 6-0 nylon for epidermal sutures.

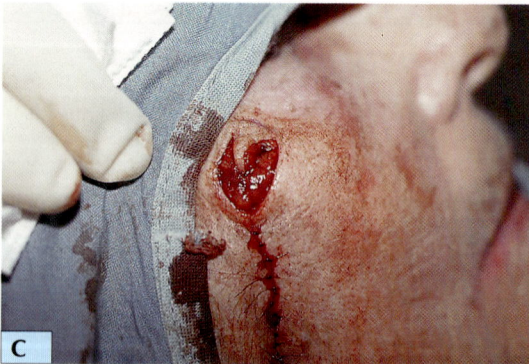

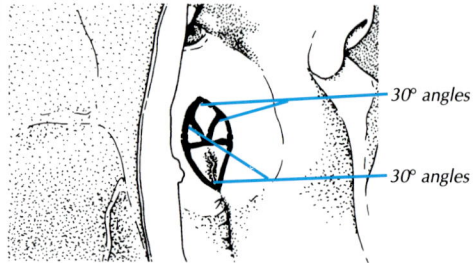

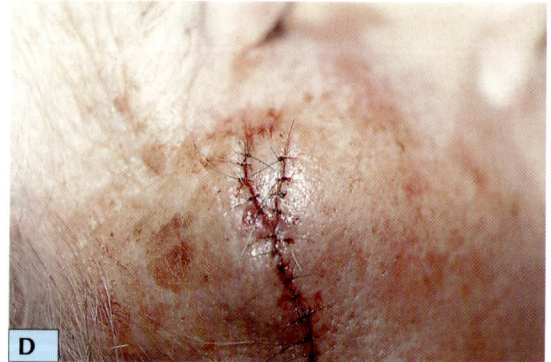

chapter 17

SCLEROTHERAPY

Unwanted varices of the lower legs are a common affliction that can be treated by injection of sclerosing solutions. Although the practice of sclerotherapy is quite common and sophisticated in Europe, the technique only recently has become popular in the United States and Canada. Increasing attention to it led to the formation in 1988 of the North American Society of Phlebology. Not surprisingly, many of the society's members are cutaneous surgeons.

With interest, knowledge, and experience in the area growing, some cutaneous surgeons have begun to develop the expertise and facility for treating larger veins and varicosities. At present, however, sclerotherapy most often is used to treat small "sunburst" vessels under 1 mm in diameter. The treatment of such telangiectases by sclerotherapy is the subject of this chapter.

SCLEROSING SOLUTIONS

A number of sclerosing agents have been used over the years, which, when injected into telangiectases, cause endothelial damage and swelling followed by thrombosis. Over time the organized thrombus becomes recanalized or progresses to fibrosis and vessel obliteration. For vessels in which the former has occurred, further treatment is necessary. Retreatment of unresponsive telangiectases can occur at 6 weeks, which is the time when the process leading to either recanalization or vessel scarring is complete.

The most commonly used agents for treating varices of the lower legs are hypertonic saline, sugar-salt solutions, polidocanol, sodium tetradecyl sulfate, and morrhuate sodium. All of these are used in essentially the same manner but differ in their potential sequelae and complications. Most can give rise to the development of macular hyperpigmentation at treatment sites, presumably due to vessel breakage with release of hemosiderin into the skin (Figure 17.1A–C). The pigmentation tends to fade in about 6 to 9 months, although permanent hyperpigmentation following sclerotherapy has been

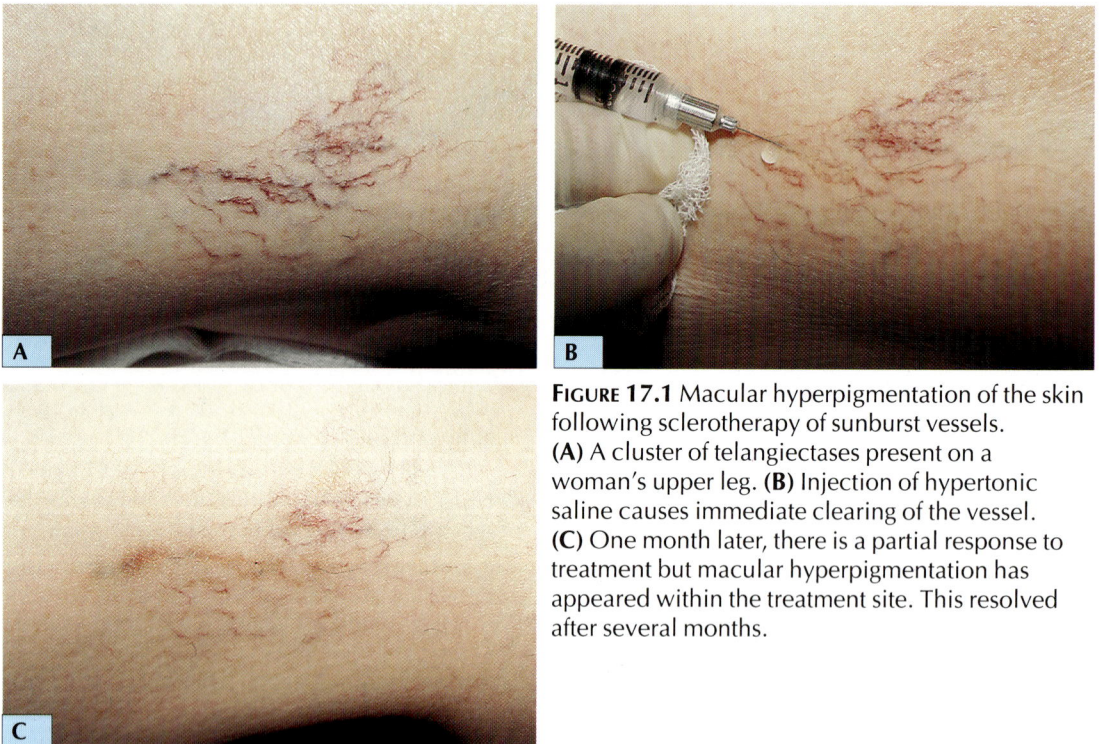

FIGURE 17.1 Macular hyperpigmentation of the skin following sclerotherapy of sunburst vessels.
(A) A cluster of telangiectases present on a woman's upper leg. (B) Injection of hypertonic saline causes immediate clearing of the vessel. (C) One month later, there is a partial response to treatment but macular hyperpigmentation has appeared within the treatment site. This resolved after several months.

reported. In addition, various degrees of bruising, swelling, and redness may be present for 1 to 2 weeks following a sclerotherapy session (Figure 17.2), after which macular hyperpigmentation may appear. Since the duration of a given treatment may be limited by patient discomfort, and since a proportion of treated vessels will be unresponsive, patients are advised that a minimum of three treatments over the same number of months usually is necessary.

HYPERTONIC SALINE

Hypertonic saline is a popular and effective sclerosant for treating sunburst telangiectases. It is inexpensive, readily available, and non-allergenic. Usually it is used at a concentration of 23.4%, which is the solution available as an abortifacient. Some clinicians have diluted this solution to concentrations of 20% and 21% with equally good results. Recently, according to one investigator, a saline solution of 11.7% proved to be an effective sclerosant.

The drawbacks of hypertonic saline sclerotherapy are pain and occasional tissue necrosis. The pain is perceived as a burning sensation that accompanies the injections and persists for an additional few minutes at the completion of a treatment session. On occasion, a skin slough can occur if the solution is injected in a perivascular location rather than into the vein. The likelihood of skin slough is minimal when tiny amounts of saline are injected around a vessel but increases when greater amounts are used. Dilution of interstitially injected solution with 1% lidocaine may prevent necrosis.

SUGAR-SALT SOLUTIONS

Sugar-salt solutions, marketed as Sclérodex and Dextroject, are hypertonic solutions containing 25% dextrose, 10% sodium chloride, and 0.8% phenylethyl alcohol. Their efficacy is probably slightly less than that of hypertonic saline solution but so too are the pain and incidence of skin slough.

POLIDOCANOL

Polidocanol, marketed in Europe as Aethoxysclerol, appears to be slightly slower than hypertonic saline in sclerosing telangiectases of the legs. For sunburst vessels, polidocanol is used in concentrations of 0.25% to 0.75%.

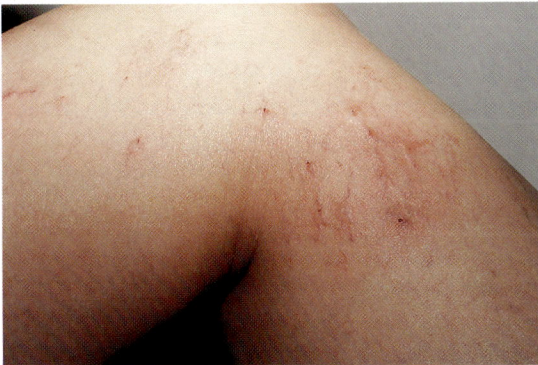

FIGURE 17.2 Swelling and irritation follow sclerotherapy treatment sessions. Bruising, swelling, and erythema can persist for up to 2 weeks.

While pain occurs with injection, it is not as severe as that seen with hypertonic saline since polidocanol was developed first as an anesthetic agent. Likewise, necrosis is reportedly less of a problem. Allergic reactions, including anaphylaxis, also have been reported, though rarely.

SODIUM TETRADECYL SULFATE

Sodium tetradecyl sulfate, marketed as Sotradecol, is an effective sclerosant but it is associated with a much greater rate of significant complication including necrosis, anaphylaxis, and generalized urticaria. Reportedly it is associated with two deaths from allergic reaction and, therefore, patients with significant history of allergy should be treated with caution. The agent is used in concentrations of 0.33%.

MORRHUATE SODIUM

Morrhuate sodium, marketed as Scleromate, is a mixture of sodium salts that is made of fatty acids found in cod liver oil. Since perivascular injection of this product carries a high likelihood of skin necrosis, it is not used in the treatment of sunburst vessels. Anaphylaxis also has been reported to occur.

TECHNIQUE

Sunburst vessels are extremely close to the skin surface. Therefore, to cannulate them, the operator must insert the needle in such a way that it is more parallel than perpendicular to the skin surface. Some clinicians find that bending the needle slightly (with the bevel up) makes injection easier (Figure 17.3). Usually a 30-gauge disposable needle on a 3-mL Luer-Lok syringe is used, although reusable 32- or 33-gauge needles also have proven effective. Magnification by loupe, magnifying glass, or a visor is helpful. The skin is cleansed with isopropyl alcohol prior to injection.

The pain associated with sclerotherapy limits the number of vessels that can be treated at a single session. Therefore, prior to injection, the surgeon should ask the patient to identify those vessels that he or she feels are most troubling so they can be treated first. The patient then lies on the treatment table with the therapist seated at the foot end. The skin is stabilized by the operator's fingers and each individual vessel is cannulated and injected in turn, usually beginning with the largest vessel in the cluster.

As the needle is inserted, a slight amount of pressure is placed on the plunger

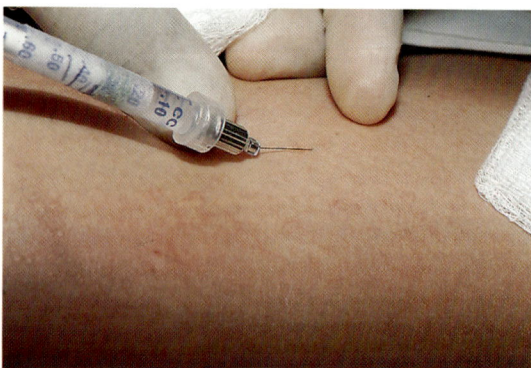

FIGURE 17.3 Bending of the needle prior to sclerotherapy sometimes makes it easier to enter the skin in a parallel fashion. The bevel is directed upward.

of the syringe. While perfect intravascular placement of the needle is not always possible, when it does occur the sclerosant begins to flow as a result of the decreased resistance offered by the vascular lumen. The sclerosing agent is then injected slowly in a volume of a few tenths of a milliliter. If the sclerosant is injected rapidly, with the attendant buildup of high pressure, bursting of the blood vessel and consequent macular hyperpigmentation are more likely to occur.

Successful injection of one of the telangiectases results in immediate "clearing" of the vessel as blood is pushed out by the colorless sclerosing agent. Blanching may be seen to extend through an entire arcade of telangiectases (Figure 17.4A,B). Because the sclerosant has little effect beyond a centimeter or so of the injection site, longer vessels are injected at 1- or 2-cm intervals along their length. The direction in which the vessel is injected is probably not critical in the low-pressure sunburst vessels of the legs. However, most clinicians try to inject in the direction of blood flow as it could potentially result in more efficient and complete vessel clearing, allowing for better contact between the sclerosing solution and the endothelium.

Occasionally, as the plunger is being depressed, it becomes immediately apparent that the needle is not in the vessel as a small wheal begins to appear. Usually this occurs when the needle is inserted too deeply and has failed to enter the vessel. It also can occur when the needle slips out of the vessel after successful entry. Since greater volumes of extravasated sclerosant are more likely to cause slough, it is important to cease injection of material immediately upon noting the appearance of the wheal. To minimize the risk of interstitial injection, a small amount of air in the syringe may be used to clear the vessel prior to injection of the sclerosing agent. This technique allows the therapist to be certain that the vessel is cannulated before fluid is injected. However, many surgeons have abandoned this technique because it is tedious and, in the case of the commonly

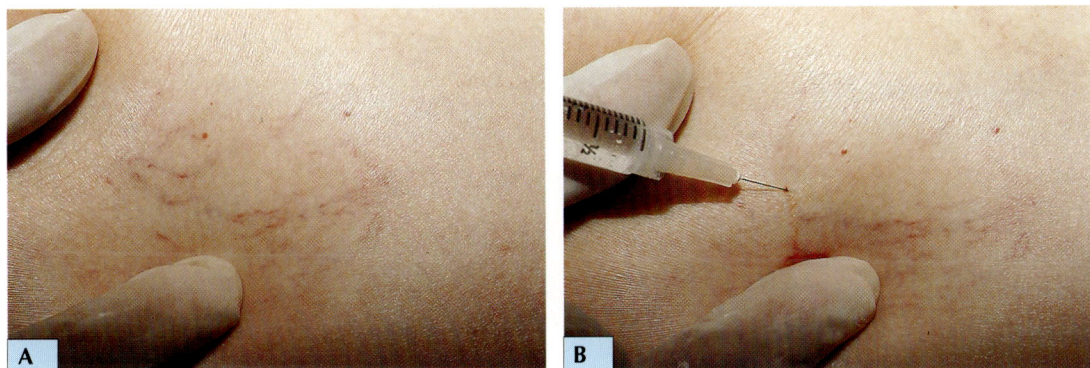

FIGURE 17.4 Successful injection with hypertonic saline of a group of "spider veins" on a woman's leg. (A) The skin is stabilized by the operator's fingers. (B) The vessel is cannulated and immediate "clearing" is noted as the saline is injected.

used sclerosants, offers little long-term advantage.

Another practice not universally followed is the use of compression following sclerotherapy of sunburst vessels. Without doubt, "compression sclerotherapy" is necessary for effective treatment of larger vessels. However, the use of compression following injection of small-caliber vessels is unsubstantiated in practice and most clinicians do not use prolonged compression in the treatment of such vessels. Many will apply elastic wraps to the treated leg(s) for a period of 24 to 72 hours following the injection of sclerosant.

Theoretically, the use of compression alters the way in which sclerosants cause obliteration of veins. The delivery of external pressure adequate to collapse a vessel results in more direct apposition of the treated vein walls, which, having been injured, will "fuse" as they heal. Because less thrombus formation occurs, the likelihood of recanalization with treatment failure is diminished. The incidence of postsclerosis pigmentation also may be less as is the incidence of telang-

iectatic mattes (discussed later). It seems reasonable, therefore, that the value of compression sclerotherapy in the treatment of small-caliber vessels should be re-evaluated.

COMPLICATIONS

The major complications associated with treatment of lower-leg telangiectases are hyperpigmentation (noted earlier), tissue necrosis and scarring, edema of the lower leg, and appearance of telangiectatic mattes. Also noted previously, anaphylaxis has been seen on occasion with morrhuate sodium and Sotradecol.

Hyperpigmentation, due to hemosiderin, likely occurs as a result of vessel rupture during sclerotherapy (see Figure 17.1). It tends to appear as discrete macules measuring a few millimeters in diameter that are seen a few weeks following therapy. Macular hyperpigmentation usually clears slowly, persisting for up to 9 months.

Tissue necrosis with a full-thickness skin slough, though infrequent, usually occurs when a relatively large volume of scle-

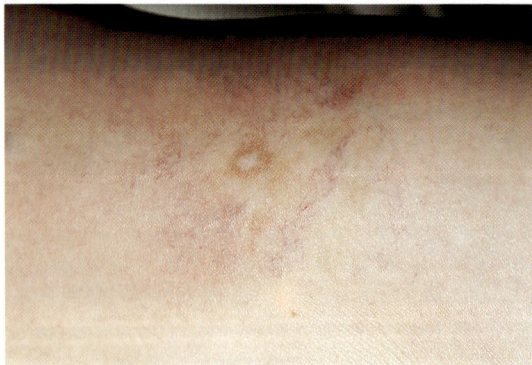

FIGURE 17.5 Scar on the leg subsequent to a full-thickness slough after hypertonic saline sclerotherapy.

rosant is injected interstitially. Small sloughs heal rapidly and leave minimal atrophic scarring. Larger sloughs can result in more significant fibrosis (Figure 17.5). Pedal edema also may be seen following sclerotherapy, particularly when the ankles have been treated. It generally resolves uneventfully and resolution can be hastened by elevation of the feet and use of ace bandage wraps.

Many clinicians have noted the appearance of telangiectatic mattes at the periphery of areas treated previously for spider telangiectases. The vessels are of extremely fine caliber (0.03 to 0.05 mm) and usually appear several weeks after treatment. While the etiology of these mattes is unclear, Ouvry believes that they arise as a result of the use of excessively strong sclerosants and a lack of compression. Although the mattes are less conspicuous than sunburst vessels, they can cause concern to the patient, who therefore should be forewarned of their potential development. Quite often, the mattes will disappear spontaneously in 3 to 6 months, although they may be permanent. When they do persist, telangiectatic mattes are difficult to obliterate. Occasionally, they will respond to sclerotherapy. The needle is injected superficially into the middle of the cluster and, with luck, the entire matte will blanche. However, even when blanching does occur, the response is variable and persistence is common.

SUGGESTIONS FOR FURTHER READING

Bodian EL. Sclerotherapy: a personal appraisal. J Dermatol Surg Oncol. 1989;15:156-161.

Bodian EL. Techniques of sclerotherapy for sunburst venous blemishes. J Dermatol Surg Oncol. 1985;11:696-704.

Duffy DM. Sclerotherapy: an overview. In: Callen J, Dahl M, Golitz L, et al, eds. Advances in Dermatology. Chicago, Ill: Year Book Medical Publishers Inc;1988;3:221-242.

Goldman MP, Kaplan RP, Duffy DM. Postsclerotherapy hyperpigmentation: a histologic evaluation. J Dermatol Surg Oncol. 1987;13:547-550.

Goldman MP, Kaplan RP, Oki LN, et al. Sclerosing agents in the treatment of telangiectasia. Arch Dermatol. 1987;123:1196-1201.

Orbach EJ. Hazards of sclerotherapy of varicose veins: their prevention and treatment of complications. Vasa. 1979;8:170-173.

Ouvry PA. Telangiectasia and sclerotherapy. J Dermatol Surg Oncol. 1989;15:177-181.

Stegman SJ, Tromovitch TA, Glogau RG. Cosmetic Dermatologic Surgery. 2nd ed. Chicago, Ill: Year Book Medical Publishers Inc; 1990:277-287.

chapter 18

INJECTABLE SILICONE, COLLAGEN, AND GELATIN MATRIX IMPLANTS

Cutaneous surgeons have led the way in developing relatively noninvasive intradermal augmentation techniques to treat facial skin irregularities. The perfect material for this purpose should be nontoxic, non-antigenic, nonirritating, nonmigratory, and should provide sustained correction. Although none is ideal, three major injectable products are currently in widespread use for the treatment of facial scars, lines, and wrinkles. They are injectable liquid silicone, bovine collagen (Zyderm/Zyplast), and gelatin matrix implant (Fibrel) (Figure 18.1).

INJECTABLE LIQUID SILICONE

The use of injectable liquid silicone for the treatment of scars and wrinkles was popularized by Dr Norman Orentreich some 35 years ago. Since then, hundreds of physicians have incorporated this procedure into their practices. A significant barrier to the more widespread use of injectable silicone in the United States has been the lack of a product in the medical marketplace with US Food and Drug Administration (FDA) approval. In the late 1960s, one manufacturer applied for FDA approval to market injectable-grade liquid silicone (polydimethylsiloxane fluid of 350 centistokes viscosity) as a medical device for soft-tissue augmentation. However, for undisclosed reasons, the application was withdrawn in 1976, prior to any action upon it.

Injectable liquid silicone is a nonimmunogenic and chemically nonreactive substance. When injected into the skin, it induces formation of a fibrous collagen capsule that is produced by local cells in an attempt to "wall off" the foreign material. Injection of multiple "microdroplets" of silicone into skin irregularities yields a nidus of large, combined surface area on which fibroplasia can take place. This selective stimulation of collagen deposition has proven to be an effective therapeutic approach to facial scars, lines, and wrinkles.

Although pure, filtered, sterilized injectable silicone fluid is held to be nonreactive in the skin, a number of instances of foreign body granulomas following silicone injection have been reported in the literature. Orentreich believes that most of these foreign-body reactions have been to impurities or additives present in the injected materials. In other cases, the problem appears to be due to reckless overcorrection with subsequent lymphatic blockage or to injection of material into inappropriate anatomic locations, such as the breast. Reports of "drifting" or "shifting" of the material also appear to relate to significant misuse of the material.

New users of silicone should seek instruction from a clinician experienced in its use, since the results obtained are technique

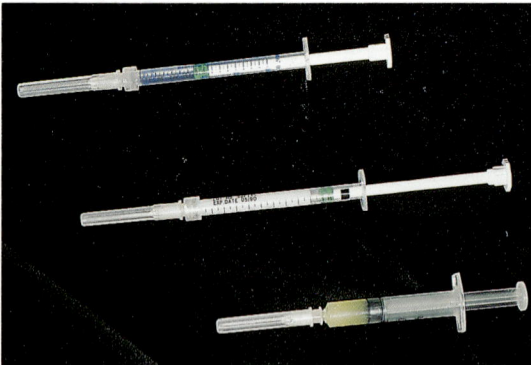

FIGURE 18.1 Three injectable soft-tissue augmentation products. From top to bottom: Injectable liquid silicone, bovine collagen (Zyplast), and gelatin matrix implant (Fibrel).

sensitive. Silicone persists indefinitely at the injection site, a fact that underscores the importance of meticulous technique. In addition to the presence of the silicone per se, it is also the delayed fibroplastic reaction to it that accounts for the augmentation seen with this treatment. Therefore, in contrast to injections of Zyderm/Zyplast or Fibrel, undercorrection rather than overcorrection is the rule. Most facial lines, wrinkles, or scars should be augmented gradually over several treatments at monthly intervals.

Silicone is injected through multiple (serial) punctures in microdroplets no greater than 0.05 mL. Injection through a 30-gauge needle on a 1-mL Luer-Lok syringe helps one to accomplish this microinjection technique (Figure 18.2A–C). The goal should be to inject discrete microdroplets of material. Each droplet induces its own fibroplastic response and results in added augmentation. For a given volume of material, a greater number of delivered microdroplets will result in greater augmentation. Only small quantities of material are injected during a given treatment session. For example, a volume of 0.3 to 0.6 mL of silicone fluid is usually more than sufficient to treat not only the nasolabial folds, but also the oral commissures and glabellar lines.

The depth of injection of silicone varies with the type of lesion being treated. Full-thickness contour defects, such as the naso-

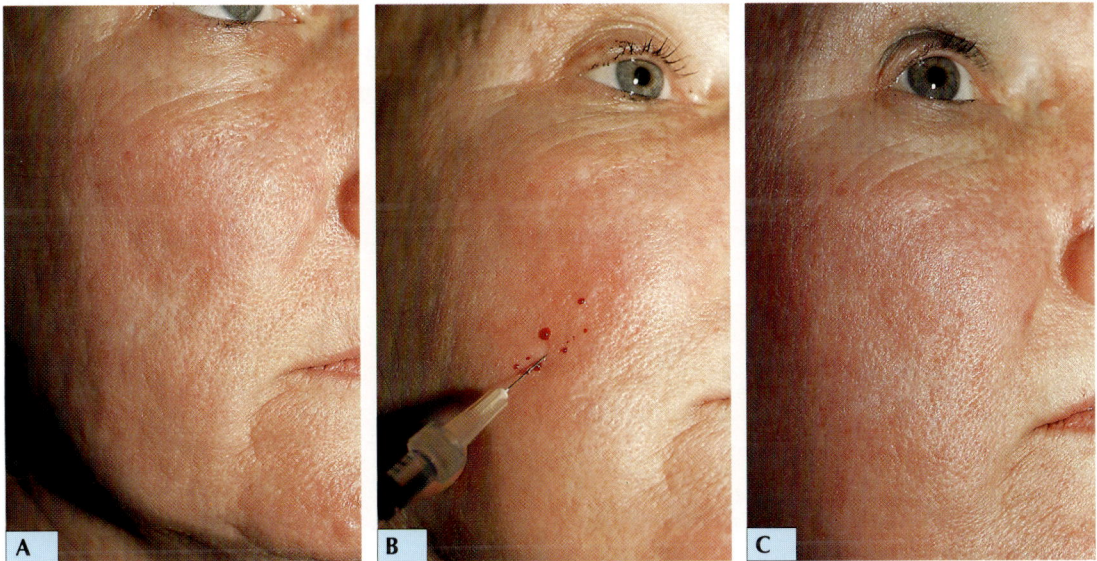

FIGURE 18.2 Treatment of acne scars with injectable liquid silicone in a woman. **(A)** Preoperative photograph shows soft, "fingerprint" scarring. **(B)** Injectable liquid silicone, delivered in microdroplets, is used to treat acne scars on both cheeks. **(C)** Follow-up photograph taken 6 months later after a total of 0.5 mL of material has been administered in two treatment sessions.

labial fold, are injected at the dermal-fat junction in an attempt to recontour the area (Figure 18.3A–C). If one injects superficially, the contour defect remains and one risks the development of superficial "beading." Intradermal injection of extremely small microdroplets (0.005 mL) is appropriate for finer, more superficial wrinkles or scars.

Occasionally, despite careful attention to injection technique, beading will develop at treatment sites. The problem is usually a temporary one that subsides spontaneously after several months. Persistent papules may be treated with intralesional injections of triamcinolone acetonide (2.5 to 5.0 mg/mL). Idiosyncratic reactions to silicone also have been reported in approximately one patient in 10,000. These reactions, which involve one or two treatment sites, appear months after injection and are characterized by swelling and slight erythema. Biopsy has revealed a nonspecific chronic inflammatory response. Treatment consists of intralesional corticosteroids and oral antibiotics.

Treatment also may be accompanied by transient erythema, swelling, and bruising but these findings generally subside within hours to days. Patients may use makeup immediately following treatment to hide these temporary sequelae.

BOVINE COLLAGEN IMPLANTS

Bovine collagen implant therapy has been the favored injectable since its approval by the FDA a decade ago as Zyderm Collagen Implant (Collagen Corporation, Palo Alto, Calif). In preparing this material, bovine dermal collagen is solubilized, purified, and reconstituted into a phosphate-buffered saline solution containing 0.4% lidocaine.

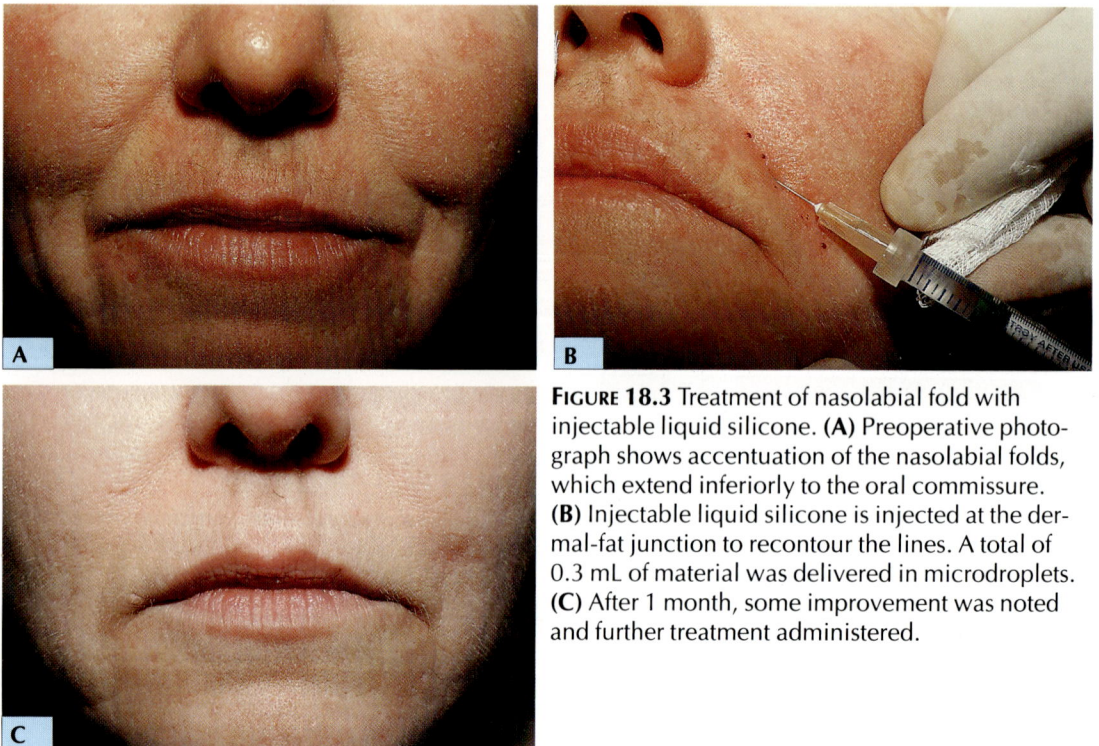

FIGURE 18.3 Treatment of nasolabial fold with injectable liquid silicone. (A) Preoperative photograph shows accentuation of the nasolabial folds, which extend inferiorly to the oral commissure. (B) Injectable liquid silicone is injected at the dermal-fat junction to recontour the lines. A total of 0.3 mL of material was delivered in microdroplets. (C) After 1 month, some improvement was noted and further treatment administered.

Zyderm Collagen Implants I and II contain collagen in concentrations of 35 and 65 mg/mL respectively.

Collagen metabolism is a dynamic process in skin. Senescent collagen fibrils are digested enzymatically by dermal collagenase while new collagen is produced by fibroblasts. Collagenase activity in the skin limits the survival of injected bovine collagen to several months. In an attempt to slow the rate of enzymatic (collagenase) digestion of injectable collagen, collagen chemists were able to cross-link bovine collagen fibrils by adding low concentrations of glutaraldehyde. This process led to the development of Zyplast Collagen Implant, which, in addition to lasting longer than Zyderm, tends to be less antigenic. Recently, The Koken Company (Tokyo, Japan) began marketing its version of injectable collagen in Canada. Because it is a natural, "biodegradable" substance, collagen is attractive to our health-conscious society although its degradation limits its longevity. The duration of correction for active expression lines of the central face is generally around 6 months. Therefore, in the treatment of facial lines and wrinkles, patients must be advised that ongoing supplemental treatments are required to maintain the correction. Most patients are prepared to accept this limitation.

The success of collagen implant therapy depends on patient selection, injection technique, and product selection. Collagen injections are not effective for treating "ice-pick" scars or otherwise fibrotic lesions. Distensible scars, superficial wrinkles, and deep contour defects all are amenable to this form of therapy (Figure 18.4A,B). Superficial, fine lines are best treated with Zyderm I or Zyderm II. Treatment of such lines with Zyplast can result in the appearance of multiple small papules (beading) along the injection line, which may persist for 6 to 8 weeks or longer. Zyplast is indicated in the treatment of coarser, deep lines such as the

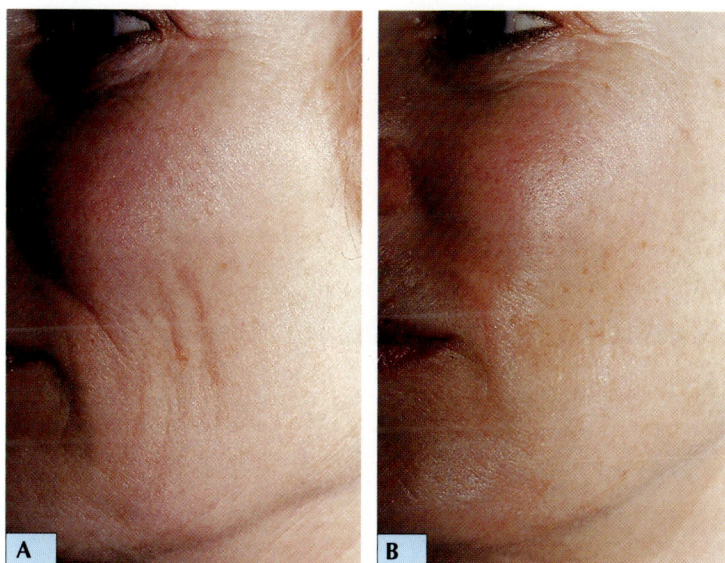

FIGURE 18.4 Treatment of facial lines with Zyplast bovine collagen implant. (A) Preoperative photograph shows secondary and tertiary nasolabial lines at the cheek. (B) Same patient shown after three treatments of 0.5 mL of Zyplast each.

nasolabial folds, forehead wrinkles, and the oral commissure (Figure 18.5A–C). Zyderm I and Zyderm II should be injected superficially and overcorrection is advised. However, Zyplast must be used with a modicum of care since it is less forgiving. It is injected more deeply (mid-dermis) and overcorrection should be limited. Careful massage of the treatment site is performed after injection to blend the interface of implanted and untreated skin.

Skin testing should be performed prior to collagen implant therapy to identify those patients most likely to experience an allergic treatment reaction to bovine collagen. Approximately 3% of all patients experience a hypersensitivity reaction to the Zyderm skin test. After excluding these patients from treatment, about 1% to 2% of individuals who did not react to the skin test will react subsequently at treatment sites. This implies that some previously nonallergic individuals

might be sensitized to Zyderm at the time of the initial skin test. Most clinicians are now performing a second skin test on the opposite arm 2 to 4 weeks after administration of the first test. This maneuver has been effective in eliminating from treatment a number of individuals who might otherwise have had an allergic treatment reaction.

Most allergic treatment reactions present as erythema and induration at the injection site, often accompanied by the presence of circulating antibodies to bovine collagen implant. The reactive sites are often pruritic and tend to wax and wane in severity as time goes on. Reactions persist until all of the implanted material has been digested by the host inflammatory response, typically from 6 to 18 months. There is no treatment that will hasten resolution of allergic reactions to collagen but symptomatic treatment with antihistamines may be useful for controlling pruritus. When necessary, a short course of sys-

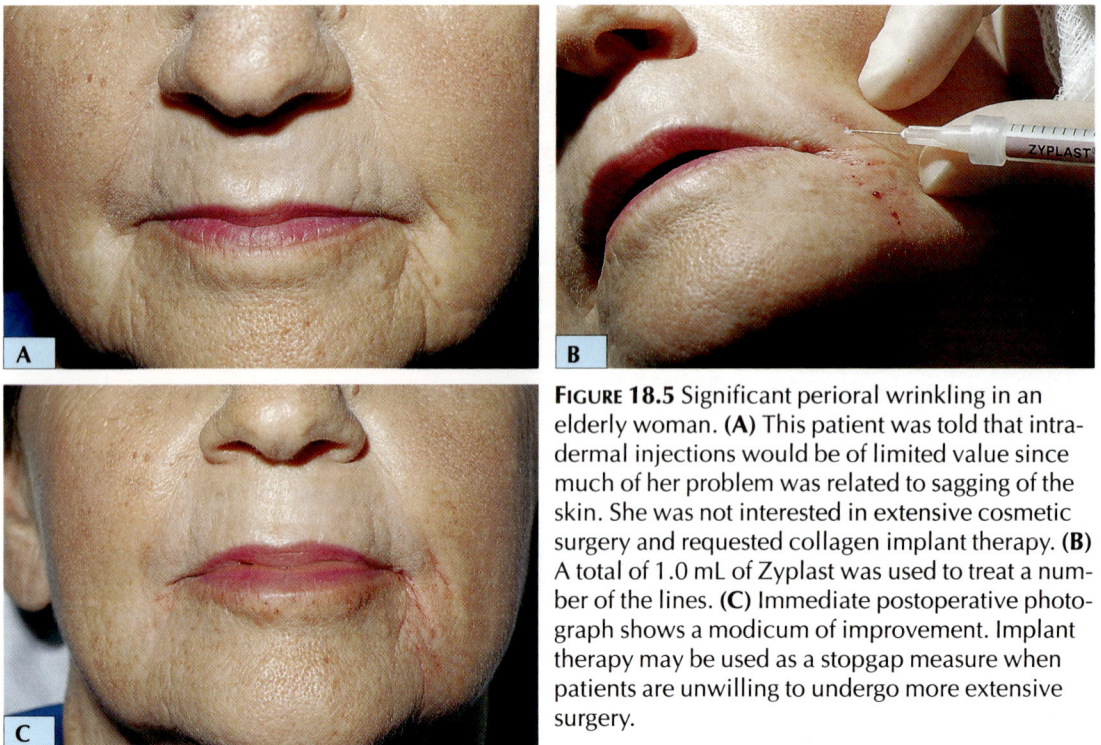

FIGURE 18.5 Significant perioral wrinkling in an elderly woman. **(A)** This patient was told that intradermal injections would be of limited value since much of her problem was related to sagging of the skin. She was not interested in extensive cosmetic surgery and requested collagen implant therapy. **(B)** A total of 1.0 mL of Zyplast was used to treat a number of the lines. **(C)** Immediate postoperative photograph shows a modicum of improvement. Implant therapy may be used as a stopgap measure when patients are unwilling to undergo more extensive surgery.

temic steroids will quiet the reaction temporarily. However, patients are advised that the inflammatory response is necessary for their skin to digest the offending substance and that interruption of this process may prolong the course of the reaction.

A nonimmunologic reaction that has been observed with collagen implant therapy is localized skin necrosis. This occurs most commonly at the glabella but also can involve other facial areas. Necrosis usually occurs at only one of several injected regions, often in patients who have had previous therapy without untoward effects. Treatment is supportive and consists of early institution of semi-occlusive dressings and antibacterials when indicated. Scarring can be expected to accompany healing. While the cause of this reaction is unknown, it is assumed to involve vascular occlusion with infarction, either due to direct injection of a vessel or to pressure placed upon it from the local injection of implant material.

Transient erythema, swelling, and bruising also may occur with collagen implant therapy. Their presentation and resolution, however, do not differ from the same responses seen with other injectable treatments.

GELATIN MATRIX IMPLANT (FIBREL)

Fibrel, an implantation product currently marketed by Mentor Corporation, evolved from work performed by Dr Arthur Spangler, a Boston, Mass, dermatologist, some decades ago. Spangler reported on the use of "Fibrin foam" for treatment of depressed scars. In this technique, patient plasma was mixed with a gelatin carrier and injected beneath scars into a pocket created with a small undermining knife. The results were impressive and the concept was eventually developed further by industry. The outcome, Fibrel Gelatin Matrix Implant, gained FDA approval in early 1988 for the treatment of scars. During the summer of 1990, the material was approved for use in the treatment of facial lines and wrinkles.

This product is individually reconstituted for each patient treatment session. A vial of blood is drawn from the patient and is spun down in a centrifuge. A small volume of plasma is added to a syringe containing highly purified, denatured porcine collagen (gelatin) and ϵ-aminocaproic acid. The gelatin acts as a temporary matrix upon which the blood plasma constituents, including fibrin, are deposited. The ϵ-aminocaproic acid interferes with fibrin digestion by inhibiting the production of fibrinolysin.

The mode of action of Fibrel is assumed to involve fibroblast activation with subsequent collagen deposition. Experimental studies have suggested that fibrin is an activator of fibroblasts. Numerous other blood constituents, such as fibronectin and a multitude of growth factors, could be involved in attracting fibroblasts into the gelatin matrix and activating them to secrete collagen. In Spangler's early work, he reported early neutrophil invasion of the fibrin-foam implant followed by phagocytosis and replacement by fibroblasts, fibrocytes, and normal collagen. The gelatin matrix reportedly is replaced in as little as 6 weeks.

The only study that reports on the efficacy of this product relates to acne scars and, thus far, has reported a 2-year persistence of correction in about 60% of patients (Figure 18.6A–C). According to unpublished data, most of these patients have now maintained correction for up to 5 years. Although Fibrel has only recently gained official approval for the treatment of facial lines and wrinkles, many clinicians have experience in treating them with this product. In this regard, Fibrel has been a useful alternative to injectable bovine collagen products, yielding comparable outcomes in the treatment of nasolabial fold, oral commissure, and glabellar lines (Figure 18.7 A–C). The material has not yet proven its effectiveness in the treatment of very fine lines or "crow's feet."

Since the porcine collagen from which

the gelatin is derived is highly denatured, very little antigenicity has been seen with Fibrel. Nonetheless, infrequent allergic reactions have been reported and therefore skin testing in the volar forearm is undertaken in all patients at least 30 days prior to their first treatment.

The amount of discomfort seen with the injection of Fibrel is greater than that accompanying Zyderm/Zyplast or silicone. Therefore, one must anesthetize the treatment sites prior to injection of the gelatin matrix implant. Plain 1% lidocaine is used, since the use of epinephrine could impede access of additional useful blood-borne elements to the treatment site. Regional nerve blocks, ring blocks, or local infiltration also may be used, although the latter may cause distortion

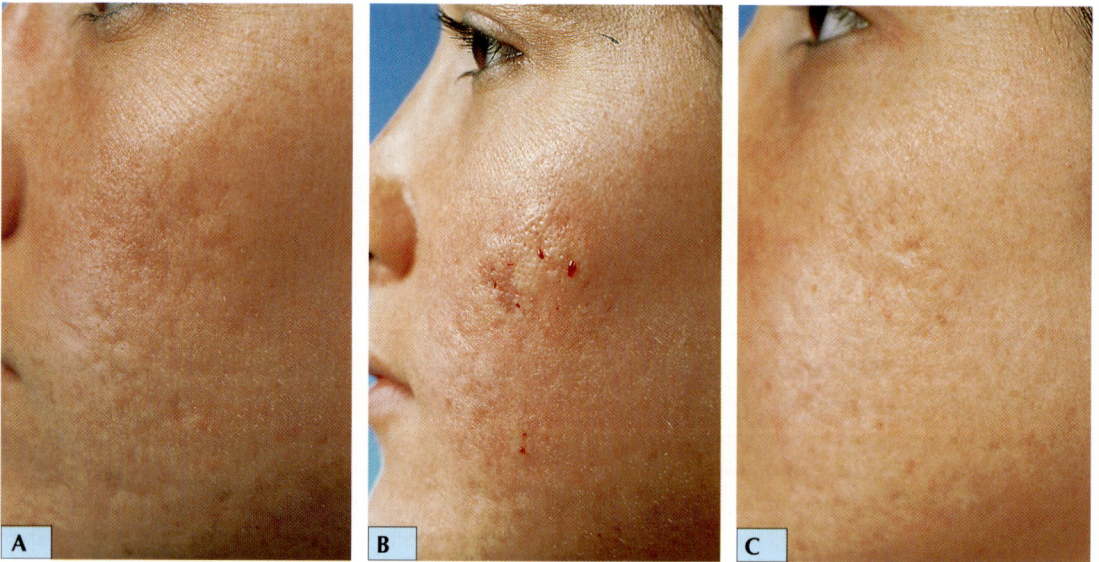

FIGURE 18.6 Treatment of acne scars with Fibrel gelatin matrix implant. **(A)** Soft, shallow acne scarring on the cheek of a young patient. **(B)** Appearance immediately following injection of Fibrel material. Note the urticarial type of swelling seen typically with this treatment. **(C)** Appearance 2 weeks later shows substantial improvement.

interfering with treatment. Massaging the site after the anesthetic is administered tends to minimize this problem. Alternatively, a topical anesthetic (Emla) has been found to be effective in minimizing the pain of injection, thereby eliminating the need for injectable anesthesia. This product, not yet marketed in North America, must be occluded for 45 minutes to achieve satisfactory results.

The injection technique for Fibrel is comparable to that for injectable bovine collagen. However, due to its increased viscosity, 1 mL of material is usually sufficient to treat both nasolabial folds and, on occasion, the glabella as well. A small- (27- or 30-) gauge needle is used to inject the material through serial punctures along the facial line.

Superficial placement of the material results in enhanced longevity, and overcorrection of about 50% is encouraged. After injection, the treatment site should be massaged gently with the fingers to blend it with the surrounding skin.

Following Fibrel implant therapy, one should expect to see transient swelling and erythema at the treatment site. Usually urticarial in nature, the response most often resembles a series of insect bites and may indicate the release of vasoactive substances by this biomaterial. Swelling and erythema usually subside in 24 to 48 hours. As with the other injectables, punctate bruising may take up to 1 week to subside completely. Patients are asked to return in 4 to 8 weeks for their second treatment. A third treatment, if neces-

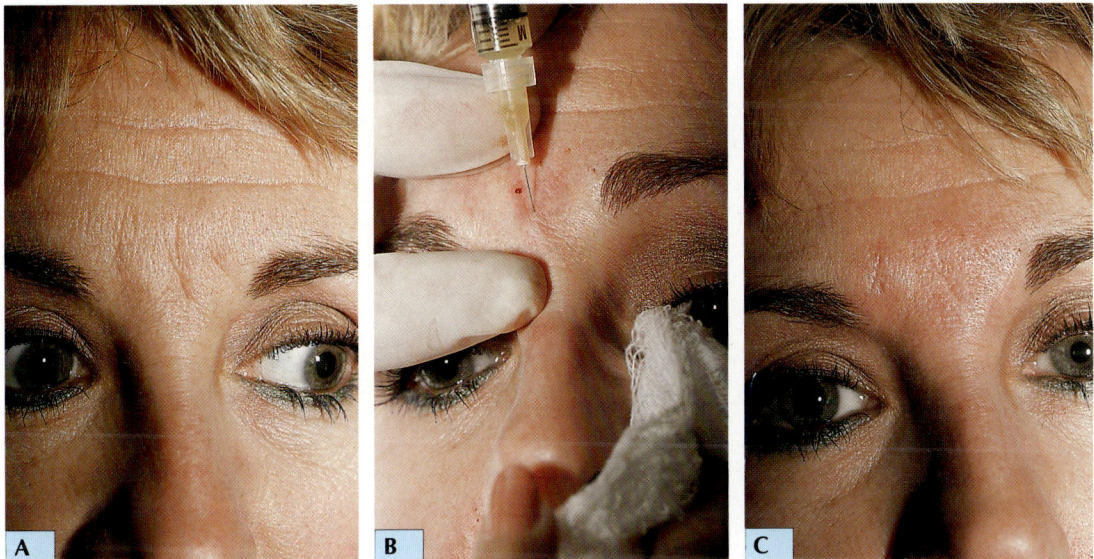

FIGURE 18.7 Treatment of glabellar lines with Fibrel gelatin matrix implant. (A) Preoperative photograph shows deep frown lines at the glabella. (B) Injection of Fibrel into facial lines. (C) Postoperatively, improvement is seen.

sary, may be administered 4 to 8 weeks after the second therapy session.

One additional concept that Fibrel borrows from Dr Spangler's original work is the "custom undermining needle" that is packaged with each kit. Essentially a 20-gauge beveled needle, it is extremely sharp and can be used to sever any fibrotic cords that may tether a scar to the underlying dermis. This modified reticulotomy has proven to be of some benefit in improving treatment results for fibrotic scars such as those seen following chickenpox, trauma, and occasionally surgery. The needle is moved in and out under the scar, and a tract or pocket is formed in the dermis (Figure 18.8). Fibrel is then injected into this opening. Some extrusion of material may occur. With subsequent treatments, the formerly bound-down scars become softer and further augmentation can be achieved more readily.

As with injectable collagens, the results seen with Fibrel have been variable suggesting that they may be, in part, technique sensitive. Superficial placement of the material improves the longevity of correction, which is comparable to that seen with Zyplast.

LIMITATIONS OF INJECTABLE MATERIALS

It is important that both clinicians and patients recognize the limitations of injectable therapy in the treatment of facial lines and wrinkles. Specific surgical techniques are a more appropriate and effective therapy than are injectables in instances where significant solar elastosis and/or cutaneous laxity is present. The yellowish plaques that characterize severe solar elastosis often have furrows running through them, between the papules of elastotic material. Some clinicians may be tempted to inject these lines with the materials discussed in this chapter. The results are usually disappointing for both therapist and patient. A more appropriate treatment is to remove the elastotic material, which is generally confined to the papillary dermis, by dermabrasion or chemical peeling. Injectables cannot be expected to counter the effects of gravity and are entirely ineffective in treating "jowls" or other problems associated with significant skin laxity. In such cases, rhytidectomy procedures should be recommended to patients.

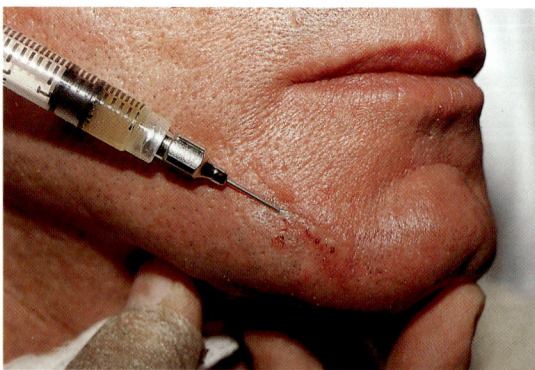

FIGURE 18.8 Use of the 20-gauge custom undermining needle to loosen the connections of a fibrotic scar prior to injection of Fibrel. This procedure is useful in improving scars that otherwise do not respond to intradermal augmentation.

SUGGESTIONS FOR FURTHER READING

Castrow FF II, Krull EA. Injectable collagen implant—update. J Am Acad Dermatol. 1983;9:889-893.

Chaplin CH. Loss of both breasts from injections of silicone (with additive). Plast Reconstr Surg. 1969;44:447-450.

Kamer FM, Churukain MM. The clinical use of injectable collagen: a three-year retrospective study. Arch Otolaryngol Head Neck Surg. 1984;110:93-98.

Kaplan EN, Flaces E, Tolleth H. Clinical utilization of injectable collagen. Ann Plast Surg. 1983;10:437-451.

Klein AW. Implantation techniques for injectable collagen: two-and-one-half years of personal clinical experience. J Am Acad Dermatol. 1983;9:224-228.

Kligman AM, Phariss BB. Injectable Collagen Implants. Introduction. J Dermatol Surg Oncol. 1988;14(suppl):10-11.

Millikan L. Long-term safety and efficacy with Fibrel in the treatment of cutaneous scars—results of a multicenter study. J Dermatol Surg Oncol. 1989;15:837-842.

Millikan L, Rosen T, Monheit G, et al. Treatment of depressed cutaneous scars with gelatin matrix implant: a multicenter study. J Am Acad Dermatol. 1987;16:1155-1162.

Orentreich DS, Orentreich N. Injectable fluid silicone. In: Roenigk RK, Roenigk HH Jr, eds. Dermatologic Surgery. Principles and Practice. New York, NY: Marcel Dekker Inc; 1989:1349-1395.

Spangler AS. Treatment of depressed scars with fibrin foam—seventeen years of experience. J Dermatol Surg Oncol. 1975;1:65-69.

Spangler AS. New treatment of pitted scars, preliminary report. Arch Derm. 1957;76:708-711.

Stegman SJ, Chu S, Armstrong RC. Adverse reactions to bovine collagen implant: clinical and histologic features. J Dermatol Surg Oncol. 1988;14(suppl):39-48.

Winer LH, Sternberg TH, Lehman R, Ashley FL. Tissue reaction to injected silicone liquids, a report of three cases. Arch Derm. 1964;90:588-593.

chapter 19

TISSUE EXPANSION IN HEAD AND NECK RECONSTRUCTION

Tissue expanders are a relatively recent addition to the field of reconstructive surgery. Introduced for clinical use by Neumann in 1959, the first expanders were Silastic blocks used to expand skin for auricular reconstruction. In the early 1960s, Radovan introduced Silastic inflatable balloons into clinical practice. The expanders currently in use consist of inflatable silicone reservoirs with injection ports that are incorporated into the reservoir or are distal to it, connected by tubing (Figure 19.1). The injectable ports are backed by a stainless steel base and are resealable, making it possible to inflate the temporary prosthesis in stages. The expanders are available through many vendors, including Mentor and Cox-Uphoff. Although many types of expanders are available, in our practice we prefer to use those with distal ports, to avoid the problem of increased pressure and tension found with expanders that incorporate the port. Integrated injection ports can cause erosion of thin facial skin during the course of expander inflation. The use of expanders with square-cornered reservoirs should also be avoided in the head and neck area, as such reservoirs can lead to pressure necrosis. Round reservoirs are preferred in the head and neck area.

The expander is placed in a subcutaneous pocket after careful hemostasis is obtained, and the skin flap is closed over the expander. Generally, larger expanders are placed with the patient under general anesthesia, while small expanders, which are useful in the recruitment of new facial skin, can be placed under local anesthesia in an outpatient setting. Once in place the volume of the expander is increased, in 20% to 30% increments over a period of 4 to 6 weeks, to create additional local tissue. When approximately 10% more epidermal tissue than required is produced, the expander is removed and the new skin is fashioned into a flap to repair the defect.

Because the donor site is in continuity with the reconstructed area, tissue expanders usually result in new skin that is well matched for local color and texture. Sensation remains intact if major sensory cutaneous nerves are not violated in the flap design, and the hair-bearing characteristics of the tissue can be tailored to the needs of the reconstruction. In addition to these local advantages, enhanced vascularity is a hallmark of tissue-expanded skin and permits increased flap-length design.

The disadvantages of tissue expansion include the potential for such complications as pain, seroma formation, pressure necrosis, and secondary infection around the capsule. Pain syndromes and pressure necrosis are more common in the latter stages of expansion. The appearance of the expander during the process of expansion is also a problem for some patients, as is the necessity for repeated office injections over a 6- to 8-week period for inflation of the expander.

CAPSULE FORMATION

The introduction of a tissue expander into its pocket always causes a capsule to be formed. The capsule is composed of active fibroblasts and its thickness increases the longer the expander is in place. The capsule also consists of a proliferation of blood vessels, which effectively increases the blood supply to the expanded tissue. The increased vascularity is due to an increase in angiogenic factors during the process of expansion and leads to a physiologic state that allows for increased width-to-length ratios in skin-flap design. It also accounts for increased survival rates in expanded cutaneous tissue, which can then be used more reliably in complex head and neck reconstruction (Figure 19.2A–D).

In addition to inducing capsule formation, tissue expanders change the morphology of the epidermis, dermis, subcutaneous tissue, and muscular tissue. The thickness of the epidermis remains the same, although its

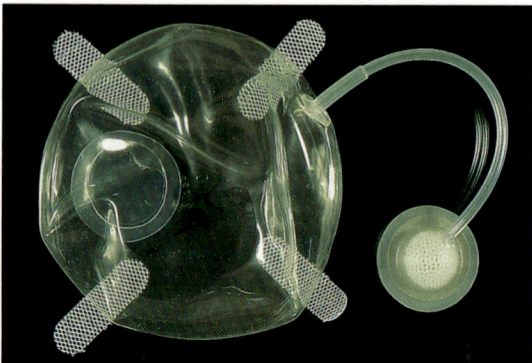

FIGURE 19.1 The injection port of this tissue expander is attached to its reservoir by Silastic tubing. Expanders with integrated reservoirs are also available but are not advisable for use in the head and neck area.

surface area is increased as a result of the expansion. While there is a general thinning of the dermis with expansion, total skin thickness remains about the same, due to the increased bulk associated with the corresponding capsule formation. Additionally, there are increases in fibroblast activity, collagen synthesis, and melanin production. The number of fat cells in the subcutaneous tissue decreases after expansion, reducing its thickness. Skeletal muscle thins significantly and the potential exists for loss of strength, or sometimes function, of the associated muscle.

CLINICAL APPLICATIONS

Tissue expanders have become an important part of the clinical repair of head and neck defects, which in the past have been difficult to reconstruct because of a relative lack of viable and appropriate tissue. They are particularly useful for reconstruction of the scalp and forehead where a paucity of subcutaneous tissue results in the inability of epidermal tissue in the area to be mobilized. In contrast to skin grafts, tissue expanders provide a better match for texture and color (as noted earlier), increased tissue bulk, and

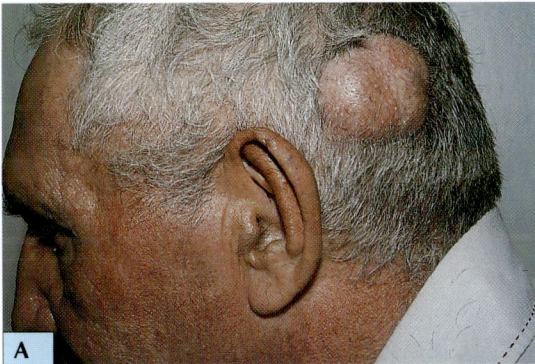

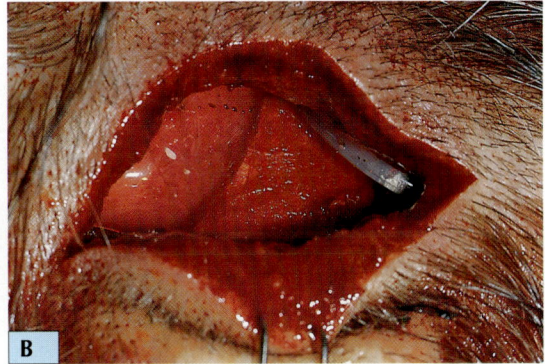

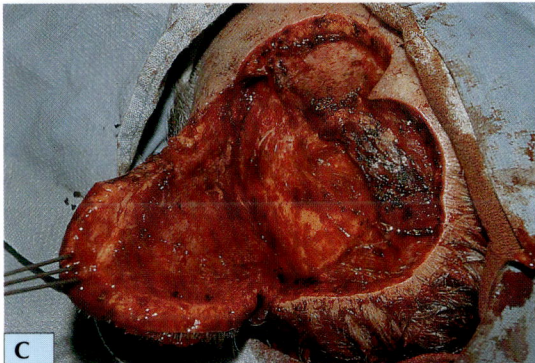

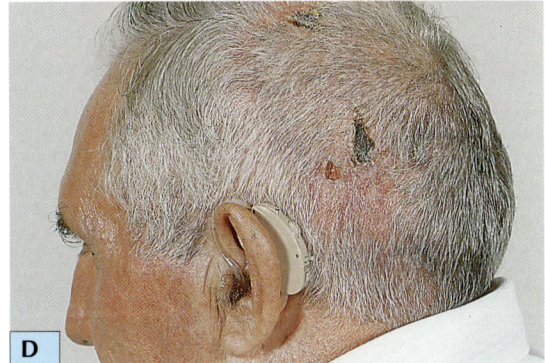

FIGURE 19.2 (A) This 55-year-old man presented with a benign dermoid cyst that had slowly been progressing in size. (B) Prior to removal of the cyst, a tissue expander was placed under the galea of the scalp. (C) After 6 weeks of biweekly expansion, a large capsule has been created by the expander. (D) Two weeks after excision of the cyst, removal of the expander, and reconstruction of the defect with a rotational flap.

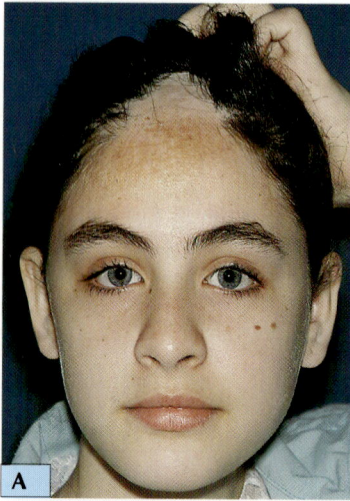

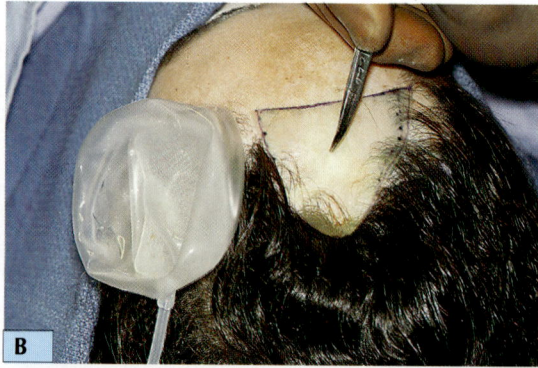

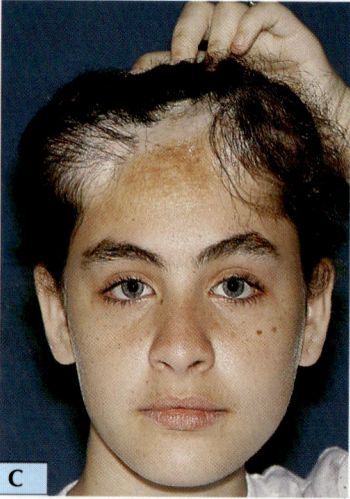

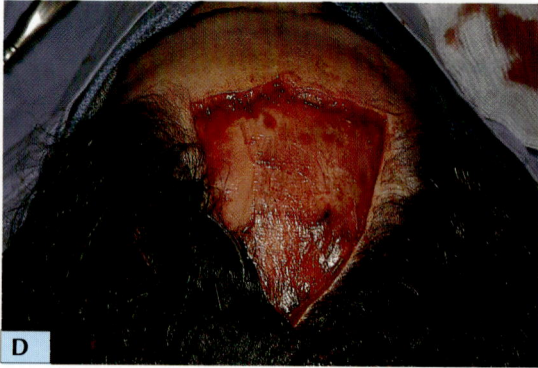

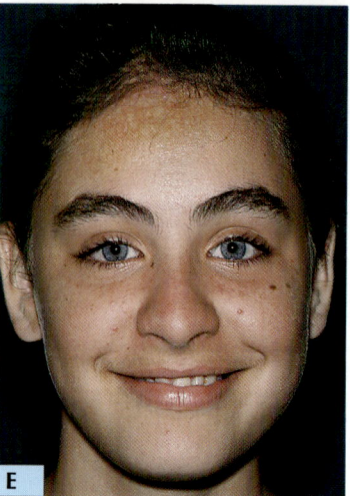

FIGURE 19.3 (A) A 16-year-old girl with third-degree burns of the fore-head. **(B)** Two expanders were placed adjacent to the scalp defect to ensure adequate mobilization of the anterior hair-bearing scalp skin. **(C)** At the end of 6 weeks, the expanders have been filled to capacity. **(D)** The tissue expanders are removed and the scar tissue is excised. The hair-bearing advancement flaps can then be mobilized to reconstruct the defect. **(E)** Two months after removal of the expanders with immediate reconstruction, the patient has active hair-bearing scalp in her anterior crown, with good hairline restoration.

greater versatility to incorporate hair-bearing tissue into the operative plan, thereby providing an improved functional and cosmetic result (Figures 19.3A–E and 19.4A–D).

Expanders can be used to create tissue in all areas of the head and neck, although if large expanders are placed in the neck the patient's airway must be carefully monitored. Expanders can also be used where cystic lesions or cutaneous masses have changed the characteristics of a previously hair-bearing region of the scalp (see Figure 19.2A–D). They are also useful in scar revision (see Figures 19.3A–E and 19.4A–D) and they are

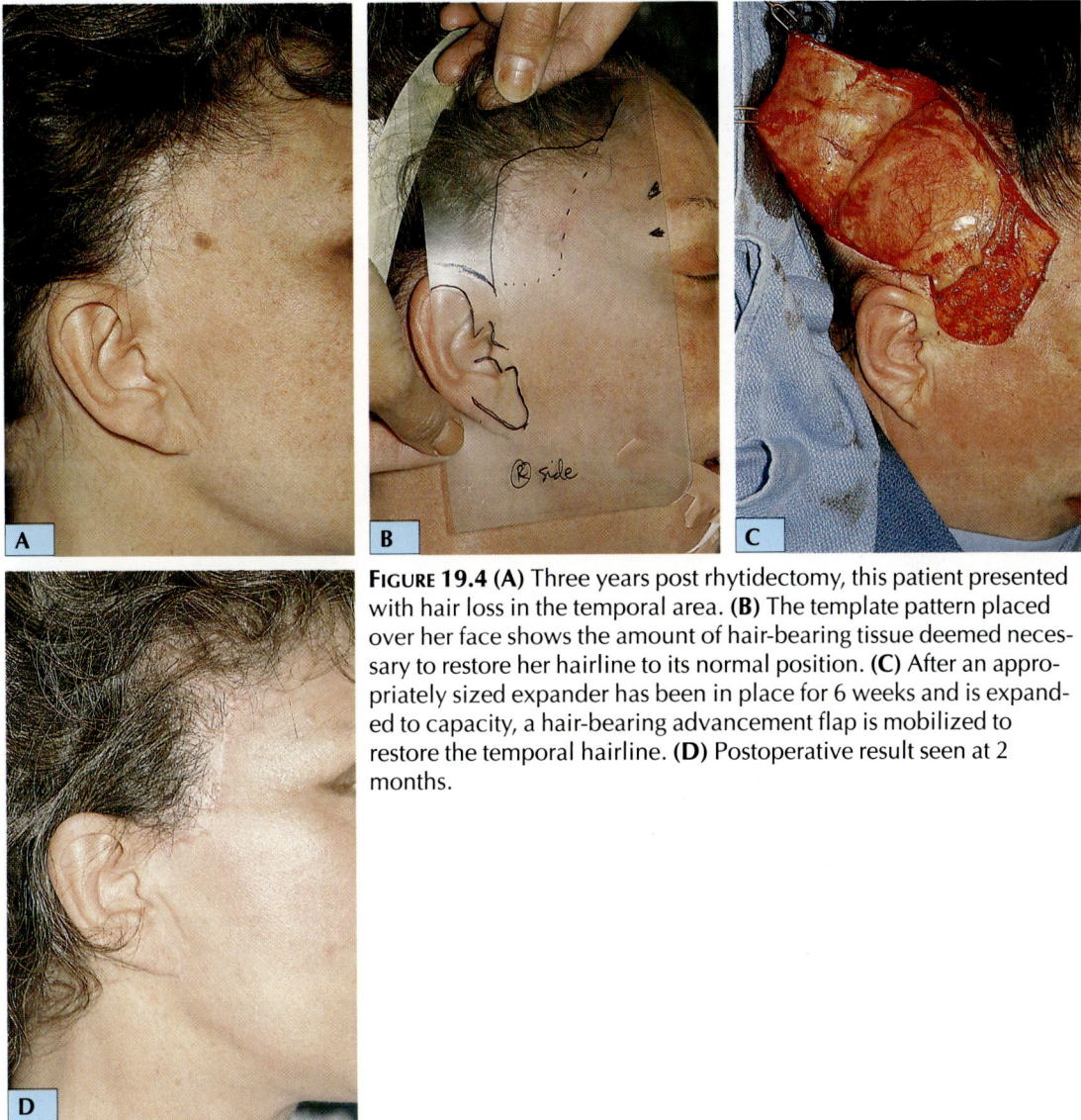

FIGURE 19.4 (A) Three years post rhytidectomy, this patient presented with hair loss in the temporal area. **(B)** The template pattern placed over her face shows the amount of hair-bearing tissue deemed necessary to restore her hairline to its normal position. **(C)** After an appropriately sized expander has been in place for 6 weeks and is expanded to capacity, a hair-bearing advancement flap is mobilized to restore the temporal hairline. **(D)** Postoperative result seen at 2 months.

particularly useful in the treatment of chronically infected wounds, where the associated increase in tissue vascularity is therapeutically beneficial (Figure 19.5A–D).

Tissue expansion is also used on an intraoperative basis, in which case the expanders are left in place for an average of 20 minutes. They are thought to decrease the collagen strength of the tissue being fashioned into a flap, thereby allowing increased mobility of the local skin (Figure 19.6A–D).

PREOPERATIVE PLANNING

The placement of a tissue expander involves careful planning and detailed patient education to create the best possible tissue for wound repair. Because the tissue undergoing

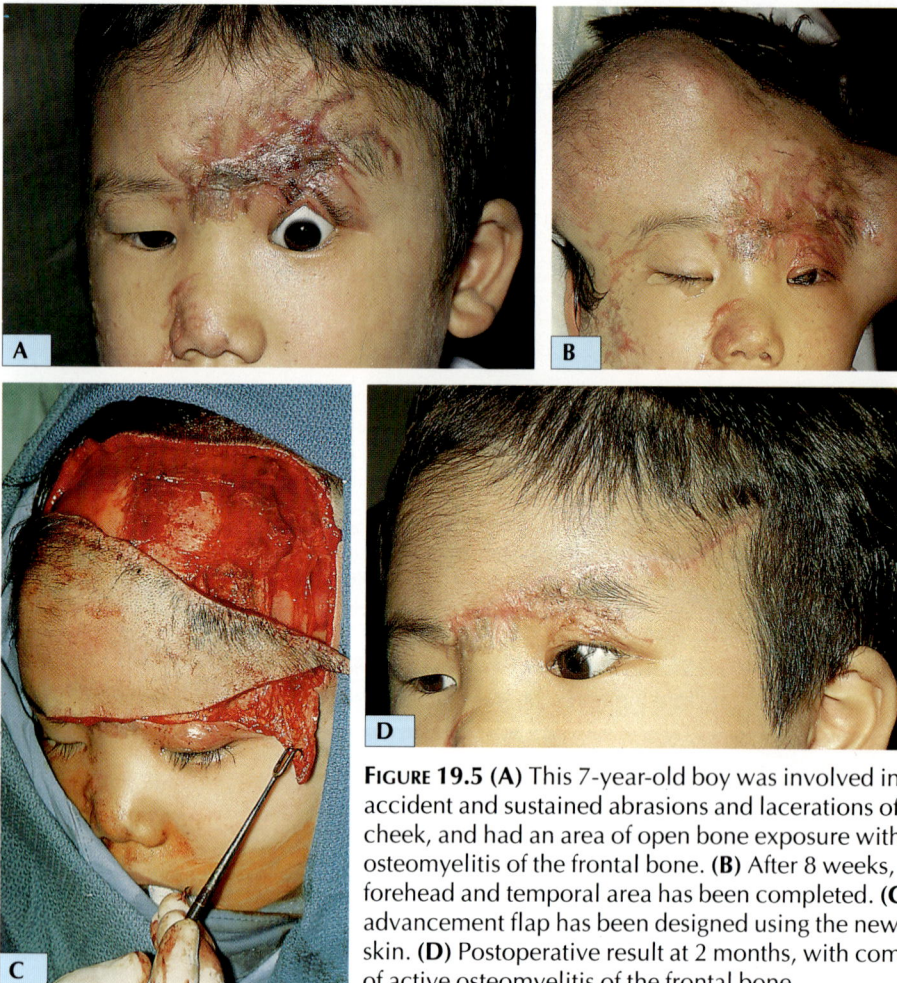

FIGURE 19.5 (A) This 7-year-old boy was involved in a motor vehicle accident and sustained abrasions and lacerations of the forehead and cheek, and had an area of open bone exposure with chronic osteomyelitis of the frontal bone. (B) After 8 weeks, expansion in the forehead and temporal area has been completed. (C) A rotational advancement flap has been designed using the newly created scalp skin. (D) Postoperative result at 2 months, with complete resolution of active osteomyelitis of the frontal bone.

expansion represents an area of increased tissue tension, careful attention must be paid to the incision used to place the expander in its pocket. Another important consideration is that of maintaining the integrity of the local flap, which will be used 6 to 8 weeks later in the definitive reconstruction.

While each reconstructive problem requires individual design, as a general rule the incision used for placement of the expander should be made along the edge of the flap to be used in the reconstruction. Choosing an appropriately sized expander is also important, as the surgeon must plan to create approximately 10% more tissue than is needed for flap repair, anticipating that an equal percentage of tissue will be lost due to contraction, when the expander is removed. The size of the expander is determined by the size of the defect. The dimensions of the proposed cutaneous incision are carefully measured and based on this measurement the appropriate

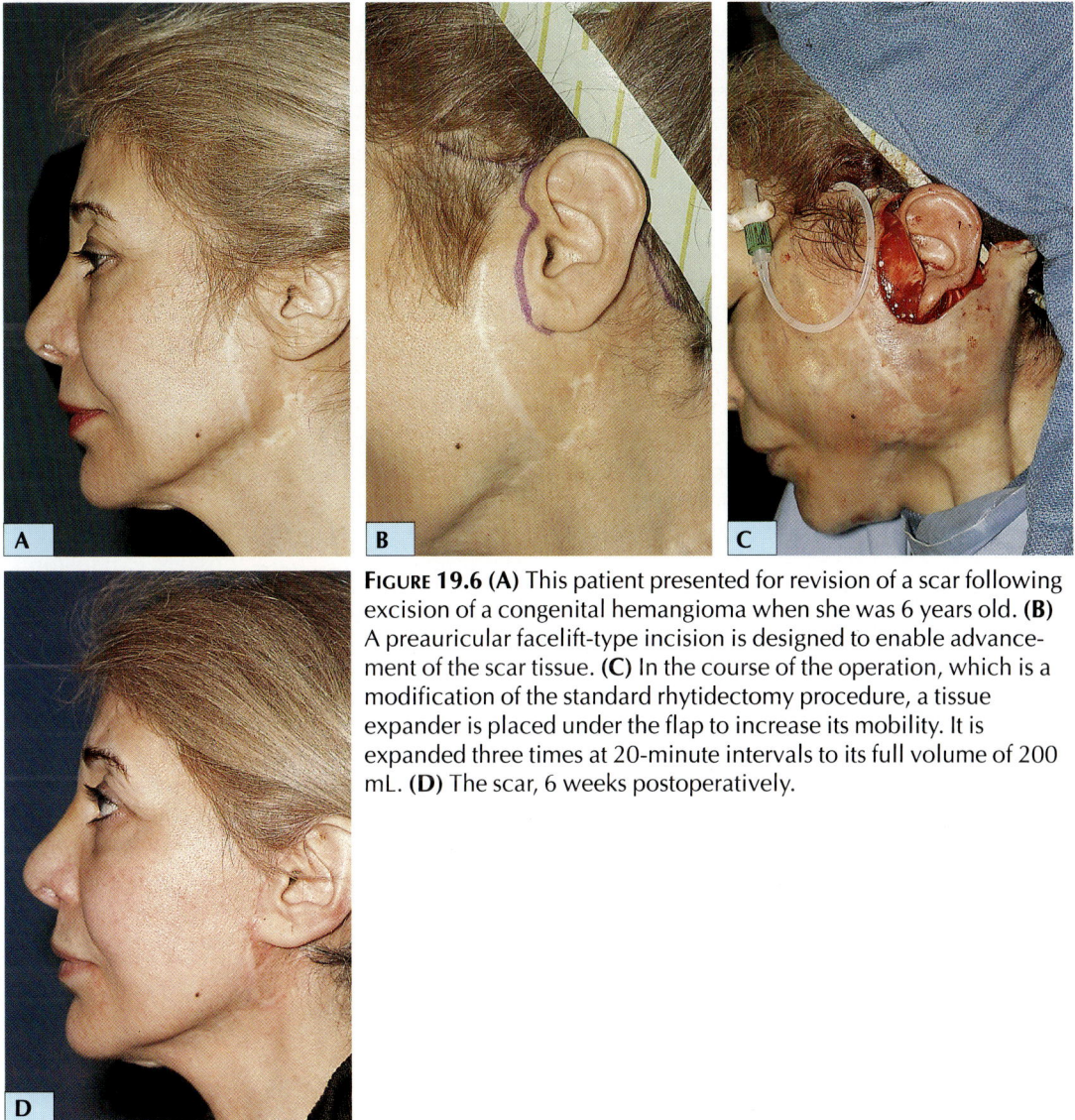

FIGURE 19.6 (A) This patient presented for revision of a scar following excision of a congenital hemangioma when she was 6 years old. **(B)** A preauricular facelift-type incision is designed to enable advancement of the scar tissue. **(C)** In the course of the operation, which is a modification of the standard rhytidectomy procedure, a tissue expander is placed under the flap to increase its mobility. It is expanded three times at 20-minute intervals to its full volume of 200 mL. **(D)** The scar, 6 weeks postoperatively.

expander is chosen, with its base being 10% larger than the base of the soft-tissue defect.

Also in the preoperative planning, the surgeon must make sure that the patient understands that there will be a 2- to 3-week period during which the expander will pose a cosmetic problem. In most cases, the expander can be covered by scarving techniques or by a hat during the late stages of inflation.

OPERATIVE PROCEDURE

After a standard preoperative history, physical examination, and appropriate laboratory testing, the patient is taken to the operating room and placed under general anesthesia. Following appropriate cutaneous preparation (Betadine scrub and solution), the predetermined incision for expander placement is made. A pocket is created, which is large enough to receive the previously sized expander, using sharp and blunt dissection techniques. A smaller pocket is created for introduction of the injection port and should be placed in a position that is easily accessible for regular injections. Meticulous hemostasis is obtained, and the pockets are irrigated with liberal amounts of bacitracin solution. In most cases, a drain is not necessary, as the expander has a local tamponade effect.

The wound is then closed in two layers, using PDS in the subcutaneous layer and Prolene in the cutaneous layer. The expander is inflated with normal saline to 10% of its total volume at the time of initial placement. (For a 200-mL expander, 20 mL of saline is used.) With the initial intraoperative expansion, the surgeon should be confident that the expander is unfolding in a manner that pro-

duces no irregularities. If irregularities do develop, they can be corrected by decreasing the volume of the expander, manipulating the expander, or by increasing the size of the pocket into which the expander has been placed. Routinely, patients are placed on a 2-week course of oral antibiotics.

POSTOPERATIVE MANAGEMENT

Postoperatively the patient is seen in the office 3 to 4 days after placement of the expander and the wound is checked for any evidence of early infection or undue tension. No expansion is done at this time.

At the next visit, 10 to 14 days postoperatively, contingent on adequate wound healing serial expansion can begin. The external port is identified and the local tissue is cleansed with alcohol. Using a 27-gauge needle, normal saline is introduced into the expander via the injection port. Generally, the cutaneous sutures are maintained for a period of 2 to 3 weeks to ensure adequate stability of the incision site.

The frequency of expansion is monitored by the subjective clinical parameters of capillary refill, pain at the site of expansion, the sensation of tension, and tissue turgor. Depending on these characteristics, expansion is either weekly or biweekly.

After full expansion has been achieved, the expander is removed and the cutaneous flap is designed and mobilized to provide immediate tissue coverage for reconstruction of the specific defect. Because of associated flap swelling and retraction, secondary touch-up procedures are best deferred for at least 2 to 3 months, until the flap is fully matured.

SUGGESTIONS FOR FURTHER READING

Argenta LC, Marks MW, Pasyk KA, et al. Advances in tissue expansion. Clin Plast Surg. 1985;12:159-171.

Cox KW, Larrabee WF Jr. Study of skin flap advancement as a function of undermining. Arch Otolaryngol. 1982;108:151-155.

Neumann CG. The expansion of an area of skin by progressive distention of a subcutaneous balloon. Plast Reconstr Surg. 1957;19:124-130.

Radovan C. Tissue expansion in soft-tissue reconstruction. Plast Reconstr Surg. 1984; 74:42-49.

Sasaki G. Intraoperative sustained limited expansion as an immediate reconstructive technique. Clin Plast Surg. 1987; 14(3):563-573.

chapter 20

FLAPS

Among the most creative and gratifying of techniques in cutaneous surgery is the use of a skin flap to close an operative defect. Many standard flaps are in common use and can be performed artfully following excision of malignant and benign lesions. Flaps have been classified variously according to movement (eg, rotation flap), shape (eg, rhomboid flap), location of donor (eg, nasolabial flap), or by eponyms (eg, Limberg flap). It is beyond the scope of this chapter to present the mechanics and design of all flaps used in cutaneous surgery. Rather, an overview of the principles operative in local skin flap surgery will be presented and some examples of advancement, rotation, and transposition flaps given. For a more detailed discussion of skin flap surgery, the reader is referred to Suggestions For Further Reading at the end of this chapter.

PRINCIPLES OF SKIN FLAP SURGERY

A flap is a segment of undermined full-thickness skin and some subcutaneous fat, which, remaining attached to the donor area at some point, is moved into a nearby defect. The point of attachment to the donor area, or pedicle, is essentially the "umbilical cord" through which the flap maintains its blood supply. Whereas in skin grafting, the transplanted skin must obtain its total blood supply from the host wound bed (see Chapter 21), skin flaps carry their initial source of nourishment with them. This allows them to be thicker than grafts and still survive. Furthermore, because skin directly adjacent to a defect can be used, the optimal color, texture, and thickness match can be achieved using this type of reconstruction.

A key to successful skin flap surgery is to ensure that there is adequate blood supply through the length of the flap. This requires that the base be wide enough to allow for adequate vascular ingress and that the length:width ratio of the flap not exceed 3:1 or 4:1. Flaps that are created without these design features in mind are less likely to survive. Also, since flaps do gain a portion of their nourishment from their beds, a wound bed containing adequate blood flow will contribute to a higher success rate. These design features are particularly important when flaps are used to cover poorly vascularized tissues such as bone, periosteum, perichondrium, or scar. Hematoma formation, which tends to lift the flap off of the wound bed and place excessive tension on the suture lines, should be prevented by careful attention to hemostasis.

The recommended thickness for flaps varies according to anatomic location. On the face, with the exception of the forehead, undermining with scissors, scalpel, or electrosection (see Chapter 9) should be performed in the upper fat. On the forehead, undermining should be in the deep fat just above the fascial plane. Similarly, on the extremities, undermining is performed in the deep fat just above muscle aponeuroses. The scalp is unique in that flaps usually are full thickness, with undermining performed in the subgaleal space. This is a relatively avascular plane that is dissected easily with a blunt instrument such as a scalpel handle or even a finger.

The initiate to skin flap surgery quickly learns that as flaps are created and defects made, the former tend to shrink while the latter expand. This is another consequence of the elastic nature of our skin. To prevent a situation in which the defect is too large for the flap, the latter should be made approximately 20% larger than the defect. Whenever possible, the flap should be oriented in such a way that incisions fall in wrinkles, facial lines, or natural skin folds. Incisions made at natural boundaries, such as the hairline, also are less conspicuous when healing is complete. When incisions are made near hair-bearing areas (eyebrow, sideburns), they should be beveled so that they are parallel to the hair shafts. This will minimize the number of hair follicles transected and limit any resultant permanent hair loss.

MECHANICAL ASPECTS OF SKIN FLAPS

Skin flaps are used, in general, when a given defect is too large to close primarily or when simple closure will result in significant tension or distortion. By use of a skin flap, tissue and/or tension can be redistributed over a given area. This is made possible by the inherent elasticity of the skin and in many cases is aided significantly by the presence of local cutaneous laxity. By assessing the prevalent skin tensions in the region of the wound and by determining where relative skin laxity or redundancy lies, one can design a flap that is either stretched, pivoted, or turned into a defect.

Two kinds of tissue movement define a skin flap repair. The primary movement is that of the flap moving into the defect. The secondary movement is that accomplished by the marginal skin of the wound advancing to meet the flap. While clinicians tend to concentrate on the movement of the flap itself, they must keep in mind that secondary movement can affect the amount of tension resulting at the suture line.

Even when tension is minimal, scar contraction at the periphery of a flap can sometimes cause its center to appear to protrude. Not uncommon, this finding is called the "trap-door effect" and is emphasized when excessive fat is present at the base of the flap. The trap-door deformity, which is at least partially due to poor venous and lymphatic outflow, often disappears gradually over a period of 3 to 6 months as wound remodeling proceeds (see Chapter 13) and fibrosis diminishes in thickness. In some cases, however, it persists and a secondary "defatting" procedure is indicated.

Although most articles and texts illustrate idealized geometric configurations for defects and flaps, these squares, triangles, and circles rarely are necessary for skin flap surgery to succeed. The skin is elastic enough to accommodate to more irregular defects, and the shape of a defect (or flap) should be altered only when it proves necessary during the course of a repair.

As mentioned earlier, skin flaps are either stretched, pivoted, or turned into a defect. These different primary movements define the three broad classes of skin flaps: advancement flaps, rotation flaps, and transposition flaps. A discussion of each of these types of flaps follows.

ADVANCEMENT FLAPS

Advancement flaps (Figure 20.1) utilize the simplest of all flap designs. The flap is moved

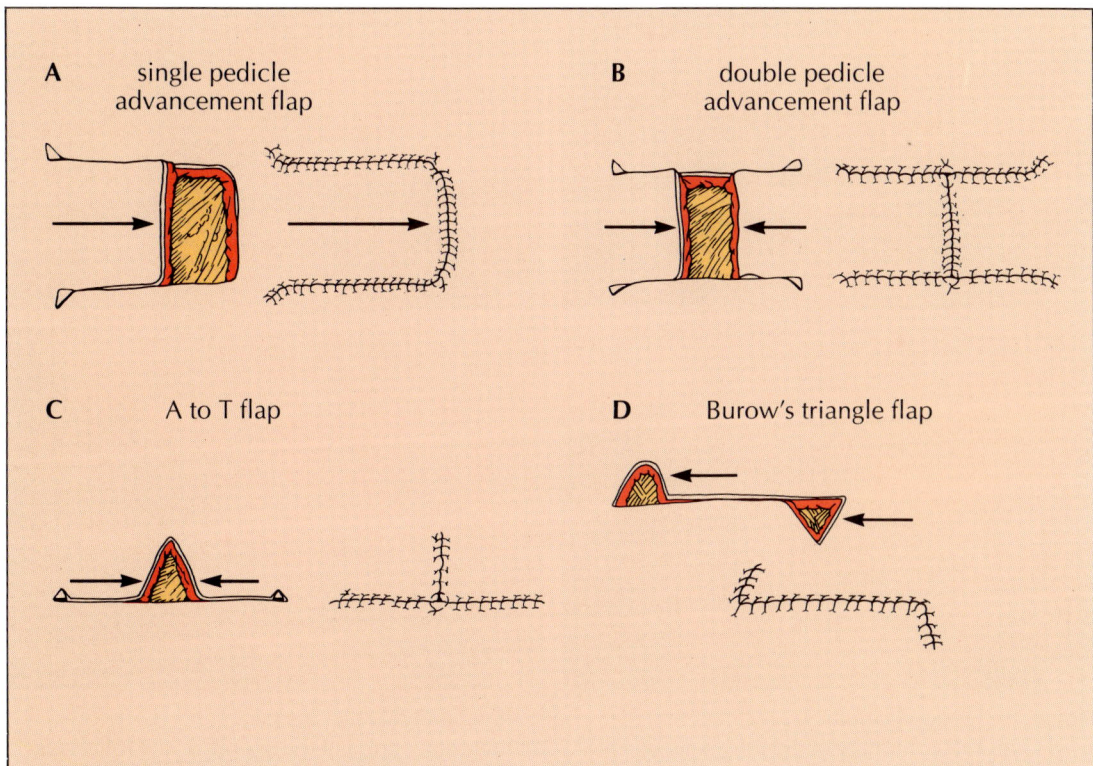

FIGURE 20.1 Schematic drawing showing advancement flaps. **(A)** Single pedicle advancement flap. **(B)** Double pedicle advancement flap. **(C)** A to T closure. **(D)** Burow's triangle flap.

forward in a straight line into the adjacent defect. The amount of undermining determines the length of the flap, which, due to the inherent elasticity of the skin, is essentially stretched to fill the defect. Some flaps included in this designation are single or double pedicle advancement flaps, the A to T flap, and the Burow's triangle flap.

SINGLE AND DOUBLE PEDICLE ADVANCEMENT FLAPS

Single and double pedicle advancement flaps (see Figure 20.1A,B) are performed easily and are particularly useful when incisions fall in natural parallel folds such as on the forehead. They are also used frequently to repair defects of hair-bearing skin in the eyebrow or mustache, where orientation of the hair shafts is important (Figure 20.2A–D). As the pedicle is advanced into the defect, some bunching of tissue or dog-ear formation may occur at the base of the flap. This is easily remedied by removal of a triangle of skin from the area (Burow's triangle). Theoretically, Burow's triangles can be made at either side of the flap base but whether one or both of these is required depends on the elasticity of the skin.

As is the case with many flaps, one or two key sutures will generally define the entire repair. In the case of a single advancement flap, the leading edge of the flap is sutured to the far wall of the defect. For double advancement flaps, the two leading edges are sutured together. The remaining wound edges are then properly oriented and easily closed.

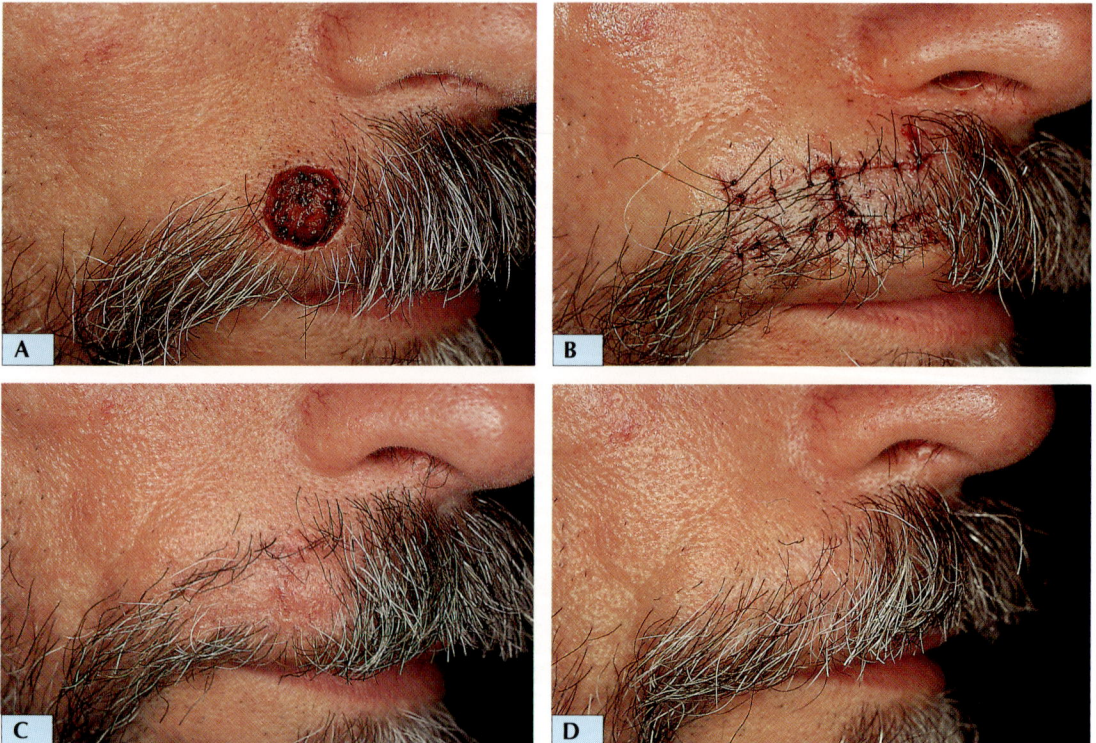

FIGURE 20.2 A double pedicle advancement flap used to restore continuity of the mustache of a 40-year-old man following skin cancer surgery. (A) Surgical defect following Mohs' surgery for a basal cell carcinoma. (B) Postoperative photograph following bilateral advancement flaps. (C) Telogen effluvium occurred at the operative site following surgery. (D) Regrowth of hair with good cosmetic outcome is seen after 10 months.

A TO T FLAP

The A to T flap (see Figure 20.1C) is a bilateral advancement flap in which incisions are made at only one end of the defect. The incision extends from the base of a triangular defect or from one side of a circular defect, allowing the adjacent tissue to be advanced and sutured in a straight line (Figure 20.3 A–F). The flap rotates slightly as it is advanced into the defect. If necessary, one or two Burow's triangles are used.

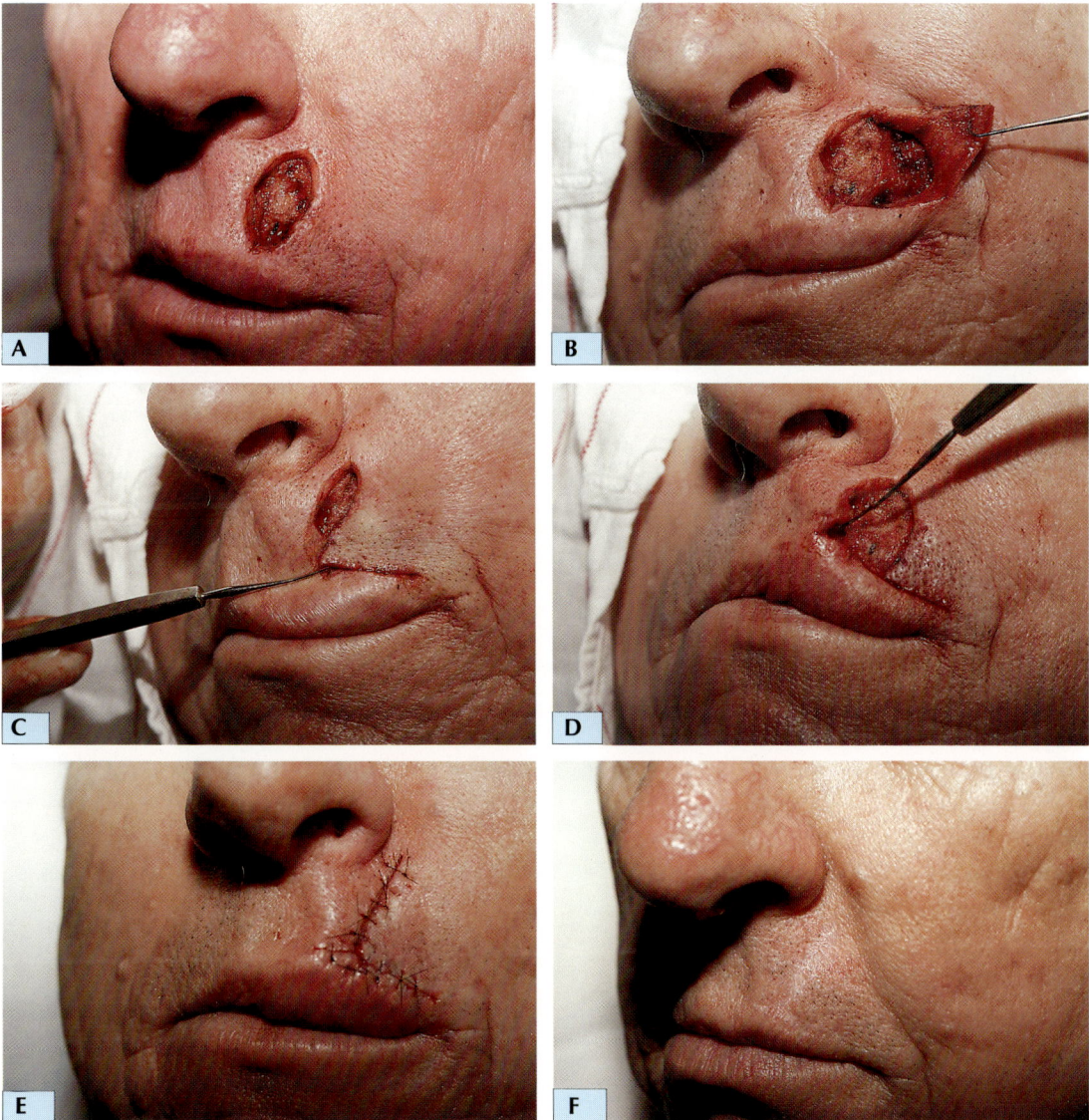

FIGURE 20.3 A to T closure with unequal sides. (A) Preoperative photograph shows a defect at the upper lip following skin cancer surgery. (B) A flap is raised at one side of the defect. (C) A small amount of tension remains as the flap is advanced into the defect. (D) A second flap, this time much smaller, is raised at the other side of the defect to relieve tension. (E) The wound is sutured closed. (F) Postoperative appearance 8 months later shows an acceptable outcome.

BUROW'S TRIANGLE FLAP

The Burow's triangle flap (see Figure 20.1D) is similar to the A to T flap except that it is a single advancement flap designed in such a way as to avoid secondary movement. It is a simple flap that can take advantage of redundant skin not immediately adjacent to the defect. If necessary, tissues can be mobilized from areas at some distance from the wound. A Burow's triangle is always used and its size will vary with the elasticity and looseness of the skin.

ROTATION FLAPS

STANDARD ROTATION FLAP

The rotation flap (Figure 20.4) is another simple flap that redistributes tissue into an adjacent defect. It is created essentially by mak-

ing an arc that extends from the base of a triangular defect. After undermining, the flap is advanced into the defect with a slightly rotational component. A Burow's triangle can be used at the distal end of the arc. Alternatively a back cut is permissible since the flap has a broad base and adequate blood supply (Figure 20.5A–D).

The rotation flap is useful for closing relatively large defects since large amounts of skin can be mobilized. If a single rotation flap will not accomplish complete closure, a second flap can be swung in from the apposing side of the defect (bilateral rotation flap). A variation on the rotation flap is the O to Z closure (see Figure 20.4B), which consists of two rotation flaps, the pedicles of which arise from opposite sides of the defect. Since the pedicles

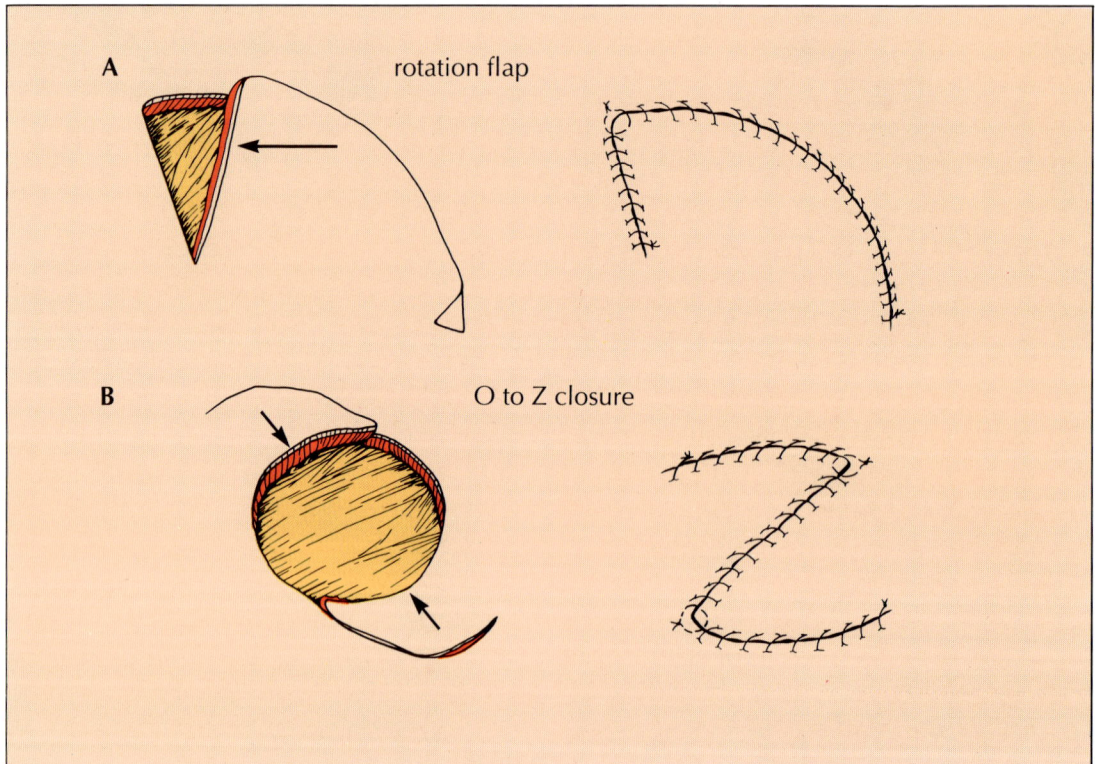

FIGURE 20.4 Schematic drawing showing rotation flaps. **(A)** Simple rotation flap. **(B)** O to Z closure.

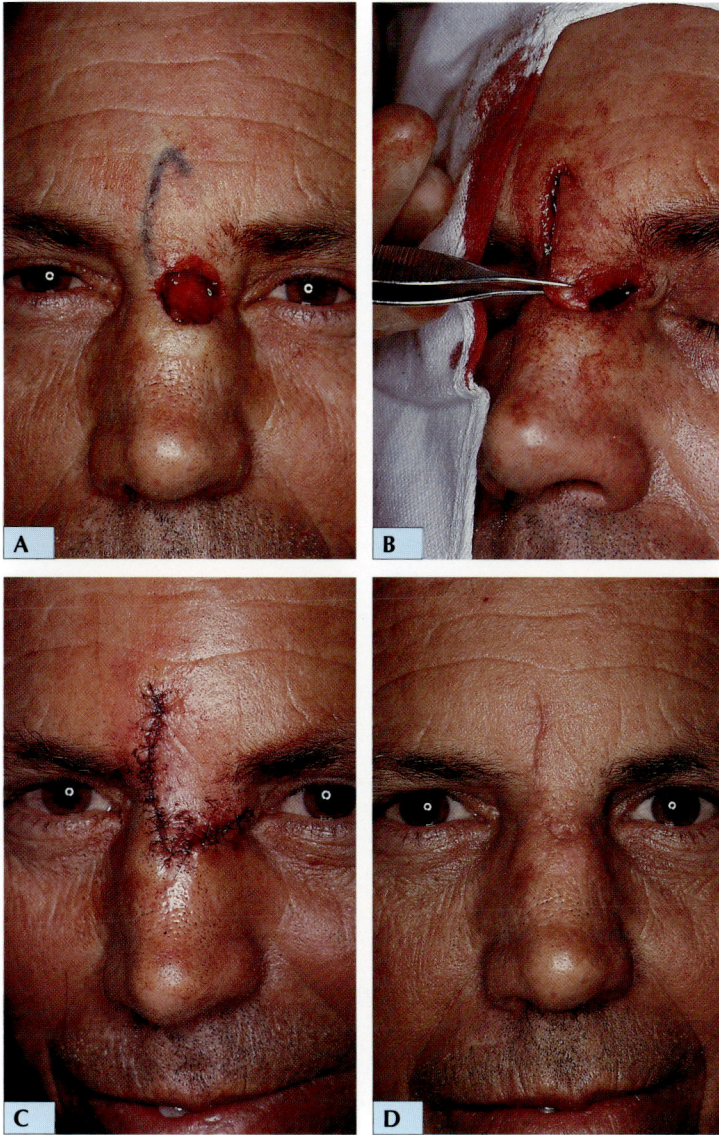

FIGURE 20.5 Rotation flap of the glabella to close a defect of the nasal root following skin cancer surgery. **(A)** The flap is planned to include a back cut. **(B)** The flap has been rotated into the defect and **(C)** sutured in place. The wide pedicle results in a high success rate. **(D)** After 8 weeks, the result is quite acceptable. Note how the major vertical scar lies in a glabellar furrow.

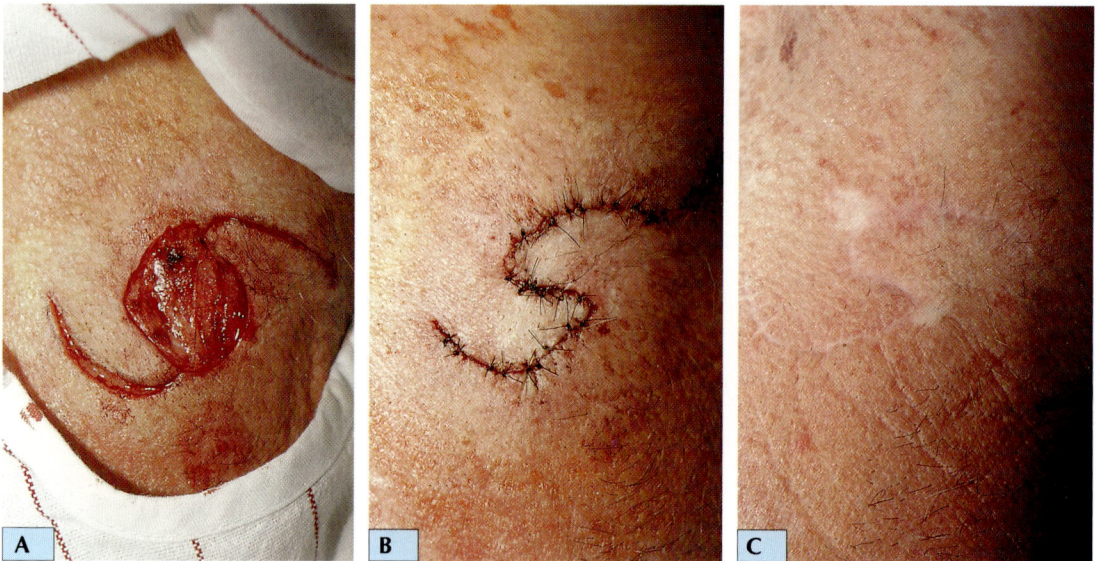

FIGURE 20.6 O to Z closure of a large defect of the neck following skin cancer surgery. **(A)** Two rotation flaps have been created at opposite sides of a circular defect in an area of relatively tight skin. **(B)** The flaps have been rotated inward and sutured in place. **(C)** The scar 4 months later.

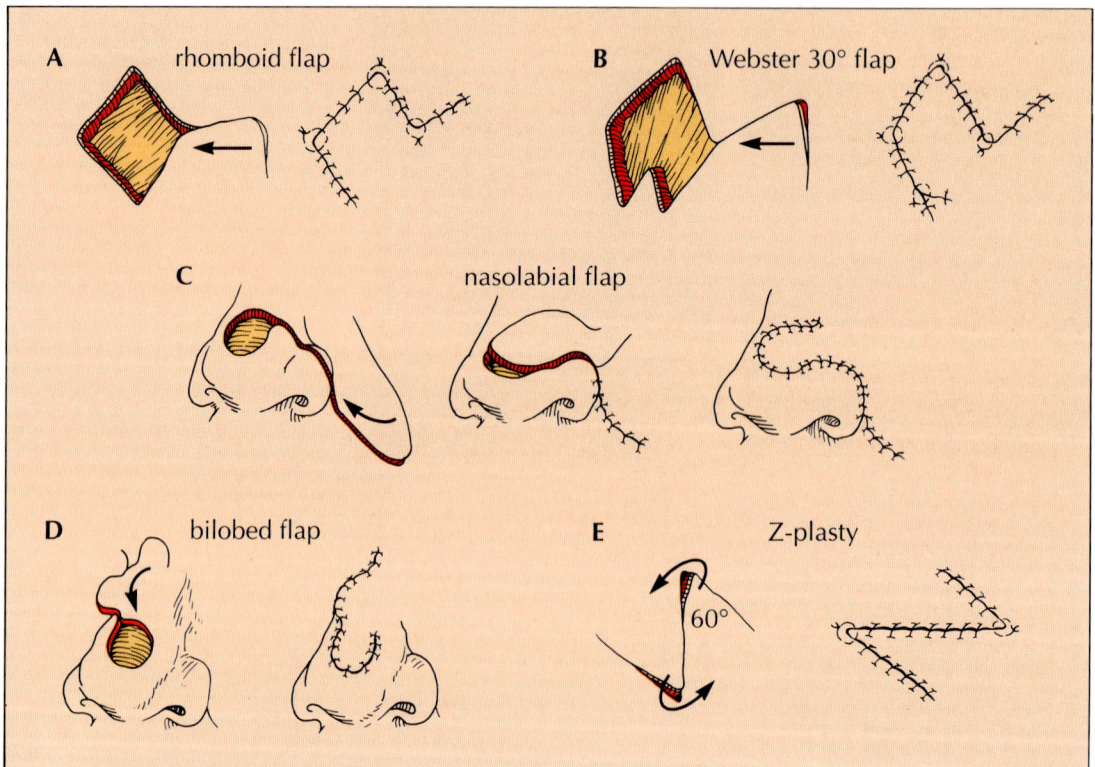

FIGURE 20.7 Schematic drawing showing transposition flaps. **(A)** Rhomboid flap. **(B)** Webster 30° flap. **(C)** Nasolabial flap. **(D)** Bilobed flap. **(E)** Z-plasty.

are quite large, flap tip necrosis is uncommon with this closure (Figure 20.6A–C).

TRANSPOSITION FLAPS

To create a transposition flap (Figure 20.7), a raised flap is transposed across normal intervening skin before it is placed in the defect. A number of common flaps are included in this category, such as the rhomboid flap and its variations, the nasolabial flap, the bilobed flap, and the Z-plasty.

RHOMBOID FLAP

The rhomboid flap (see Figure 20.7A) is very popular among cutaneous surgeons and is quite versatile since it can be designed from any corner and side of the defect. It is based on a precise geometric design (Figure 20.8 A–D). Ideally, the defect is a rhombus (an equilateral parallelogram) with angles of 60° and 120°.

The flap is created by first making a perpendicular incision, of equal length to the sides of the rhombus, from the point of the 120° angle. Another incision of the same length is made at 60°, parallel to one side of the rhombus. After undermining, the flap is transposed into the defect, thereby closing both the primary and secondary defects. The key stitch usually is the one used to close the secondary defect. Since the flap can be brought in from any direction, careful plan-

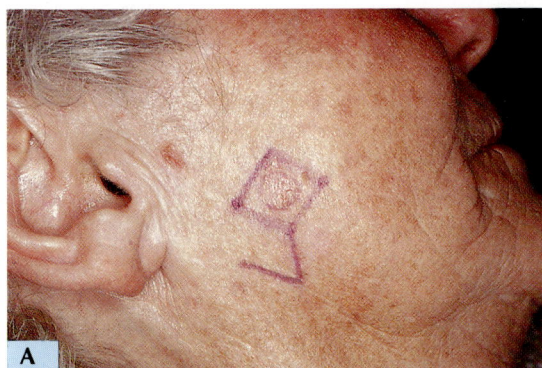

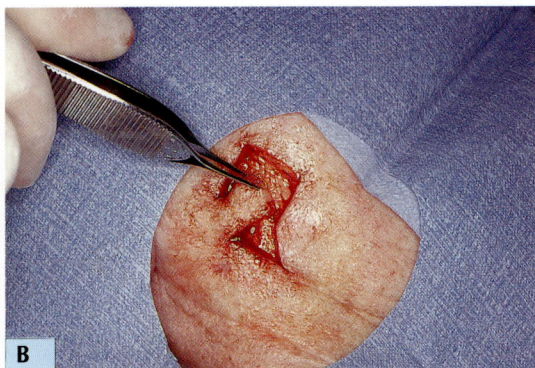

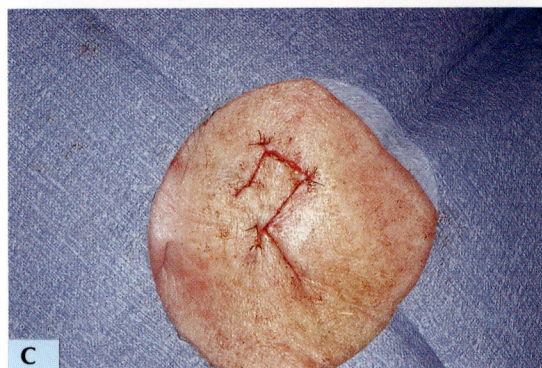

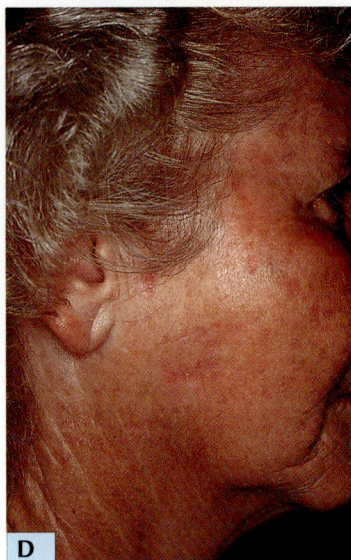

FIGURE 20.8 Rhomboid flap used to repair a defect during skin cancer surgery. **(A)** The flap is designed around a squamous cell carcinoma. **(B)** The flap has been cut, undermined, and transposed into the defect. **(C)** The flap in place. **(D)** Postoperative appearance 2 months later.

ning allows one to take advantage of local factors that may optimize flap movement or hide suture lines (Figure 20.9A–D).

WEBSTER 30° FLAP

The Webster 30° flap (see Figure 20.7B) is a variation of the rhomboid flap that uses an uneven rhomboid defect rather than a rhombus. The 60° angle at the lower portion of the defect is bisected into two 30° angles by an M-plasty. The two incisions of the flap likewise are placed at a 30° angle to one another rather than at the classical 60° angle. The defect is closed by M-plasty and transposition of the flap. The advantage of this variation is that the flap is transposed more easily through a smaller arc.

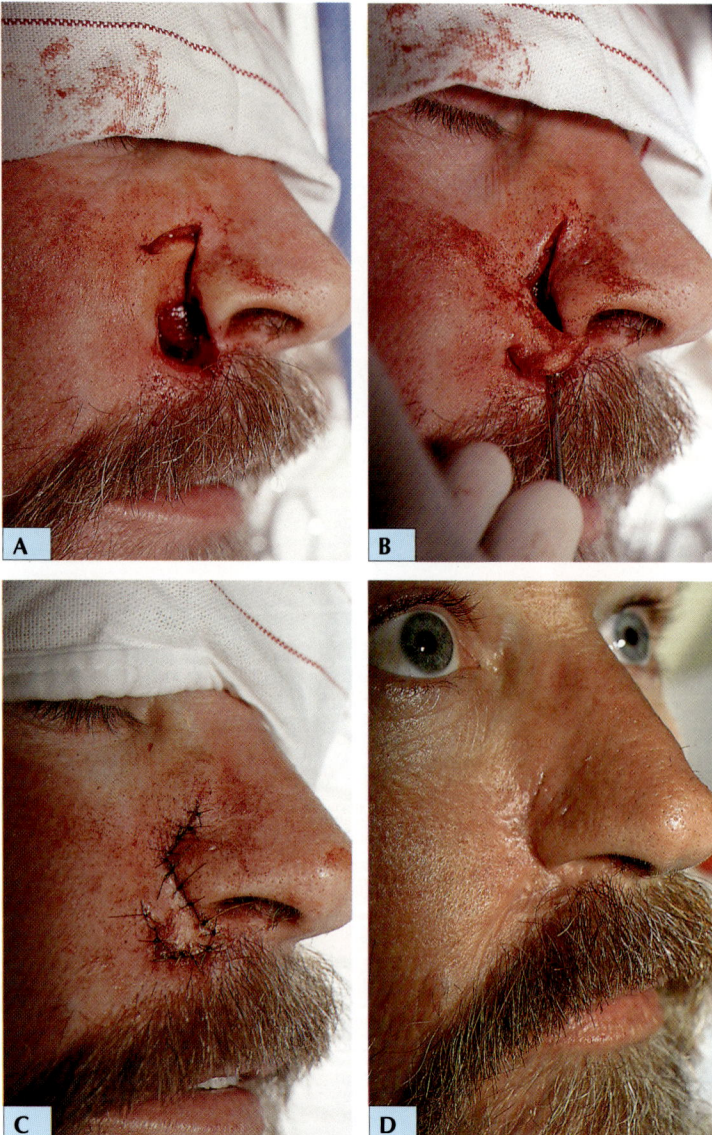

FIGURE 20.9 Rhomboid flap used to repair a defect of the alar-cheek junction. **(A)** The flap is created in such a way as to hide the scar in the nose-cheek junction. **(B)** The flap is swung into the defect. **(C)** Sutures have been placed. **(D)** After 5 months, the outcome is quite acceptable.

NASOLABIAL FLAP

The nasolabial flap (see Figure 20.7C) uses available skin along the nasolabial fold to close defects of the nasal bridge, tip, ala, and upper lip (see Chapter 32). The pedicle of the flap can be based either superiorly or inferiorly. If normal tissue is present between the defect and the base of the flap, its excision is appropriate to prevent a secondary procedure at a later date. When the flap is cut, its distal end should be tapered to a 30° angle to prevent the necessity of later having to repair a dog-ear in the area, when the secondary defect is closed.

The beauty of the nasolabial flap is that the scar from the secondary defect is camouflaged in the nasolabial fold. However, there are some drawbacks, including possible distortion of the nose-cheek crease and the trapdoor effect, which is quite common. The latter problem sometimes can be prevented by ensuring that the flap is thinned to an appropriate thickness prior to its being sutured in place.

BILOBED FLAP

The bilobed flap (see Figure 20.7D) is a large, broad-based rotation flap that is divided into two perpendicular limbs. It is especially useful in situations where relatively loose but inelastic tissue is present at the periphery of the defect. The first limb of the flap is cut to a size similar to that of the defect while the second limb usually is cut a bit smaller and fits into the secondary defect created by the first limb. The advantage of this flap is that distant loose skin can be used to aid in closure of the defect. It is particularly useful on the nose, where excess skin of the glabella can be used indirectly to close the defect. Its disadvantage is that additional scarring is produced.

Z-PLASTY

Although technically consisting of two transposition flaps, the Z-plasty (see Figure 20.7E) is not used to close defects. Rather, it is used to lengthen and reorient scars, to break them up, or to decrease tension. The classical application of Z-plasty is in the treatment of scarring, as occurs with severe burns or keloids, in which contracture has become a problem. A "Z" is prepared, consisting of two small 60° flaps that share a common limb oriented along the scar that needs to be lengthened or reoriented by 90°. The two flaps are then raised and transposed, resulting in an increase in length of up to 75%. Z-plasties are discussed in further detail in Chapter 15 of this Atlas.

SUBCUTANEOUS ISLAND PEDICLE FLAP

In the subcutaneous island pedicle flap (Figure 20.10), a fusiform excision is created that maintains the flap's attachment to the

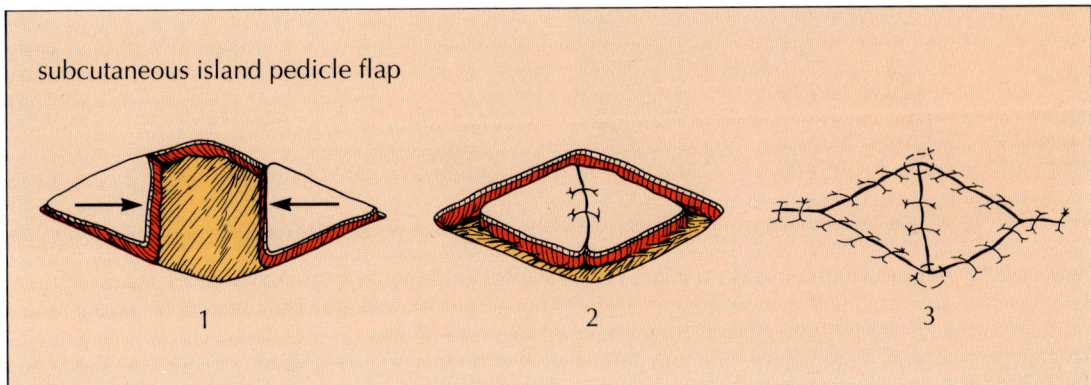

subcutaneous island pedicle flap

1   2   3

FIGURE 20.10 Schematic drawing showing a single subcutaneous island pedicle flap.

subcutaneous tissue via a pedicle. The remainder of the flap is undermined and all dermal restraints are released. The flap is then advanced into the defect on its pedicle (Figure 20.11A–D). Two flaps may be used to close larger defects. The secondary defect is closed easily.

The island flap is unique in that it retains no epidermal or dermal attachment to the donor site even though it maintains a pedicle with the underlying skin. Often, after enough undermining has been achieved to allow the flap to slide forward sufficiently into the wound, only a relatively narrow pedicle remains. Nonetheless the flap has a good rate of success, which is likely due to the fact that it combines attributes of both grafts and flaps in its survival. The flap is fre-

quently called upon in situations in which there is excessive tissue at the edge of the defect but where the prevailing tensile forces do not allow the extra skin to be utilized unless it can somehow be brought forward into the wound.

POSTOPERATIVE WOUND CARE

The mainstay of postoperative wound care is the dressing, which serves to apply slight pressure to the wound while immobilizing it. This helps to minimize postoperative bleeding and potential hematoma formation. Immobilization of the wound also is necessary for the rapid establishment of a blood supply from the wound bed. Pressure dressings usu-

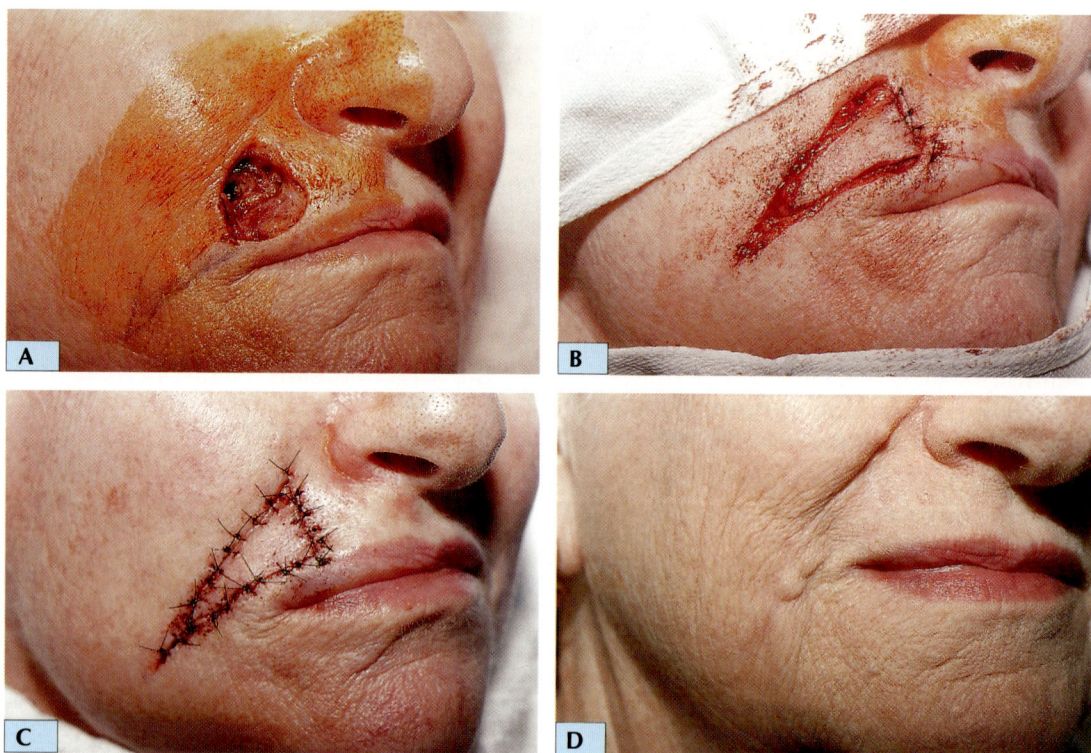

FIGURE 20.11 An island flap is used to repair a large defect at the upper lip. (A) The postoperative defect following removal of a large basal cell carcinoma. (B) The flap has been prepared, moved into the defect, and secured with key sutures. (C) Sutures have been placed. (D) The outcome 11 months later.

ally can be removed within 48 hours and a light protective dressing can be used until suture removal. Prophylactic antibiotics usually are not prescribed unless a particularly large or time-consuming procedure has been undertaken.

Patients are advised that some degree of discomfort, swelling, and erythema should be expected. They are, however, advised to call the office immediately if any of these findings becomes significant or if purulence becomes evident. Another helpful instruction is to ask patients to eat soft, semisolid foods with care for a few days following surgery, if flaps are located in regions that move freely with mastication. In such situations, vigorous chewing can cause excessive flap movement and clot dislodgment with postoperative bleeding.

COMPLICATIONS

On occasion, postoperative hemorrhage, hematoma or seroma formation, necrosis, or infection can occur. Many of these complications are for the most part avoidable. For example, strict attention given to hemostasis before the wound is closed can prevent hema-

toma formation. Likewise, aseptic technique may minimize the likelihood of postoperative infection. Regarding skin flap necrosis, the major causes of partial or total necrosis are excessive tension or poor vascular supply. An attempt should always be made to close skin flaps with the least amount of tension possible. To do so, significant undermining around the defect may be required to achieve additional secondary movement. Obviously, poor flap design also can contribute to this problem.

With regard to blood supply, it has already been stressed that the pedicle must be wide enough to support the flap through its entire length. If a narrow flap is created, flap tip necrosis is more likely to occur (Figure 20.12). The trap-door effect, as noted earlier, is not an infrequent occurrence with certain types of flaps, particularly the nasolabial and rhomboid flaps (Figure 20.13). It may resolve on its own over 6 to 9 months or a "defatting procedure" may be required, in which the edge of the flap is lifted up and excess fat and fibrotic material are removed. Some clinicians find intralesional injections of steroids to be helpful in treatment of the trap-door effect.

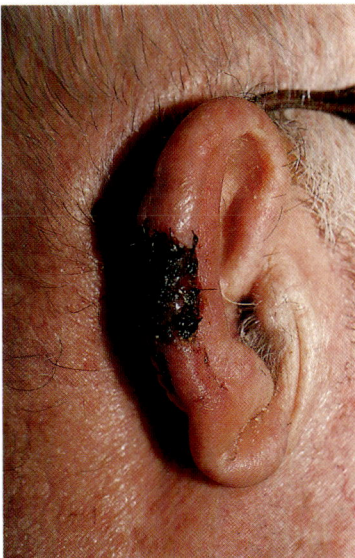

FIGURE 20.12 Flap tip necrosis occurred when a long, narrow advancement flap was used to repair a defect at the rim of the ear. Flaps with wider pedicles are more likely to survive.

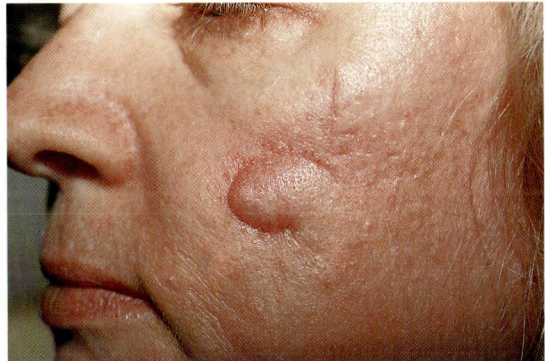

FIGURE 20.13 Trap-door effect seen after a transposition flap was used to repair a cheek defect.

SUGGESTIONS FOR FURTHER READING

Borges AF. Pitfalls in flap design. Ann Plast Surg. 1982;9:201-209.

Dzubow LM. Facial Flaps. Biomechanics and Regional Application. Norwalk, Ct: Appleton & Lange;1989.

Grabb WC, Myers MB. Skin Flaps. Boston, Mass: Little, Brown & Co Inc;1975.

Stegman SJ, Tromovitch TA, Glogau RG. Basics of Dermatologic Surgery. Chicago, Ill: Year Book Medical Publishers Inc; 1982:73-90.

Stegman SJ. Planning closure of a surgical wound. J Dermatol Surg Oncol. 1978;4:390-393.

Tromovitch TA, Stegman SJ, Glogau RG. Flaps and Grafts in Dermatologic Surgery. Chicago, Ill: Year Book Medical Publishers Inc;1989.

Wheeland RG. Random pattern flaps. In: Roenigk RK, Roenigk HH Jr, eds. Dermatologic Surgery. Principles and Practice. New York, NY: Marcel Dekker Inc;1989:265-322.

chapter *21*

GRAFTS

A knowledge of tissue grafting techniques and appropriate donor site selection can be an important part of the armamentarium of the cutaneous surgeon faced with a variety of reconstructive problems. To achieve the best possible results in a variety of situations, the ideal tissue graft should create a minimal donor-site defect, provide good cosmetic match, and function properly in the reconstruction of the defect.

Free skin grafts, such as those described throughout this chapter, are completely detached from their donor sites prior to being transferred to their recipient beds. Therefore, the recipient bed, as the sole source of nourishment for the transplanted graft, should contain adequate blood supply and underlying soft tissue to enable survival of the transplanted tissue. In situations where the recipient bed is relatively avascular, such as bone not covered by periosteum or cartilage without its perichondrium, free skin grafts are not a reconstructive option.

Skin grafts are divided into two categories: split-thickness and full-thickness. Full-thickness skin grafts consist of epidermis and full-thickness dermis and vary in thickness only in terms of the thickness of the skin from which they are harvested (Figure 21.1). Split-thickness skin grafts are composed of epidermis and a variable quantity of dermis. They are described as thin, intermediate, or thick depending on the amount of dermis included (Figure 21.2). Split-thickness skin grafts generally are harvested with a mechanical dermatome while full-thickness skin grafts are harvested by sharp dissection with a scalpel.

In general, where the characteristics of the defect allow it, the use of a full-thickness skin graft is preferred as it provides a better contour match and results in less postoperative contracture than does a split-thickness skin graft. To allow the use of a full-thickness skin graft, the defect must be characterized by a well-vascularized recipient bed and limited total surface area. For a defect that is relatively large, a split-thickness skin graft may be needed as its total potential donor area is virtually unlimited.

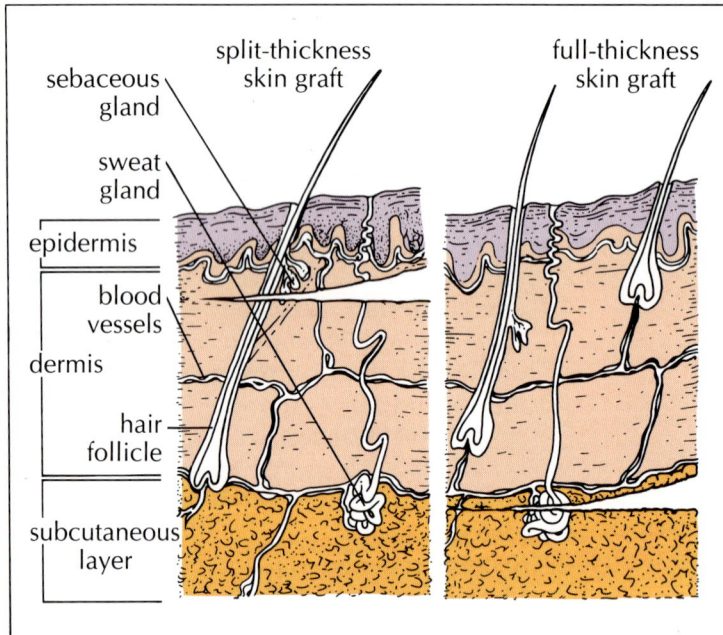

FIGURE 21.1 Free skin grafts are divided into two main types: split-thickness skin grafts and full-thickness skin grafts. This schematic drawing illustrates the constituents of each.

SPLIT-THICKNESS SKIN GRAFTS

DONOR SITES

Split-thickness skin grafts are harvested from a variety of donor sites, the most common of which are the inner aspect of the upper arm and the upper thigh. Selection of the appropriate donor site is determined by the specific needs of the defect including general color match, the hair-bearing characteristics of the skin, and the quantity of tissue required. As a rule, the inner aspect of the upper arm offers the surgeon hairless skin that is lighter in color than normal facial skin and has a limited total quantity available. By contrast, the region of the upper thigh is often hair-bearing, has darker cutaneous pigmentation, and offers extensive donor site surface area. It should be noted that split-thickness skin grafts can be expected to contract on the order of 10% to 20% of their total surface area. In areas where such contracture will produce distortion of important facial landmarks, other techniques should be considered.

For our purposes, the Padgett dermatome has provided a reliable and safe meth-

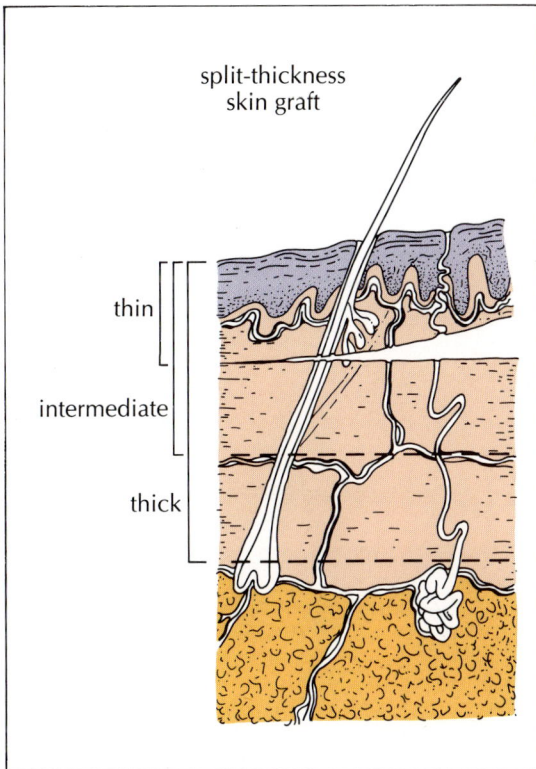

FIGURE 21.2 Schematic drawing showing the varying degrees of thickness of a split-thickness skin graft that may be harvested by adjusting the setting on the dermatome.

od of harvesting split-thickness skin grafts ranging in thickness from 0.005 to 0.03 inches (Figure 21.3A–D). For harvesting of the graft, a local field block may be used or the patient may be placed under general anesthesia. After successful harvesting of the graft, hemostasis is obtained at the donor site by the application of topical epinephrine and local pressure. The donor site is then covered with Tegaderm and wrapped with Kerlix. The Tegaderm dressing is maintained for 7 to 10 days, at which time the patient is advised to remove the dressing in the shower or bath and bacitracin ointment is applied for 5 to 7 days until total re-epithelization is obtained.

RECIPIENT BED

After harvesting of the graft and prior to its placement in the recipient bed, meticulous hemostasis is obtained using bipolar cautery. Hemostasis at the recipient bed is particularly important to prevent the formation of hematomas and/or seromas, which compromise adhesion of the graft to its bed.

The graft is then placed in its recipient bed and stabilized at its margins using either sutures or stainless steel staples. An additional measure, that of pie crusting, may be taken to prevent the formation of hematomas and/or seromas in relatively large skin grafts. The technique is accomplished by gentle lifting of the graft and excising of 3- to 6-mm slits in an irregular pattern throughout the graft. A bolster dressing is then applied, which enhances the survival of the split-thickness skin graft by providing stable approximation of the graft to the recipient bed (Figure 21.4A–I).

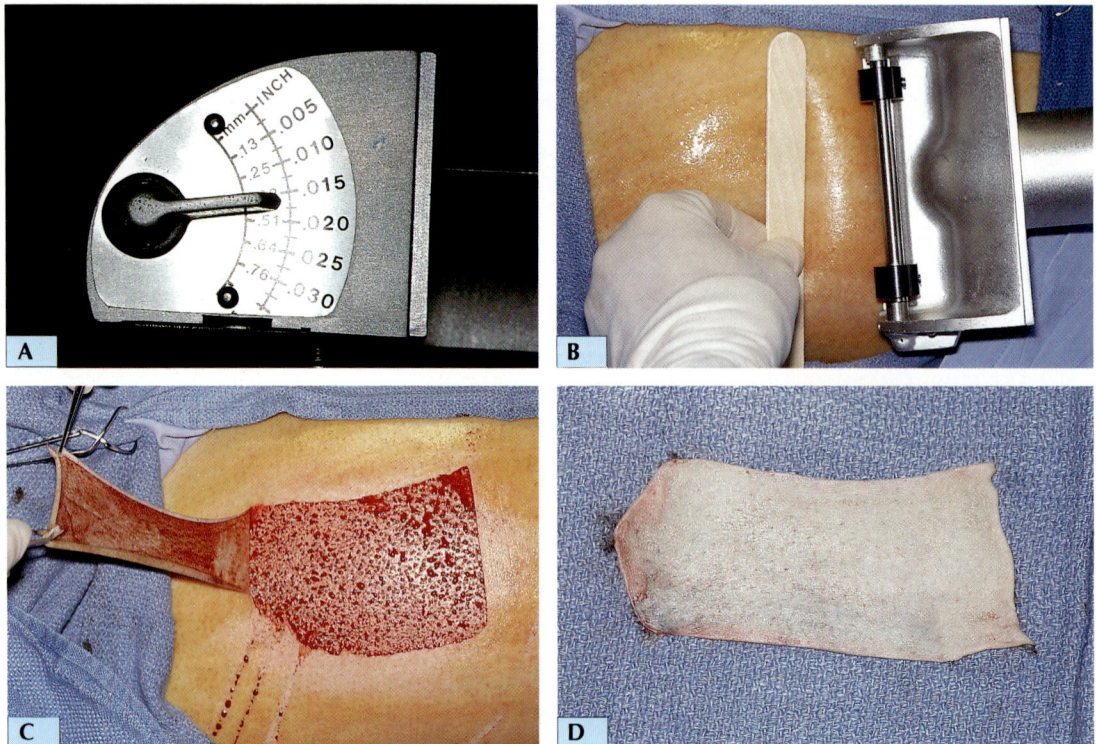

FIGURE 21.3 (A) Padgett dermatome with adjustable settings ranging from 0.005 to 0.03 inches. (B) An intermediate split-thickness skin graft is harvested from the upper thigh using the Padgett dermatome. The skin is prepared with betadine solution and mineral oil and gentle downward pressure is applied with a tongue blade to facilitate harvesting. (C) The graft is harvested and amputated at its base. (D) Appearance of the 5 x 9-cm split-thickness intermediate skin graft at the completion of harvesting.

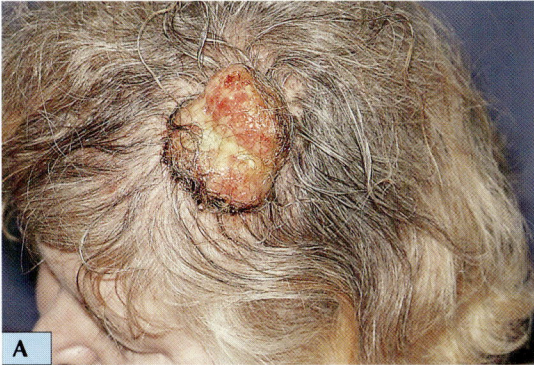

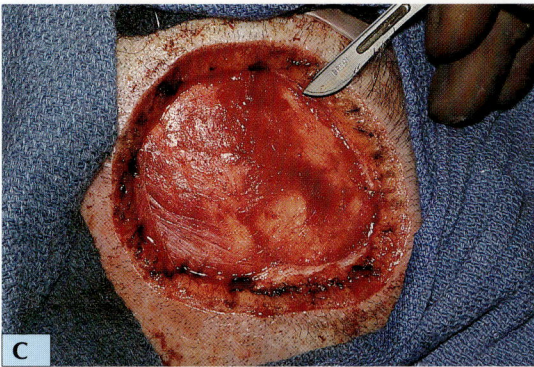

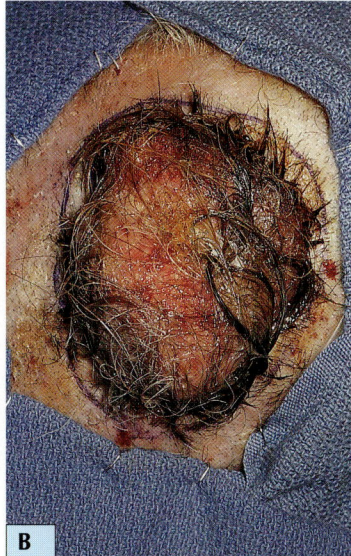

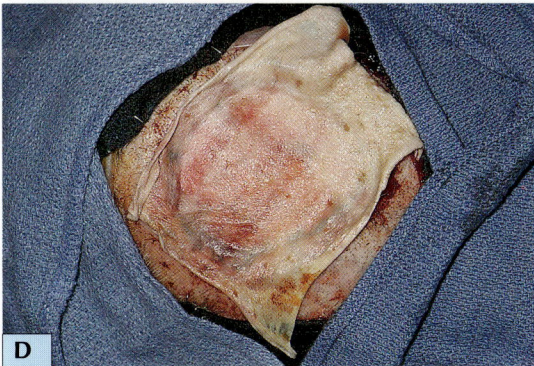

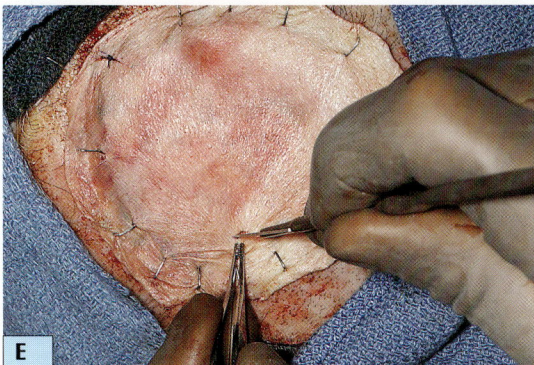

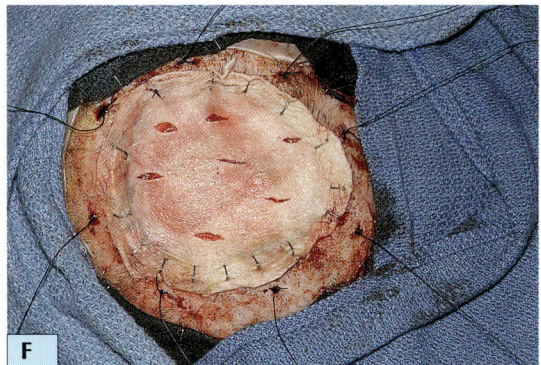

FIGURE 21.4 (A) A 62-year-old woman with a slowly progressive 7 x 7-cm scalp lesion. **(B)** The lesion is prepared and ready for surgical excision. **(C)** It is excised with careful attention to preservation of the pericranium and a beveled excision technique is utilized to increase the total surface area of the vascular bed for placement of the split-thickness skin graft. **(D)** The skin graft has been harvested from the upper thigh and placed into the recipient bed. **(E)** The skin graft is then overlapped at the margins of the defect, stabilized with staples, and a pie-crusting technique is used to minimize the risk of hematoma and/or seroma formation. **(F)** Eight bolster sutures of 3-0 silk are positioned approximately 2 cm from the periphery of the margins of the defect. The sutures are placed through the full thickness of the skin and do not incorporate the graft.

(continued on next page)

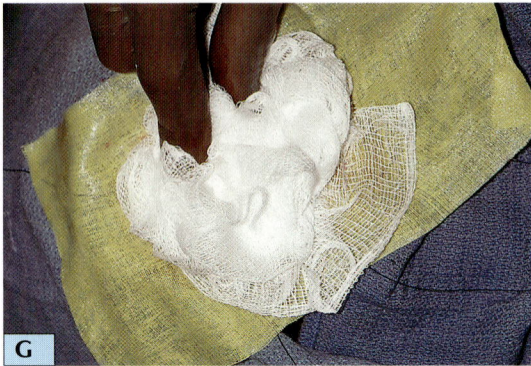

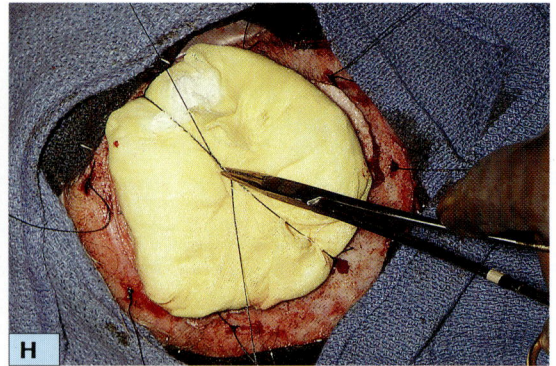

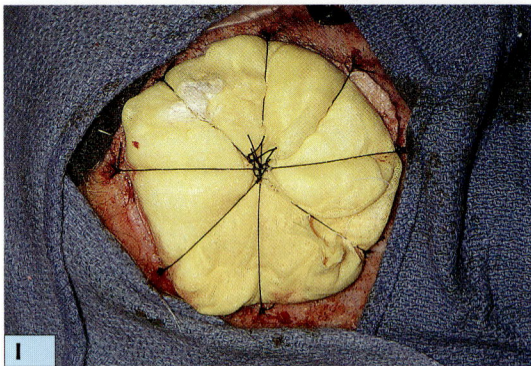

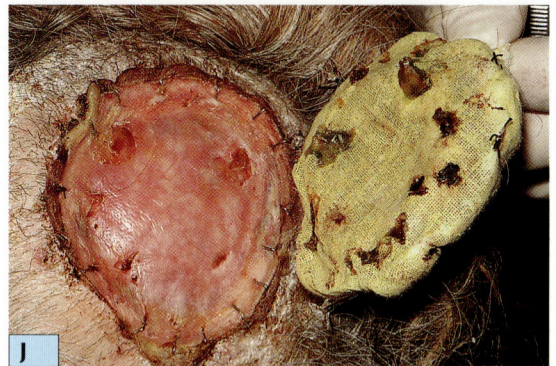

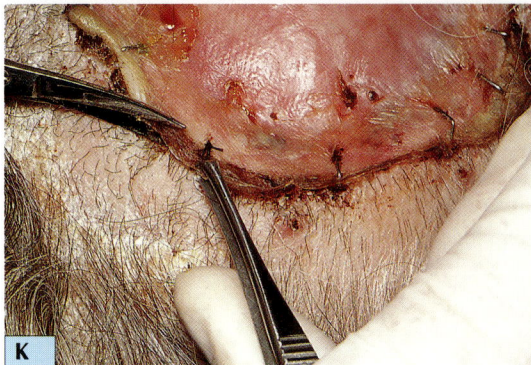

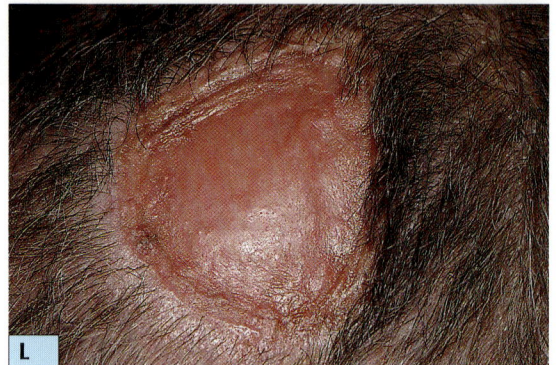

(G) Xeroform gauze is placed over the skin graft and cotton fluffs are packed within the Xeroform. **(H)** The Xeroform/cotton fluff dressing is stabilized utilizing a tie-over technique that employs the previously placed 3-0 silk. A surgeon's knot is placed, which is secured by the use of a Webster needle holder to grasp the first knot until it can be secured with a second throw. **(I)** The bolster dressing is secured in place over the split-thickness skin graft to minimize the risk of hematoma and/or seroma formation. **(J)** Appearance of the split-thickness skin graft after 10 days of stabilization by the bolster. Note crusting at the margins of the graft and the pinkish coloration, which are typical of the healthy split-thickness skin graft at this stage. **(K)** With the bolster removed, the necrotic overlapping margins of the split-thickness skin graft are debrided. **(L)** Appearance of the graft at 6 weeks post surgery. The patient will be followed every 8 to 12 weeks for 1 year to monitor skin graft viability.

For split-thickness skin grafts, overlapping of the graft across the margins of the defect (see Figure 21.4E) is a reliable technique that helps to simplify accurate graft placement. The technique anticipates necrosis of the skin graft to the recipient bed margin and ensures accurate tailoring when the bolster dressing is removed. Removal of the bolster dressing and sutures occurs at 7 to 10 days (Figure 21.4J–L).

FULL-THICKNESS SKIN GRAFTS

DONOR SITES

Full-thickness skin grafts may be harvested in the head and neck region from the preauricular, postauricular, or supraclavicular areas (Figure 21.5). The preauricular area has proven useful for the reconstruction of nasal

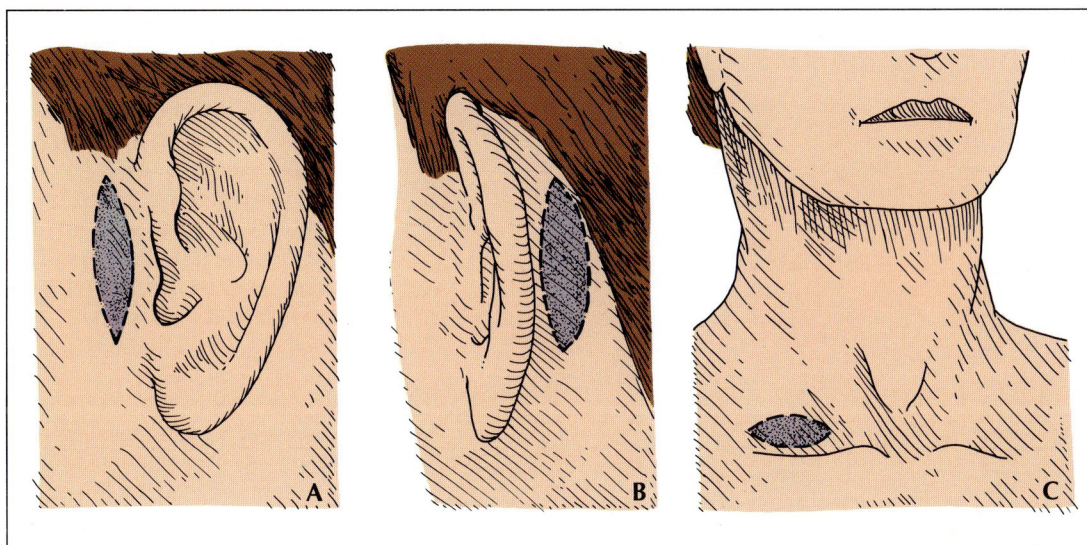

FIGURE 21.5 Full-thickness skin graft donor sites: (A) preauricular skin; (B) postauricular skin; and (C) supraclavicular skin. In general, the donor sites are excised to a specific pattern based on an x-ray template of the defect, to which modifications are made to enable appropriate closure.

defects in that the thickness and color of the skin are well matched. In addition, the donor site incision may be camouflaged in the preauricular crease (Figure 21.6A–D). For the full-thickness reconstruction of auricular defects, the postauricular area is useful as its color and skin texture are similar. For defects requiring thicker full-thickness grafts, the supraclavicular area is most suitable as it has inherent, thick epidermal and dermal components as well as an abundant subcutaneous layer, which if necessary may be harvested with the full-thickness skin graft. Again, it

should be kept in mind that the suitability of any of these donor sites to yield a full-thickness skin graft is limited by the quantity of tissue needed for reconstruction of the defect. If the defect is large, it may be better served by a split-thickness skin graft, whose potential donor area is much greater.

The most important step in the harvesting of a full-thickness skin graft is the creation of an accurate pattern or template of the defect. The template is best made using clear x-ray film, which can be customized to reflect the specific surgical defect (Figure 21.7A–C).

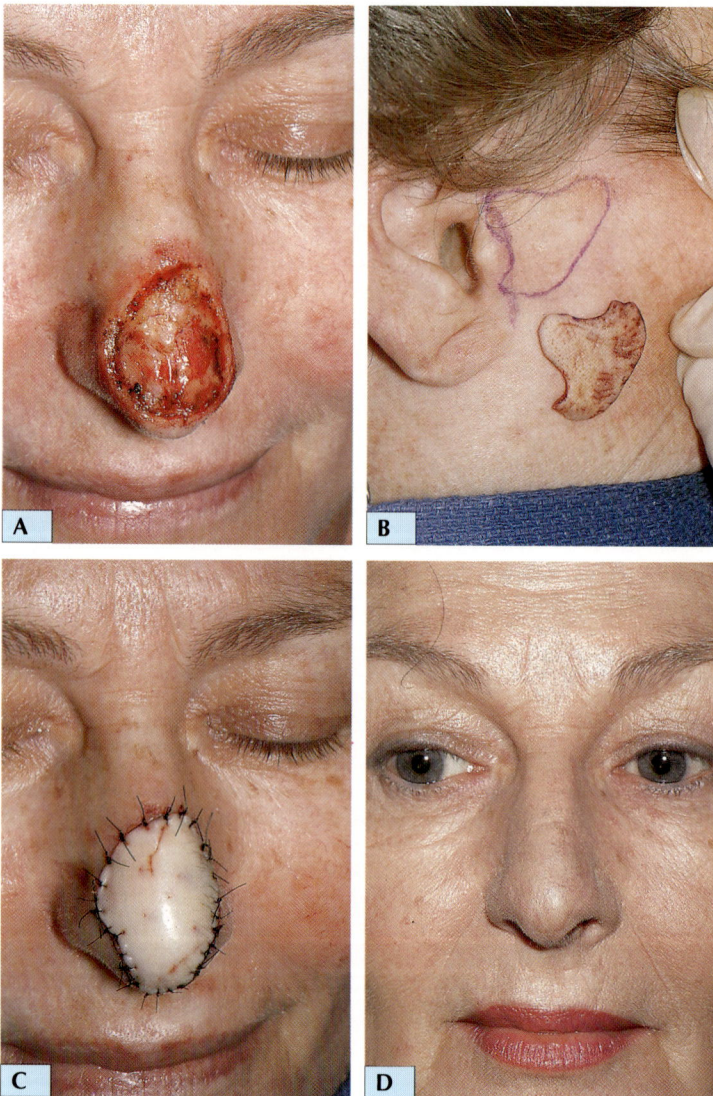

FIGURE 21.6 (A) Patient with a basal cell carcinoma at the tip of the nose, excised by Mohs' technique, who presented for reconstruction of the nasal subunit. **(B)** A preauricular full-thickness skin graft is harvested based on an x-ray template. **(C)** The graft is sutured into position using 6-0 nylon. **(D)** Result after 1 year. It should be kept in mind that full-thickness skin grafts may undergo color changes for a period of 12 to 18 months and that refinement at the skin graft margins may in some cases require the use of dermabrasion, usually 6 to 12 months after graft placement.

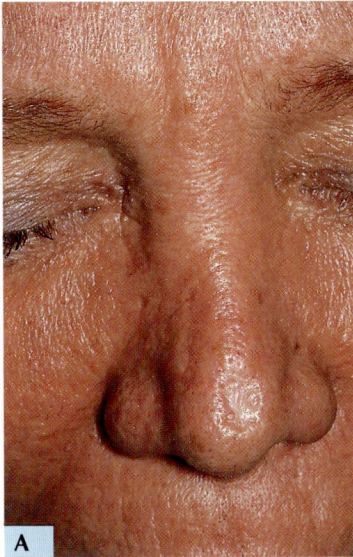

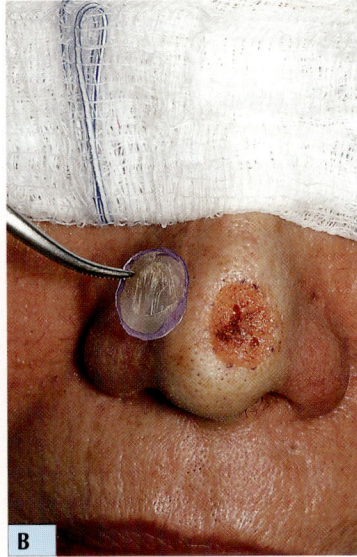

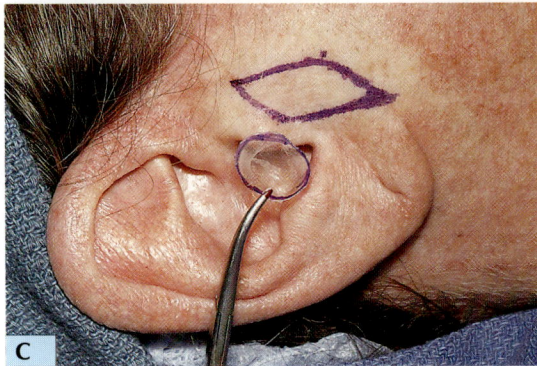

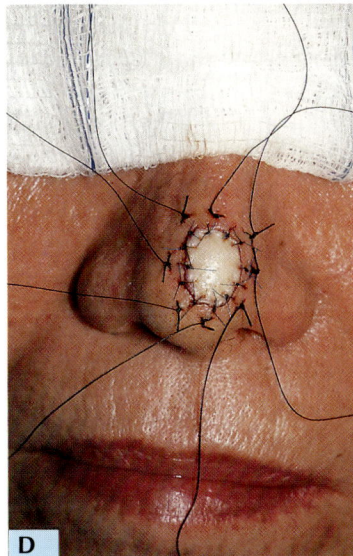

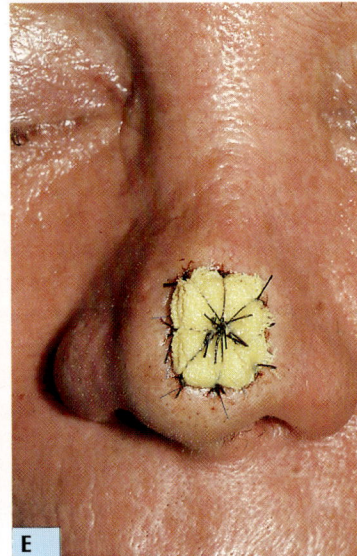

FIGURE 21.7 (A) A 55-year-old woman, 1 year post excision of a lentigo maligna excised by Mohs' technique that was allowed to heal secondarily. The patient was unhappy with the depressed and irregular nature of the scar. (B) The scar tissue is excised and an accurate pattern of the defect is obtained using clear x-ray film as a template. (C) A full-thickness preauricular skin graft is harvested based on the x-ray template, after appropriate injection of 1% lidocaine with epinephrine 1:100,000. (D) The full-thickness skin graft is carefully tailored and suture stabilized at the periphery using 6-0 nylon and 4-0 silk sutures placed circumferentially in preparation for bolster application. (E) A bolster dressing of Xeroform gauze is fashioned and stabilized utilizing a tie-over technique that employs the previously placed 4-0 silk.

A full-thickness skin graft, specific to the defect, can then be harvested from the donor site after it has been injected with local anesthetic with epinephrine to reduce small vessel bleeding and the risk of post-excision hematoma.

After 10 to 15 minutes, the graft is harvested using a combination of sharp and blunt dissection with a #15 knife blade and sharp soft-tissue scissors. The technique of harvesting in most cases will minimize the removal of subcutaneous tissue by careful adherence to the plane between the subcutaneous tissue and the subdermal vascular plexus. However, if the defect demands added soft-tissue bulk, additional subcutaneous tissue may be harvested along with the full-thickness graft. The donor site defect should then be closed in two layers, using 4-0 Vicryl or PDS subcutaneously and 5-0 or 6-0 nylon externally, after adequate hemostasis has been obtained using bipolar cautery. The sutures are left in place for 5 to 7 days.

RECIPIENT BED

Once harvested from the donor site, the graft may be defatted. It should then be accurately positioned and suture stabilized to the margins of the defect using 5-0 or 6-0 nylon. Meticulous hemostasis is a prerequisite for successful graft survival and in our experience is best obtained using bipolar cautery, which minimizes thermal damage while maximizing vessel coagulation. The key difference between the placement of a full-thickness skin graft and that of a split-thickness skin graft is that the full-thickness graft demands accurate and detailed tailoring at the time of placement while the split-thickness graft may overlap the margins of the defect. Stabilization of the full-thickness skin graft is optimized by use of a bolster dressing, described previously for the split-thickness skin graft. The bolster dressing and sutures should remain in place for a period of 7 to 10 days, after which time they are removed (Figure 21.7D,E).

COMPOSITE GRAFTS

Composite grafts by definition consist of cutaneous and cartilaginous components. They are especially useful for the repair of nasal alar defects resulting from facial burns or tumor excisions. The helical crus of the auricle provides the ideal donor site for the harvesting of composite grafts of varying sizes. This anatomic area provides a graft composed of cartilage with cutaneous coverage on either side and it has the appropriate thin edge and gentle curvature necessary for sophisticated reconstruction of the nasal alar margin (Figure 21.8A–E). The donor site can be closed primarily with minimal defect.

The limiting factor in this technique is the size of the defect. For defects greater than 1.5 cm in length across the alar margin, the graft is at risk because of its reliance on the margins of the recipient bed for its blood supply. Additionally, the blood supply may be compromised and survival rates reduced in patients who smoke, as smoking has been shown to affect small vessel perfusion of the facial skin.

COMPLICATIONS

The complications encountered with skin grafting relate primarily to problems in appropriate selection of recipient beds and in stabilization of the skin grafts. Hematoma formation may lead to skin graft necrosis and generally is the result of inadequate attention to hemostasis and/or inadequate immobilization of the graft. Immobility for a period of 7 to 10 days minimizes the risk of hematoma or seroma formation, both of which deprive the skin graft of its adhesion to the recipient bed and thereby reduce skin graft survival for both split-thickness and full-thickness grafts. Related to the need for proper immobilization, skin graft infection rates also are minimal in those grafts in which hematomas and/or seromas do not develop.

Specific anatomic areas that do not lend themselves well to bolster placement include

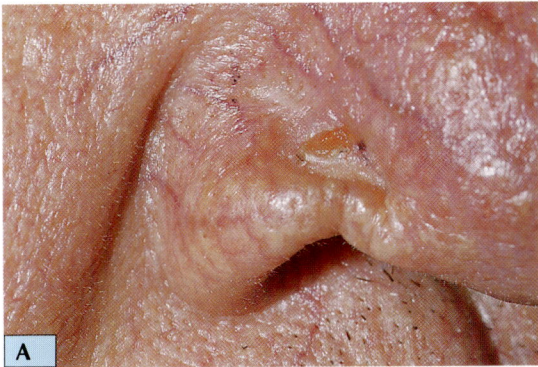

FIGURE 21.8 (A) This patient presented with a recurrent basal cell carcinoma of the nasal ala. **(B)** A wide full-thickness resection of the recurrent disease was performed. **(C)** An auricular composite graft is planned for harvesting from the auricular helix. **(D)** The composite graft is sewn into position for immediate reconstruction of the alar defect. **(E)** Result of the reconstruction at 2 months.

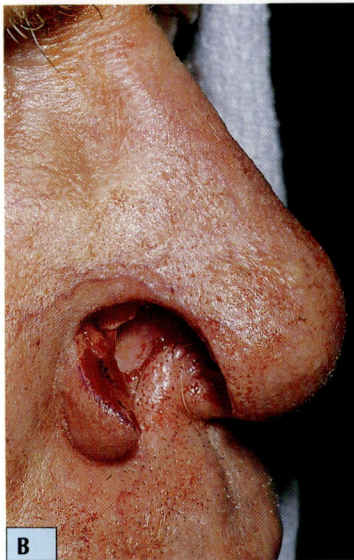

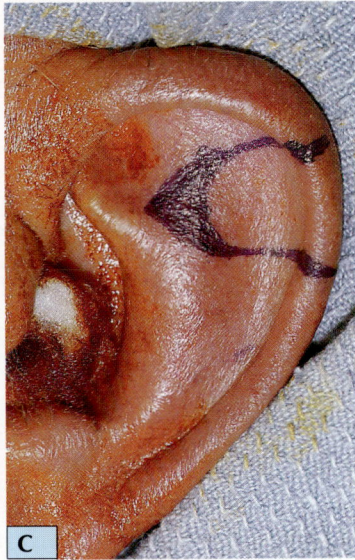

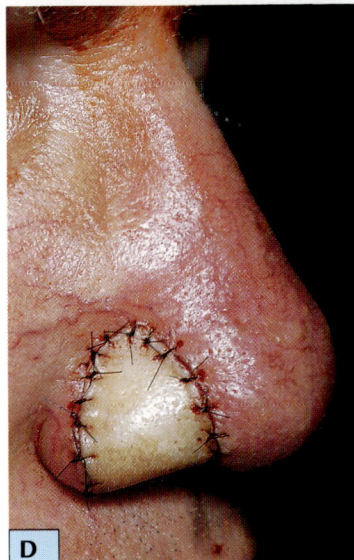

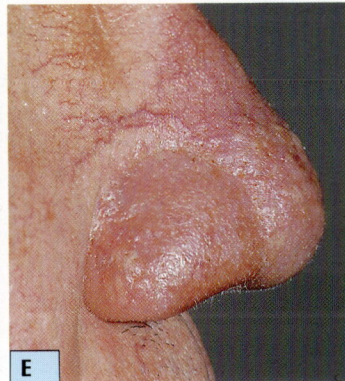

the oral cavity, the nasal mucosa, and the hypopharynx. For stabilization of split-thickness or full-thickness skin grafts to cover defects in these areas, a mattress suture technique may be used, which requires stabilization of the graft at the margins of the defect. Additional mid-graft stability is obtained by the utilization of running mattress sutures of absorbable material to approximate the graft to the recipient bed.

Split-thickness and full-thickness skin grafts, as well as composite grafts, provide the cutaneous surgeon with an effective and reliable means of coverage of cutaneous defects. Surgeons, however, should bear in mind that the techniques described herein are limited by the specific recipient bed encountered and its suitability for the particular reconstructive problem at hand. For example, when the defect involves a large or an exposed area of facial skin, other options such as local flaps or tissue expansion should be considered, as color and contour match may be less than ideal (Figure 21.9).

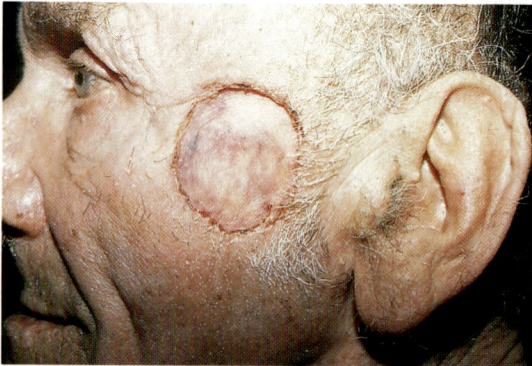

FIGURE 21.9 A 62-year-old man following excision of a basal cell carcinoma of the cheek and temporal region reconstructed immediately with a split-thickness skin graft. This patient's result illustrates a common problem of split-thickness skin graft usage in that the repair provides a poor color and contour match. In this situation, local flaps and/or tissue expansion would have been appropriate alternatives to consider.

SUGGESTIONS FOR FURTHER READING

Barrett GE, Koopmann CF. Skin grafts: physiology and clinical considerations. In: Otolaryngologic Clinics of North America. Symposium on Wound Healing. 1984; 17(5):335-352.

Brown JB, McDowell F. Skin Grafting. 3rd ed. Philadelphia, Pa: JB Lippincott Co; 1958.

Hirokawa RH, Stark TW, Pruet CW, Stucker FJ Jr. Skin grafts. In: Otolaryngologic Clinics of North America. Symposium on Plastic Surgery of the Face. 1982;15(1):133-145.

McCarthy JG. Skin grafts. In: Rudolph R, Ballantyne DL Jr. Plastic Surgery. General Principles. Philadelphia, Pa: WB Saunders Co; 1990;1:1221-1274.

Vecchione TR. A technique for obtaining uniform split-thickness skin graft. Arch Surg. 1974;109:837.

chapter 22

SURGICAL TREATMENT OF KELOIDS

Keloid scars are among the most perplexing of disorders treated by dermatologic surgeons. Caused by the formation of excessive amounts of collagen in the corium during tissue repair, keloids are most likely to afflict those of black heritage. The major difficulty in their treatment is their propensity for recurrence after otherwise unsupplemented surgical removal. Essentially 100% of keloids can be expected to recur within 4 years of such therapy. For this reason, maintaining an extended remission after keloidectomy is a formidable challenge for dermatologic surgeons.

In the treatment of keloids, several factors must be kept in mind when surgical outcomes are predicted. First, certain locations are often associated with more rapid keloid recurrence after surgical excision. These include areas of high skin tension, particularly those overlying bony prominences (eg, presternal area and shoulders). Lesions in areas of minimal tension, such as the earlobes, are less prone to rapid recurrence after surgery. Nevertheless, remissions tend to be prolonged only when adjuvant therapy, such as intralesional injection of steroids, is combined with surgical keloidectomy.

Some keloids exhibit greater clinical activity than others. Those characterized by claw-like peripheral extensions, often dumbbell-shaped, are among the most resistant to therapy (Figure 22.1). These tend to be located in anatomic sites of high skin tension, such as the presternal area, and exhibit the greatest tendency to recur after surgical excision, even when adjuvant therapy is administered. Because of this high failure rate, we prefer to avoid surgery on these particular lesions.

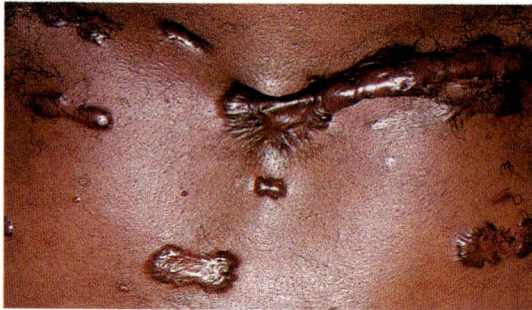

TYPES OF SURGICAL THERAPY

Our preferred treatment modality for keloids is cold steel surgery. Alternative treatments include cryosurgery, CO_2 laser surgery, and electrosurgery but we have found these modalities no more effective than scalpel surgery. All methods of treatment must be supplemented with intralesional steroids or other adjuvant measures. If laser or electrosurgery is used, the thermal damage that may occur adjacent to the incision can act as a stimulus for renewed keloid formation.

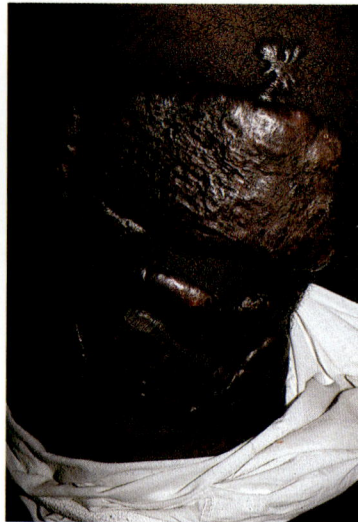

FIGURE 22.1 Multiple dumbbell-shaped keloids present at the presternal region. Note that the tumors are oriented along the lines of greatest local tension. This type of keloid tends to recur promptly after surgical procedures, even when adjuvant therapy is administered. Surgery in these lesions should therefore be avoided.

FIGURE 22.2 Massive keloid formation at skin graft donor sites on the left buttock and thigh of a 38-year-old man. The patient had undergone excision of another keloid with a split-thickness skin graft, harvested from this location, used for repair.

Surgical treatment may involve simple excisions, skin grafts, or skin flaps. The choice of a specific treatment method should be based on the size, location, and anticipated resultant skin tension. Whenever possible, simple excision is usually the best alternative. However, this is possible only for relatively small lesions in areas where skin tension is minimal. Excessive tension on the suture line will stimulate fibroblast activity, leading to increased fibrosis and a greater probability of renewed keloid formation.

When simple excision and closure resulting in a relaxed incision line are not possible, tension-relieving procedures, such as skin grafts or skin flaps, may be required. Unfortunately, keloid formation occurs at skin graft donor sites in approximately 50% of cases (Figure 22.2). One way to avoid this complication is to harvest the graft from the skin overlying the keloid, thus creating no additional site of skin trauma. This technique is particularly appropriate for treatment of very large keloids (Figures 22.3A–C and 22.4A–E).

Skin flaps are very useful for smaller

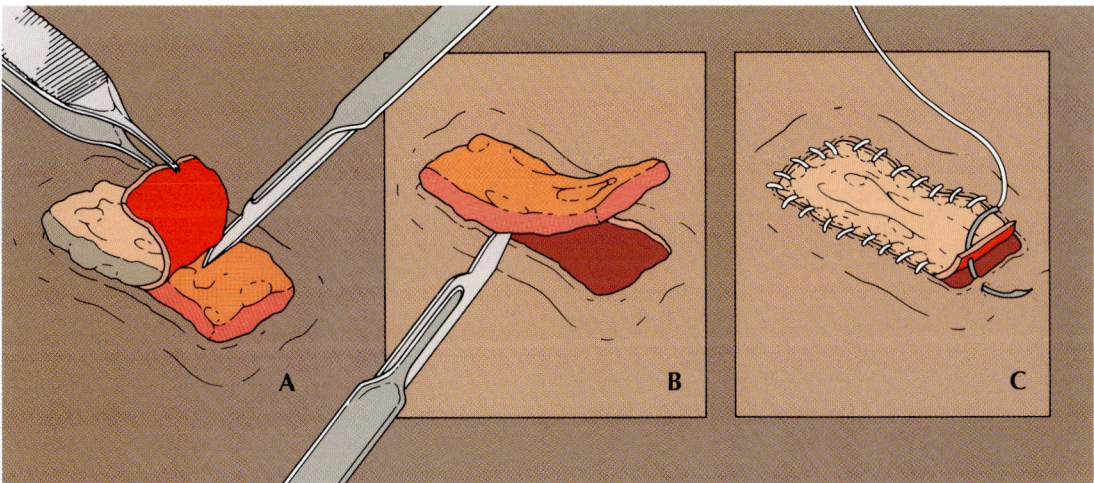

FIGURE 22.3 Diagrammatic representation of procedure for using epidermis overlying a keloid as a skin graft for resurfacing the defect. **(A)** Surface skin is resected from the keloid using scissors or scalpel. **(B)** The keloid is resected. **(C)** The harvested skin is sutured into the defect as a skin graft.

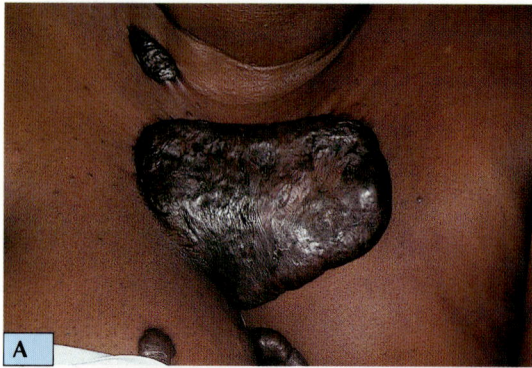

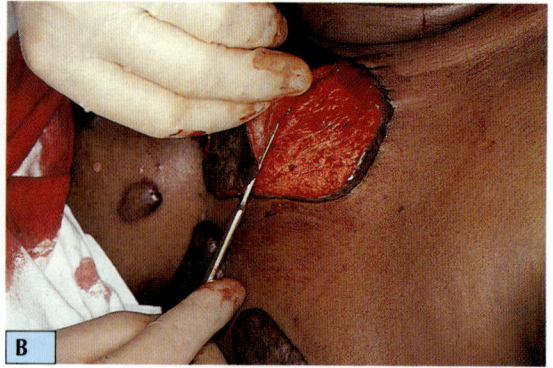

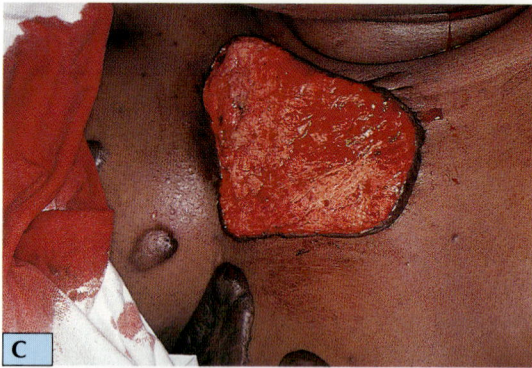

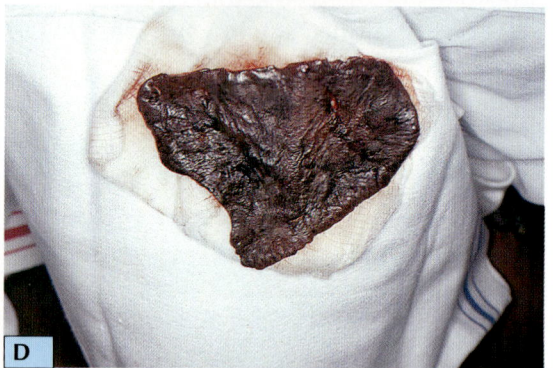

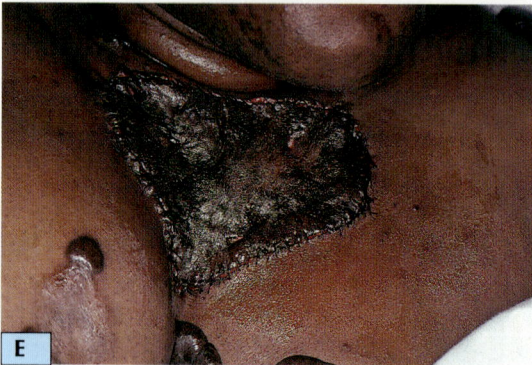

FIGURE 22.4 (A) Preoperative frontal view of a large presternal keloid. **(B)** Dissection of the epithelium and upper dermis overlying the keloid. **(C)** Appearance of the keloid after removal of the surface skin. **(D)** Appearance of the harvested skin graft. **(E)** Appearance of the skin graft in place after excision of the keloid to a plane level with or slightly lower than the surrounding skin. Postoperative intralesional steroids were required to prevent regrowth of the keloid.

lesions and are used frequently on the earlobes. At this location, we often attempt to preserve the epidermis and some dermis overlying the keloid, reflect this out of the operative field while the underlying keloid bulk is removed, and then suture it back into its original site to repair the defect (Figures 22.5A–D, 22.6A–F, 22.7A–C). Alternatively, for anterior–posterior earlobe keloids, in which keloidal growths are evident at

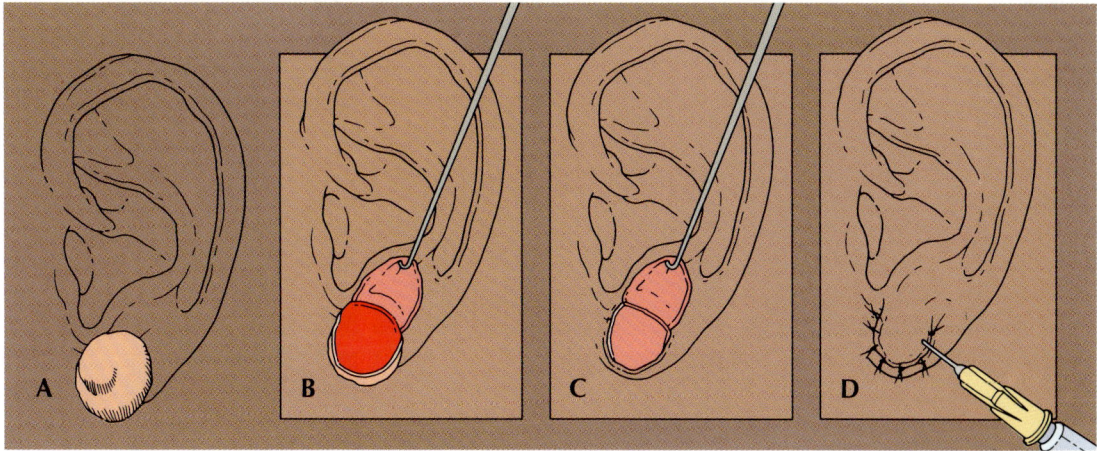

FIGURE 22.5 Diagrammatic representation of surgical excision of an earlobe keloid followed by skin flap repair. (A) Preoperative view of an earlobe keloid. (B) A skin flap is developed from the surface of the keloid and reflected upward. (C) The bulk of the keloid has been excised. Care must be taken to avoid cutting the flap during keloid excision. If necessary for support or contouring, some of the keloid tissue can be left at the base of the excision without increased risk of keloid regrowth. (D) The skin flap has been reflected downward into the operative defect and sutured in place using interrupted fine nylon sutures. No subcutaneous sutures are used, to minimize foreign body reaction to the prolonged presence of absorbable sutures. Postoperatively, corticosteroids are injected into the wound bed before application of a pressure dressing.

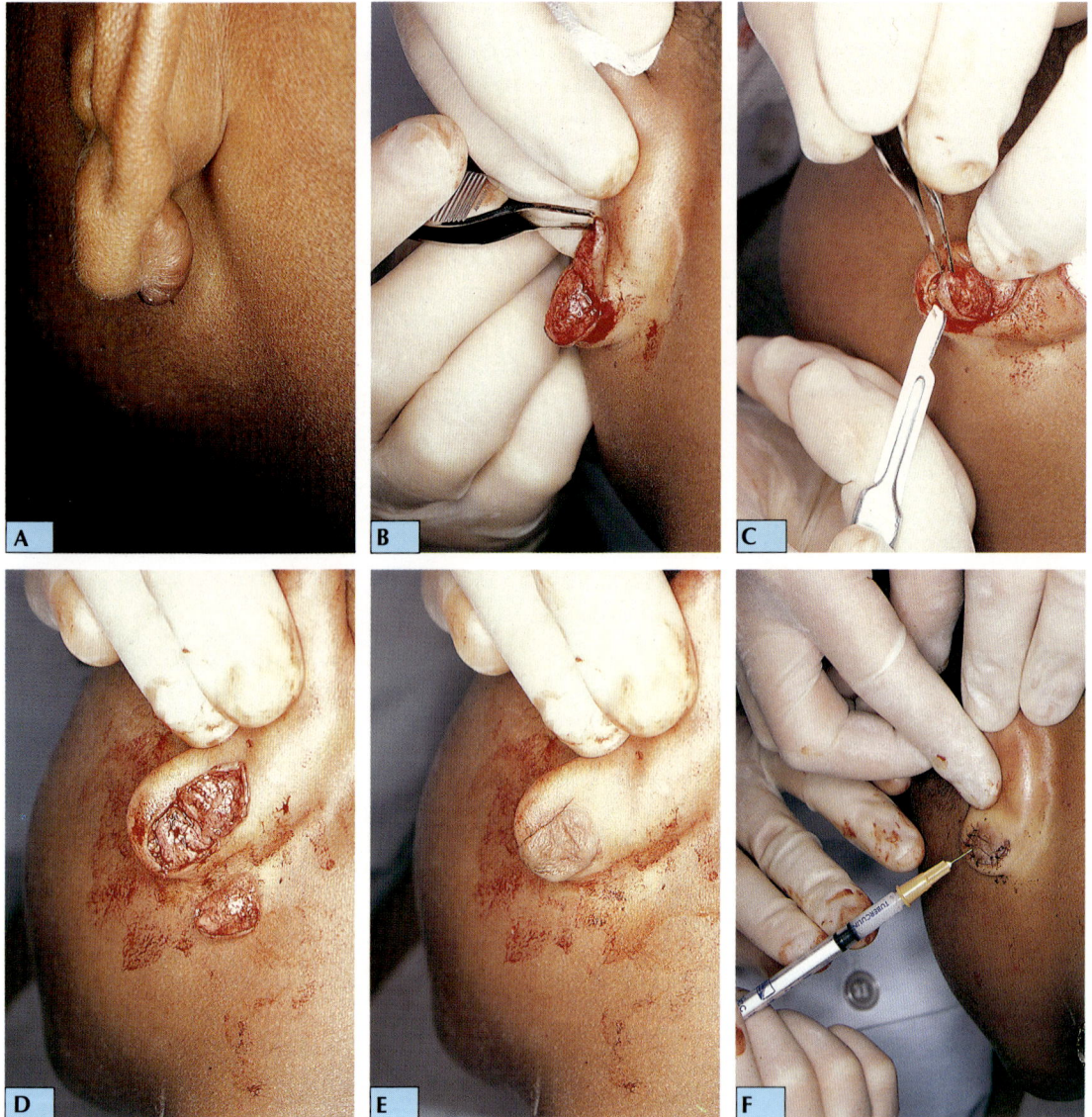

FIGURE 22.6 (A) Preoperative view of a keloid on the earlobe of a young woman after ear piercing. **(B)** Creation of a skin flap by dissection of the surface skin from the keloid surface. This has been reflected upward out of the operative field. **(C)** Appearance of the wound bed after surgical excision of the bulk of the keloid. At this point, it is often possible to identify an epithelialized tract from previous ear piercing. This should be cannulated with a needle and excised, to minimize the chance of recurrence. A suture may be required at the anterior earlobe surface if this tract extends through the earlobe. **(D)** The skin flap has been reflected downward into the surgical defect. **(E)** After trimming of the excess skin, the flap is sutured in place with interrupted 5-0 nylon suture. **(F)** Before application of a pressure dressing, the wound bed is injected with approximately 0.2 mL of 40 mg/mL triamcinolone acetonide. Patients are instructed to leave the pressure dressing in place for at least 24 hours.

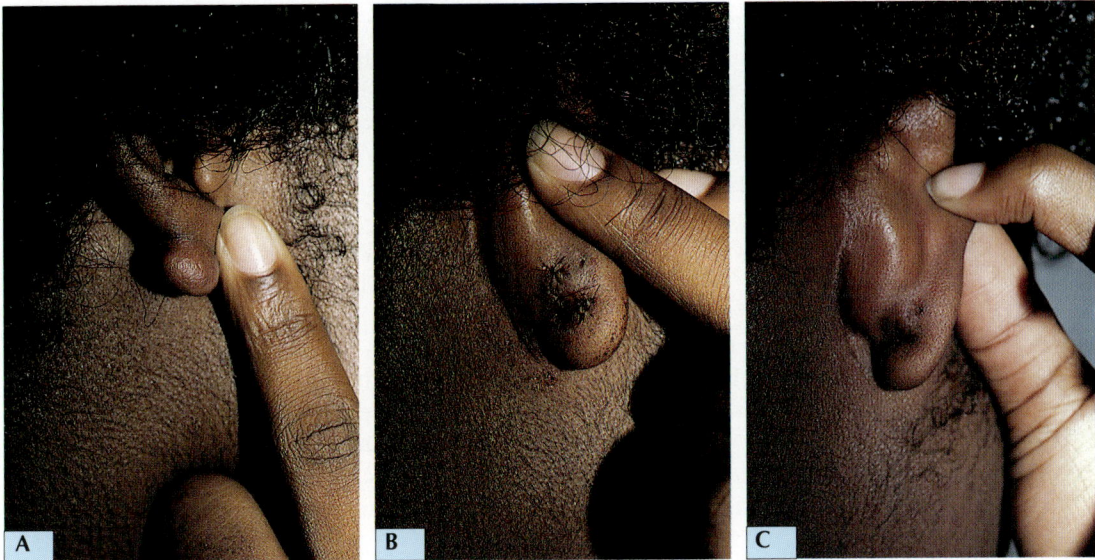

FIGURE 22.7 (A) Preoperative photograph of a nodular keloid of the earlobe in a teenage woman. **(B)** Same earlobe after excision of the keloid and skin flap repair. **(C)** Same patient 3 months after surgery. The operative site was injected with triamcinolone acetonide (40 mg/mL) at the time of suture removal and at monthly intervals thereafter.

both sides of the earlobe, dumbbell-shaped through-and-through excision has yielded excellent results (Figures 22.8 and 22.9A–C). In general, such lesions form at both ends of an epithelialized tract which has been created by ear piercing. This tract is believed to act as a nidus for keloid growth and is removed as part of the dumbbell-shaped surgical excision.

During performance of these procedures, care must be taken to minimize tissue damage and the number of sutures used, thus reducing inflammation resulting from foreign body reactions and decreasing the likelihood of further keloid development. Whenever possible, hemostasis should be obtained through pressure, to limit the thermal damage that accompanies electrocoagulation. Particularly on the earlobes, we prefer to use only nonabsorbable skin sutures of low reactivity (nylon) and to dispense with buried absorbable sutures, which can give rise to a foreign body reaction and thus act as a nidus for keloid regrowth. Pressure dressings are also helpful in avoiding the potential complications of seroma and hematoma formation.

Occasionally a keloid is so extensive that its total removal results in a significant degree of local deformity. This is particularly true in cases where there has been a previous unsuccessful surgery. Of note to

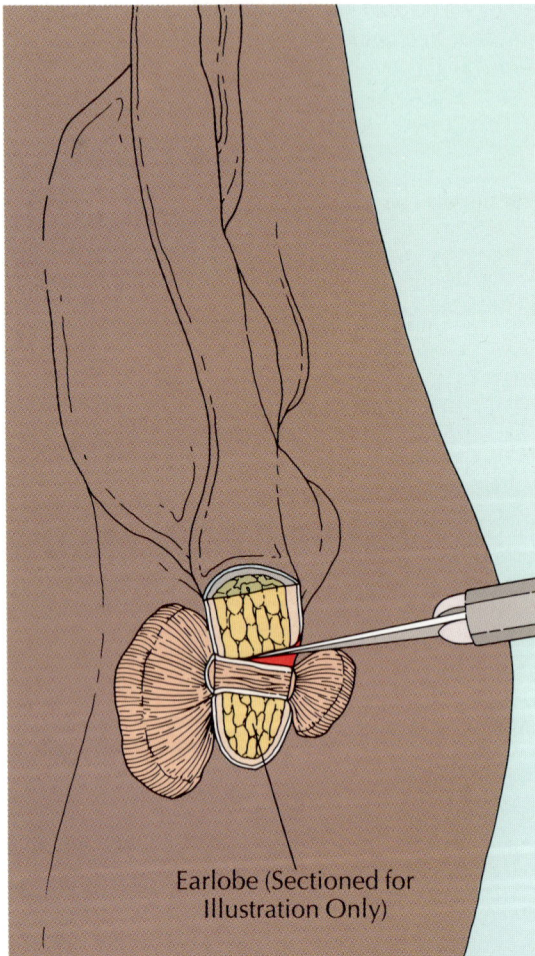

FIGURE 22.8 Diagrammatic representation of "dumbbell" excision of an anterior–posterior earlobe keloid. The epithelialized tract from ear piercing is removed as the core of the excision.

Earlobe (Sectioned for Illustration Only)

dermatologic surgeons is the fact that *subtotal* excision of such a lesion can be performed without a greater likelihood of its recurring. Therefore, portions of a keloid can be left undisturbed for purposes of contouring or support.

ADJUVANT THERAPY

As mentioned above, adjuvant therapy is necessary to prevent recurrence of keloids after all surgical procedures. Although radiotherapy, pressure therapy, and a variety of systemic pharmacotherapies have been reported to be helpful, the most common form of supplemental postoperative therapy consists of intralesional injections of corticosteroids.

Depending on the size of the defect, we generally instill from 0.2 to 1.0 mL of 40 mg/mL triamcinolone acetonide—enough to infiltrate the entire lesion or operative site —into the operative bed at the completion of keloidectomy, after the placement of sutures. Because such a high local dosage of steroid retards local wound healing, with potential dehiscence of the suture line, sutures are generally left in place for 12 to 14 days. Steroids are reinjected at the time of suture removal and monthly thereafter. After 3 to 6 months of such therapy, if no signs or symptoms of keloid regrowth are evident, we gradually lengthen the interval between follow-up injections to 2 months, 3 months, 4 months, and 6 months. At this point, patients are asked to return for annual checkups, during which additional injections are normally administered to maintain remission. Of course, patients are advised to return prior to their scheduled follow-up visits if pruritus or thickening of the operative site develops.

We have found that lower concentrations of triamcinolone are ineffective in preventing keloid regrowth. Moreover, if the

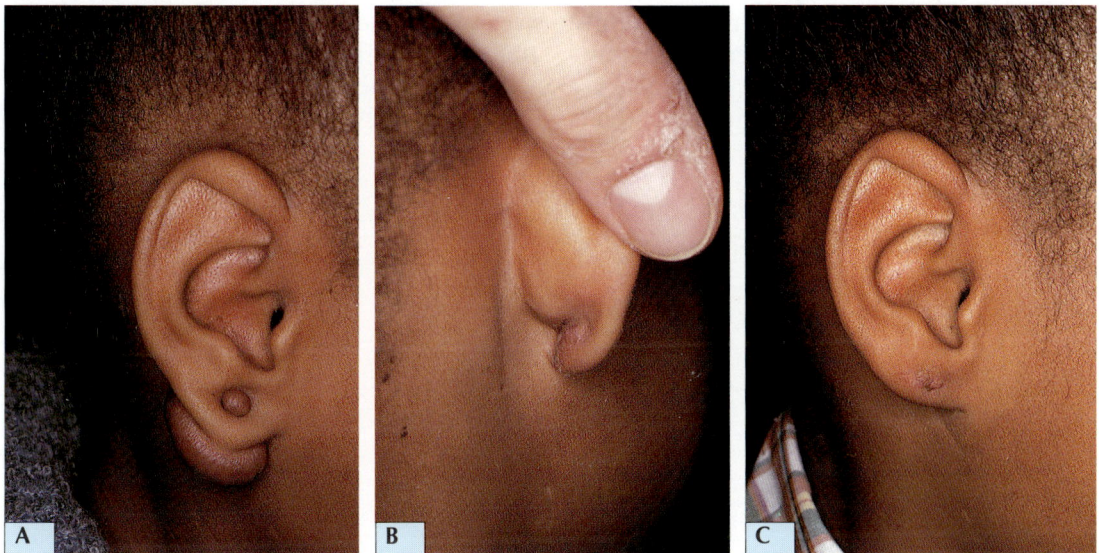

FIGURE 22.9 (A) Preoperative view of an anterior–posterior keloid of the earlobe in a 9-year-old black female. Surgical removal of this lesion involved a dumbbell-shaped excision with removal of both the anterior and the posterior keloid, as well as the intervening epithelialized tract. The anterior defect was repaired by primary closure, while a small flap of skin overlying the keloid was used to repair the posterior earlobe defect. (B) Posterior aspect of earlobe 3 weeks after keloidectomy. (C) Anterior aspect of earlobe 3 weeks after keloidectomy.

postoperative injection regimen described above is not strictly maintained, keloids usually recur within a few months. Ninety percent of the recurrent earlobe keloids we encounter are in patients who failed to present for postoperative therapy. For this reason, we require our patients to make a commitment to the postoperative follow-up regimen before we agree to perform keloidectomy. However, of note is the fact that Golladay has recently described the success of a single intraoperative injection of betamethasone sodium phosphate and betamethasone acetate suspension (Celestone Soluspan) in preventing regrowth of keloids in a pediatric population. (See "Suggestions for Further Reading," at the end of the chapter.) If this observation is confirmed, keloid management may become infinitely simpler in the future.

When supplemental intralesional corticosteroid therapy is used, the surgeon should anticipate hypopigmentation as a complication. This problem can be minimized by injecting the steroid directly into the keloid mass rather than into the overlying or surrounding skin. The problem generally reverses itself over several months, but patients should be warned of this complication before undergoing surgery.

ACNE KELOIDALIS NUCHAE

Acne keloidalis nuchae, which despite its name is not a true keloid, is worthy of mention here as a condition that we have found is best treated by electrosurgical excision. Excisions must extend into the deep subcutaneous layer beneath the hair follicles, as the etiology of this condition is fibrosis resulting from a foreign body reaction to ingrowing hairs. Electroresection, using a combined cut–coagulation current, can be rapidly performed and offers the advantage of providing a significant degree of immediate hemostasis in this highly vascular location (Figure 22.10A–C). Since removal of the hairs is curative, supplemental treatment is usually not required. We have found that the optimal cosmetic outcome is achieved when these deep wounds are allowed to heal to the surface by second intention. Skin grafting of these deep defects tends to result in a step deformity, which is less acceptable.

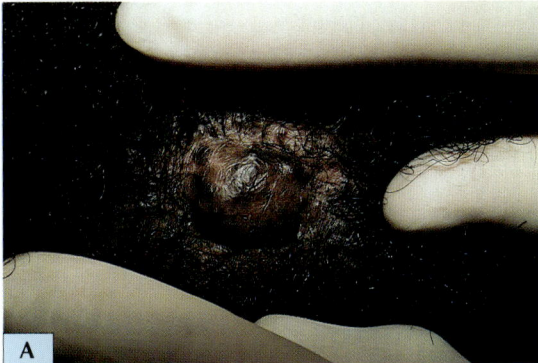

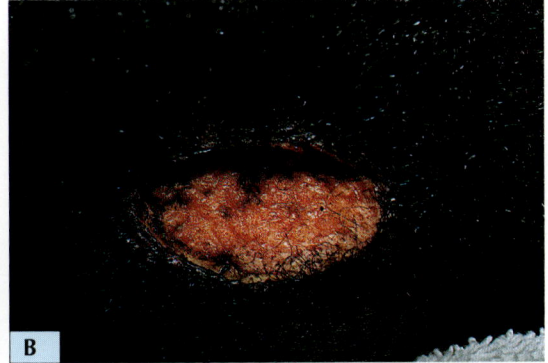

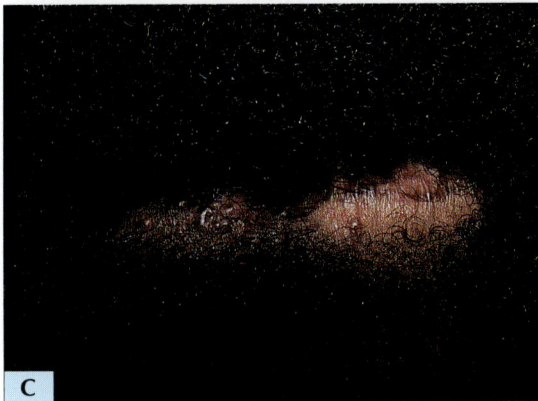

FIGURE 22.10 (A) Preoperative photograph of a long-standing lesion of acne keloidalis nuchae in a 23-year-old black male. (B) The surgical defect after electrosurgical excision of the fibrotic tissue to a level deep to the hair follicles. (C) Postoperative photograph taken 6 months after surgery. The wound was allowed to heal by second intention under semi-occlusive wound dressings. Postoperative steroid injections (triamcinolone 40 mg/mL) were given at the time of surgery to reduce inflammation. However, treatment of acne keloidalis nuchae does not require postoperative monthly injections of corticosteroids as in the case of true keloids.

SUGGESTIONS FOR FURTHER READING

Apfelberg DB, Maser MR, Lash H. The use of epidermis over a keloid as an autograft after resection of the keloid. J Dermatol Surg Oncol 1976;2:409–411.

Apfelberg DB, Maser MR, Lash H, White D, Weston J: Preliminary results of argon and carbon dioxide laser treatment of keloid scars. Lasers Surg Med 1984;4:283–290.

Brown LA, Pierce HE: Keloids: scar revision. J Dermatol Surg Oncol 1986;12:51–56.

Golladay ES: Treatment of keloids by single intraoperative perilesional injection of repository steroid. South Med J 1988; 81:736–738.

Murray JC, Pollack SV, Pinnell SR: Keloids: a review. J Am Acad Dermatol 1981; 4:461–470.

Pollack S: Keloids. In Provost TT, Farmer ER (eds), Current Therapy in Dermatology 1985–1986. Philadelphia, BC Decker, Inc, 1985, pp 255–258.

Pollack SV, Goslen JB: The surgical treatment of keloids. J Dermatol Surg Oncol 1982; 8:1045–1049.

Salasche SJ, Grabski WJ: Keloids of the earlobes: a surgical technique. J Dermatol Surg Oncol 1983;9:552–556.

Weimer VM, Ceilley RI: Treatment of keloids on earlobes. J Dermatol Surg Oncol 1979; 5:522–523.

chapter 23

NAIL SURGERY

The nail is a functional epidermal structure located on the dorsal surface of the distal phalanx of each digit. It increases the delicate manipulation ability of the fingertips, it protects the underlying soft tissue and bone, and it acts as a weapon and a tool.

The nail is susceptible to disease whether it be an underlying skin cancer or fungal infection, a superficial abnormality reflecting a widespread systemic or cutaneous disorder such as psoriasis or thyroid disease, or a distortion as caused by an adjacent periungual infection, mucoid cyst, or fibroma. Thus, at times it is necessary to remove the nail, to obtain a biopsy of it, or to repair it. An understanding of the various parts of the nail is crucial in identifying where the disease process lies and in enabling proper choice of sampling or excisional technique (Figure 23.1).

Nails grow at a rate of about 0.1 mm/day, with fingernails growing at a faster rate than toenails. The longer the finger, the faster its growth rate. On average, following avulsion, it takes 3 months to replace a finger-nail whereas a toenail takes 6 months or longer to replace.

PREPARING FOR SURGERY

Informed consent must be obtained as for any surgical procedure, and for nail surgery it must include the possibility of nail-plate distortion and therefore the possibility of functional loss. The patient should also be questioned specifically as to a history of Raynaud's disease, peripheral vascular disease, or diabetes. Also at this time, a radiograph should be obtained to rule out an underlying disease process in the bone such as an exostosis or osteomyelitis, if either is clinically indicated.

The nail and the digit are prepared as described in Chapter 3. The instruments used in nail surgery are important (Figure 23.2 A–C) and include the Penrose drain, which may be used as a tourniquet. Since no epinephrine is used with the anesthetic, the surgical site will bleed. A tourniquet also can be fashioned using finger cots, rubber bands, or surgical tubing. Whichever is used, it must be left in place no longer than 15 minutes (Figure 23.3), after which time it can be loosened. Blood is then allowed to perfuse the digit and the tourniquet is retightened to allow continuation of the procedure.

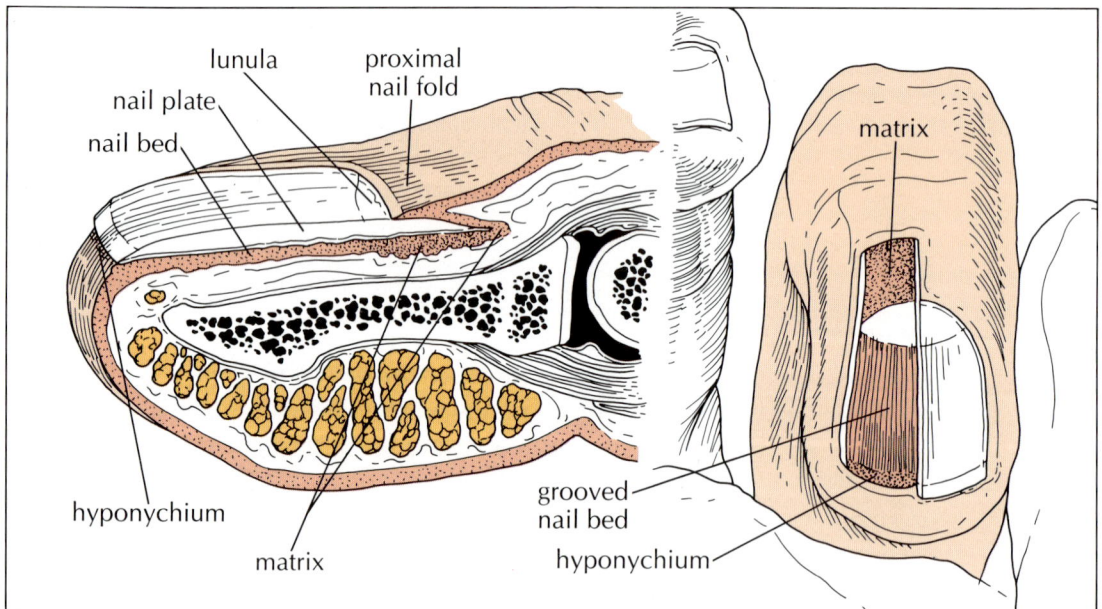

FIGURE 23.1 Schematic drawing showing the various elements of the nail and the tissue it abuts. The nail plate has ridges on its undersurface that correspond to ridges in the nail bed. This tongue-in-groove system provides a strong attachment. The nail matrix is the source of the nail plate. It extends proximally from the lunula to 1 to 2 mm proximal to the beginning of the nail plate. Disruption of the matrix may lead to a permanently dystrophic nail plate.

ANESTHESIA

Most nail surgery is performed using a digital block. Because the anesthetic takes several minutes to work, the patient is asked to arrive at the office 15 to 30 minutes prior to the anticipated time of surgery. It must be remembered that since a finger or toe is a closed space, the volume of injected anesthetic must not cause constriction or vaso-spasm in the vessels or nerves contained therein.

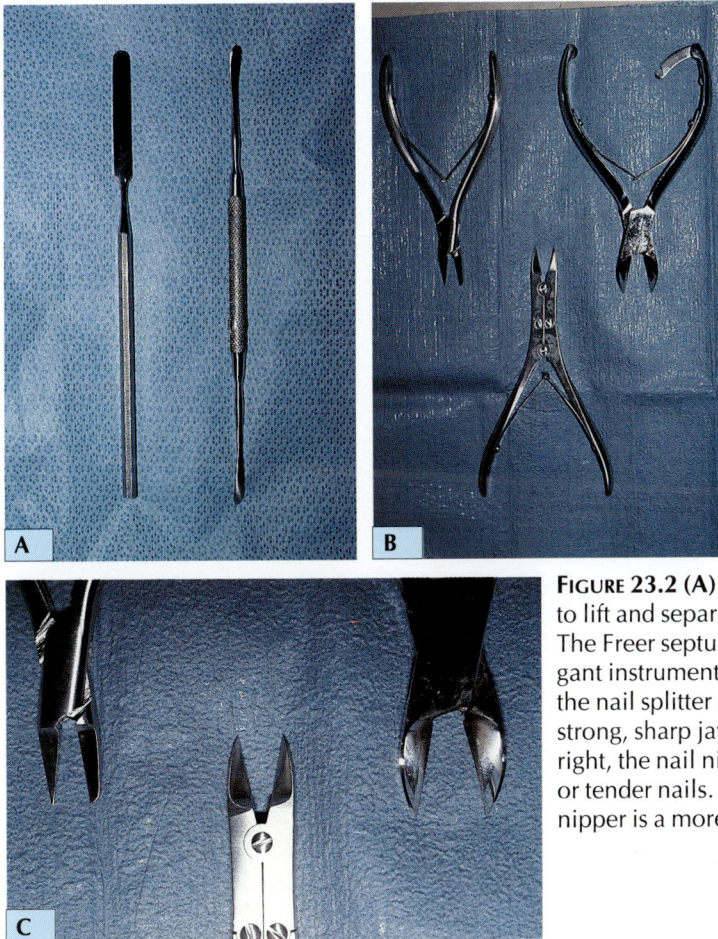

FIGURE 23.2 (A) A dental spatula, at left, works well to lift and separate the nail plate from the nail bed. The Freer septum elevator, at right, is a more elegant instrument for the same purpose. (B) At left, the nail splitter can slide under the nail and with its strong, sharp jaws cut the nail without injury. At right, the nail nipper is useful for cutting thickened or tender nails. At center, the double-action nail nipper is a more elegant variety. (C) Close-up of tips.

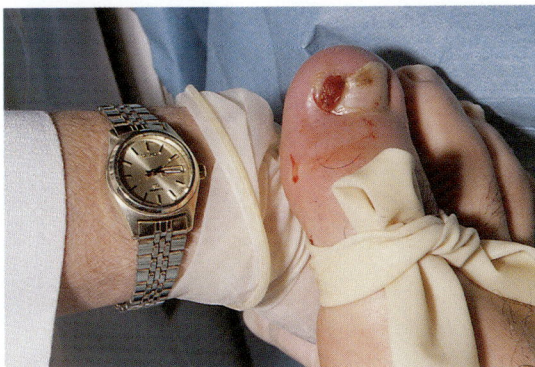

FIGURE 23.3 A Penrose drain may be tucked under itself to tighten it or a hemostat can be used to secure it. It should not be left in place for more than 15 minutes.

The first injection may be made in the web spaces on either side of the involved digit or on either side of the proximal digit, using 1% or 2% plain lidocaine injected with a 30-gauge needle. The needle is placed midway between the dorsal and plantar surfaces of the digit and a small bleb is raised. The needle is then advanced until it touches the periosteum, after which it is pulled back about ¼ inch. A small amount of anesthetic is injected with the needle angled toward the nerves running to the tip (Figure 23.4A,B). This same procedure is then carried out on the other side of the digit. The total amount of anesthetic used should be less than 0.5 mL. No epinephrine should be used. Injection can, of course, be done more distally by injecting an arc of anesthetic just proximal to the proximal nail fold. This, however, may require a more cooperative patient.

The digit is then placed in a dependent position. After 3 to 5 minutes, the skin is tested with needle pricks to determine how far the anesthesia has advanced distally. A small amount of lidocaine is then injected on both sides of the digit, at the leading edge of the numbness, in the manner just described. The nail is once again held dependently and the procedure is repeated as necessary. The desired degree of numbness should be achieved in about 15 minutes, after 2 to 3 bilateral injections (Figure 23.5). Anesthesia without epinephrine may last only 20 minutes and since digits are extremely sensitive to pain, the procedure should not be delayed.

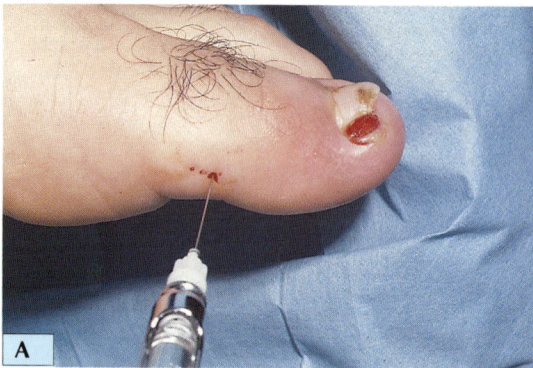

A

FIGURE 23.4 (A,B) Fingers and toes are well innervated and require time to numb. Placement of the anesthetic closer to the nerves will necessitate less volume and produce faster results.

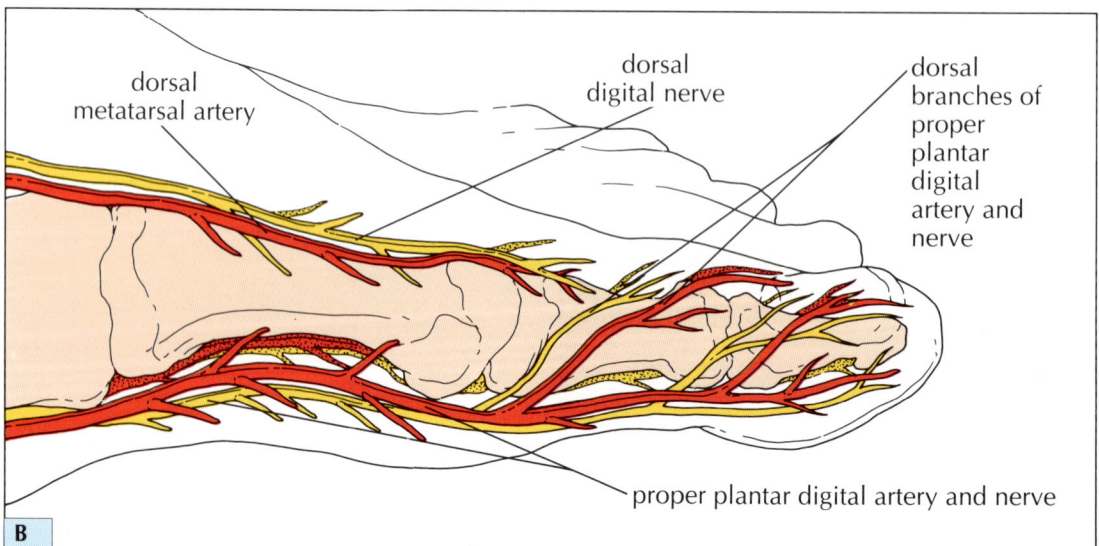

dorsal metatarsal artery

dorsal digital nerve

dorsal branches of proper plantar digital artery and nerve

proper plantar digital artery and nerve

B

BIOPSY TECHNIQUES

There are several ways to perform a nail biopsy. First, it is critically important that an attempt be made to identify the part of the nail involved by the pathology. If the lesion is in the nail plate and/or the nail bed, it is best to perform a punch biopsy, using a sharp trephine to pass through both structures (Figure 23.6). Hemostasis may be achieved by packing the defect with a collagen or gelatin sponge. This technique, which avoids removal of the entire nail plate, is not recommended if the nail matrix (including the lunula) is involved, as it may lead to permanent nail distortion.

A slight variation of this technique, which removes a portion of the nail plate and the underlying nail bed, is described in Chapter 5. It uses a larger punch to remove the nail plate and a smaller one to sample the exposed nail bed. If an incisional biopsy of the nail bed is to be done, extending as far back as the matrix in order to sample it, it should be oriented longitudinally and be less than 3 mm wide.

To sample only the matrix, an incisional biopsy is recommended to prevent permanent damage to the plate. First, the plate is removed. Next, an elliptical excision is oriented transversely to avoid disruption of the growth of the nail plate. The incision should be taken down to the bone. Sometimes it is necessary to reflect back the proximal nail fold to obtain adequate exposure of the matrix. This can be done by making two

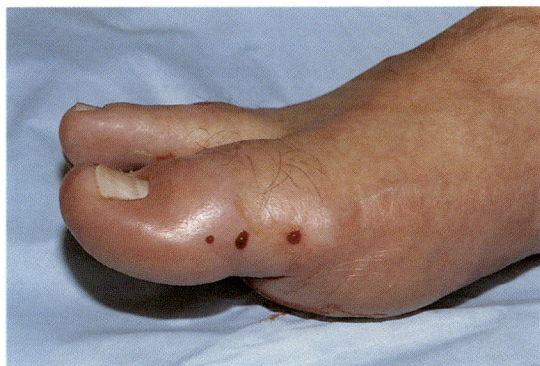

FIGURE 23.5 Drops of blood are seen at sequential injection points distally along the digit. Only three small injections were necessary to numb this entire toe.

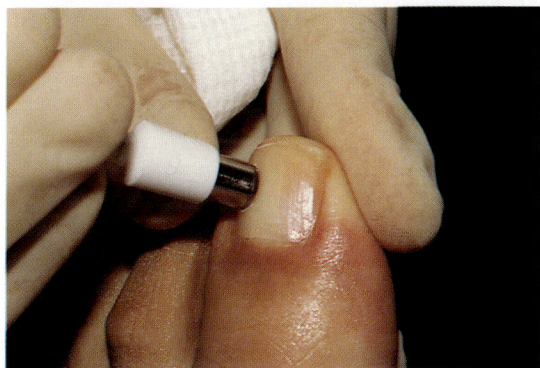

FIGURE 23.6 The punch is placed perpendicular to the surface of the nail and is advanced with firm, twisting movements.

small releasing incisions bilaterally at the junction of the lateral and proximal nail folds (Figure 23.7). The incisions are then closed with absorbable sutures.

NAIL PLATE AVULSION

Removal of the nail plate may be necessary to perform a biopsy of the nail bed or matrix, to treat a subungual lesion or infection, or to remove an ingrowing or distorted plate. The digit must be numbed completely, since it is extremely sensitive and even simple pressure may cause the patient discomfort.

The nail plate is separated from the nail bed using a dental spatula, which is pushed proximally and from side to side. The spatula should rest against the underside of the plate. Since the longitudinal grooves on the bed and the plate attaching them to one another are well formed, firm movements may be necessary to detach them. As the spatula moves laterally toward the lateral nail folds, where the plate dips down and becomes

more convex than flat, it should be angled 45° to lift the plate out of the folds. This movement is especially important where the lateral and proximal nail folds meet. Here, the nail can be difficult to detach (Figure 23.8A–C).

Once the plate is completely detached from its bed, a hemostat is used to grasp the distal end of the nail and to remove it. For complete removal of the nail, sometimes it is necessary to wiggle it back and forth or to twist it (Figure 23.9). Partial avulsions also may be done.

INGROWN NAILS

Ingrown nails can be a difficult and annoying problem for the patient. The most commonly involved digit is the hallux, or big toe, and its lateral nail fold. Trauma from shoes and/or stance causes pressure that pushes the nail plate into the fold and causes it to increase in convexity. This triggers a cycle of irritation, infection, and resultant hypertrophy of the nail fold (Figure 23.10).

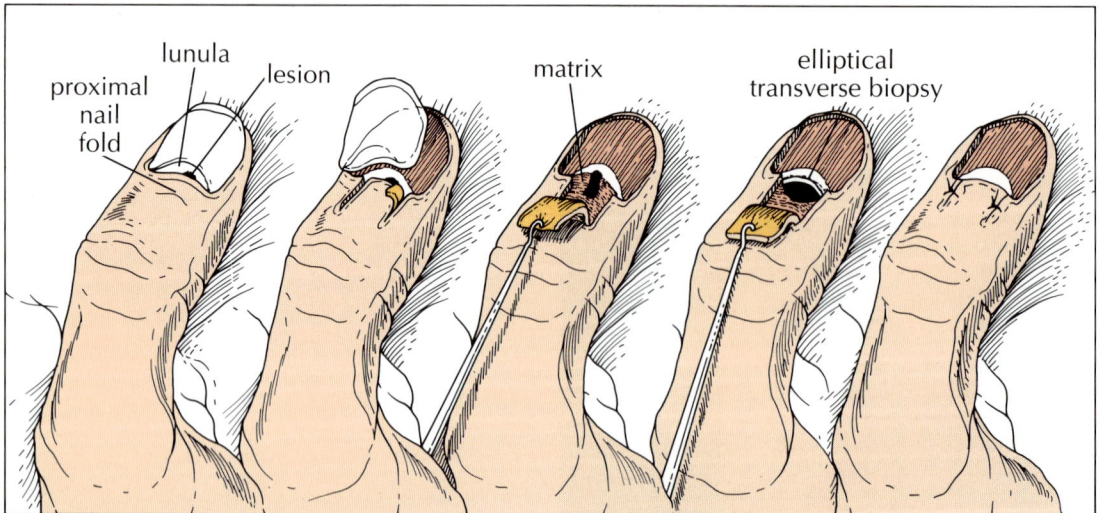

FIGURE 23.7 Schematic showing an incisional biopsy of the nail matrix. The matrix extends from the lunula to a point several millimeters proximal to the edge of the proximal nail fold. A biopsy of the area should be oriented transversely and closed primarily. Sometimes it is necessary to elevate the proximal nail fold by placing two releasing incisions, as shown, to expose the underlying matrix. The incisions are then resewn.

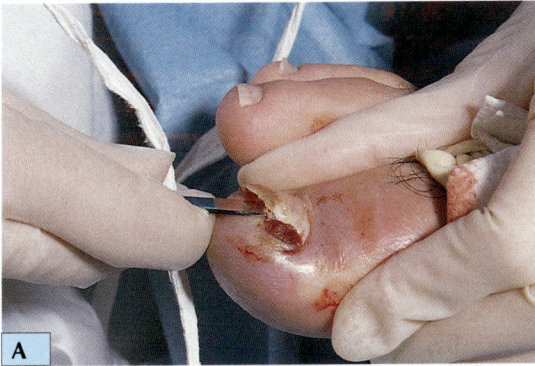

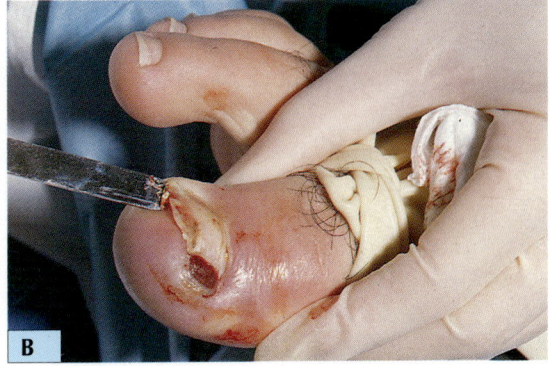

FIGURE 23.8 (A) The dental spatula is held tightly and advanced forcefully. **(B)** As the spatula is slid from side to side, it is angled 45° as it approaches the lateral nail folds. **(C)** Detachment of the proximal nail fold from the plate also may be necessary to obtain complete removal.

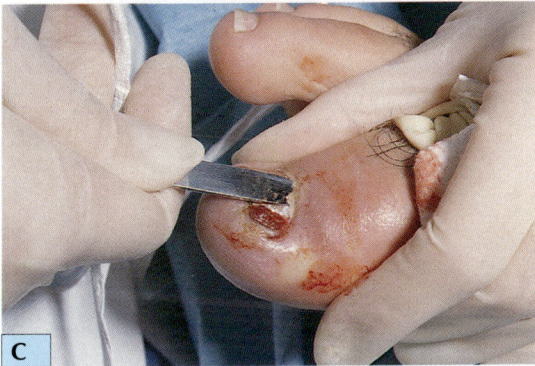

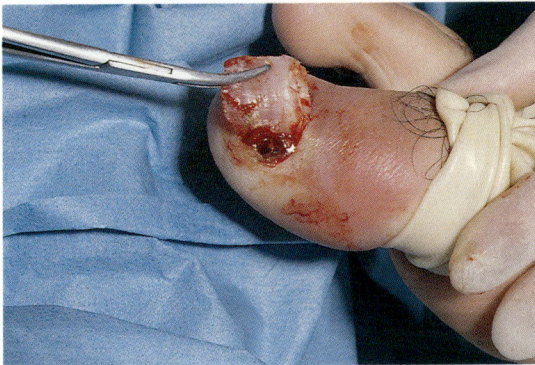

FIGURE 23.9 This nail plate is being twisted up off the nail bed to remove it from the lateral nail fold.

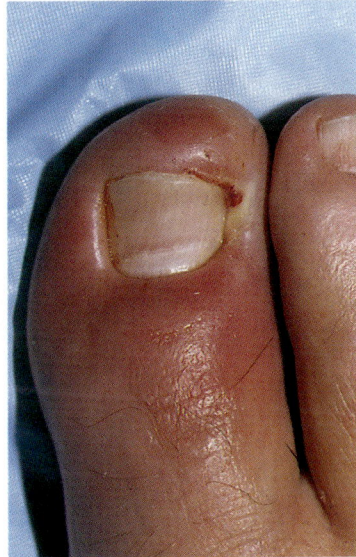

FIGURE 23.10 Note the hypertrophied tissue distally and laterally on this toe in response to chronic irritation. This is a long-standing problem leading also to thickening and fibrosis of the lateral nail fold (whitish area).

In cases that are not far advanced, the problem can be corrected by removal of the nail plate followed by regrowth of the nail. Placement of a firm substance, such as a thin piece of cardboard, under the nail will enable it to slide over any hypertrophied tissue as it grows out. Most commonly however it is necessary to ablate the part of the matrix responsible for the offending portion of nail, which may be done most easily by nail avulsion, exposure of the nail matrix, and application of an 88% phenol alcohol solution. Destruction of the matrix also may be achieved by electrodesiccation, laser surgery, or scalpel excision. With frequent recurrence, however, these methods become less reliable and also somewhat more complicated.

POSTOPERATIVE WOUND CARE

Once the procedure is finished, hemostasis is achieved using electrocautery. As the nail bed is highly vascular and bleeds readily, pressure and topical hemostatic agents rarely suffice. Next the area is cleansed with hydrogen peroxide and is covered with an antibacterial ointment and a nonadherent pad and tubular gauze (Figure 23.11A–C). A gentle but firm pressure dressing is applied for 48 hours postoperatively. It is important that there be adequate perfusion to the digit under the bandage. In some instances, a splint is used to limit movement, to protect the area, or simply to make the patient more

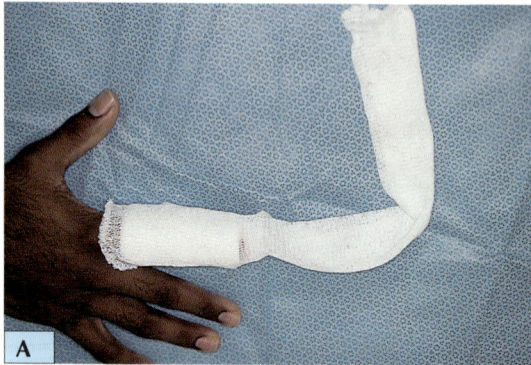

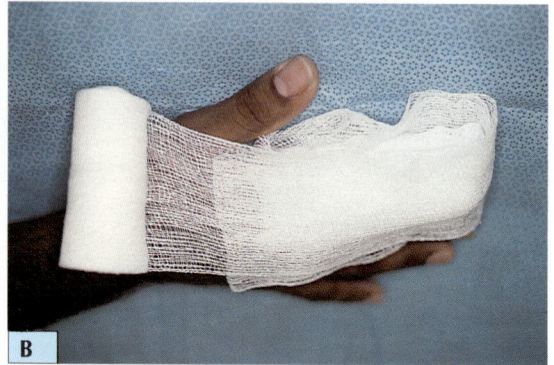

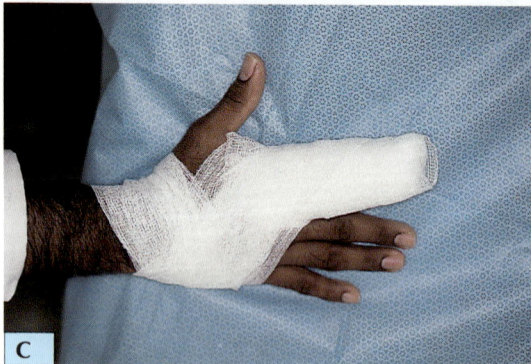

FIGURE 23.11 (A) Tubular gauze is slipped over the splint and a single layer of gauze. **(B)** Next, a roll of gauze is layered to provide cushioning and absorbency. **(C)** The final configuration of the bandage is seen.

comfortable. The patient is advised to keep the hand or foot elevated, immobile, and dry for the first week following surgery before returning for a wound check.

Since surgery in this area can be painful postoperatively, analgesics are prescribed. Antibiotics are also prescribed, since digits are closed spaces in which infection is dangerous. The patient is instructed to clean the wound with hydrogen peroxide 48 hours postoperatively, to dry it, and to apply an antibacterial ointment daily until the wound is healed.

Nail surgery is sometimes viewed as more difficult than other types of cutaneous procedures and therefore it is avoided by some. However, once the proper tools are at hand and the anesthetic technique is mastered, nail surgery can be rewarding. Correction of nail deformity, sampling of suspicious lesions, confirmation of a disease that may be manifest only in the nails, treatment of diseases well protected in the nail bed, and easing of painful conditions all serve to provide essential services to the patient.

SUGGESTIONS FOR FURTHER READING

Bennett RG. Technique of biopsy of nails. J Dermatol Surg Oncol. 1976;2:325-326.

Bureau H, Baran R, Hancke E. Nail surgery and traumatic abnormalities. In: Baran R, Dawber RPR, eds. Diseases of the Nails and their Management. Boston, Mass: Blackwell Scientific Publications Inc;1984:347-402.

Salasche SJ. Surgery. In: Scher RK, Daniel CR, eds. Nails: Therapy, Diagnosis, Surgery. Philadelphia, Pa: WB Saunders Co; 1990:258-280.

Siegle RJ, Harkness JJ, Swanson NA. The phenol alcohol technique for permanent matricectomy. Arch Dermatol. 1984;120: 348-350.

Siegle RJ, Swanson NA. Nail surgery: a review. J Dermatol Surg Oncol. 1982;8: 659-666.

Zaias N. The longitudinal nail biopsy. J Invest Dermatol. 1967;49:406-408.

chapter 24

SURGICAL REPAIR OF RHINOPHYMA

Rhinophyma, a disfiguring condition caused by hypertrophy and hyperplasia of the sebaceous glands of the nose, derives its name from the Greek *rhino* (nose) and *phyma* (growth). The patient is usually a Caucasian male (12:1 male predominance) over age 40, who experiences a gradual enlargement of the nose, beginning distally with recurrent redness and/or edema. Eventually it becomes permanent. The tip of the nose becomes more bulbous, and the sebaceous glands may ooze sebum. If there is an accompanying active rosacea, pimples may be present. Oral antibiotics may provide some relief of the latter, but they have no effect on the rhinophymatous component.

The patient experiences distress because of the unsightliness of the nose and the odor caused by constantly draining sebaceous glands. In addition, nasal obstruction may occur, caused by the weight of the rhinophymatous tissue collapsing the columella and/or nares or by hypertrophy of the tissue surrounding the opening (Figure 24.1A,B).

During consultation for the repair of rhinophyma, it is very important to assess the patient's motivations for surgery. It is equally important to explain exactly what the surgery can accomplish. Most techniques used today do not completely remove all seb-aceous glands, and recurrence is therefore possible. Nevertheless, this is one of the most gratifying procedures the surgeon can perform. Not only do the patients achieve dramatic clinical improvement; they also feel more comfortable socially.

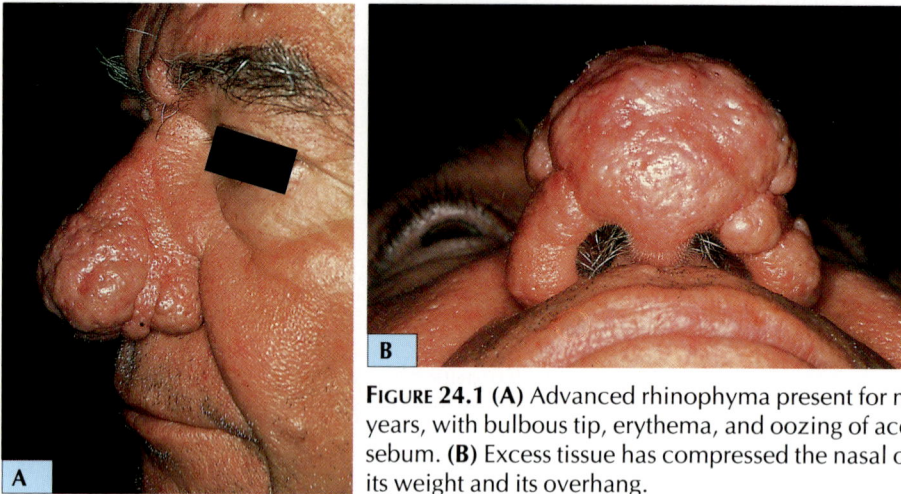

FIGURE 24.1 (A) Advanced rhinophyma present for more than 20 years, with bulbous tip, erythema, and oozing of accumulated sebum. **(B)** Excess tissue has compressed the nasal openings by both its weight and its overhang.

FIGURE 24.2

TECHNIQUES USED TO CORRECT RHINOPHYMA

TOOLS & TECHNIQUES USED TO REMOVE RHINOPHYMATOUS TISSUE	TECHNIQUES USED TO REPAIR RHINOPHYMA
1. Electrosurgery	1. Complete excision of all sebaceous material (decortication) with
2. CO_2 laser surgery	*a. flap reconstruction*
3. #15 blade scalpel	*b. full-thickness skin grafts*
4. Razor blade	*c. split-thickness skin grafts*
5. Shaw scalpel	2. Partial removal of sebaceous material
6. Dermatome	
7. Dermabrasion	
8. Cryosurgery	

TYPES OF SURGICAL THERAPY

Many techniques are available for correction of rhinophyma (Figure 24.2). We prefer electrosurgery, the advantages of which are listed in Figure 24.3. We use a Bantam Bovie machine (Figure 24.4A,B). It is set in the "cutting" or "cutting with hemostasis" mode at a medium position. The other machine

FIGURE 24.3
PROS AND CONS OF POPULAR METHODS OF RHINOPHYMA REPAIR

	CO_2 LASER SURGERY	ELECTROSURGERY	COLD STEEL SURGERY
Tissue destruction beyond actual cutting line	yes	yes	no
Ease of use	no	yes	yes
Tissue sculpting ability	yes	yes	no
Hemostasis	yes	yes	no
Odor/plume	yes	yes	no
Speed	no	yes	yes

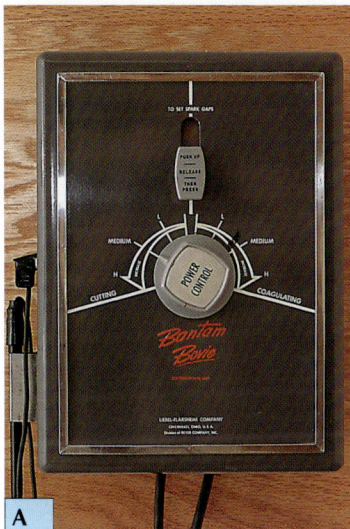

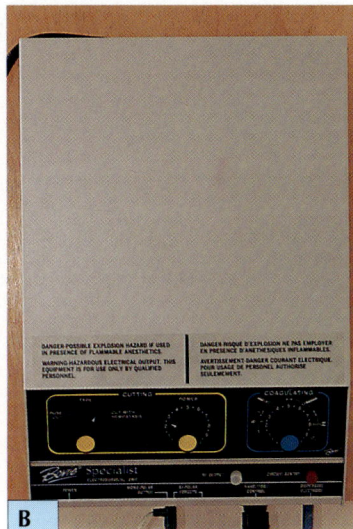

FIGURE 24.4 (A) Original Bantam Bovie. (B) New model Bovie Specialist.

used is the Ellman Surgitron (Figure 24.5). Its dials are set on "cut and coagulate," which provides a fully rectified current, and the intensity is set between 3 and 6.

When either machine is set in the "cutting" mode, the electrode will cut and achieve moderate hemostasis at the same time. Occasionally it is necessary to touch a larger vessel several times to obtain adequate hemostasis. For the electrode tip, either a wire loop or a hockey stick configuration or one of the newer bendable straight wires (Figure 24.6) is used.

PREOPERATIVE PREPARATION

The standard setup tray for rhinophyma repair using electrosurgery includes Hibiclens for preoperative cleansing, gloves, a 3-mL syringe filled with 2% lidocaine with epinephrine, gauze for blotting and wiping away the removed tissue, and the electrode tips.

We ask the patient to bring in a photograph that shows the original shape and size of the nose. A guide of this type is very help-

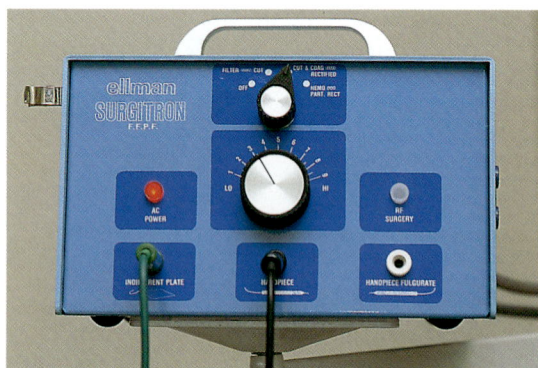

FIGURE 24.5 Ellman Surgitron.

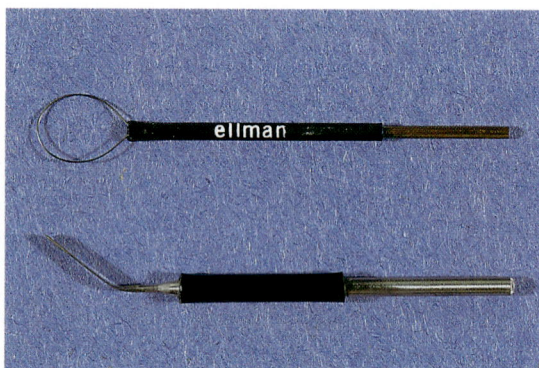

FIGURE 24.6 Wire loop configuration and hockey stick, or angled straight-wire, electrode tips.

FIGURE 24.7 This patient's high school graduation picture gives a good idea of the basic structure of his nose.

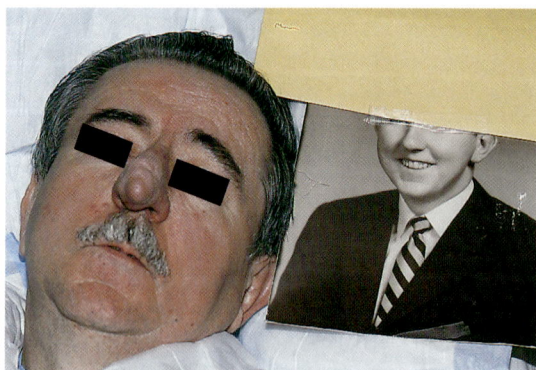

ful, as the original shape of the nose has often been completely distorted by the rhinophymatous tissue (Figure 24.7).

The patient is placed supine on the table, with his or her photograph taped to the pillow next to the patient's head or on the wall just behind the table. We explain to the patient that although we cannot re-create the nose in the photograph, it does give us an idea of its original size and form. The entire nose and the surrounding face are prepared for surgery; we clean the area with Hibiclens, which is then wiped off.

ANESTHESIA

We use no preoperative sedation and have not found it necessary. A nasal block is achieved using 2% lidocaine with epinephrine 1:100,000. Because repair of a very large rhinophyma may take an hour or more, it is sometimes necessary to use a long-acting anesthetic agent such as 0.5% bupivacaine.

The nasal block is intended to anesthetize mainly the infraorbital and infratrochlear nerves, as well as the external branches of the ethmoid nerves (Figure 24.8). The needle is placed alongside the ala and the injection is

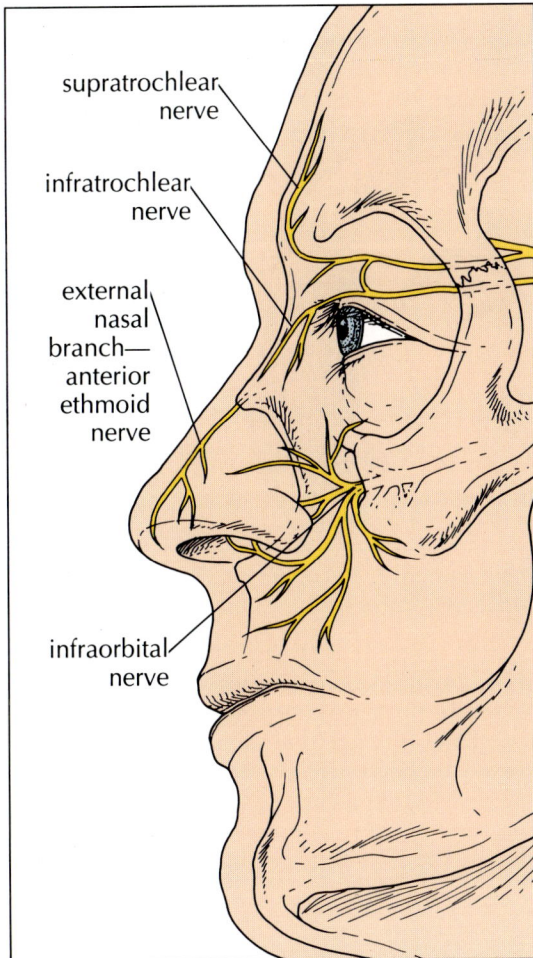

FIGURE 24.8 Anatomic location of major sensory nerves to the nose.

supratrochlear nerve

infratrochlear nerve

external nasal branch— anterior ethmoid nerve

infraorbital nerve

made along the nasofacial sulcus. If a long 1-inch, 30-gauge needle is used, it can be partially withdrawn, but not completely removed, and then redirected toward the infraorbital foramen and then the upper lip toward the columella, where more anesthetic is injected. The second injection site is the nasal bridge where anesthetic is directed laterally and slightly superiorly to catch the trochlear nerves. A third injection is given at the distal end of the nasal bone where the ethmoid nerve exits (Figure 24.9). In principle, after these blocks the nose should be numb. However, occasionally the columella and tip may not be entirely anesthetized. Therefore, if excess tissue is to be removed at these locations, a fourth injection can be made into the tip and toward the columella (Figure 24.10). Cotton plugs can be placed in the nares to minimize the patient's awareness of odor.

SURGICAL PROCEDURE

The surgeon should begin removing the rhinophymatous tissue from the area of greatest concentration. Using smooth, gliding strokes along the nose, moving from distal to

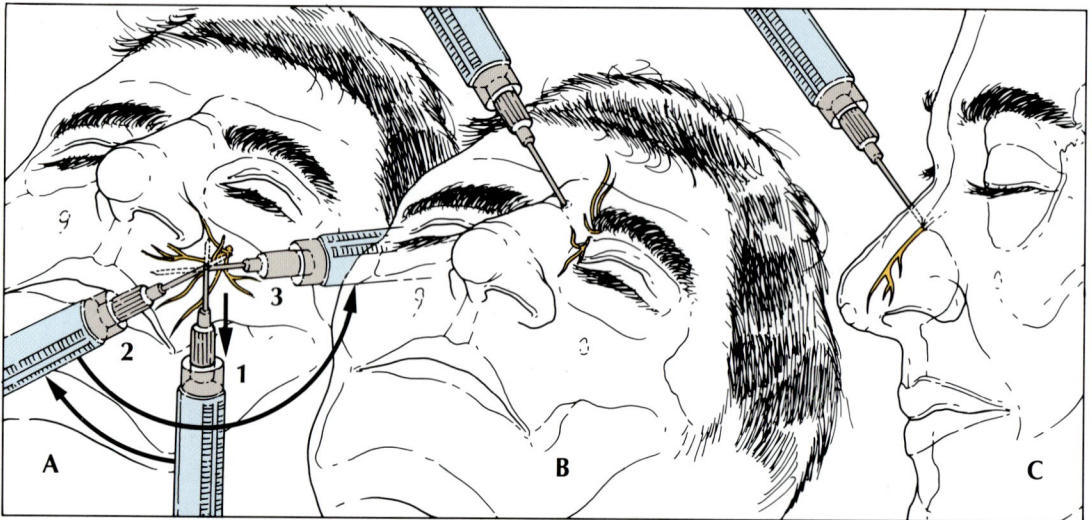

FIGURE 24.9 To anesthetize the infraorbital and infratrochlear nerves, three major injections are made: **(A) 1,** The nasofacial sulcus; **2,** The infraorbital foramen; **3,** The upper lip. **(B)** The nasal bridge. **(C)** The nasal bone (distal end).

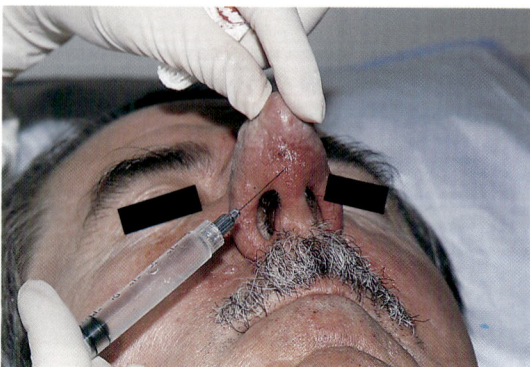

FIGURE 24.10 Since significant excess tissue is present on the tip of this patient's nose, the standard nerve block may not have numbed it completely, so extra anesthetic is injected directly into it.

proximal or proximal to distal, the tissue is elevated and removed in very thin (1- to 2-mm) slices (Figure 24.11A–C). As the enlarged sebaceous glands are unroofed, sebum will ooze out, acting as a guide against cutting too deeply (Figure 24.12). The process is then repeated, using a series of parallel strokes, until the bulk of the excess rhinophymatous tissue is removed from all areas, including the underside of the tip (Figure 24.13). It is important not to leave ridges between the parallel strokes. Smoothing of

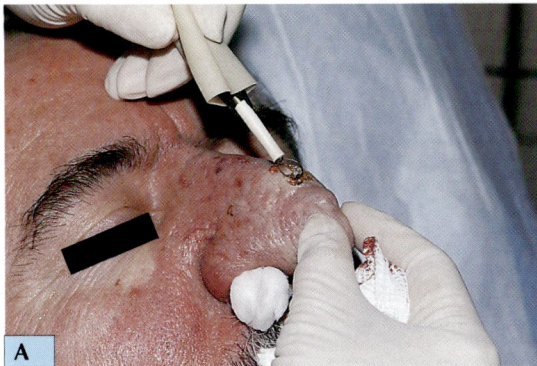

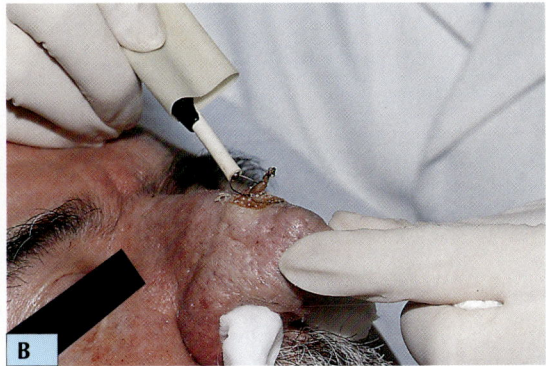

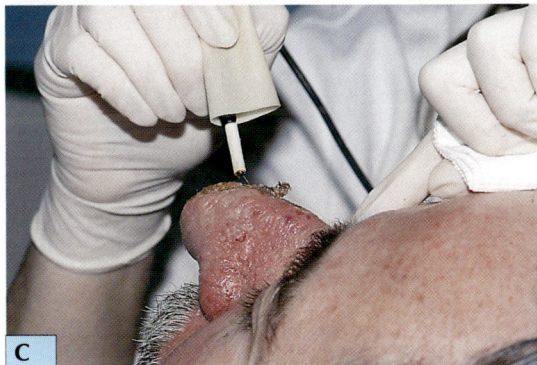

FIGURE 24.11 (A) The proper angle of electrode tip to cutting surface in the distal to proximal direction for electrosurgical removal of rhinophymatous tissue. **(B)** Elevation of strip of tissue. **(C)** The proper electrode angle in the proximal to distal direction.

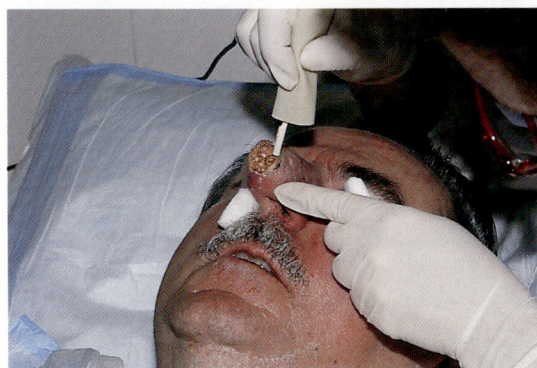

FIGURE 24.12 The central drops of yellowish-white sebum that ooze out after tissue removal indicate that we are cutting within the sebaceous glands and therefore not deep enough to cause scarring.

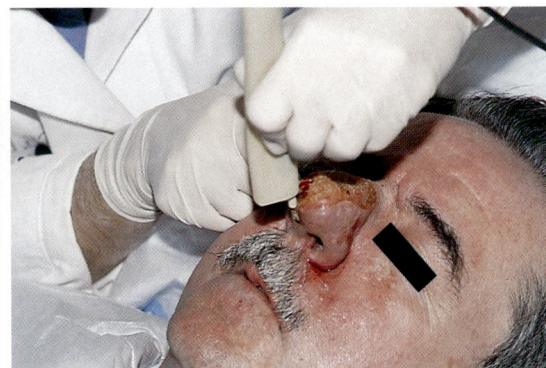

FIGURE 24.13 When removing rhinophymatous tissue, it is important to pay attention to the underside of the tip, which in most noses is flat, not rounded.

any ridges must be done with shallower and lighter strokes (Figure 24.14A,B). The critical idea is *less is best*. If too much tissue is removed, two problems can result: the nose may be too small to fit the patient's face, and/or scarring may occur.

The surgeon should walk around the patient and view the nose from many different angles, thus making it easier to sculpt a symmetrical nose and to cut from different vantage points. As the rhinophymatous tissue grows, the distal part of the nose becomes bulbous with loss of alar definition. Particular attention should be given to restoration of the alar groove, which is even more important to the overall cosmetic appearance of the resculpted nose than is its actual size (Figure 24.15).

After completion of surgery, the wound is cleansed with hydrogen peroxide, and the

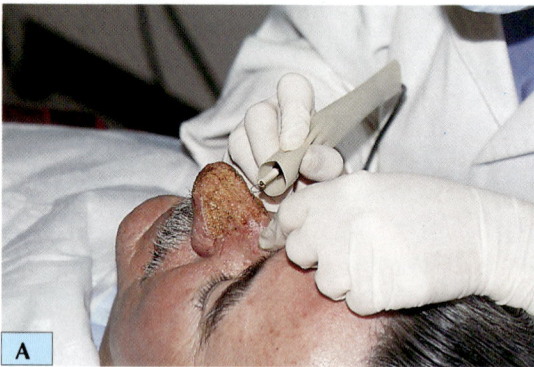

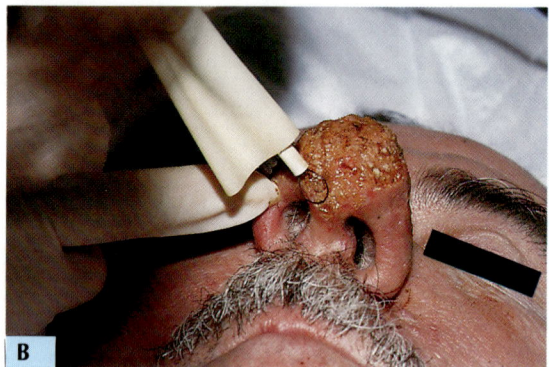

FIGURE 24.14 (A,B) The ridges created on the nose by non-overlapping parallel strokes.

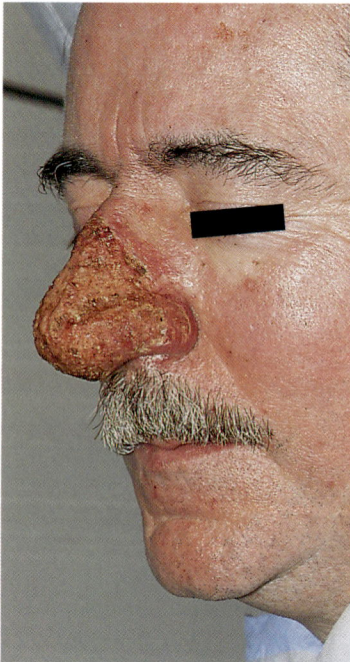

FIGURE 24.15 It is important to accentuate the alar groove after the rhinophymatous tissue has been removed. This definition is a critical feature of a well-reshaped nose. The procedure is complete when the size of the nose fits the patient's face and the limit of unroofing of sebaceous glands has been reached.

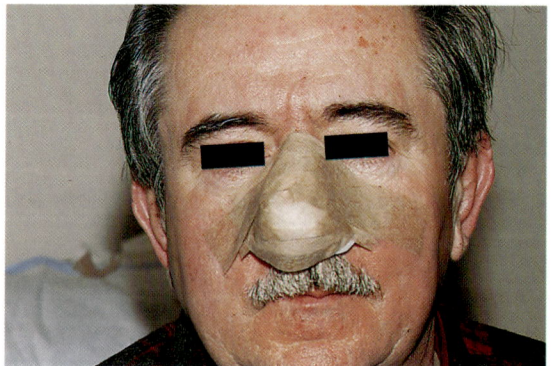

FIGURE 24.16 The patient's nose should be generously bandaged, but he or she should be able to breathe through the bandage, since some find it difficult to mouth-breathe.

area is dressed with Betadine, Telfa, and gauze (Figure 24.16). Postoperative wound care should consist of daily cleansing with hydrogen peroxide, drying, and application of an antibacterial ointment. Healing is usually complete in 3 to 4 weeks (Figure 24.17A–D).

Scarring, which may not become evident until after the wound is completely healed,

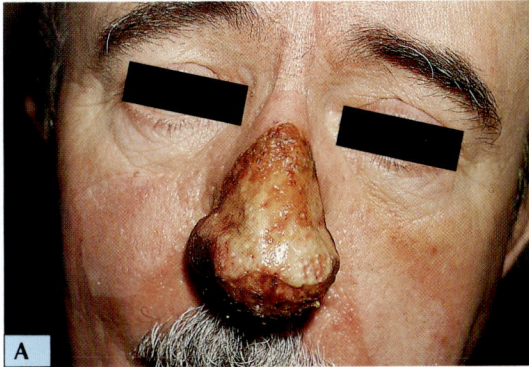

FIGURE 24.17 (A) Postoperatively, rhinophymatous lesions can be very exudative, especially during the first week, requiring frequent dressing changes and dressing reinforcement with layers of gauze. (B) At 2 weeks. Rapid improvement takes place once the patient understands the need for vigorous wound cleaning and debridement. (C) At 3 weeks. Wound is re-epithelized but still red. Wound care now requires only normal facial washing and application of the topical antibacterial several times a day. (D) At 3 months. Note normal-appearing skin and texture thereof.

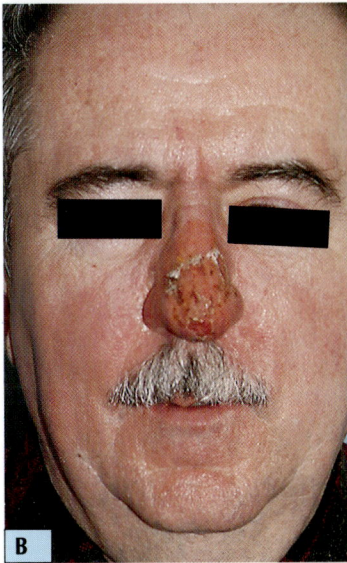

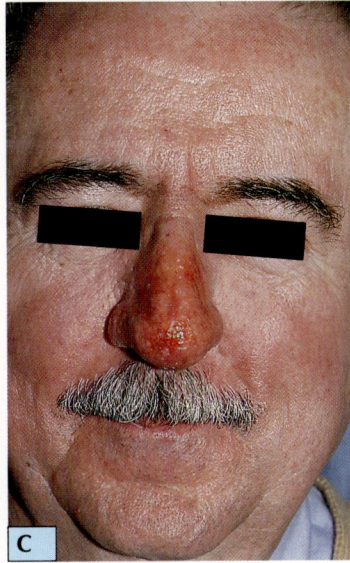

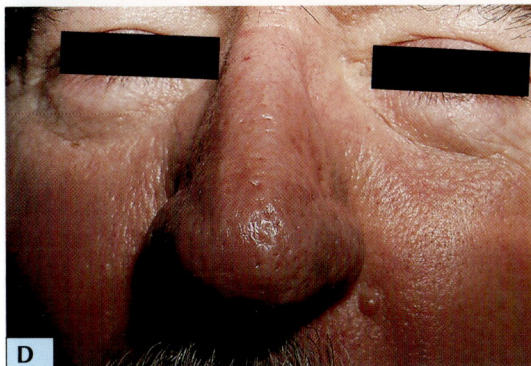

will appear as a shiny, smooth, pink area that lacks the normal texture of the nose. Occasionally, scarring occurs only in a small area where the tissue was cut too deeply, and may not detract from the overall improvement. However, scarring near the tip or the alar rim, or over a significant portion of the entire nose, may cause distortion (Figure 24.18).

Electrosurgery can be used for both large rhinophymas and localized growths to good effect (Figure 24.19A–H). Note in these examples that we have removed the rhinophymatous tissue that caused the most distortion and shaped each nose for that individual's face and underlying nasal structure.

SUGGESTIONS FOR FURTHER READING

Albom M. Electrosurgical treatment of rhinophyma. J Dermatol Surg. 1976; 2:89-191.

Fisher WJ. Rhinophyma: its surgical treatment. Plast Reconstr Surg. 1970;45:466-470.

Greenbaum SS, Krull EA, Watmick K. Comparison of CO_2 laser and electrosurgery in the treatment of rhinophyma. J Am Acad Dermatol. 1988;18:363-368.

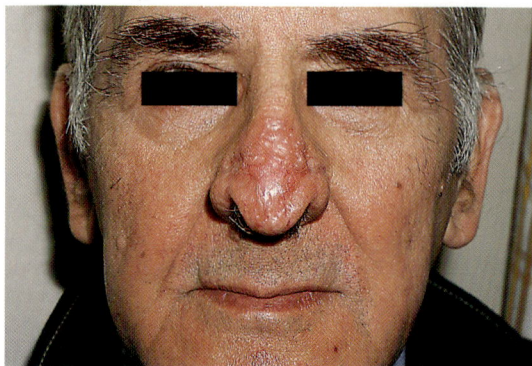

FIGURE 24.18 Significant scarring as a result of rhinophymatous tissue removal is apparent across this patient's entire nose. The smooth, shiny skin lacks follicles; consequently, both alae and the midportion of the nose have contracted.

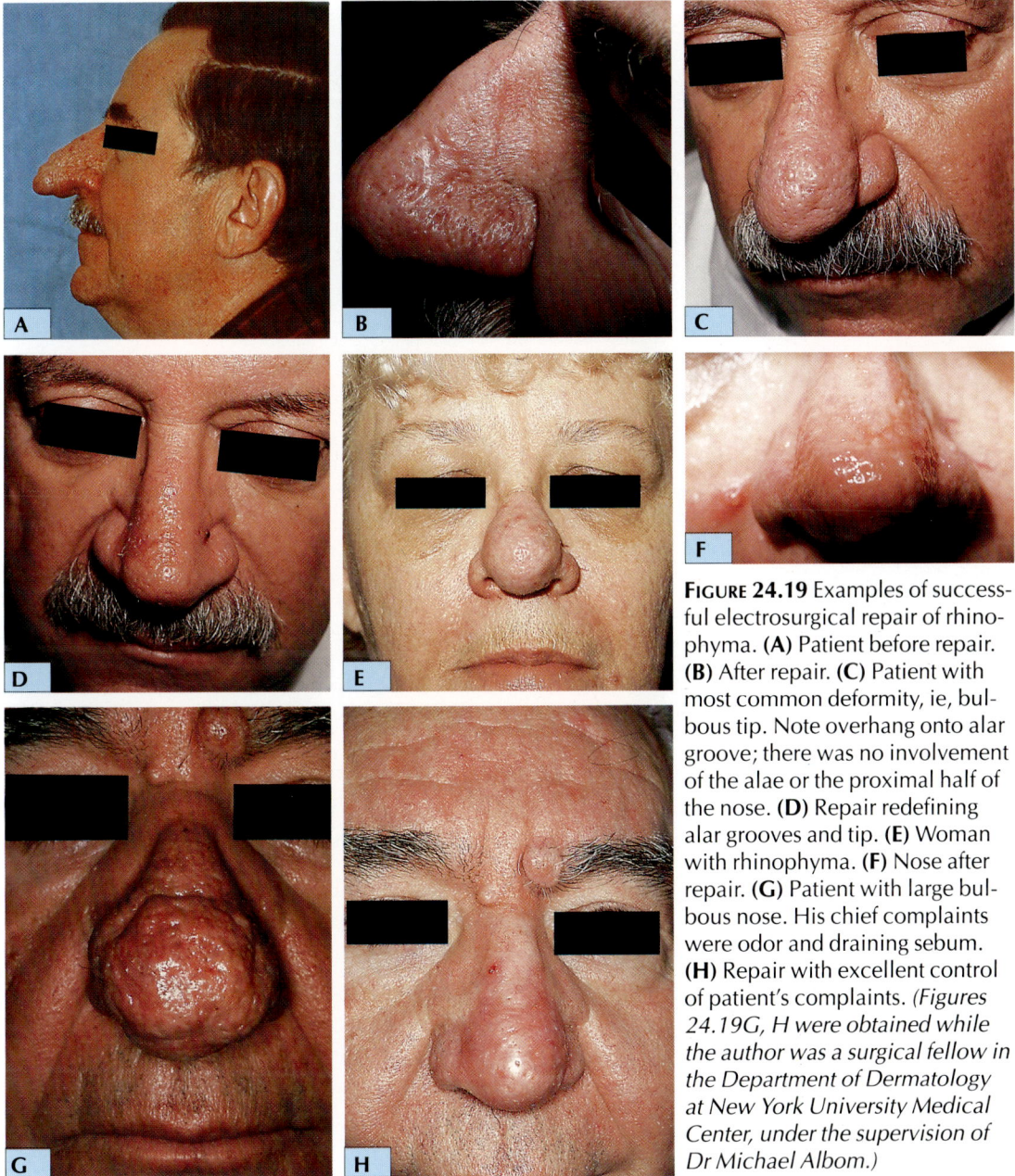

FIGURE 24.19 Examples of successful electrosurgical repair of rhinophyma. (A) Patient before repair. (B) After repair. (C) Patient with most common deformity, ie, bulbous tip. Note overhang onto alar groove; there was no involvement of the alae or the proximal half of the nose. (D) Repair redefining alar grooves and tip. (E) Woman with rhinophyma. (F) Nose after repair. (G) Patient with large bulbous nose. His chief complaints were odor and draining sebum. (H) Repair with excellent control of patient's complaints. (Figures 24.19G, H were obtained while the author was a surgical fellow in the Department of Dermatology at New York University Medical Center, under the supervision of Dr Michael Albom.)

SECTION FOUR

ADVANCED TECHNIQUES

chapter 25

CARBON DIOXIDE LASER SURGERY

A variety of medical lasers, including carbon dioxide, argon, neodymium–YAG, copper vapor, and pulsed dye models, have been used in cutaneous surgery, with other lasers such as ruby and excimer systems currently under study for cutaneous applications. Among these systems, the CO_2 laser has provided the widest range of application over a relatively long period of time. Virtually all skin tumors and many nevoid conditions have been treated at one time or another using CO_2 laser surgery, with many such conditions managed most effectively by this modality (Figure 25.1). A relatively high percentage of cutaneous surgeons use CO_2 lasers, in contrast to some of the newer lasers that are not in widespread use due to their limited indications and high cost. As a result, this chapter is devoted to a brief discussion of CO_2 laser surgery.

GENERAL FEATURES AND CAPABILITIES

The CO_2 laser emits invisible infrared light with a wavelength of 10,600 nm. Light of this wavelength cannot be transmitted by fiberoptics so it must be delivered to tissue through an operating microscope or via an articulated series of mirrored tubes attached to a surgical handpiece containing a focusing lens. To facilitate aiming, a visible red helium–neon laser beam of very low intensity is usually employed in commercial CO_2 laser systems, similar to the laser pointer systems available to lecturers in many auditoriums.

CO_2 laser light is selectively absorbed by water. Since water comprises 75% to 90% of soft-tissue content, the damage caused by the CO_2 laser is nonspecific. The rapid absorption of this energy in the skin prevents

FIGURE 25.1
DERMATOLOGIC CONDITIONS MOST FREQUENTLY TREATED BY CO_2 LASER SURGERY

VAPORIZATION

Widespread condyloma acuminatum
Recalcitrant verrucae
Lymphangioma circumscriptum
Adenoma sebaceum
Angiokeratomas
Epidermal nevus
Erythroplasia of Queyrat
Oral florid papillomatosis
Sublingual keratosis
Actinic cheilitis
Balanitis xerotica obliterans
Bowenoid papulosis
Nail plate/matrix ablation
Syringomas
Tattoos

CUTTING

Keloids
Acne keloidalis nuchae
Bone perforation
Rhinophyma*
Giant condyloma acuminatum*
Multiple giant appendageal tumors*

*Cutting used in combination with vaporization

significant thermal injury to surrounding structures.

CO_2 laser surgery has the same general capabilities as does electrosurgery (see Chapter 9). Tissues can be ablated superficially, destroyed deeply, or incised. The extent of thermal damage caused by the CO_2 laser depends on the duration and intensity of the exposure. Intensity at the skin surface is referred to as power density and is measured in watts per square centimeter (W/cm^2). With focusing or defocusing of the laser beam, the power density changes dramatically, altering the type and amount of tissue damage (Figure 25.2). High power densities, such as those achieved when a minute beam of 0.1 to 0.2 mm spot size is combined with a relatively high-power (15- to 25-W) beam, result in high tissue temperatures, vaporization, and tissue cutting. Lower power densities, such as those achieved with a larger beam of 1 to 2 mm combined with a low-power (4- to 10-W) setting, result in superficial tissue vaporization.

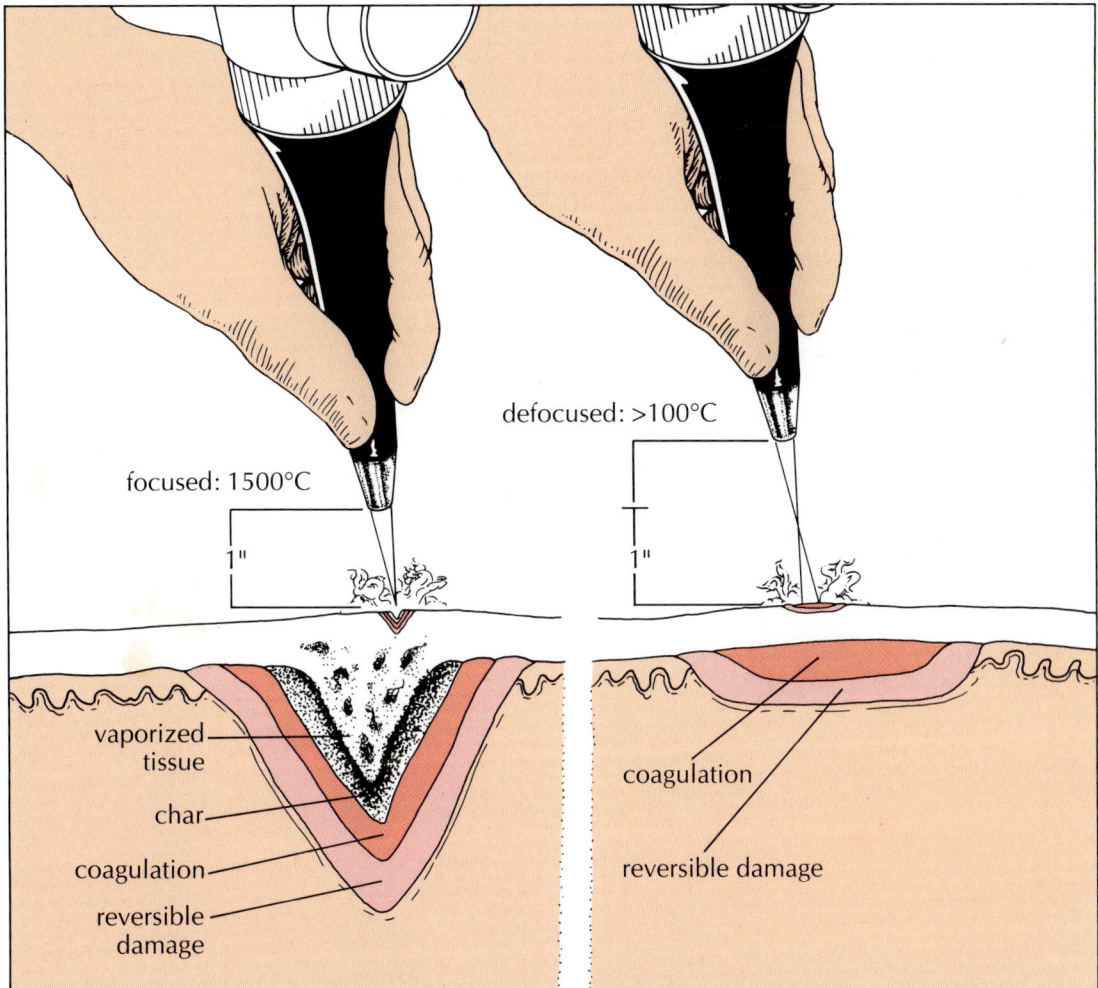

FIGURE 25.2 Precise focusing of the laser beam results in the production of high power densities that cause tissue cutting through cellular vaporization. When the beam is defocused, lower power densities result and more superficial tissue coagulation occurs over a larger skin area.

The longer the duration of the exposure, the greater the penetration of thermal damage into the skin. The duration of the beam can be controlled mechanically by the operator using a foot switch or electronically by the machine through a shuttering device. Superpulsing, discussed later in this chapter, causes the laser beam to be delivered in successive short bursts of energy.

The amount of heat generated during CO_2 laser surgery is sufficient to cause patient discomfort, requiring that local anesthesia be used. Although local infiltration of lidocaine with or without epinephrine generally is sufficient, nerve blocks can be used when appropriate, particularly in the treatment of larger lesions.

VAPORIZATION OF SOFT-TISSUE LESIONS

CO_2 laser energy causes vaporization of the water contained in the skin, resulting in the production of a vapor–smoke plume (Figure 25.3). Carbonization also occurs at the surface, and during ablation of skin lesions the carbon must be removed intermittently from the wound surface, with water or saline, to allow the laser beam to continue to interact with water-containing tissue. In the absence of such removal, the light heats the carbon particles at the surface to a high temperature causing thermal coagulation rather than vaporization of the underlying tissue.

Application of a relatively low power

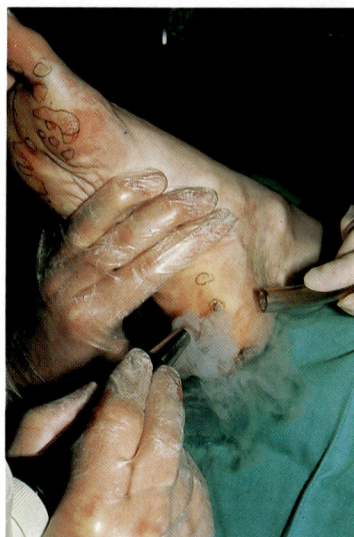

FIGURE 25.3 Vapor–smoke plume produced while ablating plantar verrucae with the CO_2 laser in a defocused mode. The plume is removed safely by the use of a smoke evacuator system, as seen to the right.

density (150 to 500 W/cm^2) using a defocused laser beam results in superficial ablation at the skin surface. Small, superficial lesions can be treated with a single pulse while larger lesions can be destroyed using a series of overlapping pulses or with a continuous brushlike motion. Deeper lesions are destroyed by repetition of this procedure sequentially, with removal of carbon deposits between laser beam passes.

VAPORIZATION TECHNIQUE

Vaporization ablation of tissues is performed using a defocused laser beam. The handpiece is held at a distance from the skin that is greater than the focal length of the lens (see Figure 25.2). As noted earlier, the amount of tissue vaporization that will occur depends on the power output, the spot size, and the duration of exposure. By withdrawing the handpiece from the skin surface and defocusing the beam further, the spot size increases and the same amount of power is distributed over a larger area. This maneuver decreases the power density, resulting in less penetrative damage suitable for the treatment of superficial skin lesions.

The defocused beam is moved over the area to be vaporized using smooth, slow, brushlike movements. For the treatment of deeper lesions, multiple passes are undertaken with serum, blood, char, and surface moisture removed between passes.

Slow vaporization of a given lesion at a low power density produces greater coagulative necrosis of adjacent tissue than does rapid vaporization of the same lesion at a higher power density. Postoperative edema, pain, and perhaps scarring also may be greater with slow vaporization. The optimal power density, therefore, is that which produces the fastest vaporization to the desired depth. Such power densities generally are achieved when power outputs of 15 to 20 W (5 to 8 W for superficial lesions) are used.

Of the cutaneous lesions that have been ablated effectively by CO_2 laser vaporization

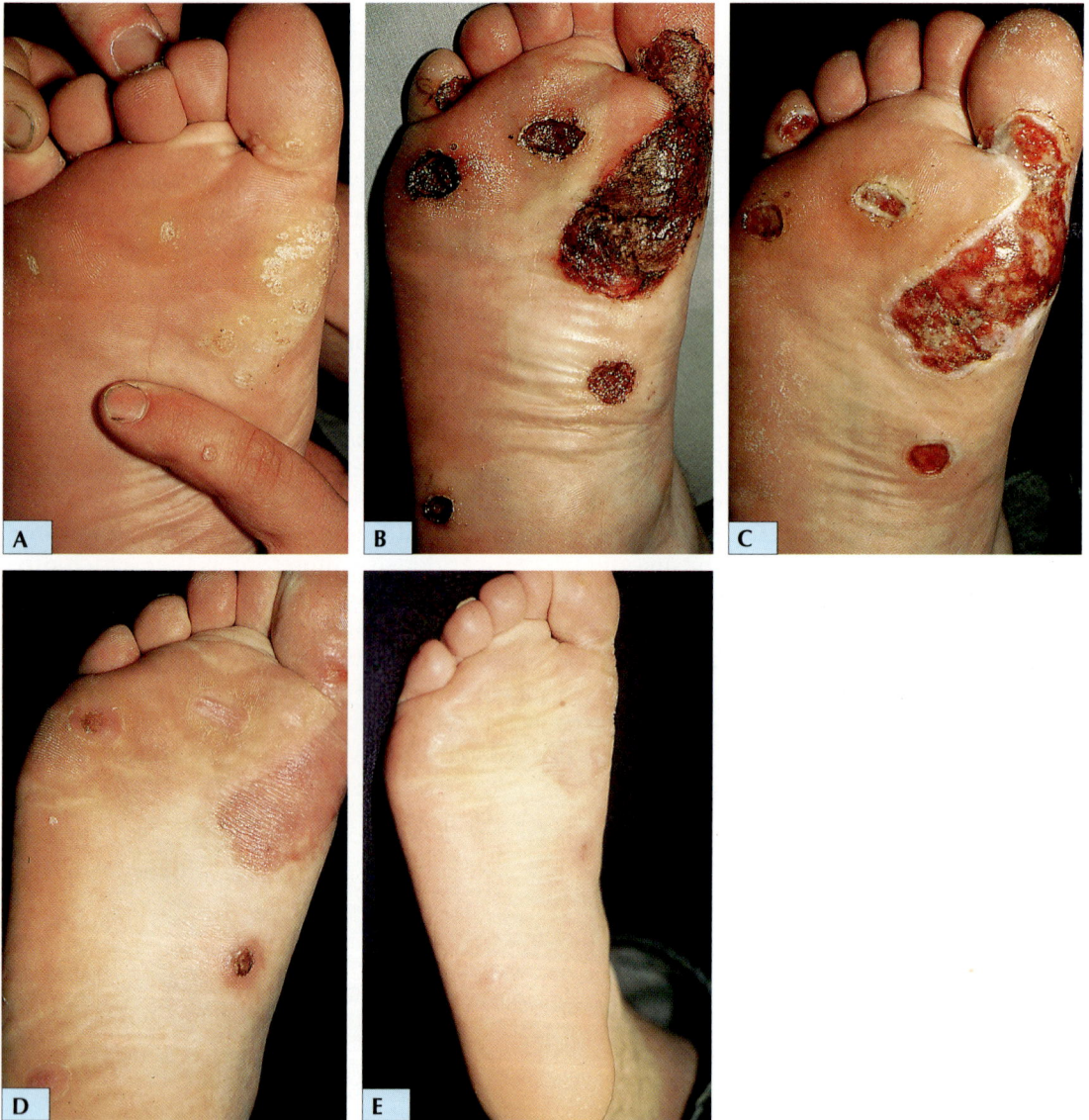

FIGURE 25.4 Recalcitrant plantar verrucae treated by CO_2 laser surgery. **(A)** Preoperative photograph of multiple recurrent plantar verrucae that have been unresponsive to previous treatment. **(B)** Photograph immediately following ablative treatment using the CO_2 laser in a defocused mode. Multiple surface ablations were performed, with the carbon at the surface removed vigorously between passes using saline-soaked gauze. The final layer of carbonization is evident. **(C)** At 1 week post surgery, the wound is healing normally. **(D)** Six weeks following surgery, the wounds are almost entirely healed. **(E)** The outcome at 3 months post surgery is excellent, without evidence of abnormal scar formation or other complication. The stratum corneum overlying the treatment site can be expected to reach its usual thickness 6 months later. Until then, the operative site remains subject to blistering with shearing injury.

(see Figure 25.1), those that have been found to be particularly responsive to this type of therapy include recalcitrant verrucae, tattoos, and actinic cheilitis. These are discussed briefly below.

Recalcitrant Verrucae

Recalcitrant verrucae such as plantar warts probably account for the greatest single group of lesions treated by CO_2 laser ablation. Since the human papilloma virus tends to be confined to epidermal tissue, vaporization into deep papillary dermis generally provides sufficient treatment depth. However, wart virus genome has been found in normal-appearing skin up to 1 cm from the visible edge of the wart, necessitating that a

margin of peripheral skin of up to 1 cm be treated around a given wart (Figure 25.4A–E). CO_2 laser ablation treatment of plantar verrucae generally is contraindicated in patients with a history of poor wound healing, diabetes, peripheral vascular disease, or peripheral neuropathy.

Tattoos

Tattoos also are treated frequently by CO_2 laser ablation (Figure 25.5A,B), which allows for the precise removal of all tattoo pigment. However, given the deep thermal damage necessary to ablate deeply placed pigment, some degree of scar formation usually occurs. Such scars may be atrophic or hypertrophic, depending on the location of the treatment

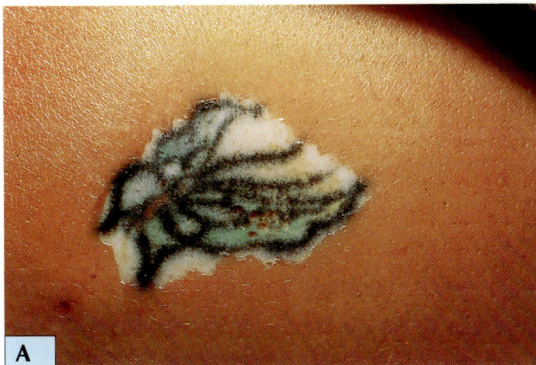

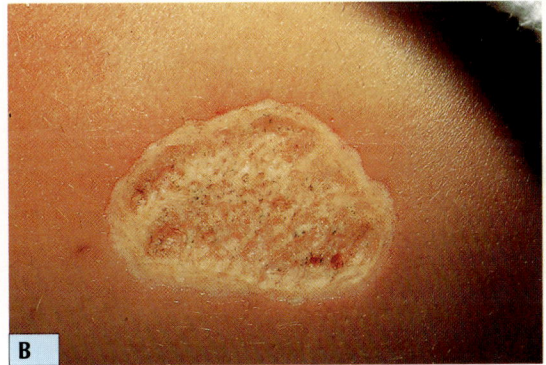

FIGURE 25.5 CO_2 laser treatment of a tattoo. **(A)** After initial surface vaporization, most of the pigment remains in the skin. **(B)** Following several surface ablations, all of the tattoo pigment has been removed. Due to the depth of coagulation required for complete removal, significant fibrosis should be anticipated and its likelihood discussed preoperatively with the patient.

site. Patients must be forewarned of their likelihood prior to surgery.

Actinic Cheilitis

Actinic cheilitis is a common condition that is managed most easily, quickly, and effectively by CO_2 laser ablation (Figure 25.6A–C). Coagulation of the lip mucosa generally can be achieved in one pass, using a power output of 5 to 10 W. The lip surface will bubble and blister as an epidermal–dermal split occurs. This is the desired end point since the pathologic process is limited to the epidermis. Vaporization of the vermilion border should be avoided as it can result in unacceptable

scarring. Healing occurs in 2 to 4 weeks and the outcome is often a "rosy red" lip, which appears healthier than did the lip preoperatively.

INCISION/EXCISION OF TISSUE

The CO_2 laser beam also can be used as a "light scalpel" when high power densities (greater than 25,000 W/cm²) are used (Figure 25.7). This is accomplished by reducing the beam diameter to its minimum size of 0.1 to 0.2 mm. Vessels of 1 to 2 mm in diameter are sealed spontaneously during surgery, provid-

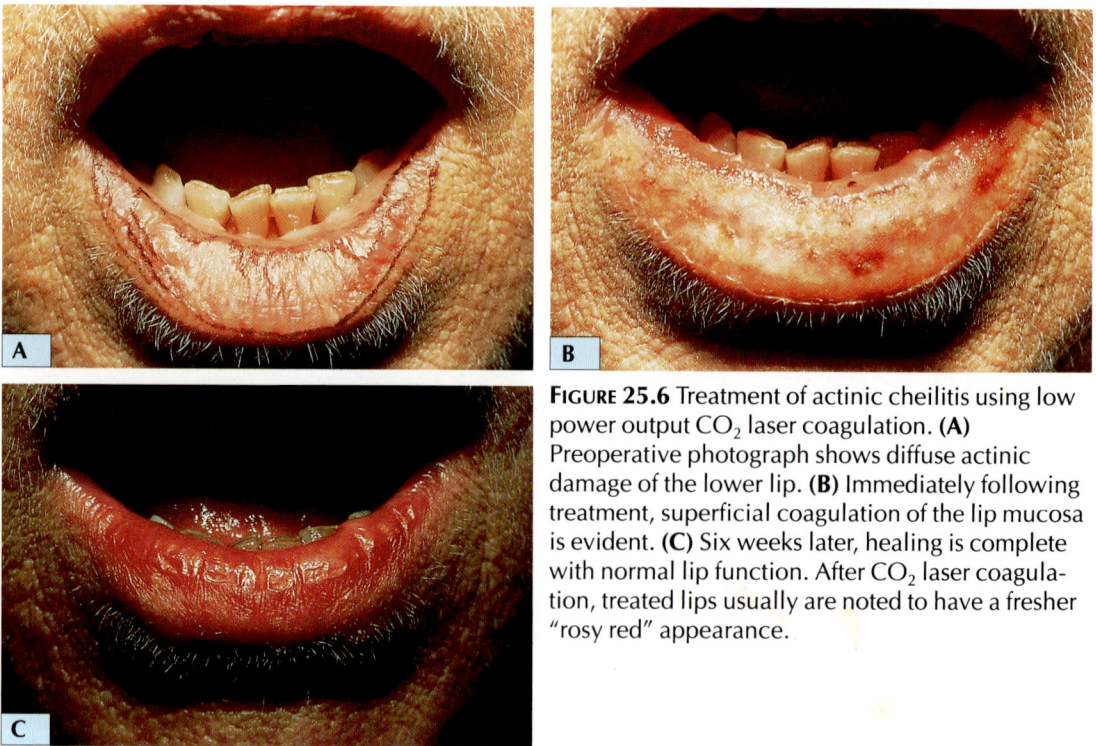

FIGURE 25.6 Treatment of actinic cheilitis using low power output CO_2 laser coagulation. (A) Preoperative photograph shows diffuse actinic damage of the lower lip. (B) Immediately following treatment, superficial coagulation of the lip mucosa is evident. (C) Six weeks later, healing is complete with normal lip function. After CO_2 laser coagulation, treated lips usually are noted to have a fresher "rosy red" appearance.

ing significant instantaneous hemostasis. Energy may be emitted continuously or it can be broken into a series of extremely short, high energy pulses of 100 to 5000 repetitions per second. The latter is termed "superpulsing." By reducing delivered energy to about 30% of normal, superpulsing minimizes thermal damage but also provides less effective hemostasis.

For the incisional mode of CO_2 laser therapy, the depth of the incision depends on the power of the beam and on its rate of movement across the skin surface. The technique is particularly useful for the treatment of anticoagulated patients and for the surgical removal of vascular lesions or other lesions in vascular anatomic locations.

INCISIONAL TECHNIQUE

Because of the necessity of using the articulated handpiece, cutting with the CO_2 laser tends to be somewhat more awkward than scalpel excision. However, the ability of the laser beam to provide simultaneous hemostasis renders this modality superior to scalpel surgery in the following situations:

1. In patients who have bleeding disorders or who are on anticoagulants;

2. In patients in whom epinephrine is contraindicated;

3. In patients with pacemakers in whom the use of electrosurgery is limited (see Chapter 9);

4. For the treatment of vascular lesions or tissues such as hemangiomas or scalp tumors; and

5. For the treatment of infected surgical sites.

The use of the CO_2 laser as a light scalpel is relatively easy. With the handpiece held at sufficient distance from the skin surface for the beam to be focused (a distance that usually coincides with the smallest helium–neon beam size), the laser beam is directed at the skin surface. The focused beam is then advanced at a smooth, steady pace of approximately 0.25 cm/s. The initial incision is limited in depth by absorption of the beam by char, serum, and blood. A slightly charred cut surface results, which is cleansed with a moistened gauze pad and patted dry before further cutting is attempted to complete the incision or excision. Following this, a standard repair is performed and the usual surgical dressing is applied. Laser wounds also may be allowed to heal by second intention.

Using this technique, a variety of benign and malignant skin tumors including skin

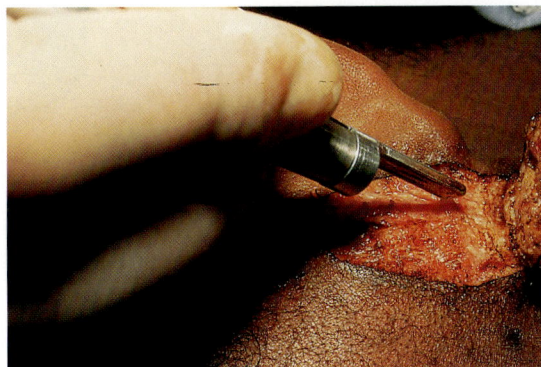

FIGURE 25.7 Tissue excision performed with the CO_2 laser. High power densities are used to cause vaporization of tissue with resultant near-bloodless incision.

cancers, keloids (Figure 25.8A–C), hemangiomas, and cysts have been treated. Rhinophyma, giant condyloma acuminatum, and multiple giant appendageal tumors (Figure 25.9A–C) also have been approached using a combination of CO_2 cutting and vaporization (see Figure 25.1).

POSTOPERATIVE CARE OF CO_2 LASER WOUNDS

In the case of laser wounds that are closed primarily or otherwise repaired (eg, flaps or grafts), the usual postoperative care is practiced as described elsewhere in this text. The remainder of laser wounds, particularly those following ablations of skin lesions, are allowed to "granulate" in. Such wounds are best maintained in a moist environment. The wounds are cleansed twice daily with soap and water or hydrogen peroxide solution followed by application of an antibiotic ointment. A semi-occlusive dressing is then applied and is kept in place continuously until the next dressing change.

Perineal and perianal wounds following laser ablation of condyloma acuminatum are difficult to cover (Figure 25.10A–C), and thin feminine hygiene pads or panty liners have been found to be useful for the coverage of such lesions. The antibiotic ointment is applied directly to the wound and the pad is held in place by the patient's underwear. Stool softeners, prescribed during the healing of such lesions, will minimize the pain that often accompanies defecation. Similarly, following the treatment of extensive facial lesions, lip lesions, or eyelid lesions, a dressing may not be practical and in such instances patients are asked to apply antibiotic ointment frequently to prevent dehydration and eschar formation.

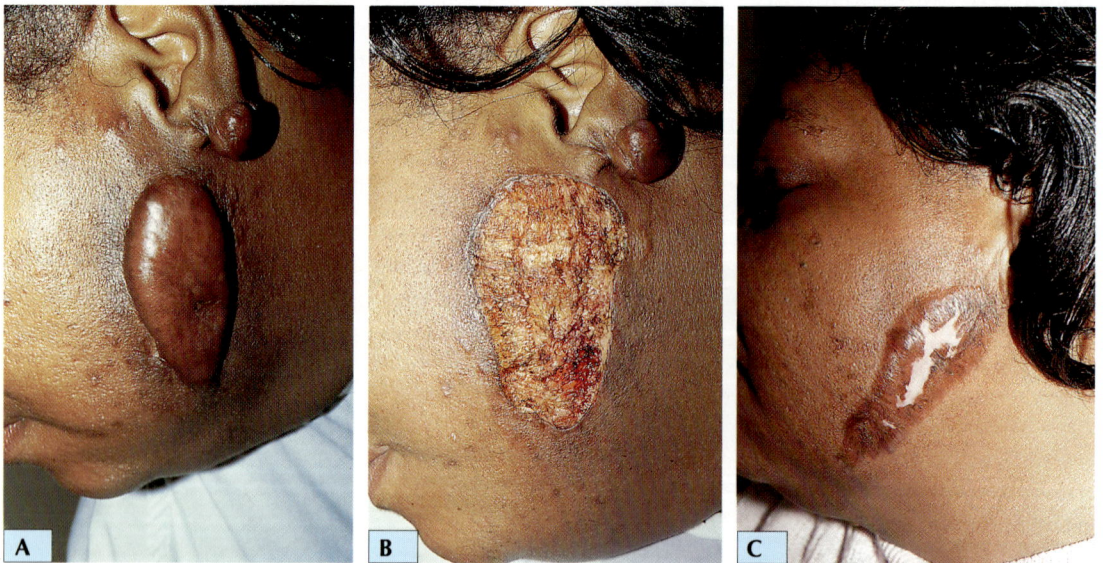

FIGURE 25.8 Excision of a facial keloid using focused CO_2 laser cutting. **(A)** Preoperative photograph of a large, thick keloid on the face of a middle-aged black woman. **(B)** The postoperative defect is seen following removal. Surface charring is produced during laser excision. **(C)** Five years later, after many post-surgical intralesional injections of triamcinolone acetonide, pigmentary alteration is seen although the keloid has not recurred.

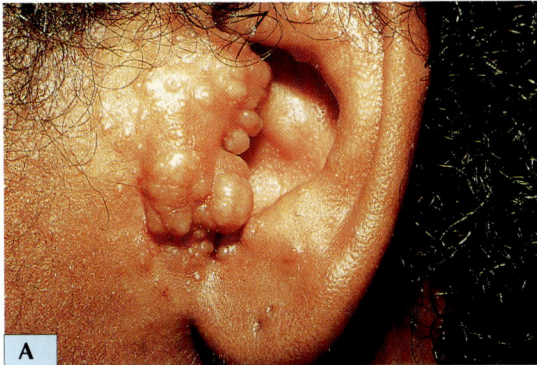

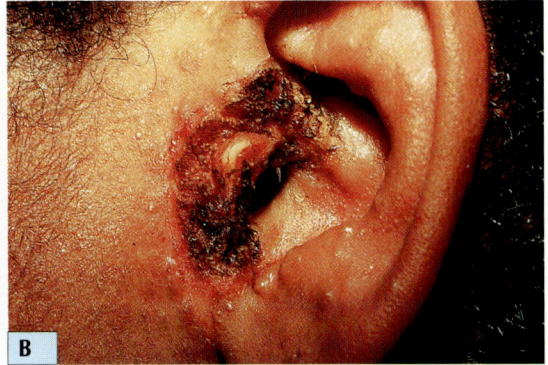

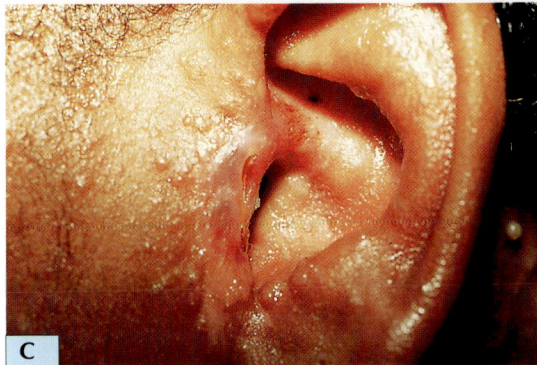

FIGURE 25.9 Treatment of multiple trichoepithelio-mata by combined CO_2 laser cutting and vaporization. (A) Preoperative photograph shows multiple coalesced papules and plaques at the left preauricular region in a black woman. (B) The large tumor mass was treated by CO_2 laser excision while the smaller peripheral lesions were coagulated with the laser in a defocused mode. (C) The result 6 weeks later shows excellent healing of the treatment site.

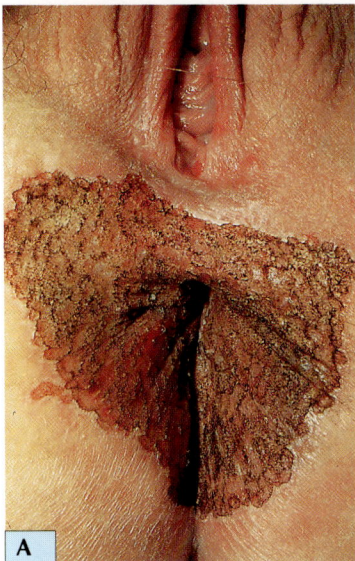

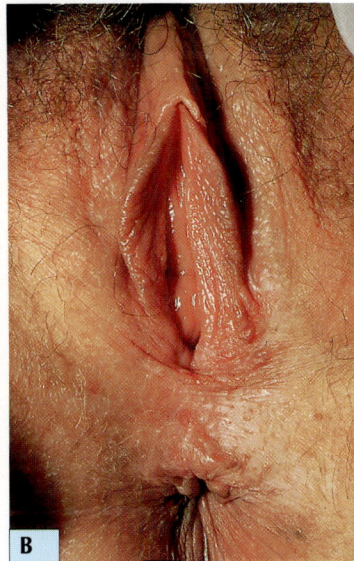

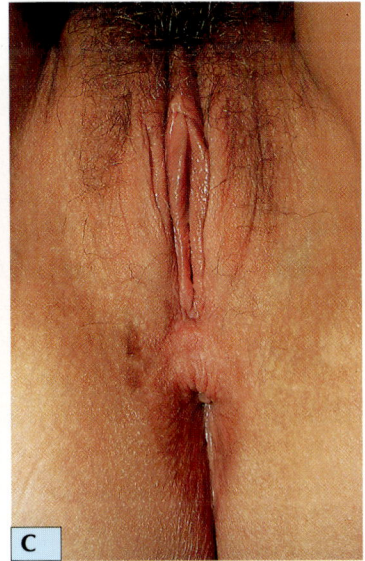

FIGURE 25.10 Healing of a perianal wound following treatment of a large lesion of Bowen's disease. (A) Following coagulation using the CO_2 laser in a defocused mode, a large perianal defect is present. The patient was instructed to cleanse the area with sitz baths twice daily, followed by the application of a thin layer of antibiotic ointment covered by a panty-liner type of feminine hygiene pad. (B) After 6 weeks, excellent early healing has occurred, with the usual slight fibrosis. (C) Six months later, the fibrosis is gone, the scar is soft, and no recurrent tumor is evident.

CO$_2$ laser wounds often heal slightly slower than other open wounds, and do so in about 4 to 8 weeks. On the plantar aspect of the foot, the normal thickened stratum corneum does not fully appear for an additional several months. Pain following CO$_2$ laser surgery is variable but usually is controlled with non-narcotic analgesics such as acetaminophen. For more severe discomfort, codeine occasionally is required.

HAZARDS OF CO$_2$ LASER SURGERY

During CO$_2$ laser surgery, significant amounts of smoke and steam are produced. This laser plume has been shown to contain carbon particulates and wart viral DNA fragments, which, upon inhalation by patient, physician, or operating room personnel, may cause pulmonary disease or spread infectious disease. Therefore, when laser surgical procedures are undertaken, smoke evacuation systems and high filtration surgical masks designed for use with laser surgery should be employed.

Corneal injuries, which may result from stray laser emissions, can be avoided by the use of protective eye goggles, glasses, or protective polycarbonate eye lenses. Everyone in the treatment room, including the patient, should use eye protection (Figure 25.11). When treatment of the immediate periorbital area is undertaken with CO$_2$ laser surgery, greater patient eye protection is provided by placement of moistened gauze pads over the eyes or by the use of a sterile concave stainless steel scleral eye shield placed over the cornea.

As an added hazard, the concentrated light beam from the laser is capable of igniting combustible dry surgical drapes. Therefore, nonflammable, disposable sterile drapes or moistened reusable cloth drapes should be used to prevent this potential hazard. In addition, most operators place moistened gauze pads around the operative site to prevent damage to surrounding tissues.

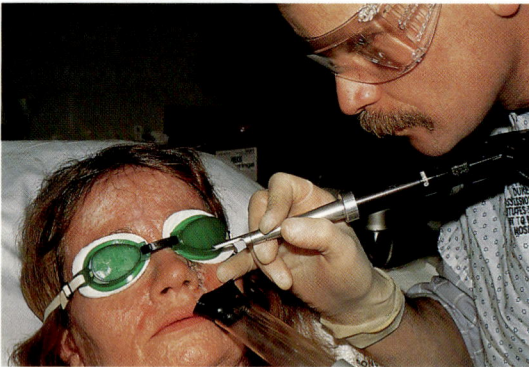

FIGURE 25.11 Photograph showing the necessary eye protection for both physician and patient during CO$_2$ laser surgery. The patient wears plastic eye shields with gauze pads underneath. The physician should also wear a surgical mask (not shown) and gloves. A smoke evacuation system is necessary to remove the vapor–smoke plume.

SUGGESTIONS FOR FURTHER READING

Apfelberg DB, Maser MR, Lash H, et al. Comparison of argon and carbon dioxide laser treatment of decorative tattoos: a preliminary report. Ann Plast Surg. 1985;14:6-15.

Dover JS, Arndt KA. Illustrated Cutaneous Laser Surgery—A Practitioner's Guide. Norwalk, Ct: Appleton & Lange;1990: 22-72.

Garden JM, O'Banion K, Shelnitz LS, et al. Papillomavirus in the vapor of carbon dioxide laser-treated verrucae. JAMA. 1988; 259:1199-1202.

Hobbs EH, Bailin PL, Wheeland RG, Ratz JL. Superpulsed lasers: minimizing thermal damage with short duration, high irradiance pulses. J Dermatol Surg Oncol. 1987; 13:955-964.

Leshin B, Whitaker DC. Carbon dioxide laser matrixectomy. J Dermatol Surg Oncol. 1988;14:608-611.

Ratz JL, ed. Lasers in Cutaneous Medicine and Surgery. Chicago, Ill: Year Book Medical Publishers Inc;1986.

Ratz JL, Bailin PL. The case for use of the carbon dioxide laser in the treatment of port-wine stains. Arch Dermatol. 1987; 123:74-75.

Van Gemert MJC, Welch AJ, Tan OT, Parrish JA. Limitations of carbon dioxide lasers for treatment of port-wine stains. Arch Dermatol. 1987;123:71-73.

Walker NPJ, Matthews J, Newsom SWB. Possible hazards from irradiation with the carbon dioxide laser. Lasers Surg Med. 1986;6:84-86.

Wheeland RG, Bailin PL, Ratz JL. Combined carbon dioxide laser excision and vaporization in the treatment of rhinophyma. J Dermatol Surg Oncol. 1987;13:172-177.

Whitaker DC. Microscopically proven cure of actinic cheilitis by CO_2 laser. Lasers Surg Med. 1987;7:520-523.

chapter 26

DERMABRASION

Dermabrasion is an effective modality for improving textural and pigmentary alterations of the skin. The conditions most often treated by this modality are scarring (due to acne, trauma, or surgery), solar elastosis, multiple actinic keratoses, extensive epidermal lesions such as large seborrheic keratoses, and tattoos. The technique can be performed safely in the office setting as an ambulatory procedure. Success, in the main, depends on appropriate patient selection and realistic patient expectations for outcome.

PATIENT SELECTION

A major determinant of success with dermabrasion lies in patient selection. Although acne scarring is one of the most frequent indications for the procedure, many such patients are poor candidates for dermabrasion. Soft, undulating "fingerprint"-type

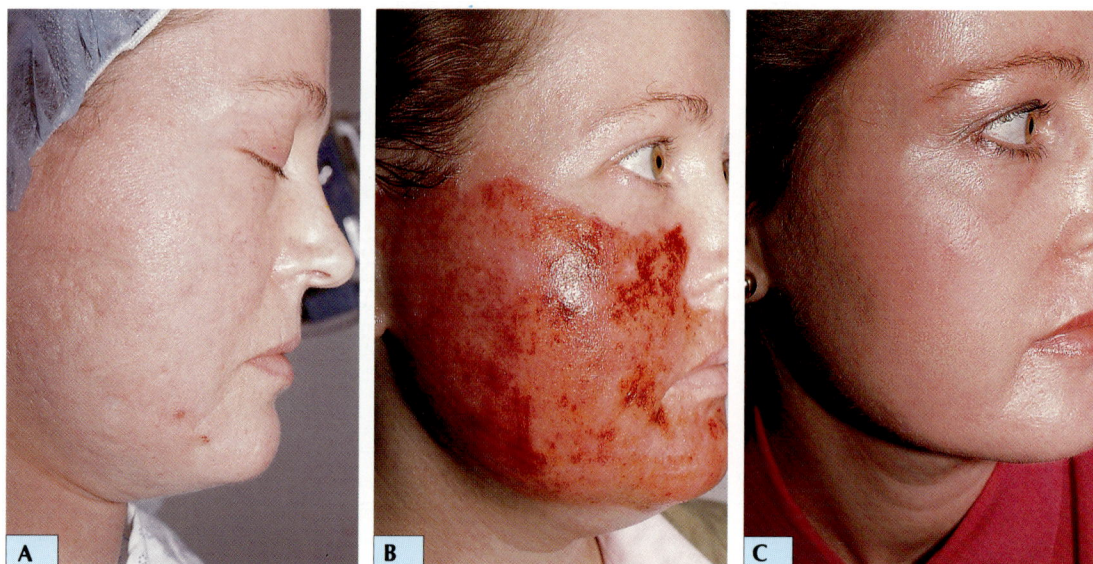

FIGURE 26.1 Treatment by dermabrasion of superficial acne scarring in a young woman. **(A)** Preoperative photograph shows shallow facial scarring. **(B)** The malar and perioral regions were dermabraded with a coarse diamond fraise. **(C)** After 3 weeks, significant improvement is noted. There is still some swelling evident at this point, and as it subsides further residual scarring may become evident.

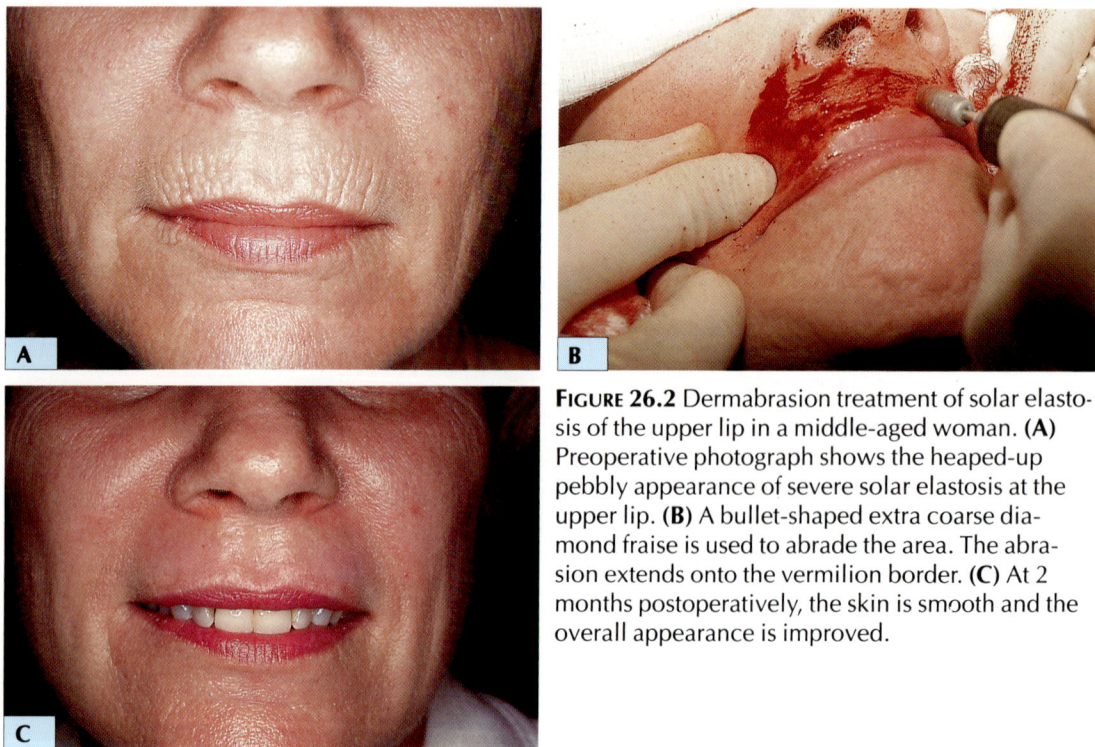

FIGURE 26.2 Dermabrasion treatment of solar elastosis of the upper lip in a middle-aged woman. **(A)** Preoperative photograph shows the heaped-up pebbly appearance of severe solar elastosis at the upper lip. **(B)** A bullet-shaped extra coarse diamond fraise is used to abrade the area. The abrasion extends onto the vermilion border. **(C)** At 2 months postoperatively, the skin is smooth and the overall appearance is improved.

scarring does not tend to improve appreciably with dermabrasion and often requires supplemental intradermal augmentation (see Chapter 18). Deep "ice-pick" scarring, likewise, usually does not improve appreciably because only the surface of the scar is removed and significant scar depth persists after healing. A more effective treatment for this type of scarring is punch excision, elevation, or grafting of individual scars followed by dermabrasion.

Relatively shallow fibrotic or ice-pick scarring is the optimal type of acne scarring to be treated by dermabrasion. Shallow scars can be made considerably less apparent through substantial alteration of their total depth and optical properties (Figure 26.1 A–C). On occasion, a second dermabrasion can be performed 3 to 6 months after the first treatment and further improvement can be achieved.

Traumatic and surgical scars also can be made less conspicuous by dermabrasion. For- merly it was held that wounds should be allowed to mature for several months prior to their being treated by dermabrasion. More recently, however, Dr John Yarborough has demonstrated that optimal results can be obtained when dermabrasion is performed approximately 6 to 8 weeks following suture removal.

Dermabrasion also can be used to achieve rejuvenation of aging skin. Fine lines and wrinkles are improved by dermabrasion as is the pebbly appearance seen with severe solar elastosis (Figure 26.2A–C). Patients, however, must be advised that significant sagging of skin (jowls) due to loss of elasticity cannot be improved by dermabrasion. Dermabrasion is also a rapid and effective way to deal with multiple epidermal skin lesions such as actinic or seborrheic keratoses, which otherwise must be dealt with individually or by prolonged topical chemotherapy (Figure 26.3A–C). Although tattoos can be obliterated by dermabrasion, the resultant scarring is

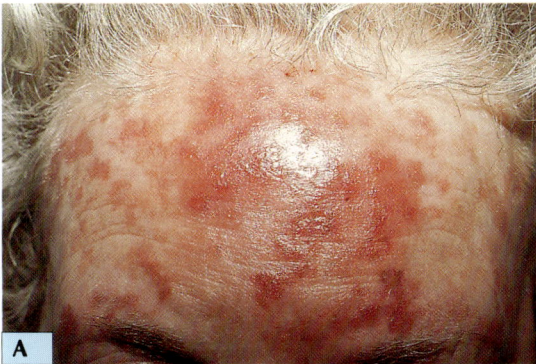

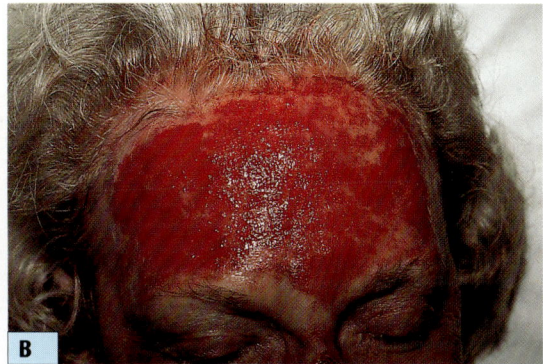

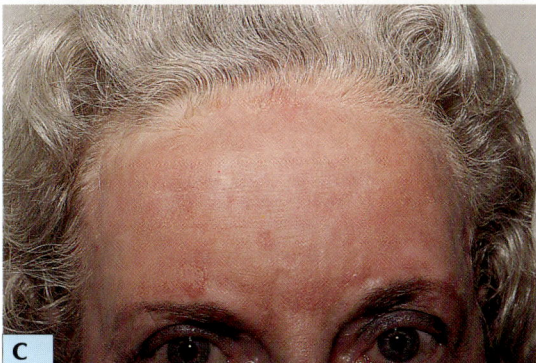

FIGURE 26.3 Treatment, by dermabrasion, of multiple actinic keratoses in an elderly woman. (A) Preoperative photograph demonstrates dozens of actinic keratoses of the forehead. (B) The forehead was treated with a coarse diamond fraise. (C) Two months later most but not all of the lesions are gone. The remaining lesions were treated by cryosurgery.

usually less acceptable than that following surgical excision of such lesions.

Preoperative work-up for patients undergoing dermabrasion includes a medical history with particular attention paid to previous history of herpes labialis, hepatitis, or other transmissible disease. Results of prior surgery also should be evaluated to determine whether wound healing is normal. Patients who have taken isotretinoin (Accutane) in the months preceding dermabrasion may be at increased risk of developing healing problems and abnormal hypertrophic scarring. The reasons for this are unclear. However, most clinicians advise patients to wait 6 to 12 months after cessation of isotretinoin therapy before undergoing dermabrasion. Preoperative laboratory investigations vary from one clinician to another and most often include bleeding time, hepatitis B antigen, and HIV antibody titers.

EQUIPMENT

In dermabrasion, the epidermis and the superficial dermis are physically removed using either a rapidly rotating wire brush or a diamond fraise. The wire brush is a stainless steel wheel upon which multiple beveled wires are arranged that protrude at an angle (Figure 26.4). The wires cut deeply and rapidly into frozen skin. In the diamond fraise, diamond chips of different grades of coarseness (regular, coarse, or extra coarse) are bonded to the surface of a stainless steel wheel (Figure 26.5). Most clinicians use the latter instrument, which is easier to control and less likely to cause gouging of the skin, even when extra coarse fraises are used. Once appropriate experience has been achieved with the fraise, many clinicians "graduate" to wire brush dermabrasion, which they find to be more effective.

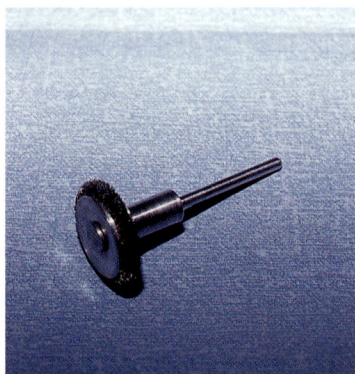

FIGURE 26.4 A wire brush is used for dermabrasion when deeper injury is desired. The possibility of skin gouging with scar production exists if extreme care is not taken.

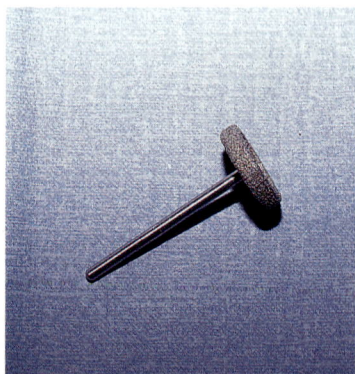

FIGURE 26.5 A diamond fraise is suitable for performing shallow dermabrasions. Mild to moderate downward pressure may be applied without risk of gouging the skin.

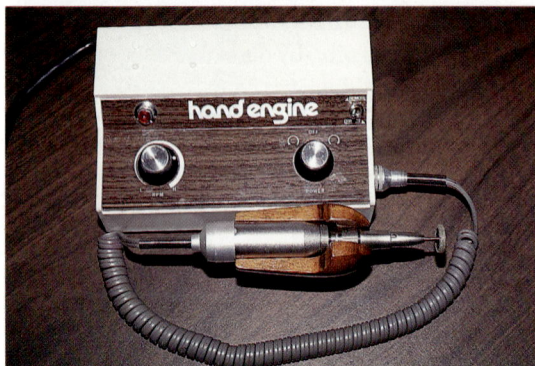

FIGURE 26.6 The hand engine (Bell International Machine Company) is a compact unit that is popular for dermabrasion.

For powering the fraise or the brush, a variety of types of motorized equipment is available, which over the years has become more compact and portable. Such engines are characterized by high torque, which means that the rotations per minute (rpm) do not diminish in response to friction caused by the operator exerting downward pressure on the skin. The machinery varies in terms of rotary speed, ranging from 12,000 rpm to 40,000 rpm or greater. One clinician with extensive dermabrasion experience has suggested that optimal results can be obtained only with the fastest equipment. This observation, however, is not entirely consistent with the excellent results seen routinely with the Bell hand engine (Figure 26.6), which rotates the abrader at approximately 20,000 rpm.

Since dermabrasion results in the generation of blood-borne particles in the environment, the operator and assistants should take appropriate measures to protect themselves from exposure to blood-borne hazards, including hepatitis and HIV infection. This involves wearing of an operative gown, a face mask, a face shield, and surgical gloves (Figure 26.7).

Some controversy appears to exist regarding the perceived necessity for freezing of the skin prior to dermabrasion. Although a number of topical refrigerants are available for cryoanesthesia, not all practitioners use them. However, most cutaneous surgeons believe that topical refrigerants have a role in dermabrasion and that their use contributes to an improved ultimate outcome. The refrigerant is thought to "freeze" the topographic features in place so that they are not distorted by the fraise or brush during the procedure. In this way, the "peaks" of the irregularities are removed while the "valleys" are left intact, resulting in a smoother outcome. Topical refrigerants also provide anesthesia. The most common cryoanesthetic agents in use are Frigiderm and Fluro-Ethyl, which are Freon 114 and Freon 114 plus ethyl chloride, respectively (Figure 26.8). Overly aggressive freezing can result in cryonecrosis, particularly over mandibular bone.

AESTHETIC UNITS

With the exception of surgical or traumatic scars, which are often treated on their own,

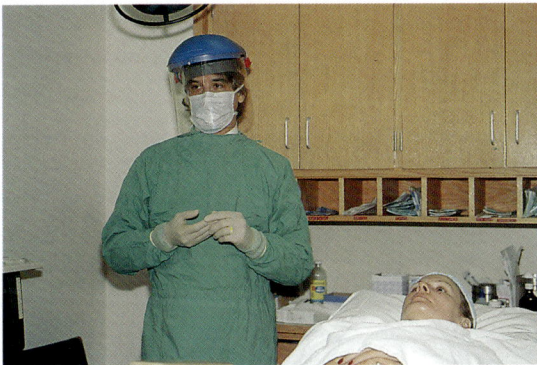

FIGURE 26.7 The operator and assistants should wear gowns, gloves, masks, and face shields during dermabrasion.

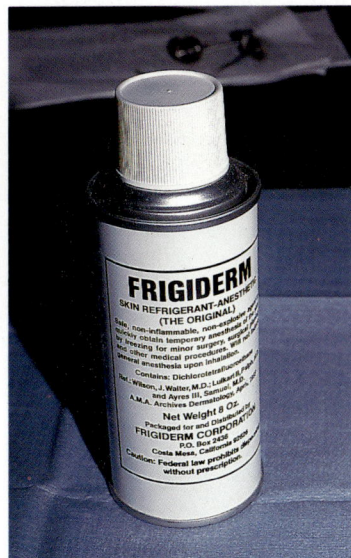

FIGURE 26.8 Frigiderm is one type of cryoanesthesia used for dermabrasion. Fluro-Ethyl (not shown) is another popular brand.

most cosmetic dermabrasion is performed so that it includes an entire "aesthetic" or anatomic unit (Figure 26.9). The usual boundaries of such units are the natural folds of the face, such as the nasolabial fold, the hairline, or the orbital rim. At the periphery of the face, dermabrasion is extended approximately 1 cm over the mandibular rim to a submandibular location to avoid any obvious lines of demarcation. If only a portion of a unit is treated, a color mismatch can result after healing. Therefore, rather than treat isolated scarring at the malar eminence, for example, the entire malar region is treated to achieve better blending of the result.

PREOPERATIVE PREPARATION

Most cutaneous surgeons perform dermabrasion without general anesthesia. Patients wear a treatment gown during the procedure and their hair is covered by a surgeon's cap or is wrapped in a sterile towel. To allow them to dress more easily following the procedure, patients are instructed to wear a blouse or a button-down shirt to the office rather than a pullover. A typical preoperative medication regimen, administered intramuscularly 30 minutes beforehand, is 50 to 100 mg of Demerol and 25 mg of Phenergan, although

other agents may be used. The face is washed with soap and water and the patient is asked to be sure that all makeup has been removed.

Using 1% lidocaine with epinephrine, most clinicians administer nerve blocks of the appropriate branches of the trigeminal nerve and of the supratrochlear and temporofacial nerves for forehead planing (Figure 26.10). These blocks anesthetize only the mid-portion of the face. The lateral portions of the cheeks are numbed by blocking the temporozygomatic nerves using a long needle and fanning medially from the preauricular area.

PROCEDURE

Within 30 minutes of the Demerol/Phenergan injection, patients feel relaxed and for the most part are able to endure with ease the modicum of discomfort associated with the procedure. The patient is told what to expect and is allowed to hear both the sound of the refrigerant spray and the dermabrasion engine before the start of the procedure.

Also in advance of the procedure, it is helpful to outline with a marking pencil the boundaries of the regions to be abraded. These regions are then treated in a series of overlapping silver dollar-sized segments. The most dependent areas are treated first so that bleeding from above does not occur as treat-

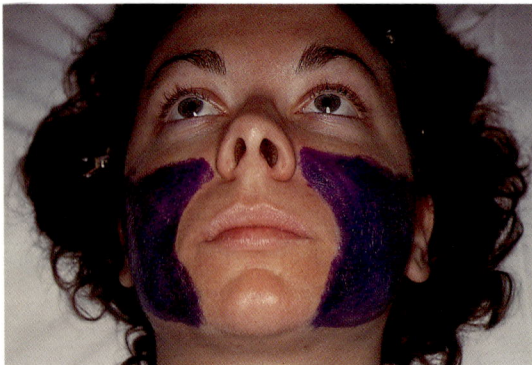

FIGURE 26.9 Gentian violet is used to demarcate matching cosmetic or "aesthetic" units of the face. These areas were dermabraded for treatment of bilateral acne scarring of the malar eminences.

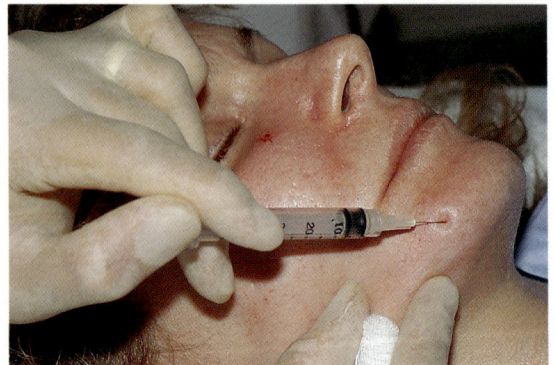

FIGURE 26.10 A few minutes after the preoperative injection of Demerol and Phenergan, nerve blocks are performed. Here the mental nerve is being blocked using 1% lidocaine with epinephrine.

ment proceeds. A skin refrigerant is sprayed in a circular motion for approximately 10 seconds to freeze the area evenly. The appearance of frosting at the surface indicates that the area is frozen firmly and is ready to be abraded (Figure 26.11).

The skin is stabilized by traction applied by both the operator and the assistant. With the opposite hand, the operator holds the abrader in a manner similar to that used in holding a tennis racquet. Most operators extend the thumb distally along the shaft of the handle to achieve added control. The frozen area is abraded while the fraise or brush is kept in motion, usually perpendicular to the direction of rotation of the abrader (Figure 26.12). Some downward pressure

can be exerted when fraises are used but a very light touch is required when wire brush dermabrasion is performed.

The skin remains frozen for approximately 5 seconds, which is long enough to abrade each silver dollar-sized treatment area. When skin segments at the periphery of the face are treated, the mandibular rim should be treated first since it derives its entire anesthesia from the skin refrigerant, which loses its effectiveness as thawing occurs. Adjacent areas are frozen and dermabraded in succession until the entire region has been completed (Figure 26.13). The matching region on the contralateral side is then treated in the same manner.

Some specialized fraises are useful for

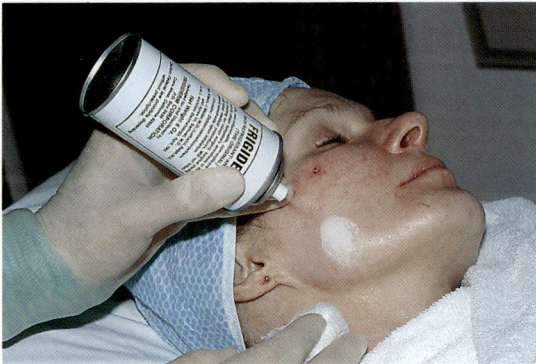

FIGURE 26.11 A silver dollar-sized area in the most dependent part of the face is sprayed with cryoanesthetic.

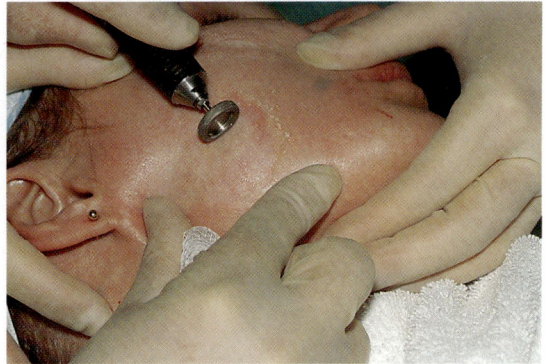

FIGURE 26.12 The frozen segment of skin is abraded with an extra coarse diamond fraise. The skin is held taught by the operator and assistant, while the fraise is moved back and forth in a direction perpendicular to the rotation of the wheel.

FIGURE 26.13 Adjacent skin segments are frozen and abraded. The abrasion should overlap into neighboring segments.

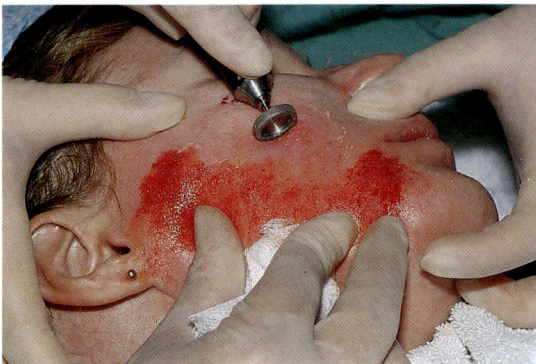

particular anatomic locations or functions. Bullet- and pear-shaped fraises are useful for re-abrading individual scars after the bulk of the abrasion has been performed (Figure 26.14). They are also helpful for abrading in and around structures such as the philtrum and nose and also for treating the upper lip. Effective dermabrasion of the latter should extend slightly onto the vermilion border to avoid accentuation of the lip margin (see Figure 26.2B). When abrading at the lip margin or near the eyelids, the rotating abrasion tip should be adjusted so that it rotates toward the opening, rather than away from it, to avoid accidental pulling or tearing by the instrument.

POSTOPERATIVE CARE

Immediately upon completion of the procedure, 1% lidocaine with epinephrine is sprayed on the abraded skin, which is then covered with sterile towels (Figure 26.15). The lidocaine provides immediate relief from the mild burning discomfort while the epinephrine helps to control any bleeding that may be present. After several minutes an antibacterial ointment is applied (Figure 26.16), followed by application of an absorbent nonadherent dressing. A face mask of the dressing is commercially available and is secured in place with rolled gauze (Figure 26.17).

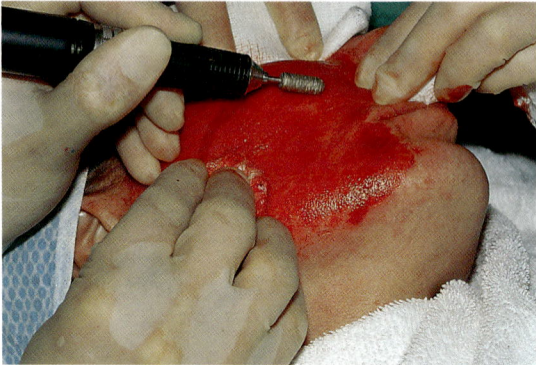

FIGURE 26.14 An extra coarse bullet-shaped fraise is used for individual treatment of some of the deeper scars at the malar eminence.

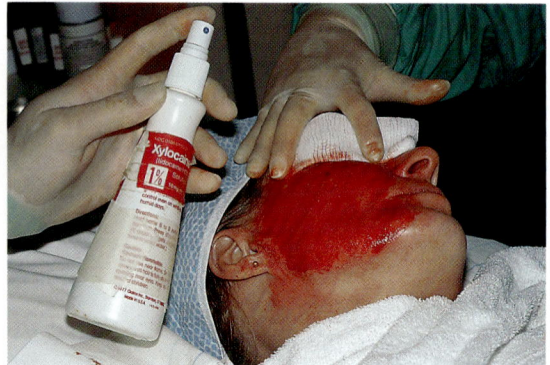

FIGURE 26.15 The abraded areas are treated with 1% lidocaine with epinephrine in a spray-pump container, thereby providing instant relief from the burning sensation felt after dermabrasion.

FIGURE 26.16 A thin layer of antibacterial ointment is applied to the abrasion.

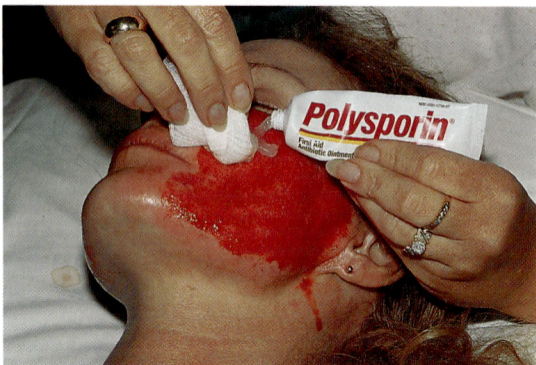

Patients are instructed to leave the face mask in place for 24 to 36 hours. Upon its removal, a straw-colored serous exudate becomes evident, which will gel on the skin surface within minutes. The patient is then instructed to apply a thin layer of antibiotic ointment to the entire abraded surface to prevent desiccation. The coating of ointment should be reapplied several times daily as well as at bedtime. Desiccation will prolong healing time, which generally takes 7 to 10 days for completion. During this time, the patient may wash the treated area with plain water and may get into the shower and allow water to run over the face as often as is desired. Washing and showering help to remove the exudate and also serve to relieve the itching that commonly follows dermabrasion. A film of antibiotic ointment is reapplied after each wash or shower.

A number of absorptive semi-occlusive dressing materials have been reported to be useful in dermabrasion healing. Vigilon, a hydrogel dressing, is particularly popular in this regard and is reported to hasten wound healing. The dressing is applied once daily. Another new semipermeable dressing, Omiderm, offers the advantage of allowing topical medicaments to permeate the dressing without disturbing it.

During the healing phase, some degree of swelling and inflammation can be expected to occur. A 7-day course of systemic prednisone, beginning at 40 mg/day and tapering by 5 mg/day, is often administered in the hopes of minimizing edema and discomfort. Patients are advised to avoid direct sun exposure during this time and for several months afterward. Pain is usually minimal and can be controlled with over-the-counter acetaminophen or ibuprofen preparations, although codeine occasionally is necessary. Postoperative antibiotics are not used routinely. Once epithelization is complete, the patient may begin to use nonmedicated makeup and a nondetergent soap. The treated skin may remain pink for a period of weeks to months following epithelization but gradually fades, usually within 6 weeks.

Milia formation is a common occurrence following dermabrasion and is not a cause for alarm (Figure 26.18). The lesions seem to occur most frequently following superficial abrasions rather than deeper ones. They are likely the result of epidermal fragments becoming embedded in the upper dermis dur-

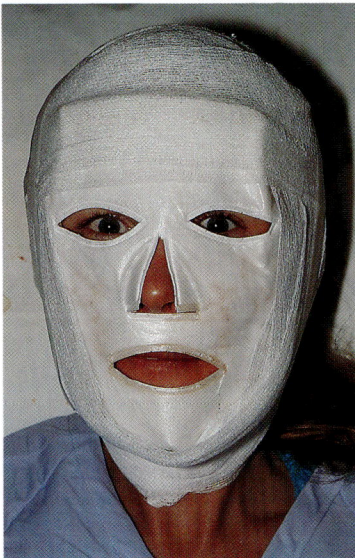

FIGURE 26.17 A special face-mask dressing containing an absorptive non-adherent dressing is applied over the antibacterial ointment. The patient is instructed to remove the dressing in 24 hours.

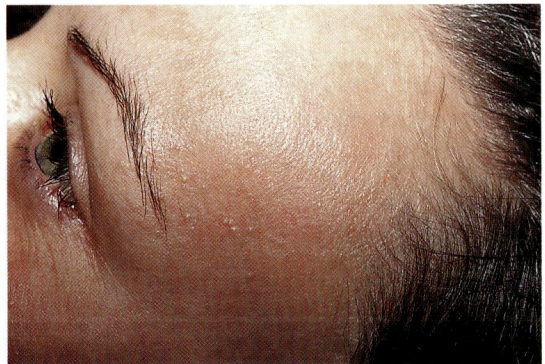

FIGURE 26.18 Milia formation is common following dermabrasion. These lesions appeared approximately 1 month following surgery and were manually evacuated with a 30-gauge needle and comedo extractor.

ing the procedure, to form small inclusion cysts. Two waves of milia are often seen. The first occurs within a week or two after dermabrasion and consists of multiple, thin-walled lesions, many of which resolve on their own in subsequent weeks. No treatment is recommended at this point. A second wave of milia is seen at about 1 month following the procedure, and tends to require manual incision with a fine-gauge needle and drainage with a comedo extractor. It has been suggested that use of topical retinoic acid for several weeks preoperatively may reduce the incidence of postoperative milia formation and enhance wound healing. Cohen has suggested that scrubbing of the abraded skin with copious amounts of saline at the completion of dermabrasion will prevent milia formation.

Patients are advised that for a year following treatment, treated skin is a little thinner than normal and is more likely to sunburn or be sensitive to temperature fluctuations. Therefore, sunscreens are advised during outdoor activities, as well as avoidance of temperature extremes when possible, during the year following surgery.

COMPLICATIONS

Occasional complications may accompany dermabrasion and relate mainly to pigmentary alteration, scarring, and infection. Both hyperpigmentation and hypopigmentation may occur, particularly in dark-skinned individuals. The pigmentary alterations usually are temporary but, on occasion, may persist indefinitely. At the first sign of post-inflammatory hyperpigmentation, many clinicians institute the use of a topical hydroquinone preparation (Melanex), which if administered early is usually very effective. Some hypopigmentation of the treatment site occurs in up to 50% of patients undergoing dermabrasion, although usually it is mild and easily covered by makeup. A greater problem is persistent severe hypopigmentation which, fortunately, is uncommon.

Scarring is also uncommon following dermabrasion. Obviously, it may accompany overly aggressive abrasion in which the operator has entered the deeper dermis. With few epidermal appendages at this level, healing must occur via scar formation. More often, scarring occurs without apparent reason in certain anatomic locations, primarily in the perioral area or over the mandibular rim. A contusive injury due to underlying bone and/or teeth in the area may account for additional inapparent tissue damage that later results in hypertrophic scar formation. Injections of triamcinolone acetonide 2.5 to 5 mg/mL are usually effective in flattening the scars to normal levels.

Infection following dermabrasion may be due to virus, bacteria, or yeast. The most worrisome of these is postoperative herpes infection in patients who are prone to occa-

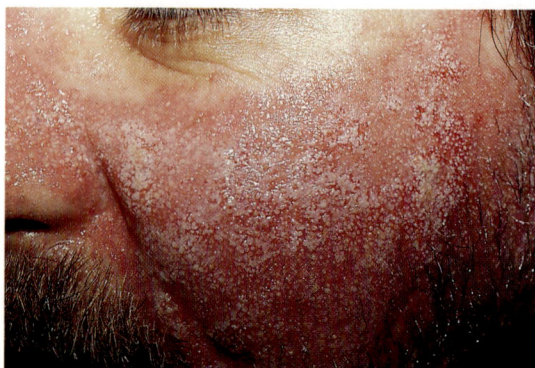

FIGURE 26.19 *Candida* species infection of the skin is seen 2 weeks following dermabrasion for acne scarring. It resolved rapidly after 1 week of oral ketoconazole (Nizoral) therapy.

sional herpes labialis. The entire operative site can be involved, with the possibility of scarring. Therefore, patients with a history of herpes labialis are prescribed prophylactic oral acyclovir (Zovirax) 200 mg five times daily, beginning 3 days prior to dermabrasion and continuing until epithelization is complete. Secondary bacterial infection of dermabraded skin may result in delayed healing and should be treated promptly with appropriate systemic antibiotics.

Not uncommonly, dermabrasion sites become infected with *Candida* species, particularly when a patient has been taking a broad-spectrum antibiotic just prior to the procedure. The infection usually manifests as significant erythema persisting several days after the procedure (Figure 26.19). The degree of redness seen is beyond that seen normally and often telltale pustulation is present. Treatment with either topical or systemic ketoconazole (Nizoral) is rapidly effective.

SUGGESTIONS FOR FURTHER READING

Cohen BH. Prevention of postdermabrasion milia (letter). J Dermatol Surg Oncol. 1988;14:1301.

Dzubow LM. Histologic and temperature alterations induced by skin refrigerants. J Am Acad Dermatol. 1985;12:796-810.

Hanke CW, O'Brian JJ, Solow EB. Laboratory evaluation of skin refrigerants used in dermabrasion. J Dermatol Surg Oncol. 1985;11:45-49.

Hanke CW, Roenigk HH Jr, Pinski JB. Complications of dermabrasion resulting from excessively cold skin refrigeration. J Dermatol Surg Oncol. 1985;11:896-900.

Pinski JB. Dressing for dermabrasion: occlusive dressings and wound healing. Cutis. 1986;37:471-476.

Robbins N. Dr. Abner Kurtin, father of ambulatory dermabrasion. J Dermatol Surg Oncol. 1988;14:425-431.

Roenigk HH Jr. Dermabrasion. In: Roenigk RK, Roenigk HH Jr, eds. Dermatologic Surgery. Principles and Practice. New York, NY: Marcel Dekker Inc;1989.

Roenigk HH Jr. Dermabrasion: state of the art. J Dermatol Surg Oncol. 1985;11:306-314.

Rubenstein R, Roenigk HH Jr, Stegman SJ, et al. Atypical keloids after dermabrasion of patients taking isotretinoin. J Am Acad Dermatol. 1986;15:280-285.

Siegle RJ, Chiaramonti A, Knox DW, Pollack SV. Cutaneous candidosis as a complication of facial dermabrasion. J Dermatol Surg Oncol. 1984;10:891-895.

Yarborough JM Jr. Dermabrasion by wire brush. J Dermatol Surg Oncol. 1987;13:610-615.

chapter 27

CHEMICAL PEELS

Chemical peeling is a controlled wounding in which peeling agents are painted on the skin to produce superficial exfoliation. With healing, irregularities of contour, texture, and coloration become less apparent. The technique is used for a variety of conditions but primarily for the treatment of wrinkles, solar damage, hyperpigmentation, and keratoses. The procedure can achieve many of the favorable results of dermabrasion (see Chapter 26) without the need for actual abrasive surgery. There is no spraying of tissue or blood to contend with and outcomes are fairly consistent.

The key to understanding chemical peeling is to appreciate that various chemicals, in particular concentrations or formulations, will penetrate and injure the skin to variable predictable depths. In performing chemical peeling, the cutaneous surgeon must determine to what depth the skin irregularity extends and match the appropriate peeling agent with the condition. Light chemical peels, which remove stratum corneum and nonadherent epidermal cells, traditionally have been used in the treatment of acne and excessive oiliness of the skin. Medium-depth peels, which extend into the papillary dermis, are effective in the management of the textural and pigmentary changes that accompany early photoaging of the skin. Superficial wrinkling, scattered lentigines, and early actinic keratoses all are managed effectively by peeling agents that injure the upper dermis. Deep chemical peeling, which extends into the reticular dermis, is used to treat the more advanced changes of photoaging, in particular deep wrinkles and severe solar elastosis.

Over the years, a variety of chemical agents have been used for peeling skin. At present, cutaneous surgeons use various preparations of phenol and trichloroacetic acid (TCA) for most of their light, medium, and deep chemical peeling.

PHENOL PEELS

Liquefied phenol has been used for decades as a peeling agent. Careful formulation, efficacy, and toxicity studies by Dr Thomas J Baker established chemical peeling with phenol as a safe and effective treatment modality for the management of significant skin photoaging. The formula proposed by Baker in the early 1960s, which is still in use today (Baker's formula), is:

phenol USP	3 mL
distilled water	2 mL
croton oil	2 drops
Septisol soap	5 drops

In Baker's formula, full-strength phenol (88%) is diluted down to roughly a 50%

aqueous solution. Baker was the first to realize that phenol is most penetrating when formulated at this concentration. Whereas Baker's formula is used for deep chemical peeling, full-strength phenol achieves only a medium-depth peel. Croton oil, an epidermal irritant, is used in Baker's formula to enhance the penetration of phenol into the skin.

TOXICITY

Because phenol is readily absorbed percutaneously, blood levels of phenol rise during chemical face peeling with phenol-containing agents. Rapidly rising phenol blood levels can cause cardiac arrhythmias, some of which have been known to result in sudden death during peeling procedures. The speed with which the phenolic agent is applied is directly related to the development of arrhythmias. The mixture, therefore, should be applied over a prolonged period of time. In performing a full-face phenol peel, the face is divided into eight or ten segments, each of which is treated individually, at 10-minute intervals. The segments are slightly overlapped to ensure that all interfaces are peeled. Cardiac monitoring is recommended during the procedure so that the surgeon can detect quickly any changes in heart rate or rhythm. This allows for the immediate institution of measures to reduce the amount of phenol absorption, such as adjustment of the size of the segments treated, the amount of material applied, and the time span between segments. An intravenous line should be in place in the event that intravenous lidocaine is required to control an arrhythmia.

Although hepatic and renal toxicity are frequently cited in discussions of phenol, neither has been reported to occur with the small doses of phenol used for face peeling. Nonetheless, it is probably wise to consider the use of a different peeling agent in treating patients with significant renal or hepatic impairment.

COMPLICATIONS

The major complications associated with phenol face peeling are pigmentary alteration and scarring. Deep peeling characteristically results in hypopigmentation, which patients should be made aware of since the peeled skin will be lighter than adjacent skin of the unpeeled neck and upper trunk, necessitating the daily use of face makeup. In the treatment of melasma, hyperpigmentation rather than hypopigmentation may occur, suggesting that the factors responsible for the initial hyperpigmentation remain operative. Alternatively, areas of hyperpigmentation may persist following peeling, while adjacent "normal" areas become hypopigmented, causing further accentuation of the initial pigmentary alteration. On occasion, if the chemical focally penetrates more deeply than is usual, areas of scarring can occur. Patients should be apprised of these possibilities during initial discussions about chemical peeling.

The histological changes observed following deep chemical peeling with Baker's formula include replacement of some or all of the dermal elastosis, creation of a new and thickened papillary dermis, and production of a more orderly epidermis. These microscopic changes appear to persist and clinically are related to more youthful-looking skin (Figure 27.1A,B).

TECHNIQUE

A similar technique is used for performing either Baker's formula peeling or full-strength phenol peeling. The patient washes the face with soap and water to remove surface oil and all remnants of facial makeup. Preoperative medications vary from surgeon to surgeon, ranging from 75 to 100 mg of meperidine (Demerol) hydrochloride and 10 mg of prochlorperazine (Compazine) given intramuscularly to twilight anesthesia. Deep burning and pain that lasts for approximately

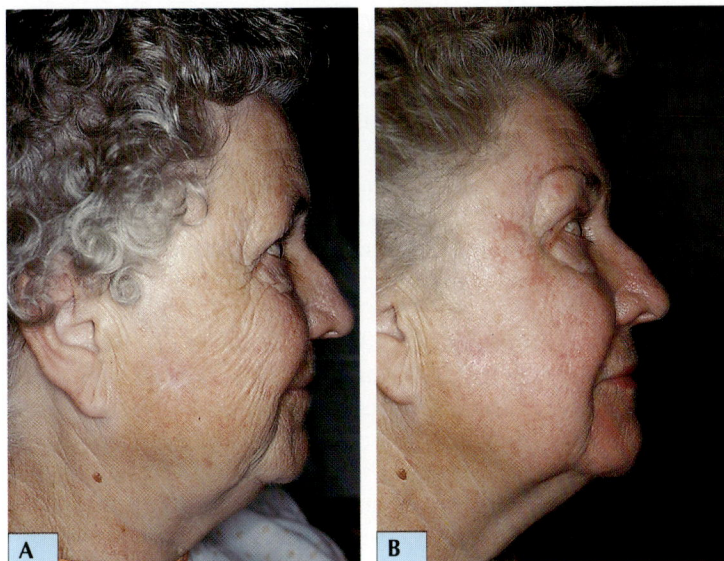

FIGURE 27.1 Phenol face peel in a woman in her 60s. (A) Preoperative photograph shows significant actinic damage with wrinkling and solar elastosis. (B) Photograph taken 3 weeks following Baker's formula face peel shows smoother, more youthful-looking skin.

6 hours is usual with phenol face peels. One way to diminish or even to avoid this problem is to provide local field-block anesthesia of the face using a mixture of plain lidocaine and bupivacaine (Marcaine) hydrochloride prior to peeling. The long-acting bupivacaine is usually sufficient to keep the patient pain free during the immediate postoperative period. Since epinephrine can exacerbate cardiac arrhythmias, McCollough and Langsdon have suggested that epinephrine-containing local anesthetic not be used.

While some surgeons suggest vigorous degreasing of the skin prior to surgery with either isopropyl alcohol or acetone, others omit this step or wipe the skin only lightly with acetone. The concern is that vigorous cleansing of the skin will disrupt the epidermal barrier, allowing for greater penetration of the peeling agent and the increased likelihood of scarring.

As mentioned earlier, the face is peeled in overlapping segments to avoid the development of cardiotoxic levels of phenol in the bloodstream. Another way to lessen the dosage of phenol delivered over time is to apply very small amounts of the peeling agent using cotton-tipped applicators. Baker's formula is applied using one to three cotton-tipped applicators, which also are used to stir the mixture before each application, since the constituents readily separate. The applicator is then pressed against the side of the glass container to remove all excess liquid and the skin segment is uniformly "painted" with the peeling agent.

Effort should be made to see that the phenolic mixture reaches the base of existing furrows and folds. This is achieved most easily by stretching out the skin and effacing folds and wrinkles, prior to application of the chemical. The peeling agent should extend onto the vermilion border and into the hairline. At the edges of the face, slightly less material is applied ("feathering") in an attempt to make the interface between peeled and unpeeled skin less stark. The eyelids are usually peeled last. Since the skin is thinner in this area, many clinicians use 88% phenol liquid or concentrations of TCA up to 35%, rather than Baker's formula, to peel this region. Since full-strength phenol becomes stronger with dilution, an assistant blots away any tears that may form to prevent them from diluting the chemical. This action also prevents the peeling agent from being drawn into the eye via the tear itself.

Within seconds of applying the peeling agent, the skin begins to frost. Phenolic agents cause a frosting that is a much deeper white than that seen with TCA (see Figure 27.4C). The intensity of frosting appears to correlate with the depth of peel achieved. Some clinicians "neutralize" the peeling agent after a given period of time by application of water or alcohol. An informal survey by one of us (SVP) at a recent meeting of the American Society for Dermatologic Surgery revealed that not 1 of 20 experienced cutaneous surgeons performing chemical peeling was aware of any scientific evidence that validates the concept of such "neutralization" for either phenol or TCA. Similarly, many clinicians will apply gauze squares soaked in cold water to each segment immediately after it is peeled. This may relieve the initial burning that accompanies penetration of the chemical. An electric fan blowing air across the treatment site also is helpful in relieving this sensation.

Occlusion of the peeled skin with adhesive tape increases the depth of the peel. Some or all of the peeled skin may be occluded, at the surgeon's discretion. Strips of occlusive adhesive tape usually are applied with an irregular, scalloped margin to break up the interface of the occluded and nonoccluded skin. The tape mask is left in place for 24 to 48 hours, depending on the depth of peel desired (Figure 27.2A–F). In recent years, many clinicians have abandoned the practice of tape occlusion with phenol peeling, without apparent compromise of clinical outcomes.

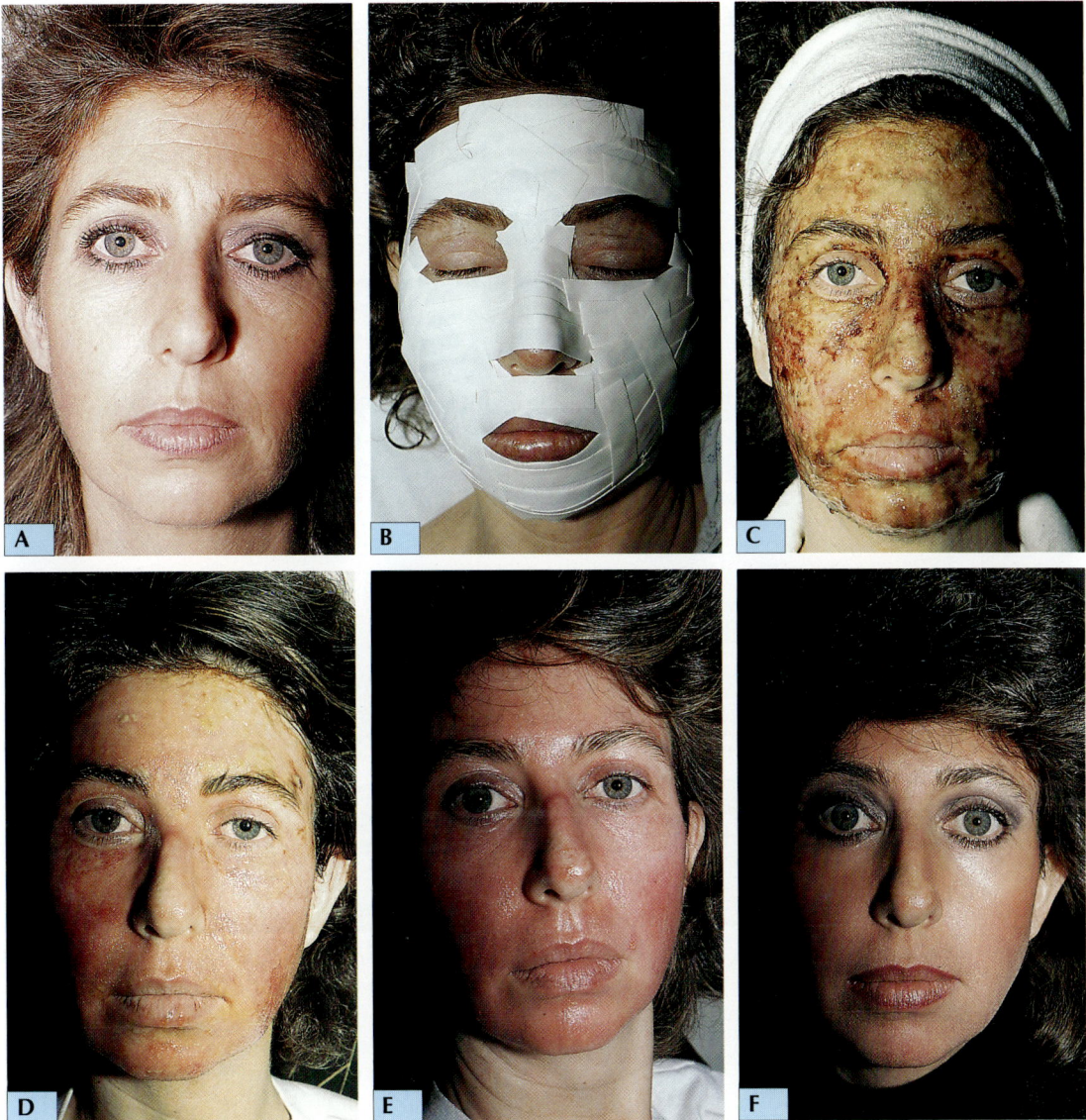

FIGURE 27.2 Baker's formula face peel in a 38-year-old woman. (**A**) Preoperative photograph shows moderate actinic damage with accentuation of perioral and periorbital wrinkling. (**B**) Following application of Baker's formula to the entire face, an adhesive tape mask is applied. This was removed in 24 hours. (**C**) On postoperative day 2, a great deal of serous exudate is noted. (**D**) Healing is proceeding well by postoperative day 4. (**E**) By day 9, healing is complete and erythema persists. (**F**) Three weeks after face peel, wrinkling is much improved. Makeup is able to cover the remaining erythema, which may persist anywhere from weeks to months.

POSTOPERATIVE CARE

Severe pain begins approximately 30 minutes postoperatively and usually requires strong analgesics and/or local anesthesia (discussed earlier) to control. A hypnotic such as 0.25 mg triazolam (Halcion) is given for 2 or 3 nights afterward to help the patient through the discomfort resulting from swelling, oozing, and crusting that occurs as healing proceeds. Whereas eschar formation was formerly encouraged by the application of thymol iodide powder, the modern concept of "moist wound healing" (see Chapter 13) has given rise to more rational, tolerable, and efficient wound-care regimens. Dr E Gaylon McCollough is credited with being the first to encourage his patients to shower several times a day to wash the peeled skin with soap and water. After each shower, the operative site is then patted dry and a thin layer of antibiotic ointment is applied. A layer of ointment is kept on the skin at all times, including at bedtime, to hasten healing by prevention of desiccation. The operative site usually has re-epithelized and is ready for makeup in 10 days as opposed to the 2 to 3 weeks necessary when eschar formation is allowed to occur. Erythema is present for a period of weeks to months after which skin lightening usually becomes apparent. Increased sensitivity to sunburn often is present following chemical face peeling.

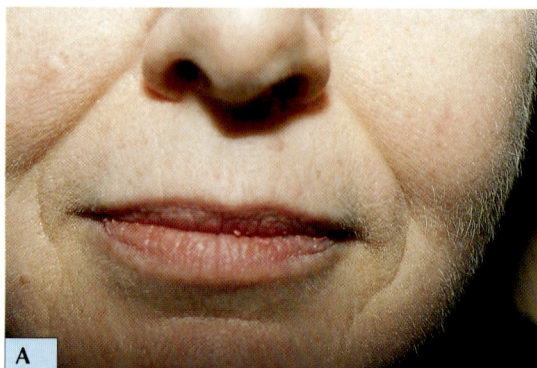

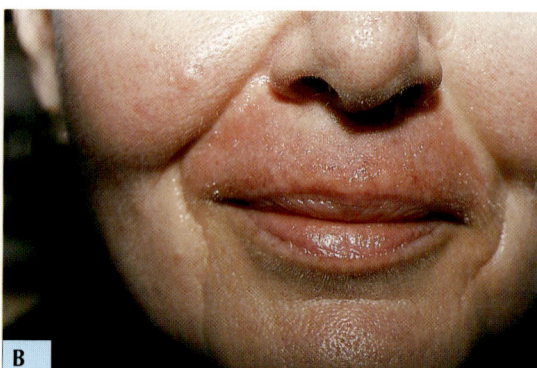

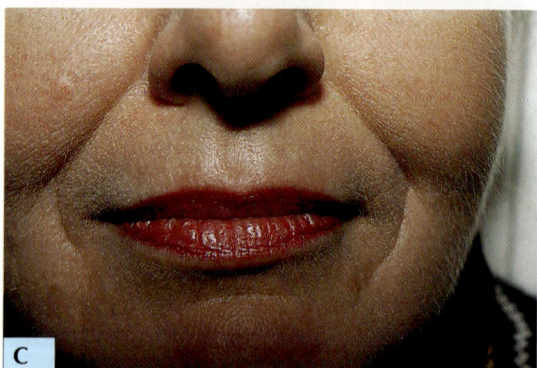

FIGURE 27.3 Treatment of upper lip wrinkling with TCA peeling. (A) Preoperative photograph shows radial wrinkles of the upper lip. (B) One week following medium-depth peeling with 35% TCA, healing is almost complete. (C) Two months following peeling, correction persists.

TCA PEELS

TCA peeling has become a popular technique for treating cases of less advanced photoaging (Figure 27.3A–C). The frequency of adverse reactions is low and the chemical is free of major side effects, particularly cardiac toxicity. The depth of penetration and resultant tissue damage vary with the concentration of TCA used. Light "freshening washes" of 10% to 20% TCA are effective in the treatment of acne or excessive oiliness. TCA used in concentrations of 35% to 45% yields medium-depth damage into the papillary dermis while 50% TCA produces a deeper peel that extends to the reticular dermis (but less deep than that seen with phenol). Concentrations of TCA in excess of 50% are more likely to cause scarring, and therefore are used infrequently. If a deeper peel is desired, adjunctive chemicals, such as dry ice or Jessner's solution (see below) are used in combination with TCA to enhance its penetration. Occlusion does not appear to increase the depth of injury with TCA, a finding recently confirmed in pig skin by Brodlund and Roenigk.

TECHNIQUE

Anesthesia generally is not used for TCA peeling, although some cutaneous surgeons administer a preoperative sedative, amnesic, or analgesic. As with phenol peeling, the skin at first is washed with soap and water and all remnants of facial makeup are removed. The skin is then thoroughly degreased with acetone, which is applied gently to the face with a gauze pad. It is likely that more vigorous cleansing of the skin and "buffing" with the gauze pad will lessen the barrier function of the epidermis and allow for a deeper peel. This can be a desirable effect for the experienced surgeon seeking slightly more penetration or an unwelcome surprise for the overly enthusiastic novice.

Once the skin has been thoroughly cleansed, the TCA is applied evenly over the skin surface. Clinicians frequently use two saturated cotton-tipped applicators for the chemical application. This obviously is a carry-over from the methodology used for phenol peels, which seeks to deliver a minimal dosage of a potentially cardiotoxic agent. Since this is not a concern with TCA, many therapists find a piece of folded gauze to be a more convenient delivery system (Figure 27.4A–C). As with phenol peeling, an effort should be made to apply a uniform amount of chemical to the entire skin surface. Since cardiotoxicity is not a threat, TCA peeling can be performed more rapidly than phenol peeling without adverse sequelae.

Within a minute or two of application of the chemical, frosting becomes evident. This is accompanied by short-lived discomfort, which is perceived by the patient as a "burning" sensation followed by a tight feeling or "drawing" of the skin. For full-face TCA peels, the discomfort persists for approximately 7 to 10 minutes and its severity varies with the concentration of acid used. As noted earlier for phenol peels, the use of an electric fan to circulate air over the face immediately after chemical application sig-

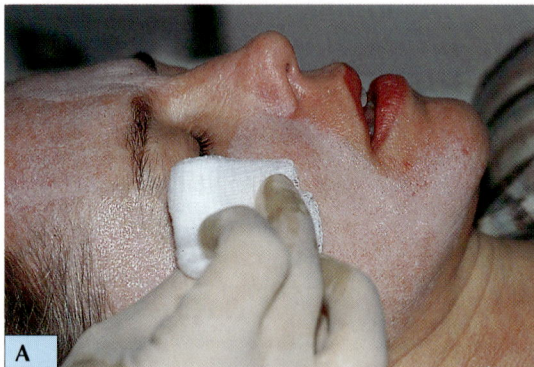

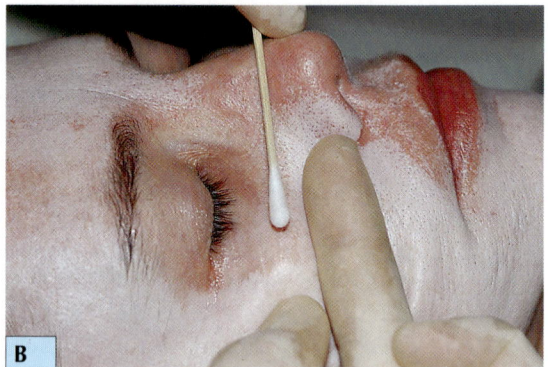

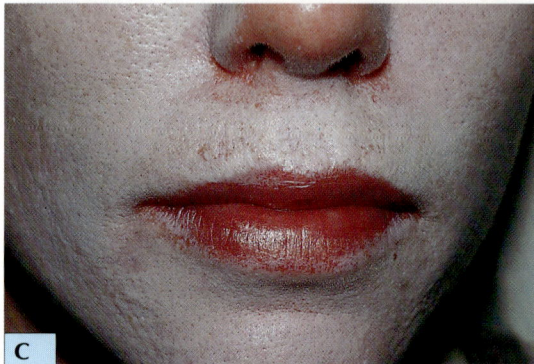

FIGURE 27.4 Application of TCA. **(A)** The use of a folded gauze pad to apply the TCA. Many surgeons prefer this delivery system to the use of cotton-tipped applicators. **(B)** Cotton-tipped applicators are used for applying the acid to the eyelids. **(C)** Frosting appears within a few minutes of applying the chemical. This should extend over the vermilion border of the lip.

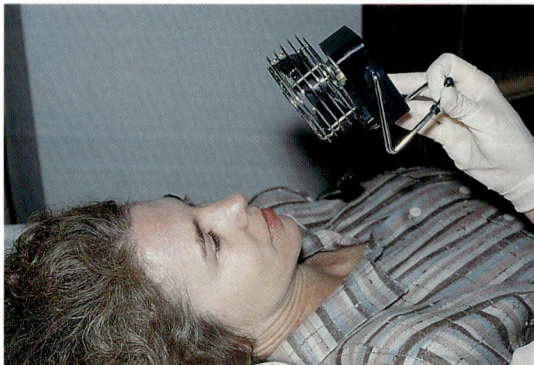

FIGURE 27.5 A small fan held by an assistant blows air over the treatment site immediately following application of the peeling agent. This is helpful for the next few minutes during which frosting proceeds to its peak.

nificantly lessens the amount of burning perceived by the patient (Figure 27.5). The feeling of tightness is rapidly and significantly reduced by the application of a thin layer of antibiotic ointment at the completion of the procedure. The immediate use of cool wet compresses on the treatment site following TCA peeling is soothing for some patients but actually may increase discomfort in others. Frosting is replaced by erythema in about 30 minutes.

SUPERFICIAL TCA PEELS

Low (10% to 20%) concentrations of TCA cause superficial exfoliation and a comedolytic action that is helpful in the management of acne. Shortly after application of the peel solution, a faint frosting of the skin will appear. A small amount of burning may occur but this discomfort is easily tolerated by most patients. Erythema and superficial desquamation are seen within the next 48 hours and healing usually is complete within 2 to 4 days. The

skin is sensitive for approximately 1 week following the peel, during which time topical acne medications should be discontinued.

Very light TCA peels of this type also are helpful for the treatment of oily skin and skin with prominent pores. The effects, as with other keratolytic and desquamating agents, are only temporary and, as a result, TCA "washes" may be repeated every few weeks or months as needed. Textural improvement may occur, over time, with repeated applications.

MEDIUM-DEPTH TCA PEELS

Medium-depth peels with 35% to 45% TCA yield improvement of skin texture, pigmentary alterations, and other changes of photoaging (Figure 27.6A–C). Early actinic keratoses also are effectively removed while hypertrophic lesions are relatively unaffected. As expected, more peeling, inflammation, and edema is seen with medium-depth peels than with superficial peels. When the perior-

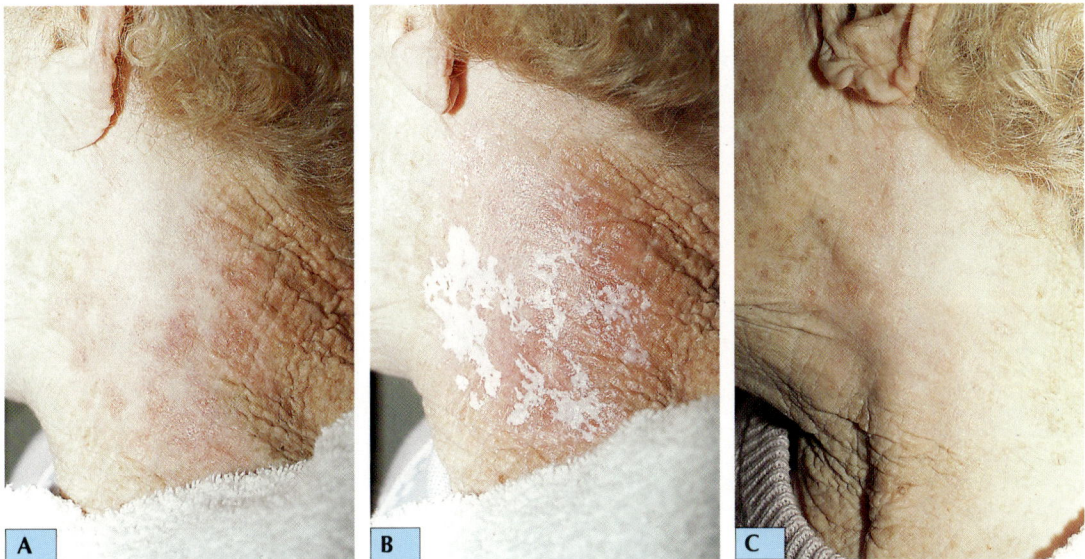

FIGURE 27.6 Treatment of areas of actinic damage on the neck with 35% TCA in a middle-aged woman. **(A)** Preoperative photograph shows actinic damage. **(B)** Following application of the chemical, uneven frosting is noted. This is common in severe actinic damage, and an attempt to achieve uniform frosting should be avoided since it can result in excessive application of chemicals. **(C)** Three months later, significant improvement is noted.

bital area is peeled, eyelid edema can be severe enough to shut the eyelids. Healing occurs in 1 week, with erythema persisting for 3 to 4 weeks afterward.

JESSNER'S MEDIUM-DEPTH TCA PEEL

Relatively low concentrations of TCA can cause deeper injury when combined with other substances that enhance the penetration of TCA into skin. Jessner's solution, used years ago as an exfoliating agent and a keratolytic for treating acne, recently has been used with success for this purpose. The solution consists of 14% each of lactic acid, salicylic acid, and resorcinol mixed in 95% ethanol.

After cleansing of the skin with acetone and prior to the application of TCA, the skin is painted evenly with Jessner's solution, using a folded gauze pad. A small amount of frosting will appear, particularly over keratotic areas. Some keratolysis is presumed to occur, allowing for deeper penetration of the

TCA, which is applied in a 35% to 45% concentration immediately following application of Jessner's solution (Figure 27.7A–C). Healing is complete in 7 to 10 days, with erythema persisting for 3 to 4 weeks afterward.

DEEP TCA PEELS

Chemical peeling with 50% TCA is used for the treatment of severe actinic damage and deeper wrinkles. In most cases of advanced photoaging, phenolic peeling agents are more effective than 50% TCA. The latter agent is chosen most often by those clinicians who do not want to risk the possible cardiotoxicity and usual hypopigmentation that accompany phenol peeling. This decision is a particularly sound one when dark-skinned individuals are treated.

The application and sequelae of the 50% solution are similar to those of the medium-depth TCA peel. To feather the interface with nonpeeled skin, it is recommended that 35% TCA be used at the mandibular rim and upper edges of the neck.

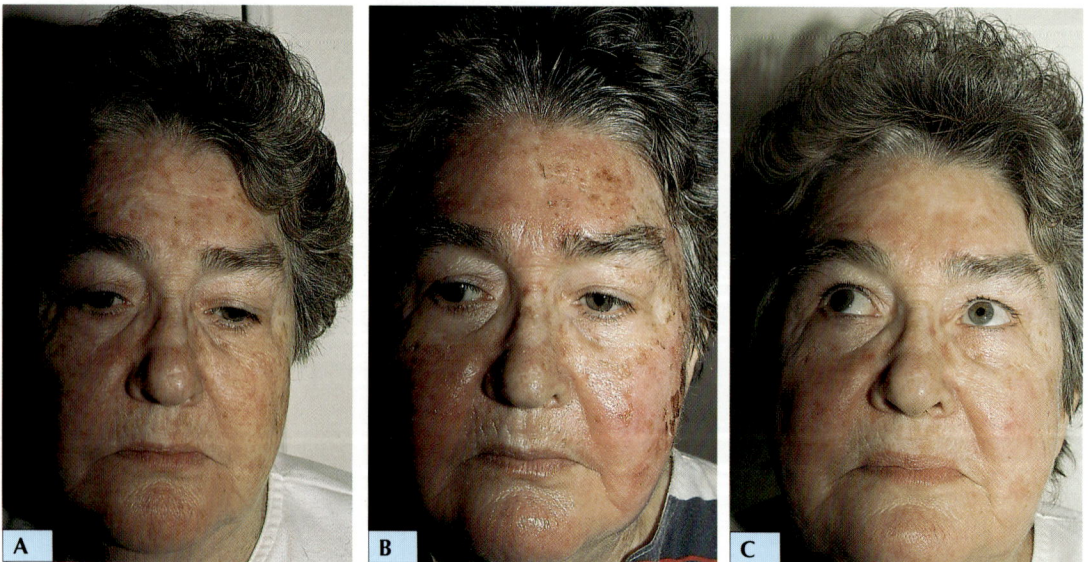

FIGURE 27.7 Treatment of actinic damage with multiple solar lentigines using Jessner's TCA peel. **(A)** Preoperative photograph shows significant sun damage and pigmentary alterations of the facial skin. **(B)** One week following face peel with Jessner's 35% TCA, healing is proceeding. **(C)** One month later, improvement of the macular hyperpigmentation is noted.

POSTOPERATIVE MANAGEMENT

Postoperative care for TCA peels is similar to that outlined earlier for phenol peels. Patients leave the office with a thin layer of antibiotic ointment applied to the treatment site. No dressing is required. They are advised that the chemical burn and accompanying pain is complete and that over the next 24 to 48 hours the skin will begin to peel much as it would following a severe sunburn. Patients are instructed to keep the treatment site covered with a thin layer of antibiotic ointment at all times including bedtime. This prevents the treatment site from drying out and crusting. Patients may get into the shower and wash the treatment site as often as they wish as long as they reapply the ointment afterward. They may gently massage away any skin that has entirely loosened but they are instructed not to attempt to peel off any adherent skin.

Many clinicians prescribe a 1-week prednisone taper to minimize swelling and discomfort, which usually takes the form of pruritus. The dosage begins at 40 mg the first day, and diminishes by 5 mg on each successive day. Patients are seen again at 7 days and, at that point, most if not all of the injured skin has separated and a pink regenerated base is present. Occasionally, focal non-healed areas may be present, signifying that a deeper injury was sustained, presumably due to uneven application of acid (Figure 27.8). Care should be taken to treat any secondary infection in these areas and to keep them covered with ointment as healing proceeds. Scarring may result in such areas but it rarely takes the form of raised hypertrophic scarring. Rather, slightly depressed scars with threadlike margins are the common sequelae. If hypertrophic scarring does occur, it should be treated immediately with intralesional injections of triamcinolone acetonide in a strength of 5 to 10 mg/mL.

All patients undergoing chemical peeling for photoaging are, of course, instructed in the use of sunscreens. They are advised to begin using sunscreens with a high sun protection factor, on a daily basis under their makeup, as soon as healing is complete. The results obtained with chemical peeling are among the most dramatic seen in cutaneous surgery. Nonetheless, there remains a great deal of inconsistency in our understanding and performance of chemical peeling. Hopefully, new insights that improve this technique even further will emerge in years to come.

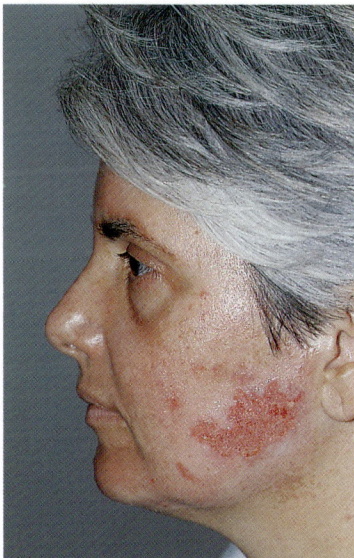

FIGURE 27.8 Area of slow healing 2 weeks following 35% TCA peeling. During the procedure, the acid was reapplied to this one area twice in an attempt to remove a large patch of hyperpigmentation. The applications were additive in their effect. Fortunately, the area went on to heal with only minimal scar formation.

SUGGESTIONS FOR FURTHER READING

Alt TH. Occluded Baker-Gordon chemical peel: review and update. J Dermatol Surg Oncol. 1989;15:980-993.

Asken S. Unoccluded Baker-Gordon phenol peels—review and update. J Dermatol Surg Oncol. 1989;15:998-1008.

Baker TJ. Chemical face peeling and rhytidectomy. Plast Reconstr Surg. 1962;29:199-207.

Brodland DG, Cullimore KC, Roenigk RK, et al. Depths of chemoexfoliation induced by various concentrations and application techniques of trichloroacetic acid in a porcine model. J Dermatol Surg Oncol. 1989;15:967-971.

Brody HJ, Chenault WH. Medium-depth chemical peeling of the skin: a variation of superficial chemosurgery. J Dermatol Surg Oncol. 1986;12:1268-1275.

Collins PS. The chemical peel. Clin Dermatol. 1987;5:57-74.

Gross BG. Cardiac arrhythmias during phenol face peeling. Plast Reconstr Surg. 1984;73:590-594.

McCollough EG, Langsdon PR. Chemical peeling with phenol. In: Roenigk RK, Roenigk HH Jr, eds. Dermatologic Surgery. Principles and Practice. New York, NY: Marcel Dekker Inc;1989:997-1016.

Monheit GD. The Jessner's + TCA peel: a medium-depth chemical peel. J Dermatol Surg Oncol. 1989;15:945-950.

Resnik SS. Chemical peel with trichloroacetic acid. In: Roenigk RK, Roenigk HH Jr, eds. Dermatologic Surgery. Principles and Practice. New York, NY: Marcel Dekker Inc;1989:979-995.

Stagnone GJ, Orgel MG, Stagnone JJ. Cardiovascular effects of topical 50% trichloroacetic acid and Baker's phenol solution. J Dermatol Surg Oncol. 1987;13:999-1002.

Stegman SJ. A comparative histologic study of the effects of three peeling agents and dermabrasion on normal and sun-damaged skin. Aesthetic Plast Surg. 1982;6:123-135.

Stegman SJ, Tromovitch TA, Glogau RG. Cosmetic Dermatologic Surgery. 2nd ed. Chicago, Ill: Year Book Medical Publishers Inc; 1990:34-58.

PUNCH HAIR TRANSPLANTATION

Autologous hair transplantation using punch transplants is another innovative technique contributed to cutaneous surgery by Dr Norman Orentreich. Through a series of experiments reported in 1959, Orentreich formulated the donor dominance theory of hair follicle growth. This, simply stated, holds that hairs from growing areas will survive when transplanted to bald areas.

We are all aware that individuals suffering from even severe male pattern baldness tend to retain a fringe of active hair throughout their lifetimes. These hairs have become "programmed" to continue indefinitely through the stages of the hair cycle and will do so even if transplanted to the top of the head, the anterior hairline, or to any other location. Over the years, it has been theorized that hair follicles, as known end target organs for androgenic hormones, are programmed via their relative sensitivities to such hormonal influences. These sensitivities appear to be genetically based, and other factors such as blood supply, hygiene, and diet play only a secondary role in the process.

The technique of punch hair transplantation, as developed by Orentreich, utilizes cylindrical dermal punches for removal of

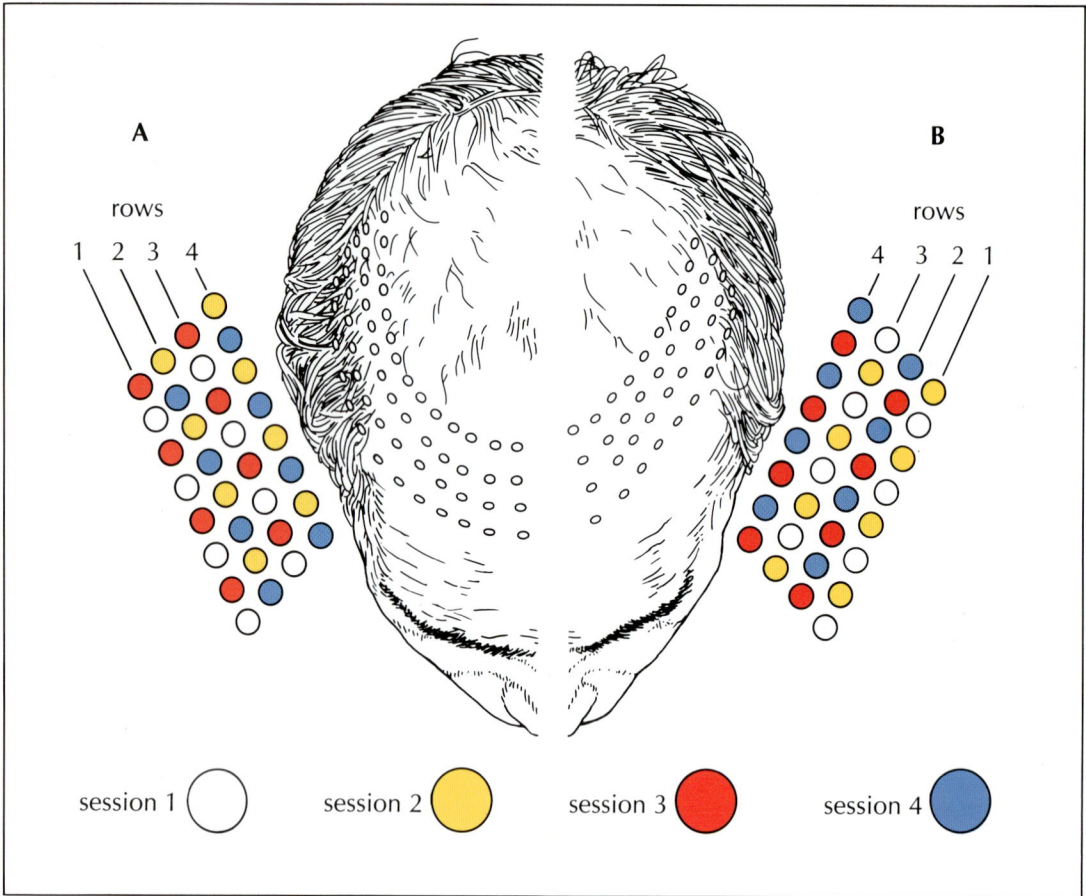

FIGURE 28.1 Schematic drawing showing common patterns used for the planning of hair transplant surgery. **(A)** In the first pattern, odd-numbered rows are transplanted during the first and third transplant sessions, while even-numbered rows are transplanted in the second and fourth sessions. **(B)** Some surgeons prefer a variation in which the odd-numbered rows are transplanted in the first two sessions with intervening even-numbered rows "planted" during the third and fourth sessions.

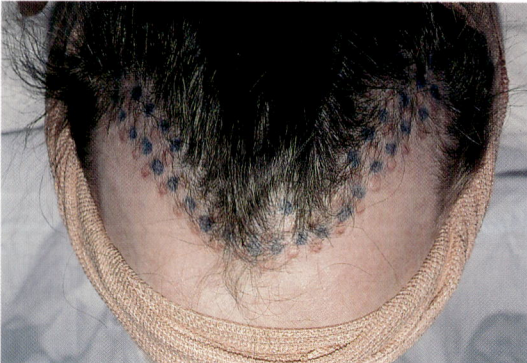

FIGURE 28.2 A patient undergoing hair transplantation at the second session, according to the plan depicted in Figure 28.1A. The plugs placed in the odd-numbered rows at the first session, while evident, are not yet growing hair. The next set of plugs will be placed in the even-numbered rows, as shown.

full-thickness plugs of hair-containing scalp. The donor plugs are then inserted into recipient holes made at the anterior scalp or vertex, using slightly smaller punches. The recipient holes are spaced apart to allow for adequate blood supply to each punch graft. Usually a minimum of four sessions of transplant surgery is required to graft a recipient site fully, with 50 to 100 plugs transplanted per session (Figures 28.1 and 28.2).

Over the years, the procedure of punch hair transplantation has been refined and expanded. Scalp reduction, minigrafting, and micrografting are now commonly performed as supplements to autologous punch grafting. In the pages that follow, an overview of punch hair transplantation is presented.

PATIENT SELECTION

The ideal patient for hair transplantation has adequate thick donor areas, does not have significant ongoing hair loss, understands the limitations of the procedure, has reasonable expectations as to outcome, and is committed to completion of the four or more sessions that make up a hair transplant. Of these factors, the presence of adequate donor areas and the commitment to proceed are the most valuable patient assets. Each hair transplant performed speaks for our collective skills as cutaneous surgeons and a poor or an incomplete result can do more to damage patients' confidence in the technique than any single excellent result can make up for. Therefore, we should do our best to avoid embarking on hair transplantation in situations where good results are unlikely. Our role, therefore, is to inform, educate, and, if need be, dissuade patients presenting for surgery.

INSTRUMENTATION

The major tool for this procedure is a collection of dermal punches, ranging in size from 3 to 4.5 mm, including both hand punches and drills that can be used with a motorized driver. The Orentreich punch was developed specifically for use as a hand punch for hair transplantation. A modification of the Keyes punch, it maintains the relatively thick wall, internal cutting edge, and external bevel of the original. The grip is grooved, allowing one to rotate the punch easily between thumb and index finger. Various hand punch modifications have been made over the years, such as thickening of the handle by Stough and the addition of knurling by Lewis and Resnik. More recent modifications have concentrated on the development of punches that will provide cylindrical grafts with the greatest number of viable follicles per plug.

Most surgeons use a motor-driven punch for harvesting of donor plugs. For creation of the recipient holes, however, many continue to use hand punches. The reasons for this vary, but a common feeling among hand punch users is that the recipient holes are more carefully placed, angled, and executed when created meticulously by hand. There is no evidence to substantiate this subjective impression. A more practical reason to consider the hand punch is that it is less likely than the power punch to attach to and pull out neighboring hairs during hair transplant surgery. The Bell hand engine is the most popular hand-held machine used for the harvesting of hair transplant plugs.

In addition to the hand engine and punches, the instrument tray for the procedure includes 4 x 4-inch gauze pads, 5-mL syringes containing 1% lidocaine with epinephrine, 5-mL syringes containing normal saline, short 30-gauge and long 25-gauge needles, a needle holder, Brown-Adson forceps, jeweler's forceps, scissors for harvesting plugs, suture scissors, and petri dishes containing saline-moistened gauze (Figure 28.3). A number of other instruments and "gadgets" designed to assist in hair transplant surgery are available but none of these is strictly required. Since a great deal of bleeding and splatter of blood is associated with the procedure, the surgeon and assistants should wear gloves, masks, face shields, and gowns.

TECHNIQUE

The technique of hair transplantation is best learned from an experienced colleague who can demonstrate its precise nuances. The most difficult part of the procedure to learn is that of planning the transplant. Hair transplant planning requires that the surgeon be able to anticipate future patterns of hair loss, predict treatment outcomes, and modify directions as the process evolves. A full discussion of hair transplant planning is well beyond the scope of this book. The reader is referred to Suggestions For Further Reading at the end of this chapter for sources of additional information on the topic.

PREOPERATIVE PREPARATION

Preoperative preparation for hair transplant surgery is not complicated. Patients don a hospital gown to protect their clothing from blood. No special surgical preparation of the scalp is necessary other than to wipe the recipient and donor areas with alcohol or with chlorhexidine followed by alcohol. Preoperative medication varies from practice to practice. Diazepam, given sublingually in a dosage of 5 to 10 mg, is probably the most commonly used preoperative drug. It calms the patient and, since it is also effective in the treatment of lidocaine toxicity, it is well to have "on board" in the event that lidocaine blood levels rise to significance.

THE DONOR SITE

Part of the planning procedure for hair transplantation involves comprehensive assessment of the donor site and potential placement of hairs from the area. The usual donor area, at the posterior scalp, should be beyond the advancing area of hair loss. Often, one must look closely to appreciate that some degree of hair thinning and miniaturization extends downward from the midocciput into potential donor sites. The useable donor area is often wider in the postauricular area. Close examination of the donor area also will reveal

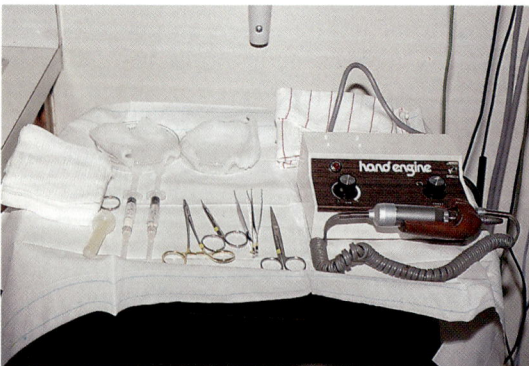

FIGURE 28.3 The instrument tray used for hair transplant surgery. The punches have not yet been selected.

a gradation of hair types, ranging from fine to thick. Plugs containing finer hairs are best used at the hairline to help soften the interface with non–hair-bearing skin. The coarser hairs, used more for coverage and to promote a look of fullness, should be reserved for use in the mid-portion of the recipient site.

Several patterns have been proposed for the harvesting of donor plugs. In the "total harvest" technique, a frequently used pattern in recent years, as many grafts as possible are taken from a relatively narrow strip of donor scalp. The remaining intervening tissue is removed completely and deeply with scissors, and can be placed on saline-soaked gauze for later use in the preparation of minigrafts and micrografts. The edges of the donor wound are scalloped, allowing for interdigitation of the edges during closure (Figure 28.4A–D).

Another popular harvest pattern consists of two rows of plugs, followed by a skip area of equal width, and a second set of two

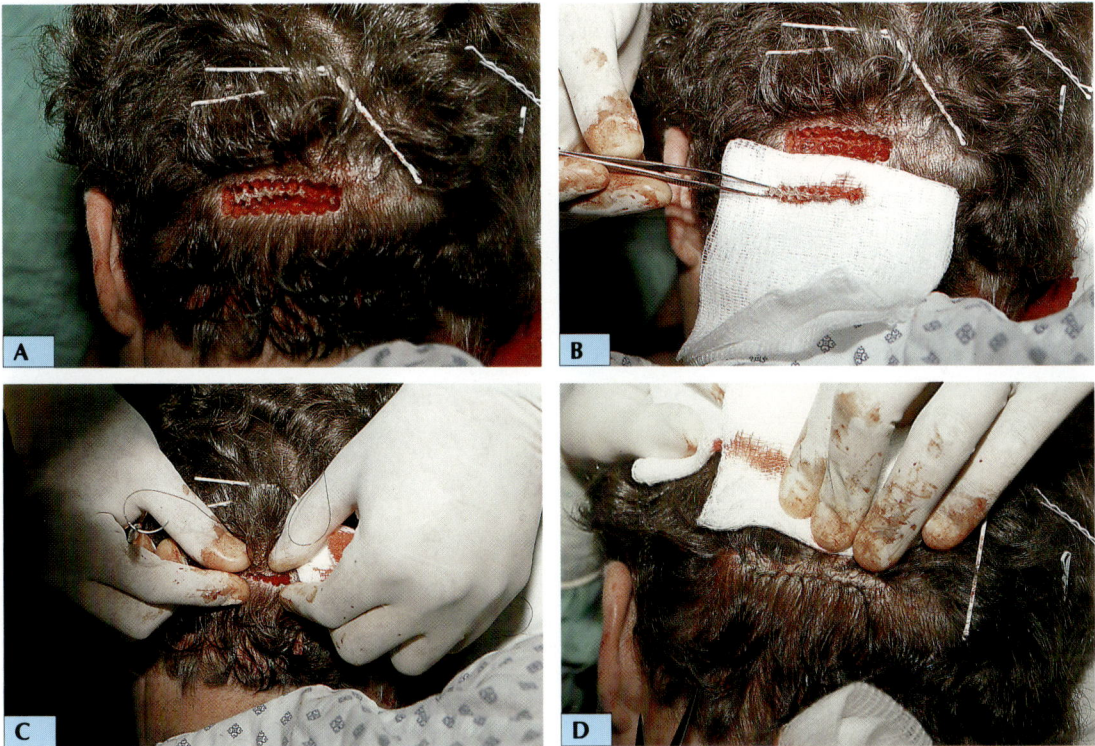

FIGURE 28.4 The "total harvest" technique of harvesting punch grafts. **(A)** The area has been harvested with a 4-mm punch. **(B)** Using scissors, the intervening skin is removed down to the galea. **(C)** The scalloped edges of the defect should interdigitate. **(D)** The defect is easily closed with 3-0 running nylon suture.

rows of plugs (see Figure 28.5D). As with the "total harvest" technique, the wound is often closed with a running suture of 3-0 nylon placed through both rows. However, it is not a problem to leave the area to heal by second intention. The skip area can be harvested later, when healing is complete in the current donor site.

Once a decision has been made as to which harvest pattern will be used, the hairs in the donor area are trimmed with scissors to a few millimeters in length. Some stubble must remain to indicate the direction of follicular growth. The hair above the chosen donor site is kept out of the operative field with either a strip of tape placed circumferen-

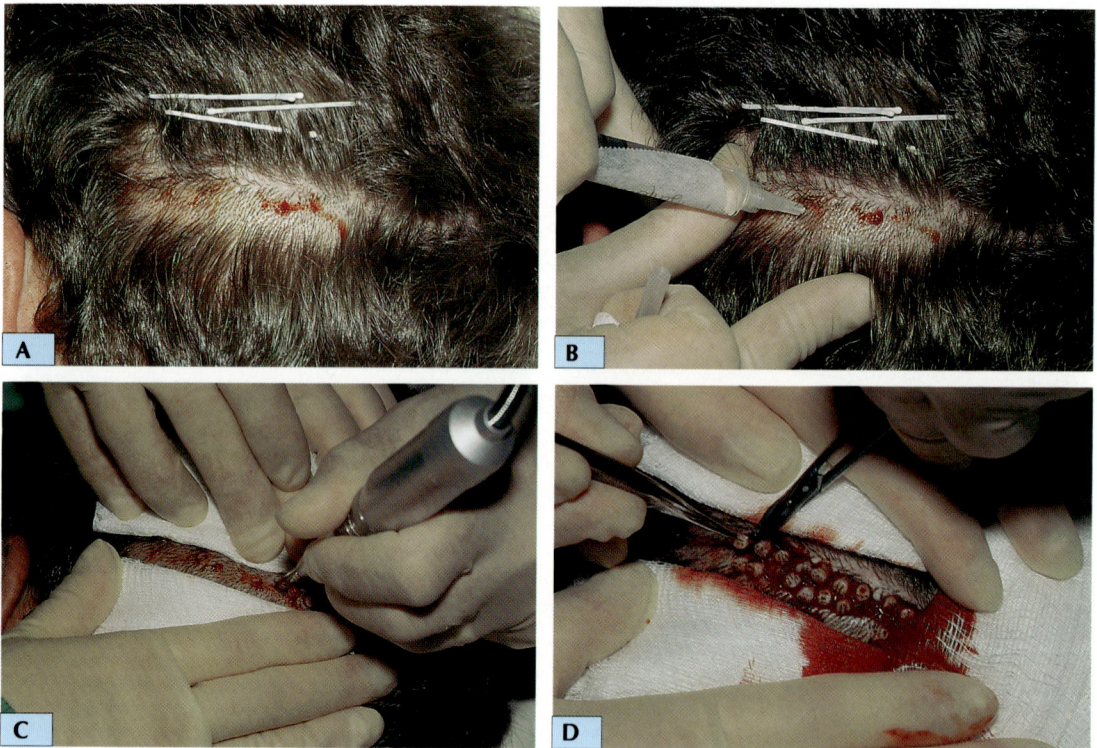

FIGURE 28.5 Method for harvesting punch grafts. (A) The hair at the site has been trimmed with scissors and the hair above it is pinned out of the way. (B) After injection of the entire donor site with local anesthetic, the first section to be harvested is made turgid by injection of normal saline. (C) This firm scalp yields excellent donor grafts. Care is taken to keep the motor-driven punch parallel to the follicular axis. (D) While the plug is grasped gently by the epidermal edge and pulled upward, an assistant cuts the fibroadipose base of the plug.

tially around the head, a sweat band, hair clips, or bobby pins (Figure 28.5A).

Using 1% lidocaine with epinephrine, the donor and recipient sites are locally infiltrated, first using a short 30-gauge needle and then a longer 25-gauge needle to infiltrate the areas thoroughly. A 5-mL syringe is used and the physician or assistant should keep track of how many syringes of anesthetic are injected. Most patients can safely receive 40 to 50 mL of 1% lidocaine with epinephrine. Some surgeons provide nerve blocks of the supraorbital nerve for the recipient site and of the retroauricular nerve for the donor site, prior to local infiltration. Others find a ring or field block sufficient. After the area has been anesthetized, a 20-minute delay, prior to surgery, allows the epinephrine to take full effect and provide maximal vasoconstriction.

Most authors agree that the 4-mm donor plug is optimal in terms of growth success, cosmetic outcome, and even postsurgical morbidity. Unger has shown that the 4-mm plug gives the best yield of hairs per surface area. Plugs of 4.5 mm are sometimes used to move a greater number of hairs into the donor area, but they are not used in the immediate hairline since they give a brushlike effect. For "fill-in" procedures, 3.5-mm plugs or even 3-mm plugs can be used. Plugs over 4.5 mm or under 3 mm do not do well and generally are not used.

Alt, through macro-lens photography, has suggested that the major determinants of a "good" donor plug are the angle of the cut, the sharpness of the punch, and the speed of its rotation. Most surgeons performing this technique agree that sharpness is by far the most important of these factors. Alt has also shown that more uniformly cylindrical plugs can be obtained if the scalp is kept firm during harvesting. To this end, he has suggested that saline be injected into a limited area of donor skin to firm it up immediately prior to the harvesting of 10 to 20 plugs from the injected segment. This is repeated for each section of the donor site until harvesting is complete (Figure 28.5B).

For the harvesting of plugs, it is essential that the long axis of the punch remain oriented exactly parallel to the follicular axis of the donor hairs. This is done by close observation of the direction of growth of the stubble. If proper orientation is not maintained, transection of follicles will occur and outcomes will be poor. From time to time during harvesting, the plugs should be inspected to make sure that they are of good quality. If they are not, it may be because the punch is dull and a sharper one is needed. During harvesting, the assistant uses gauze pads to apply pressure to the donor area to minimize bleeding (Figure 28.5C). Once all of the plugs have been cut, each one is pulled up gently by the epidermis, its fatty base is cut with sharp scissors (Figure 28.5D), and it is placed in a petri dish atop gauze that has been soaked liberally with saline. If there are any active bleeders at the site, they should be stopped with ligatures. The donor area is then cleansed of blood using hydrogen peroxide and is either sutured closed or covered with a pressure dressing.

The plugs are then cleaned, usually by an assistant. Most, but not all, of the fat at the inferior aspect of each plug is removed, along with any loose hair remnants at the edge of the plug, and any transected follicles, debris, or clots. Epidermal lipping also should be removed. As they are cleaned, the plugs are placed in another petri dish containing saline-soaked gauze. Often they are arranged in some meaningful fashion, be it hair density, thickness, or overall quality. Attention is now turned to the strip of intervening scalp that was removed from the donor site at the completion of graft harvesting. This strip can be cut into very small micrografts, each of which contains one or two hairs of good quality (Figure 28.6). In addition, larger grafts of 2 or 3 mm in diameter can be created

to serve as minigrafts, which are arranged in the petri dish along with the other grafts.

THE RECIPIENT SITE

Planning of the recipient site is a task of obvious importance that takes many factors into account: the likelihood of further progression of hair loss, the number of donor grafts available, whether excisional alopecia reduction procedures will be performed, and the patient's hair style.

Most patients are concerned with the anterior hairline and indeed it is the area most often transplanted. A realistic adult hairline does not begin at the forehead-scalp junction but, rather, above it. It is best to draw an arciform frontal hairline on the scalp with a grease pencil and to discuss this placement with the patient. The starting point for each temple is where the direction of hair growth changes. The degree to which the arc is rounded or peaked depends on the general

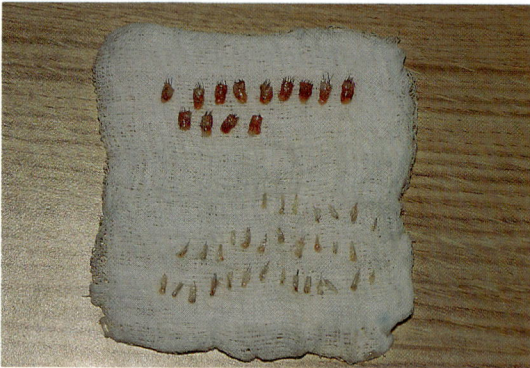

FIGURE 28.6 Micrografts are seen beneath normal 4-mm plugs.

shape of the head and on the surgeon's judgment. If scalp reductions are planned as a definite part of the treatment strategy, it is best to leave the arc a bit more rounded since one or two scalp reductions may have the effect of narrowing the frontal area to give it more of a peaked shape (Figure 28.7A–D).

During transplantation, a slight shrinkage of the donor plug occurs along with comparable gaping of the recipient hole. Therefore, a snug fit is unlikely if the same diameter punch is used at donor and recipient areas. Usually a slightly larger (4-mm) punch is used for the donor grafts with a slightly

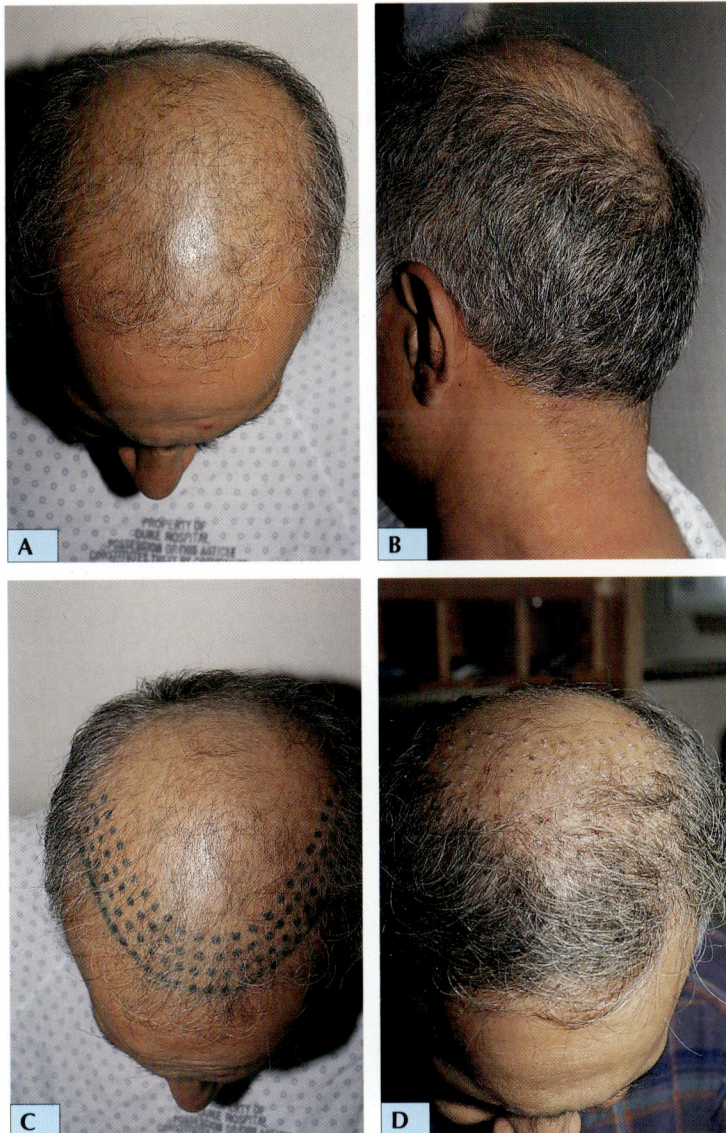

FIGURE 28.7 Hair transplantation in a middle-aged man who is no longer actively losing hair. (A) Preoperative photograph shows extreme thinning over the top of the scalp. (B) The donor sites are excellent in terms of amount, color, and texture of the hair. (C) Rebuilding of the frontal hairline is planned along with the option of future scalp reduction. (D) Following successful rebuilding of the hairline, the patient decided against scalp reduction and underwent one session of transplantation behind the hairline. This photograph was taken 2 weeks later. A total of 324 plugs were used to build the hairline, with 85 plugs placed posterior to it.

smaller (3.5-mm) punch used for the recipient holes. The recipient holes should face forward and are placed at acute angles of 30° to 45°. This gives a "shingling" effect to the new hairs, resulting in a fuller appearance (Figure 28.8).

The average frontal hairline is five or six rows deep and is transplanted in a minimum of four sessions. Minigrafts and micrografts are used to soften the hairline, which otherwise has a tendency to be abrupt rather than more natural and transitional in appearance. Minigrafts, each of which contains three to five hairs, are prepared by quartering a normal 4-mm or 4.5-mm punch graft (Figure 28.9). The minigrafts are placed between the larger grafts at the anterior hairline via stab wounds made with a #15 scalpel blade. Micrografts, which should have the appearance of random hairs found anterior to the normal hairline, consist of only one or two hairs that can be teased off the edges of standard grafts during cleaning. Recipient stab wounds for micrografts are made with a 16-gauge needle and are placed irregularly just ahead of the anterior hairline (Figure 28.10A).

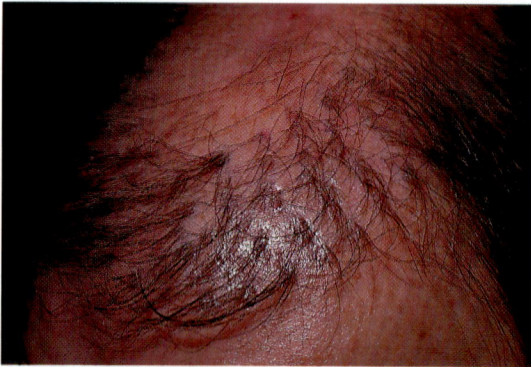

FIGURE 28.8 Hair growth after two sessions of transplant surgery. Note the "shingling" effect, in which acutely angled hairs have a tendency to overlap hairs situated more anteriorly, giving a fuller appearance.

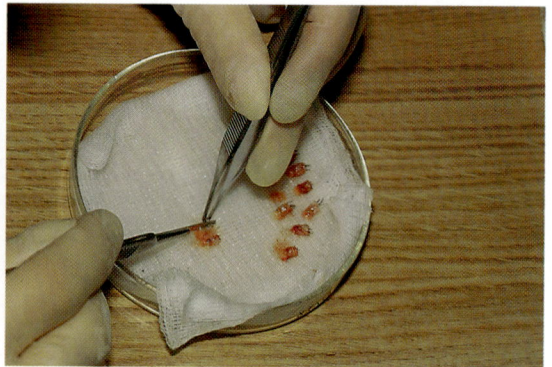

FIGURE 28.9 Minigrafts are prepared from 4-mm punch grafts. Many surgeons prefer a Gillette blue blade to a scalpel blade for cutting them.

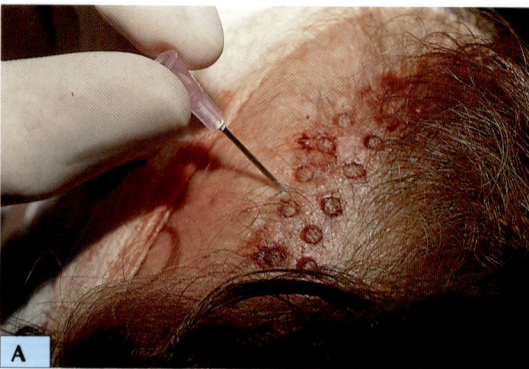

FIGURE 28.10 The use of micrografts to soften the hairline. (A) A 16-gauge needle creates the recipient wound while acting as a microdilator.

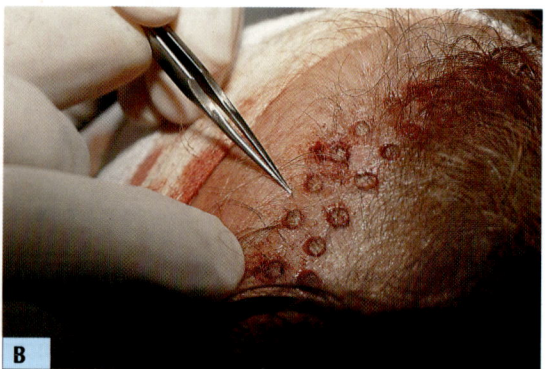

(B) After removal of the needle, the graft is quickly inserted into the defect. A single hair has been placed successfully.

It is helpful to wait until bleeding at the recipient site has stopped before an attempt is made to implant minigrafts and micrografts. Bleeding usually stops after 7 to 10 minutes, at which time the recipient sites have become slightly sticky as coagulation proceeds. During the waiting period, commercially available dilators or 16-gauge needles may be left in the recipient areas to hold them open. When the dilator or needle is removed, the wound will continue to gape momentarily as the minigraft or micrograft is slipped into place (Figure 28.10B). Alternatively, the recipient site can be held open with cross-action jeweler's forceps.

Because the implantation of minigrafts and micrografts can be tedious, it is best to implant some with each session of transplantation to break up the drudgery. The results are well worth the effort (Figure 28.11A,B).

POSTOPERATIVE CARE

At the completion of the procedure, a small amount of antibiotic ointment is placed over both donor and recipient sites, which are covered with a nonadherent absorptive dressing and wrapped with a pressure dressing such as Kling. Postoperative antibiotics are prescribed by some, but not all, clinicians. The patient returns on the following day for removal of the dressing, gentle cleansing of the scalp with hydrogen peroxide, and evaluation of the grafts. Beginning 5 days postoperatively, the patient is allowed to shampoo the area gently. Healing of the recipient sites generally is complete in about 3 weeks. The donor sites, if left to heal secondarily, usually do so in about 4 weeks.

During the first 4 weeks following surgery, telogen effluvium will occur, in which

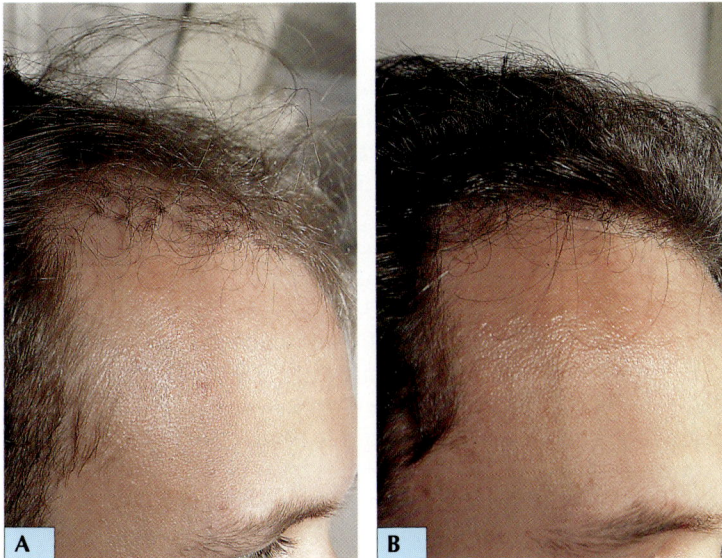

FIGURE 28.11 Thickening of the hairline in a young man using 4-mm plugs, minigrafts, and micrografts. (A) Photograph taken 6 months after the first transplantation session performed in another city. (B) Same patient 1 year later. A total of 184 4-mm plugs and 75 micrografts and minigrafts were placed throughout the hairline.

hair is shed from the grafts. While normal and predictable, it is important that patients be forewarned of its occurrence. The hair begins to reappear at 12 to 14 weeks. Some believe that telogen effluvium following hair transplant surgery can be minimized by the application of minoxidil during the postoperative period.

COMPLICATIONS

Significant complications are unusual after hair transplant surgery. Some patients experience significant swelling of the forehead accompanied by discomfort. These same patients also may develop periorbital swelling or "black eyes," which resolve over a week or so. Patients who experience these complications are good candidates for postoperative steroids following subsequent hair transplant sessions.

Persistent bleeding may occur from the donor site and is easily controlled by a ligature. Arteriovenous malformations have been reported to accompany healing in both recipient and donor areas. Poor growth, scarring, or scalp tissue necrosis can occur if too many grafts are placed and vascular supply is compromised. Sparse growth usually is the result of poor technique, and is correctable by further hair transplant surgery.

SUGGESTIONS FOR FURTHER READING

Alt TH. Evaluation of donor harvesting techniques in hair transplantation. J Dermatol Surg Oncol. 1984;10:799-806.

Hill TG. Closure of the donor site in hair transplantation by a cluster technique. J Dermatol Surg Oncol. 1980;6:190-191.

Keenan BS, Meyer WJ III, Hadjian AJ, et al. Syndrome of androgen insensitivity in man: absence of 5 α-dihydrotestosterone binding protein in skin fibroblasts. J Clin Endocrinol Metab. 1974;38:1143-1146.

Kuster W, Happle R. The inheritance of common baldness: two B or not two B. J Am Acad Dermatol. 1984;11:921-926.

Marritt E. Single hair transplantation for hairline refinement: a practical solution. J Dermatol Surg Oncol. 1984;10:962-966.

Orentreich N. Autografts in alopecias and other selected dermatological conditions. Ann N Y Acad Sci. 1959;83:463-479.

Pinski JB. Hair transplantation. In: Roenigk RK, Roenigk HH Jr, eds. Dermatologic Surgery. Principles and Practice. New York, NY: Marcel Dekker Inc;1989:1047-1078.

Sadik NS, Hitzig GS. Adjuvant techniques in punch graft hair transplantation. J Dermatol Surg Oncol. 1986;12:700-705.

Stegman SJ, Tromovitch TA, Glogau RG. Cosmetic Dermatologic Surgery. 2nd ed. Chicago, Ill: Year Book Medical Publishers Inc; 1990:83-143.

Stough DB, Mendoza F, Freilich IW. Surgical procedures for the treatment of baldness. Cutis. 1986;37:362-365.

Sturm H. The benefit of donor site closure in hair transplantation. J Dermatol Surg Oncol. 1984;10:987-990.

Unger WP, Baran R. Hair Transplantation. New York, NY: Marcel Dekker Inc;1979.

Unger WP, Nordstrum REA, eds. Hair Transplantation. 2nd ed. New York, NY: Marcel Dekker Inc; 1987.

chapter 29

MOHS'
MICROGRAPHIC
SURGERY

Mohs' micrographic surgery is a technique that combines tissue removal with microscopic examination of 100% of the tissue margins. Its success lies in three critical points that distinguish it from standard excision with frozen section margin control. First, the tissue is removed in the shape of a pie pan with its sides cut at a 45° angle to its base. Second, once the tissue is excised in this manner, its entire cut surface can be examined for margin control, in contrast to the "bread-loaf" technique used by most pathologists, in which only a percentage of the margin is sampled (Figure 29.1). Third, the surgeon and the pathologist are one and the same person.

The technique was first introduced in the 1930s by Dr Frederic Mohs at the University of Wisconsin at Madison. At that time it was called chemosurgery, its name having been derived from the use of a chemical paste containing 20% zinc chloride, which was applied to cancerous tissue to fix it in situ. The fixed tissue was then excised and its margins were examined under the microscope. If the margins were found to be positive, the paste was reapplied to the remaining cancerous area and the entire procedure was repeated, thus allowing tissue removal with complete microscopic control.

In the 1970s, Drs Theodore Tromovitch and Samuel Stegman experimented with the technique, but omitted the fixation of tissue with zinc chloride paste, which was found to cause inflammation, swelling, and pain, and was poorly tolerated around the eyes, nose, and mouth. The fixed-tissue technique was also found to be time consuming, since several days of repeated paste application were sometimes needed to remove large or complex tumors.

The modified, fresh-tissue technique proved useful in several ways. Since it did not use any fixative, it permitted removal of all tumor-containing tissue in one day, as it

was no longer necessary to wait up to 24 hours for the fixative to work. Also, less tissue was destroyed because there was no surrounding rim of inflammation. In addition, patients did not need to be hospitalized for analgesic therapy due to pain from use of the zinc chloride. Finally, any resulting defects could be repaired immediately following the procedure, as the wounds were fresh. Today, almost all Mohs' surgeons prefer the fresh-tissue technique, although Dr Mohs still recommends use of the fixative for special cases, such as for large tumors or for tumors involving bone or the erectile tissue of the penis. It has also been recommended for use in patients carrying the human immunodeficiency virus.

INDICATIONS

Mohs' technique is best suited for removal of difficult tumors whose clinical margins are least likely to reflect the true extent of the

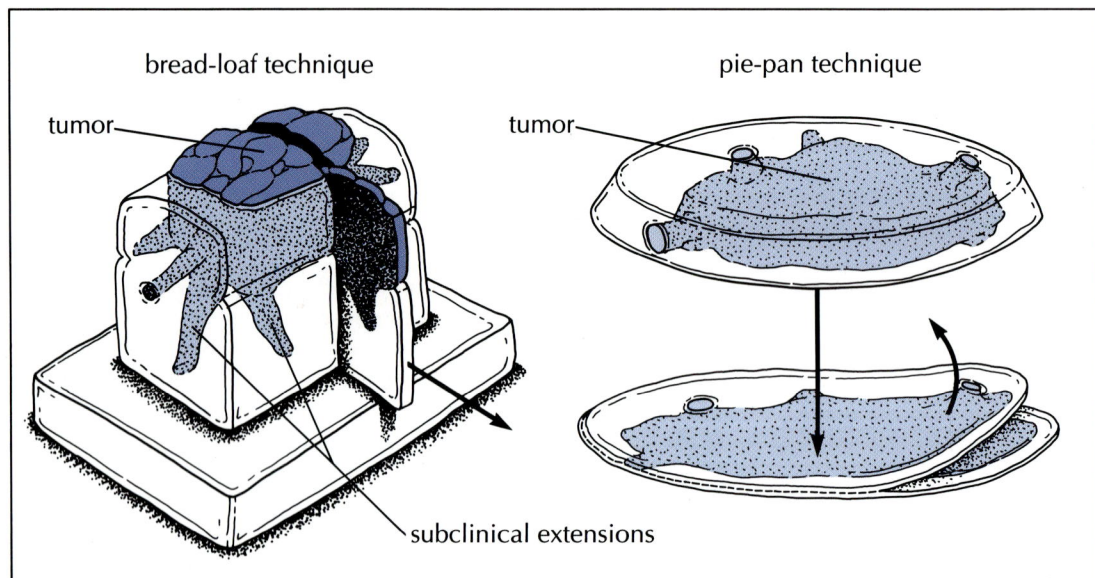

FIGURE 29.1 Schematic drawing showing pie-pan versus bread-loaf technique. The former configuration allows complete examination of the cut surface of the tissue.

cancer. Figure 29.2 lists the most common situations in which this might occur. Clinical margins may also be obscured by scar tissue, such as may be produced by cryosurgery, radiation therapy, electrodesiccation, and excisional therapy for an existing tumor.

Since tumors generally take the path of least resistance, recurrent tumors may grow at length down into fat and around the sides of scars, before becoming clinically apparent. Similarly, flaps and grafts may lay full-thickness skin on top of any residual tumor, which may further delay detection of recurrence (Figure 29.3A,B). Even with Mohs' technique, large tumors greater than 2 to 3 cm in diameter have a higher recurrence rate (8%) than do their smaller counterparts (2%). For such larger lesions, Mohs' technique can help to seek out subclinical extensions.

Mohs' technique is also useful for lesions in cosmetically important areas, such as those abutting the eyelid or the vermilion

FIGURE 29.2
INDICATIONS FOR USE OF MOHS' SURGERY

Recurrent tumor

Large tumor

Location of tumor adjacent to a critical structure

Indistinct clinical borders present

Morpheaform or sclerosing tumor

Tumor present in a young adult

Location of tumor in area of high recurrence

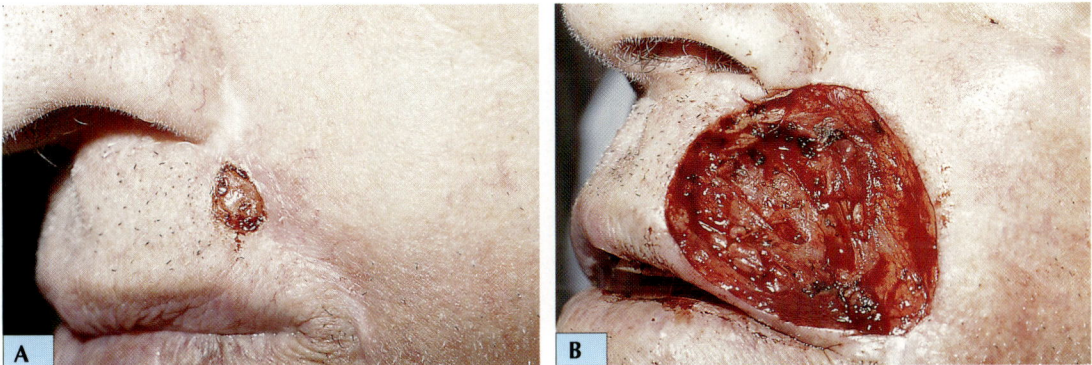

FIGURE 29.3 Lateral cheek advancement flap scar concealing recurrent tumor. **(A)** At first appearance of clinical recurrence. **(B)** After Mohs' surgery.

border, where cosmetic or functional distortion may result if an entire tumor is removed using larger, standard excisional margins (Figure 29.4A,B). However, if the actual extent of the tumor includes such an area, sacrifice of that area because of its actual involvement by the cancer usually helps the patient and the surgeon to accept any resulting deformity.

A tumor that falls in the midface (Figure 29.5A,B) may also have subclinical extensions. Because of fusion planes in the developing embryo, the tumor may intercalate between these planes, such that tumors that appear small superficially may actually run very deep. Other areas with fusion planes, such as the ear, are also associated with a high tumor recurrence rate, and since it is best to cure a cancerous lesion at the initial time of removal, Mohs' should certainly be considered for primary tumors in these locations. Other areas of high recurrence are the periorbital region and the scalp (Figure 29.6A,B).

The use of Mohs' technique for such tumors allows maximum preservation of nor-

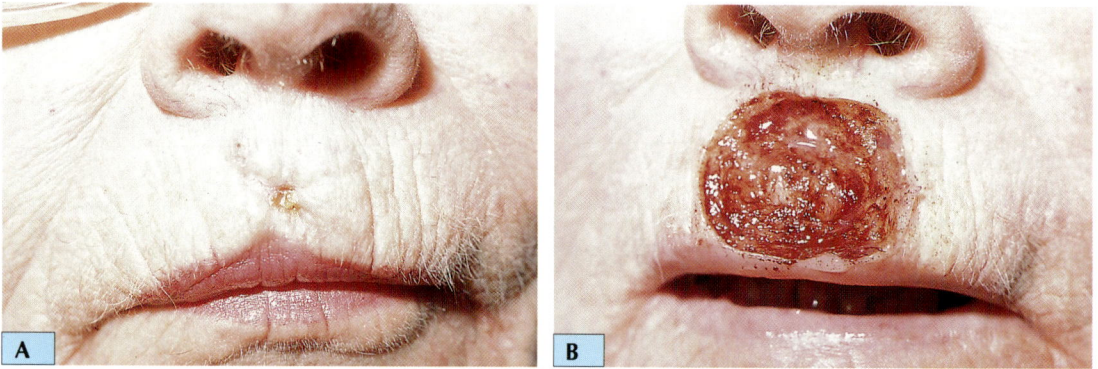

FIGURE 29.4 (A) A tumor adjacent to the vermilion border, which was maximally spared because the tumor was followed laterally. **(B)** Extent of actual spread of the tumor.

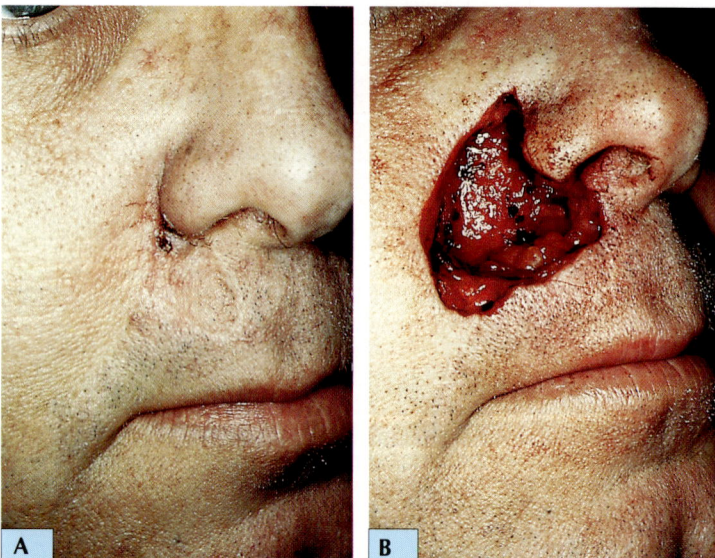

FIGURE 29.5 (A) A midface lesion appears as a crust in the nasolabial fold pocket. **(B)** Its true extensions to facial musculature and maxilla.

mal tissue. Since all margins are examined, as soon as no tumor is seen microscopically, no more tissue is removed. The fact that the Mohs' surgeon is also the pathologist is equally important. For example, if a tumor has clear margins but looks aggressive histologically, the surgeon might choose to extend the margins anyway to decrease the chance of recurrence (Figure 29.7A,B).

The subtle judgments made by the Mohs' surgeon, in combination with the unique method of tissue handling, are responsible for the low recurrence rates achieved with this technique. In the largest studies published, recurrence rates using Mohs' for all types of tumors approach 2%. Recently, a statistical analysis of recurrence rates in the literature over the past 40 years has shown recurrence rates of 1.4% (less than 5 years) and 1% (5 years) for primary basal cell carcinomas treated with Mohs' technique. Surgical excision in the same study produced recurrence rates of 2.8% and 10.1%, respectively.

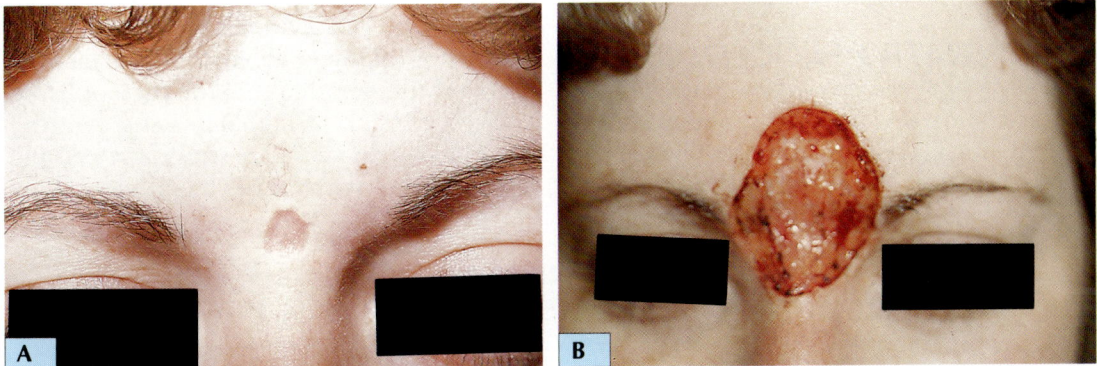

FIGURE 29.6 (A) A primary morpheaform basal cell carcinoma in a young adult. **(B)** The true extensions of the tumor.

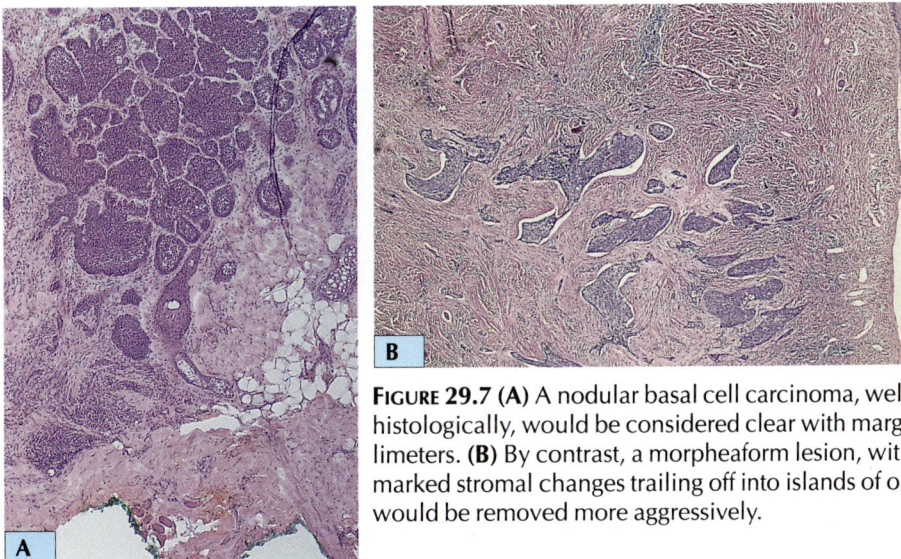

FIGURE 29.7 (A) A nodular basal cell carcinoma, well-circumscribed histologically, would be considered clear with margins of a few millimeters. **(B)** By contrast, a morpheaform lesion, with surrounding marked stromal changes trailing off into islands of only a few cells, would be removed more aggressively.

Figure 29.8 shows the wide range of tumors treated by Mohs' technique. Its unique characteristics make it applicable to many different tumor types. Contiguously growing tumors lend themselves best to the technique. Obviously, skip areas will decrease the high cure rate, although they are usually handled by removal of another rim of tissue, once negative margins are found, in an attempt to account for any skips. Although this technique may impinge on the maximal conservation of surrounding tissue, prevention of recurrence should be the major goal of any tumor-removing technique.

OPERATIVE PROCEDURE

The actual procedure is planned and performed much like a standard excision. First the patient is assessed as to his or her suit- ability for the technique. One or more of the indications listed in Figure 29.2 should apply. The procedure is then explained to the patient in detail, with adequate emphasis placed upon the "waiting time" during which the tissue is prepared, as this aspect of the procedure differs from most patients' concept of surgery.

The procedure is performed on an outpatient basis under local anesthesia in an office setting, a hospital operating room, or a specialized surgical suite. Although the procedure should normally take only 2 to 3 hours, the patient is asked to put aside an entire day, given the possibility of unsuspected subclinical tumor extensions or repairs. It is also recommended that the patient bring along a companion, snacks, and reading material to help minimize stress, anxiety, and fatigue, all of which can contribute to how

---

FIGURE 29.8
SOME OF THE TUMORS TREATED BY MOHS' SURGERY

Basal cell carcinoma	Sebaceous carcinoma
Squamous cell carcinoma	Angiosarcoma
Dermatofibrosarcoma protuberans	Amelanotic melanoma
Merkel cell carcinoma	Atypical fibroxanthoma
Microcystic adnexal carcinoma	Keratoacanthoma
Malignant fibrous histiocytoma	Lentigo maligna melanoma
Cylindroma	Nevus sebaceus
Eccrine poroma	Granular cell tumor
Metastases	Melanoma

the patient feels at the completion of the surgery. Presurgical preparation for the patient should include the avoidance of aspirin and alcohol for 5 days before the procedure, adequate rest, a light breakfast, and routine administration of any normally prescribed medications. Anticoagulants, prophylaxis, and other medical concerns should be handled on an individual basis.

On the morning of surgery, the patient's medical history should be verified and informed consent should be obtained. The patient should then be placed on the operating table and gloves donned by the surgeon.

The skin is prepared in a routine fashion (see Chapter 3).

The first stage in Mohs' technique is defining the size of the tumor, which is done by curettage. Since most tumors appropriate for Mohs' have poor clinically defined margins, use of a curet helps the surgeon to identify the extent, depth, and feel of the tumor so that the initial tissue removed for examination approaches the tumor margins (Figure 29.9A–C).

Once the lesion is defined, the next stage is excision of the tumor site with an approximately 2-mm rim of normal-appear-

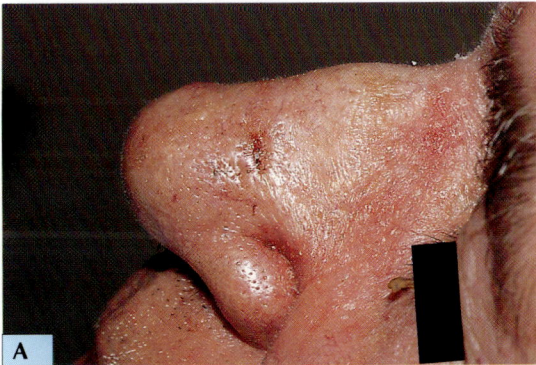

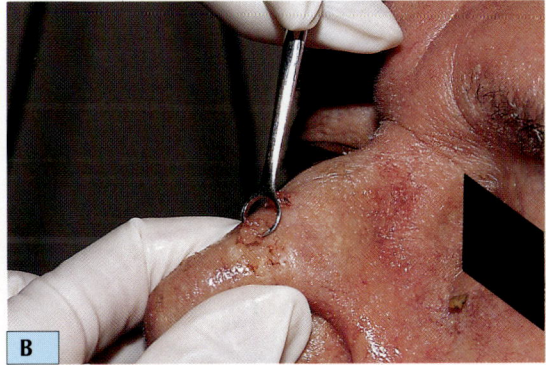

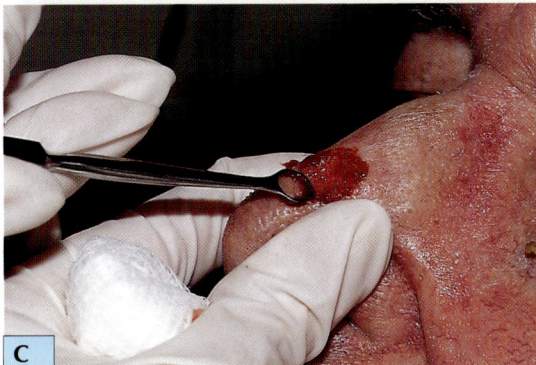

FIGURE 29.9 (A) A basal cell carcinoma on the nose shows only the biopsy site. (B) Using very little pressure, the curet easily finds the soft, friable cancerous tissue. (C) A better picture of the true extent of the tumor is now obtained.

ing tissue. The cutting instrument is held at a 45° angle for beveling (Figure 29.10), following which the piece of tissue is elevated and the scalpel or other instrument is moved across the bottom of the tissue parallel to the skin surface (Figure 29.11). If the cut is made at an angle steeper than 45°, the piece of tissue cannot be processed correctly.

The next step is critical to the proper performance of the technique. Marks must be placed on the tissue and on the patient, and a corresponding reference map must be created.

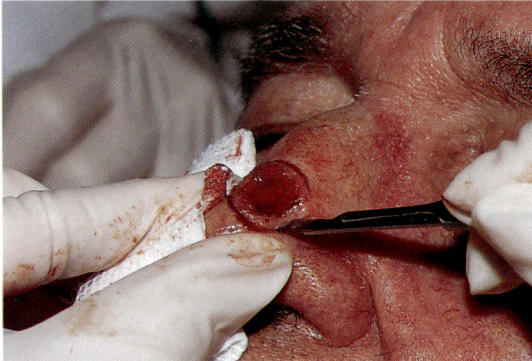

FIGURE 29.10 The rim of normal tissue and the curetted site are harvested with a scalpel angled at 45°.

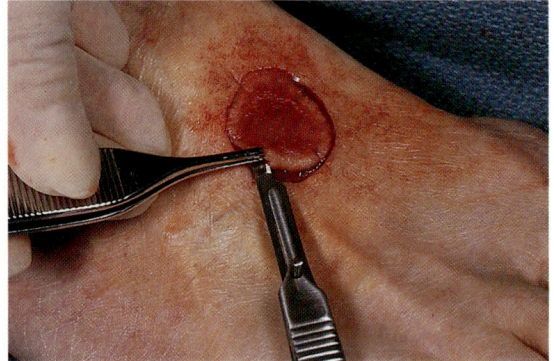

FIGURE 29.11 Toothed forceps gently raise the tissue just enough to allow the scalpel underneath to cut a flat bottom to the piece, parallel to the skin surface.

FIGURE 29.12 The tissue has been oriented on the gauze. Both the tissue and the map have been marked with hatch marks at the 6-o'clock and 12-o'clock positions.

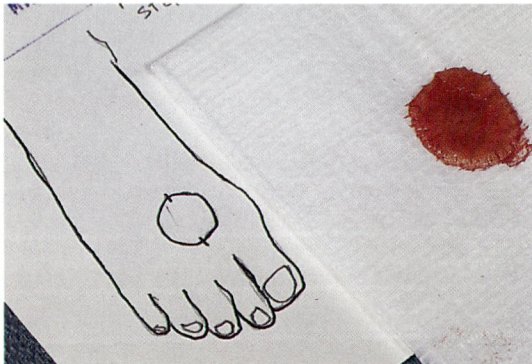

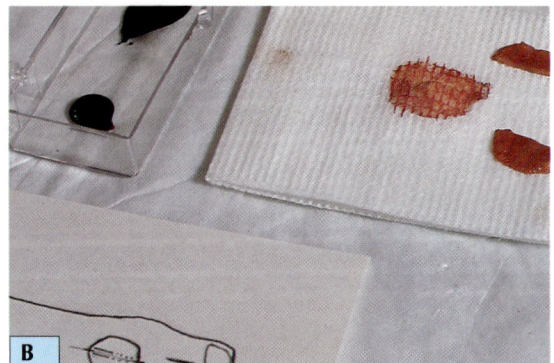

A

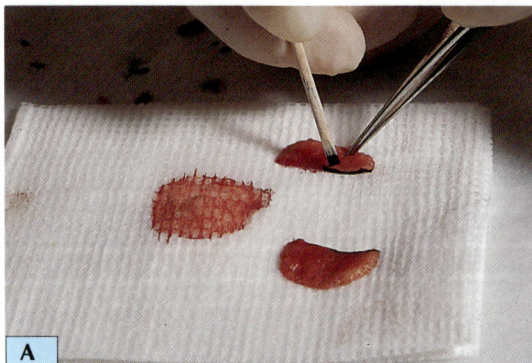

B

FIGURE 29.13 (A,B) The tissue is cut in half and marked with black and green dyes to denote right and left. The corresponding map is coded similarly using solid and dotted lines.

Many different techniques may be used. Our preference is to make hatch marks on the patient and on the piece of tissue at the time that the tissue is removed. The tissue sample is then placed on a piece of gauze with the fold of the gauze always indicating the superior edge of the tissue. At the same time, a map is drawn on a 3 x 5-mm index card to show the location of the piece of tissue as well as to re-create its exact form and the hatch marks that were placed on it (Figure 29.12). Thus, if the tissue were to be dropped, it would still be possible to orient it correctly. This painstaking attention to detail is a hallmark of Mohs' surgery and requires that the surgeon be properly trained in Mohs' technique in order to perform the surgery correctly.

The tissue is then taken to the laboratory and the patient is bandaged and allowed to return to the waiting room for approximately 20 minutes, depending on the size of the tumor, during which time the tissue is processed and examined histologically. In the laboratory, the tissue is cut into smaller, more manageable pieces that will fit on a microscope slide. Each piece is then marked to provide orientation for when it will be examined under the microscope. Such marking can be done with color dyes or it can be achieved by the orientation of the tissue. The same code that is used to orient the tissue on the slide is used to mark the corresponding map (Figure 29.13A,B).

Next, the tissue is prepared for histological examination. Each piece is flipped so that its cut surface is facing upward on a cryostat chuck. It is then fixed in an optimal cutting temperature (OCT) embedding compound for frozen specimens, while a heat extractor is pressed onto the tissue (Figure 29.14A–C). It

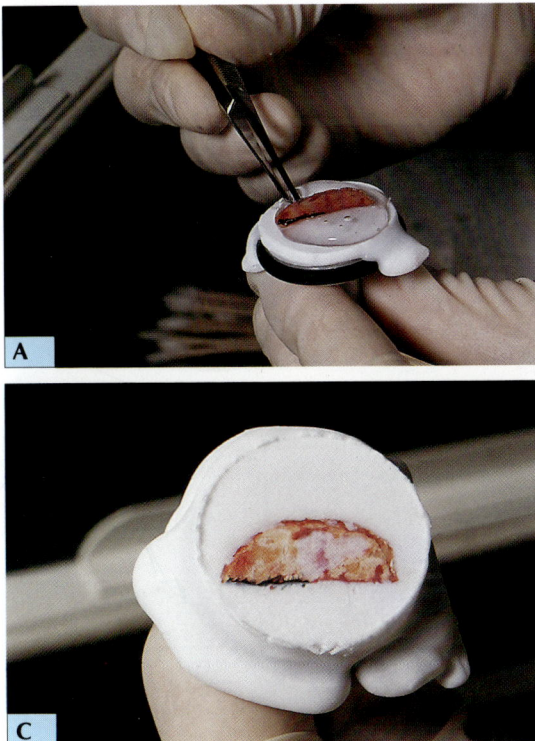

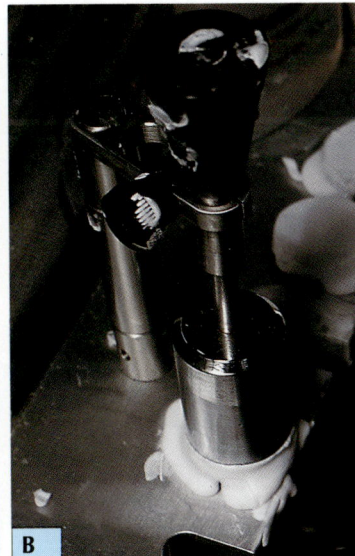

FIGURE 29.14
(A) A piece of tissue is placed in the OCT compound. Note the size of the chuck, which limits the size of each specimen.
(B) The heat extractor, a heavy weight kept in the cryostat, flattens the specimen while rapidly freezing it. (C) The final result.

is at this point that the pie-pan shape of the tissue becomes critical. When the tissue is flipped and placed on the chuck and pressure is applied, its two sides tend to flatten so that a three-dimensional piece of tissue becomes two dimensional without loss of any of its margins. If this same step were to be done with a piece of tissue cut at a 90° angle to the skin surface, as in a standard excision, the tissue would accordion and a portion of the margins of the tumor would be lost (Figure 29.15).

Each specimen, once adequately frozen, is cut into horizontal slices 6 to 10 microns thick, and placed on a microscope slide. Usually several slices from different depths are taken, allowing the surgeon to track suspicious structures throughout the piece of tissue. A small tumor about 1.5 cm in diameter will yield two slides, with each slide containing two to four cuts.

The slide is then stained using toluidine blue or hematoxylin and eosin (Figure 29.16A,B). Each slide or specimen is then examined under the microscope. Since the piece of tissue seen through the eyepiece corresponds perfectly to the reference map, the surgeon can mark on the map each area of tumor that he or she sees under the microscope. If the tumor margins are not clear, the map is so marked. The patient is now asked to return to the operating room and the map is placed next to the patient. Using the shape of the piece of tissue and the hatch marks as guides, any suspicious spot can be located with relative accuracy at the operative site. At this point, the patient may need to be reanesthetized if a long-acting anesthetic was not used initially. Further tissue is then removed only at positive sites, and the entire process is repeated until there is no remaining tumor on the slides and, in the surgeon's judgment, adequate margins have been removed (Figure 29.17).

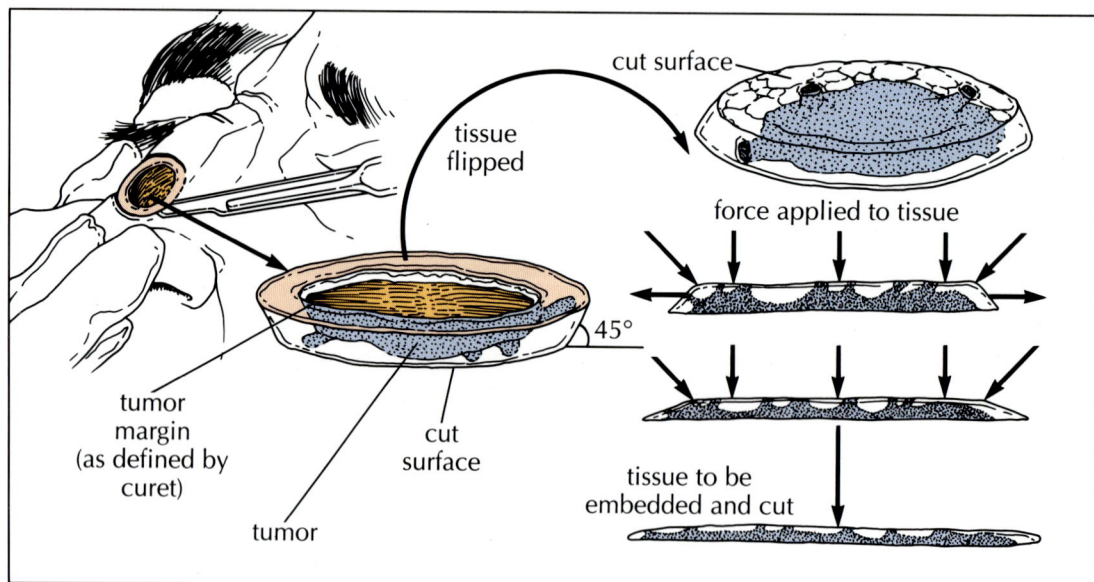

FIGURE 29.15 Schematic drawing showing how a pie-pan-shaped piece of tissue allows 100% margin control.

POSTOPERATIVE MANAGEMENT

Once the tumor has been removed, the surgeon's attention turns to repair of the defect, which in many cases has been prearranged. Some patients may have been referred by a reconstructive surgeon, and therefore will be referred back to that surgeon. In other cases, particularly where there is a large lesion or one in a critical anatomic site (periorbital, perioral), reconstruction has been anticipated during the consultation and possibly scheduled in advance to provide a smooth, organized surgical experience for the patient.

Since the wound is fresh and clean, primary closure may be performed immediately. Depending on the wound's size and location, a simple repair, flap, or graft can be chosen.

Wounds also may be left to heal by second intention. The choice of closure may also depend on the skills of the surgeon. Some Mohs' surgeons trained in reconstruction will close 75% of lesions primarily. For certain multiply recurrent tumors, large tumors, or morpheaform lesions, healing by second intention or simple closure is best. These techniques will least obscure the surgical site and allow it to be observed carefully for a year or more before the definitive repair is done. As mentioned previously, since a repair may require flaps or other methods that could "bury" recurrent tumor, it is advisable to postpone such repair for certain types of tumors or for tumors in certain areas that are associated with a high recurrence rate (see page 29.4).

Despite the uniqueness of the tech-

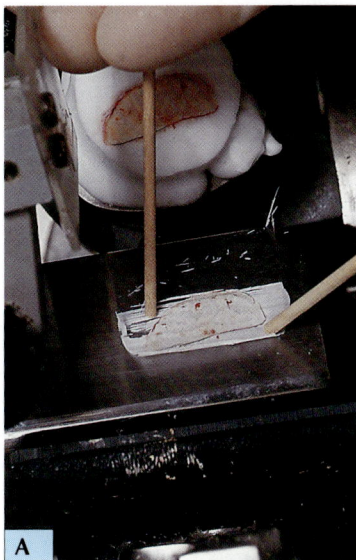

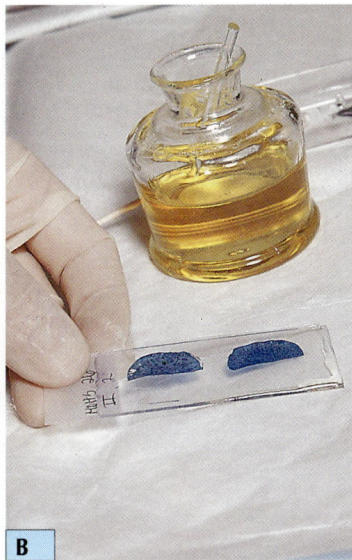

Figure 29.16 (A) Thin sections cut with a cryostat. (B) Sections stained with toluidine blue. Because these pieces were large, only two could fit on a microscope slide.

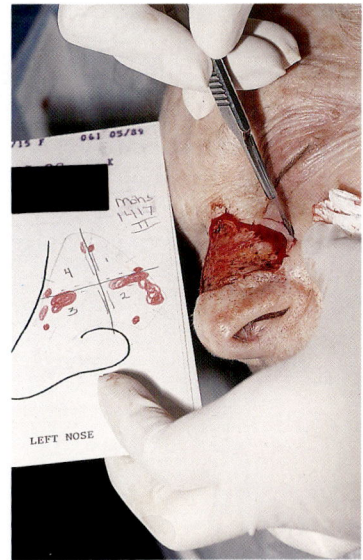

Figure 29.17 The map has been marked and is used to guide the surgeon to the areas that need further excision. The rest of the defect will not be touched, leading to maximal conservation of normal tissue and a resultant defect that reflects the tumor's true extent.

nique, postsurgical wound management for Mohs' patients is no different than that for patients who have undergone standard excision, followed by flaps, grafts, or second-intention healing. The unique features of Mohs' surgery reside in the method of tissue excision, handling, and examination of 100% of the tissue margins, which account for its high cure rate in comparison to other methods of tumor excision.

SUGGESTIONS FOR FURTHER READING

Albom MJ, Swanson NA. Mohs micrographic surgery for the treatment of cutaneous neoplasms. In: Friedman RJ, Rigel DS, Kopf AW, Harris MN, Baker D, eds. Cancer of the Skin. Philadelphia, Pa: WB Saunders Co; 1991:484-529.

Fewkes J, Mohs FE. Dermatologic surgery: microscopically controlled surgical excision (the Mohs' technique). In: Fitzpatrick TB, Eisen AZ, Wolff K, Freedberg IM, Austen KF, eds. Dermatology in General Medicine. New York, NY: McGraw-Hill Inc; 1987: 2557-2563.

Mohs F, Larson P, Iriondo M. Micrographic surgery for the microscopically controlled excision of carcinoma of the external ear. J Am Acad Dermatol. 1988;19:729-737.

Robins P. Chemosurgery: my fifteen years of experience. J Dermatol Surg Oncol. 1981; 7:779-789.

Robins P, Pollack SV, Robinson J. Immediate repair of wounds following operations by Mohs' fresh-tissue technique. J Dermatol Surg Oncol. 1979;5:329-336.

Rowe DE, Carroll RJ, Day CL Jr. Long-term recurrence rates in previously untreated (primary) basal cell carcinoma: implications for patient follow-up. J Dermatol Surg Oncol. 1989; 15:315-328.

Swanson NA, Grekin RC, Baker SR. Mohs' surgery: techniques, indications, and applications in head and neck surgery. Head Neck Surg. 1983;6:683-692.

Tromovitch TA, Stegman SJ. Microscopically controlled excision of skin tumors. Chemosurgery (Mohs): fresh tissue technique. Arch Dermatol. 1974;110:231-232.

Zitelli JA. Mohs surgery. Concepts and misconceptions. Internat J Derm. 1985; 24: 541-548.

chapter 30

RHYTIDECTOMY

The rhytidectomy, or facelift operation, has become an increasingly popular procedure in recent years. The reasons for this trend are numerous and in some ways reflect the fact that although our population is gradually aging, our society remains youth-oriented. The skin of the face can provide others with clues as to our biologic age, yet we often feel that what nature has wrought correlates incorrectly with our mental or physical age.

The toll that time and exposure to the sun take on the skin is unmistakeable. As it ages, the skin begins to relax, with a decrease in thickness and elasticity. Both the epidermis and the dermis lose their firm attachment to the underlying subcutaneous layers, with associated loss of muscle and deep tissue atrophy. All of these factors contribute to the progression of cutaneous wrinkling (Figure 30.1).

The rhytidectomy obviously cannot turn back the hands of time, but, properly performed, it can make its passage less apparent. Currently, there are several accepted methods of performing this procedure, all of which require the surgeon to have a thorough understanding of soft-tissue surgical techniques and regional head and neck anatomy (Figure 30.2). The method we use is built around an incision plan that is designed to decrease the possibility of complications involving hair loss and tragal and earlobe distortion. The incision begins in the temporal hairline, sweeping gently to the root of the helix, then extending into a preexisting skin crease in the pretragal area. From this point inferiorly, the incision courses around the lobule, to extend upon the posterior conchal bowl, with its posterior extension coursing approximately 1 cm into the hair-bearing scalp. The method varies slightly depending on whether the patient is a man or a woman (Figure 30.3). We do not vary the incision if a coronal forehead lift incision is to be performed jointly.

Apart from surgical technique, effective communication between the aesthetic surgery patient and the surgeon may be the most important factor determining the patient's ultimate postoperative satisfaction. During the preoperative period, the surgeon must establish a rapport with the patient to crystallize realistic expectations. The ultimate result of

aesthetic surgery also depends on external factors such as skin type, heredity, use of tobacco, actinic exposure, and general health, and it is the surgeon's responsibility to make the patient aware of the types of limitations that these factors can produce. The surgeon should try to screen patients with unrealistic expectations and to uncover any motivating factors that may indicate an underlying psychological dysfunction.

PREOPERATIVE PLANNING

We perform this procedure in a fully equipped operating room on an outpatient basis. Ideally, the patient should be seen on three separate occasions prior to surgery. In the initial consultation, in addition to a detailed history, the surgeon should take clinical photographs of the patient and attempt to determine his or her expectations and motivations. In the second visit, the photographs should be reviewed, and the surgeon should outline for the patient the expected preoperative and postoperative course, and clarify for the patient the goals and priorities of the surgery. During this second visit, the patient should be alerted to the problems associated

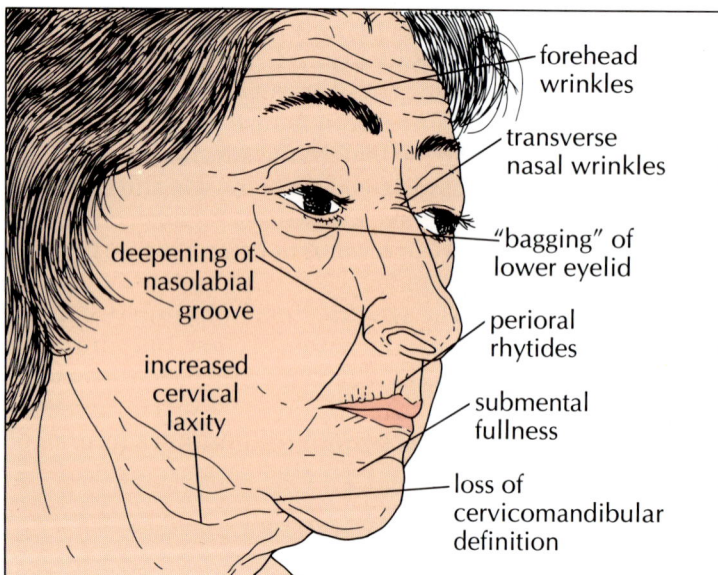

forehead wrinkles

transverse nasal wrinkles

"bagging" of lower eyelid

deepening of nasolabial groove

perioral rhytides

increased cervical laxity

submental fullness

loss of cervicomandibular definition

FIGURE 30.1 In addition to the general wrinkling and loosening of the skin associated with aging, the nose and lips are also affected.

with aspirin intake and should be started on 3000 mg/day of vitamin C in preparation for soft-tissue manipulation and in an attempt to minimize soft-tissue swelling.

The third visit should take place approximately 7 days prior to surgery. In preparation for surgery, the preoperative laboratory work should be performed, as well as a pre-

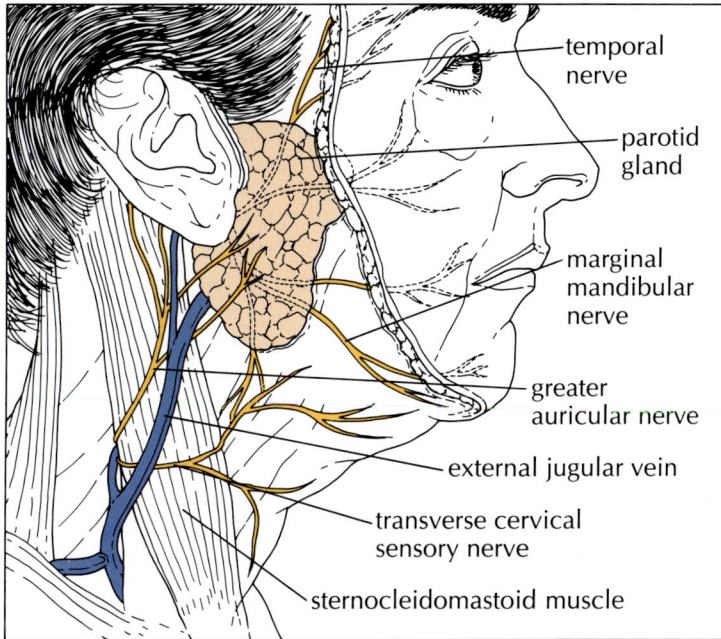

FIGURE 30.2 The surgeon performing a rhytidectomy should have a thorough knowledge of head and neck anatomy. Note that the greater auricular nerve lies at a point 6.5 cm caudal to the bony canal, where the main trunk of the nerve crosses the mid-point of the sternocleidomastoid muscle. Parallel and 5 mm ventral to it lies the external jugular vein.

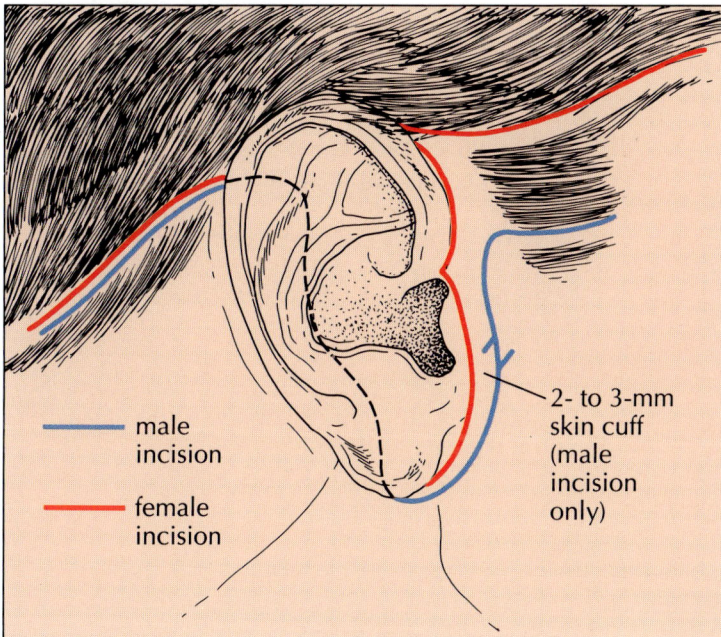

FIGURE 30.3 A variation of the incision is necessary when rhytidectomy is performed on a man. As illustrated here, beard-bearing skin should not be directly approximated with the tragus. To avoid this, a 2- to 3-mm cuff of skin is maintained in the preauricular area.

operative history and physical. Medication to be taken by the patient prior to surgery also should be dispensed. If the patient has any remaining questions, they should be answered at this time.

ANESTHESIA

Anesthesia is crucial to the success of facelift surgery, as the patient must be cooperative yet well sedated during the 2 to 3 hours necessary to perform the procedure. Effective anesthesia should provide the patient with total amnesia and should allow the surgeon to perform his or her work effectively, with no discomfort to the patient. It can also aid the surgeon in achieving hemostasis. The anesthetic agents must be carefully infiltrated

and their administration should be accompanied by close monitoring of vital signs. We recommend the course of preoperative anesthetics advocated by Johnson and Cook (Figure 30.4), which calls for medication to be taken the night before and also on the morning of surgery.

On the day of surgery, once the intravenous lines are in place and the final dose of preoperative anesthetic has been administered, the patient should be taken to the operating room and prepared for monitoring with ECG leads, blood pressure monitor, and pulse oximeter. (The pulse oximeter increases the safety of anesthesia in that it detects hypoxia in the sedated patient receiving local anesthesia significantly before ECG changes are observed.) Since intra-

---

FIGURE 30.4
JOHNSON AND COOK'S PRESURGICAL AND SURGICAL MEDICATION REGIMEN*

TIME OF ADMINISTRATION	MEDICATIONS ADMINISTERED
The night before surgery (at bedtime)	100 mg sodium pentobarbital (Nembutal) and 50 mg hydroxyzine pamoate (Vistaril) orally, with a sip of water
One hour prior to arriving at surgical unit†	250 mg trimethobenzamide HCl (Tigan) orally, with a sip of water
Upon arrival at hospital (30-45 min prior to injection of local anesthetic)	50-100 mg meperidine (Demerol) HCl intramuscularly; 50 mg hydroxyzine pamoate (Vistaril) orally, with a sip of water
When IV is started	Lorazepam (Ativan) intravenously; 1 mg if patient is going home on the same day, 2 mg if patient is to stay overnight

*From Johnson CM Jr, Toriumi DM. Open Structure Rhinoplasty. Philadelphia, Pa: WB Saunders Co; 1990:34, with permission.
†These medications are given to the patient during the last office visit prior to surgery with instructions for their proper time of administration.

venous sedation is to be administered, emergency equipment for airway management and resuscitation should be available.

A nurse anesthetist or an anesthesiologist administers the narcotic analgesic, 50 µg/mL of fentanyl citrate (Sublimaze) intravenously, in 0.5-mL increments concurrently with midazolam hydrochloride (Versed) in 0.5-mg increments. Usually, 1 to 3 mg of fentanyl is required. It is important to monitor the effect of each increment carefully, before another dose is given. The desired endpoint is general calmness, with normal blood pressure and baseline pulse; the patient should be drowsy, but arousable. When the desired degree of anesthesia has been obtained, the intravenous infusion should be supplemented with an infiltrate of 1% lidocaine hydrochloride with epinephrine 1:100,000 for local anesthesia and vasoconstriction. The pattern of infiltration of local anesthesia is discussed below. In most cases, the amnesic effects of Ativan in combination with Versed are such that the patient has little or no recollection of the procedure.

OPERATIVE PROCEDURE

In the operating room, the patient is placed in the supine position. His or her hair should be taped to keep it from interfering during the procedure and the incision site should be marked in the pretragal and post-tragal areas, as well as along the anterior temporal hairline and cervical neck. The preauricular incision is a gradual taper into the superior helix from the temporal hairline, which then follows the pretragal crease to the lobule. The postauricular incision extends onto the conchal bowl posteriorly and then courses into the hairline approximately 1 cm superior to it in the postauricular area (Figure 30.5A–C).

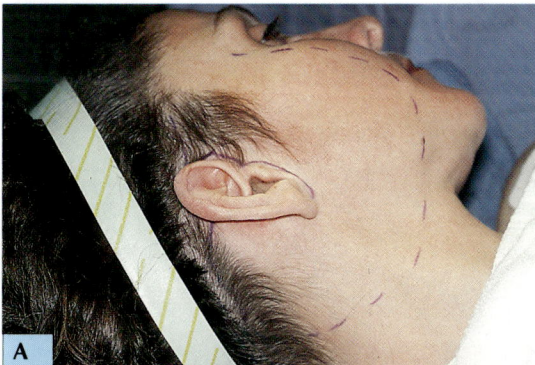

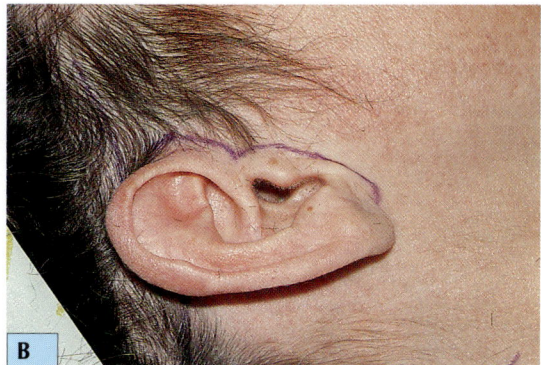

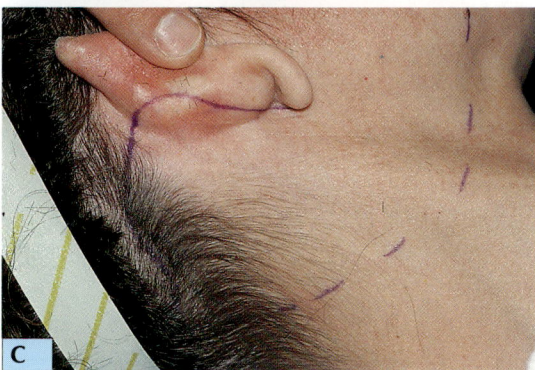

FIGURE 30.5 (A,B) The incision begins in the temporal hairline, tapers gradually into the superior root of the superior helix, and courses inferiorly in the pretragal crease to the lobule. Plans for a 6- to 7-cm skin flap are made, with appropriate facial markings to be used as landmarks during the dissection. (C) The postauricular incision extends from the lobule onto the conchal bowl and tapers approximately 1 cm into the postauricular hairline.

Prior to making each incision, we inject local anesthetic (1% lidocaine with epinephrine 1:100,000) along the incision line, creating a field block by encircling the entire flap with anesthetic (Figure 30.6A,B). The incision is begun in the preauricular area, through the dermal layer, and the skin flaps are elevated anteriorly with a #15 knife blade, with care taken to avoid the hair follicles by undermining below them (Figure 30.7). A well-defined subdermal plane is established using sharp and blunt dissection, and is carried forward anteriorly. The skin flap is created by undermining 6 cm anteriorly from the initial preauricular incision and hemostasis is obtained using bipolar cautery.

Retraction techniques are important in the development of proper skin flap thickness in both the preauricular and postauricular areas. Our technique utilizes wide retractors

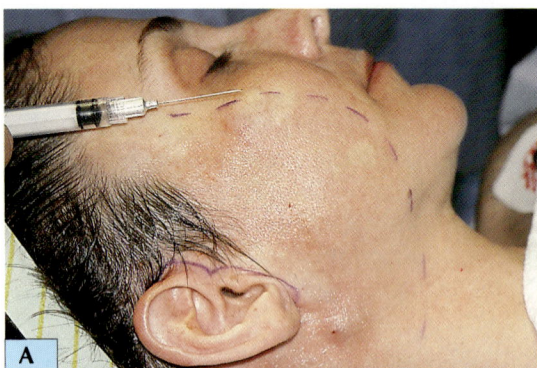

FIGURE 30.6 (A,B) One-percent lidocaine with epinephrine 1:100,000 is injected peripherally along the incision line creating a field block for local anesthesia and vasoconstriction.

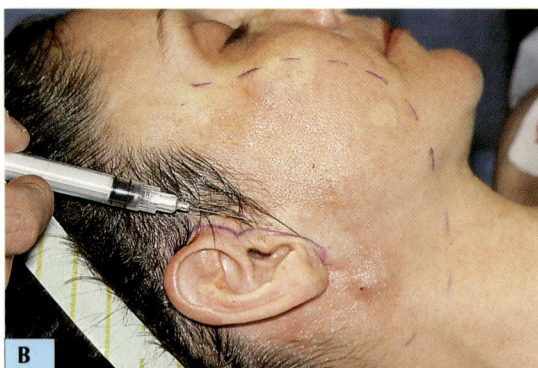

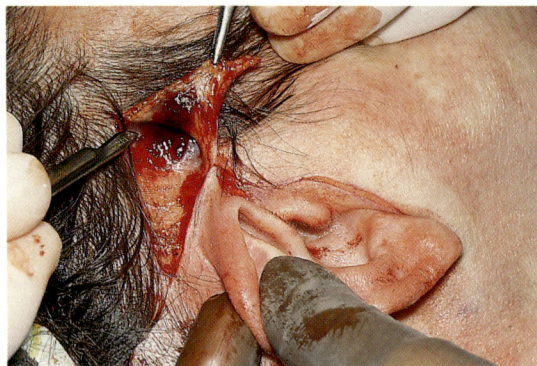

FIGURE 30.7 The skin flap is initially developed in the temporal area using sharp dissection and careful avoidance of the hair follicles in the area.

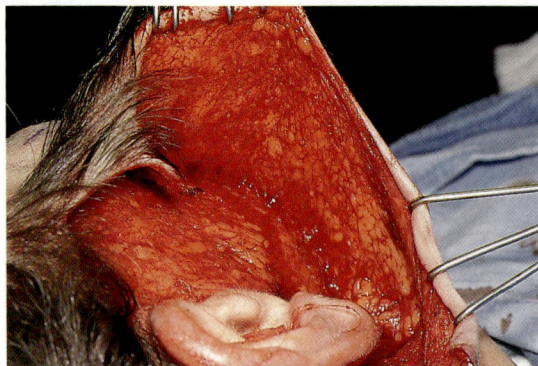

FIGURE 30.8 The anterior skin flap is developed in a surgical plane below the subdermal vascular plexus.

at the skin flap margin, which are used to provide superior traction with the surgical assistant providing inferiorly directed countertraction. This technique facilitates exposure of the proper subdermal plane and reduces the risk of damage to the subdermal vascular plexus (Figure 30.8). Next, the postauricular incision is made and the cervical skin flap is elevated. Care must be taken to avoid injury to the greater auricular nerve, as damage to this nerve can cause decreased sensation of the ear (Figure 30.9).

Once complete elevation of both the anterior and posterior flaps has been obtained with adequate hemostasis, the superficial musculoaponeurotic system (SMAS) flap elevation should be carried out in the pre-parotid fascia, elevating the tissue from the root of the zygomatic arch to a point just anterior to the sternocleidomastoid muscle (Figure 30.10).

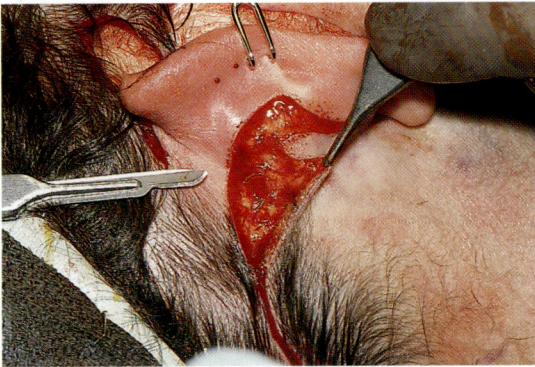

FIGURE 30.9 The postauricular skin flap is elevated using sharp dissection. Bleeding may be encountered here, as the fibers of the sternocleidomastoid muscle interdigitate with the skin at this location. In

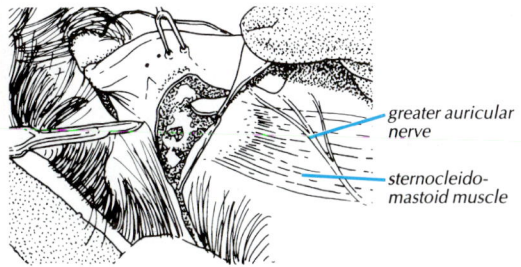

addition, as the flap is advanced, the location of the greater auricular nerve should be identified and the nerve avoided.

FIGURE 30.10 With completion of the elevation of the anterior and posterior cervical flaps to approximately 6 cm, the SMAS may be developed. A 2-cm ellipse of fascia is removed in an arc extending from the root of the zygomatic arch to the anterior border of the sternocleidomastoid muscle.

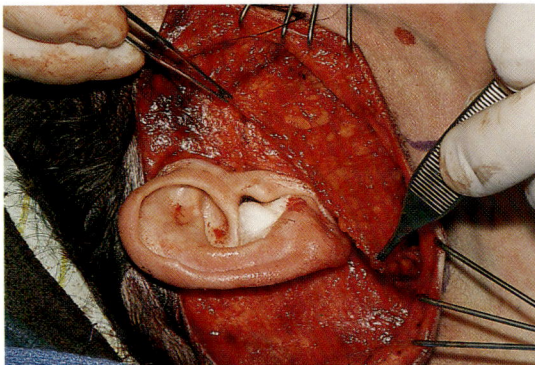

The undermining for the SMAS flap elevation should extend beyond the line for the initial elevation (Figure 30.11).

Once the SMAS has been elevated to a distance of approximately 3 cm (Figure 30.12), the flap is tailored carefully and sutured with 4-0 PDS, using an interrupted buried suture technique. The surgical knot should be buried to ensure that it is not palpable through the skin (Figure 30.13). With the SMAS in an acceptable position and stabilized, the overlying skin flaps are redraped and tailored. The initial step consists of a stab incision made at the superior point of the anterior flap (Figure 30.14). This incision is then used as a point of reference and tension for tailoring the remainder of the anterior flap.

The second step requires the establishment of a cutaneous margin at the tragus (Figure 30.15). The amount of skin removed varies depending on individual skin laxity, and is determined by establishing a new surgical margin. This allows for proper redraping of the skin flap but avoids tension at the incision. A similar procedure is performed posteriorly (Figure 30.16), with the posterior skin flap tailored into position

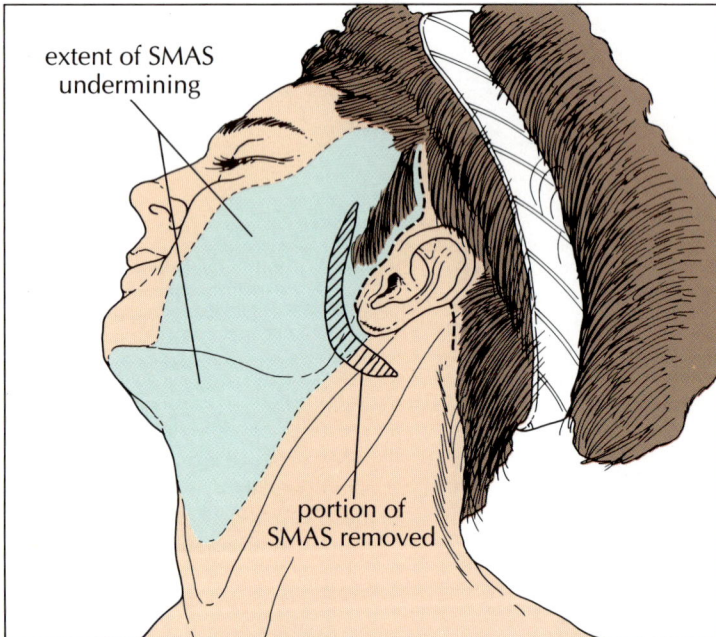

FIGURE 30.11 SMAS elevation and excision is begun at the zygomatic arch approximately 3 cm anterior to the tragus and extends posteriorly to the sternocleido-mastoid muscle.

extent of SMAS undermining

portion of SMAS removed

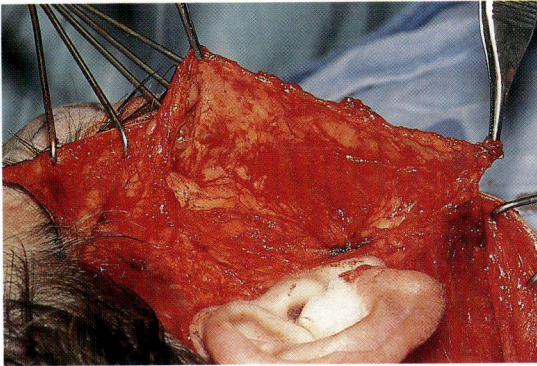

FIGURE 30.12 The SMAS flap is elevated and ready to be tailored and sutured.

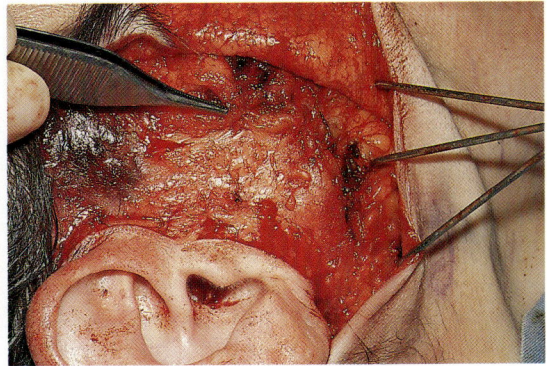

FIGURE 30.13 The flap is stabilized with interrupted 4-0 PDS, using a buried suture technique.

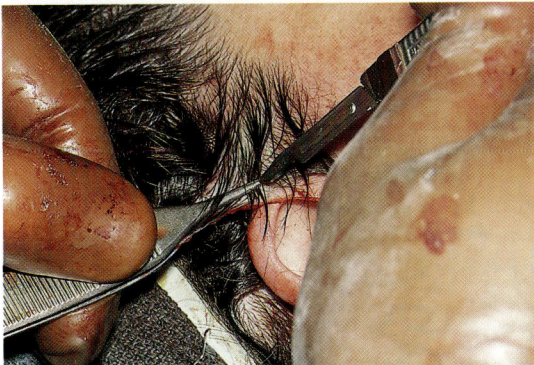

FIGURE 30.14 The preauricular flap is redraped and proper tension is established, initially at the root of the temporal aspect of the incision.

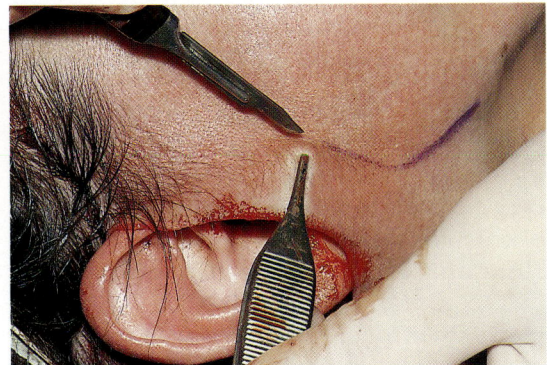

FIGURE 30.15 The next step in flap tailoring is to create a crisp, tension-free margin. After tension has been established in the temporal hairline, a preauricular skin incision is made using a #15 knife blade and Brown-Adson forceps.

FIGURE 30.16 Postauricular flap tension is established using a method similar to that for the preauricular area and excess skin is excised.

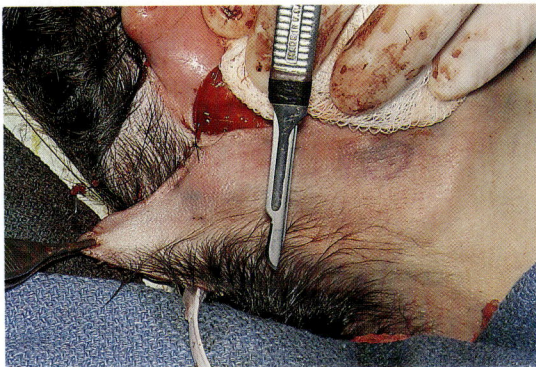

(Figure 30.17). A silicone bivalve suction drain is placed through the posterior incision, and the lobule is tailored and sutured using scissors and a single suture layer (Figure 30.18). The wound edges are then closed with a series of 4-0 nylon sutures in the hair-bearing scalp, and interrupted 5-0 nylon sutures to close the non–hair-bearing incisions. At the completion of the procedure, bacitracin ointment is applied liberally to the entire incision line. A layer of Telfa dressing is then applied over the incisions and a bulky, compressive dressing is placed from the occiput to the submental area (Figure 30.19).

POSTOPERATIVE MANAGEMENT

Postoperatively, patients are taken to the recovery room for approximately 1 hour before they are returned to the outpatient area, where they are allowed to recuperate from the effects of sedation. Once able to ambulate and tolerate oral intake, they are discharged in the care of a relative or close friend. The following morning, in an outpatient clinical treatment area, the dressings are removed, the wounds are inspected and cleaned with hydrogen peroxide, and bacitracin ointment is reapplied to the incision sites. A looser version of the pre-viously placed bandage is then applied, and should remain in place for the next 4 to 5 days. In approximately 7 days, the sutures are removed and the patient is able to shampoo the hair and resume the use of makeup.

COMPLICATIONS

Rhytidectomy is not without risk. The most common sequelae are bleeding and hematoma formation. However, adequate hemostasis at the time of surgery, appropriate preoperative education concerning the use of aspirin, and adequate application of compressive dressings minimize the risk of these complications. Despite such precautions, any patient who complains of unusual or progressive pain postoperatively should be checked for hematoma formation.

Sloughing of skin, another complication, can be caused by many factors, including failure to evacuate a hematoma, closure of skin flaps under undue tension, or heavy cigarette usage by the patient in the perioperative period (Figure 30.20). This condition should be managed with minimal debridement and local wound care, and should be allowed to heal by second intention.

Some degree of temporary sensory dep-

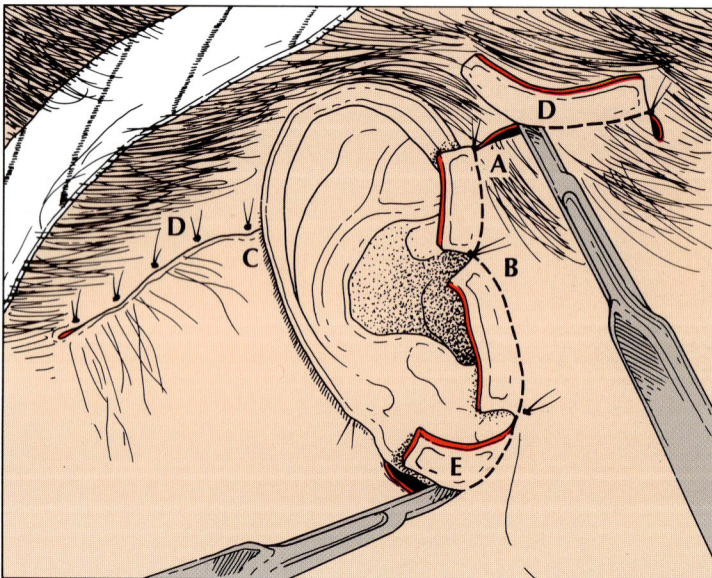

FIGURE 30.17 (A) The tension of the preauricular flap is established in the temporal hairline. (B) A crisp, tension-free preauricular incision is created. (C) Tension is established in the postauricular flap. (D) The excess skin from the anterior and posterior skin flaps is trimmed. (E) The position of the lobule is established and the skin is tailored.

rivation often occurs as a result of elevation of the cervicofacial skin flaps. Reinnervation usually occurs within a 4- to 6-month period. The patient should be informed preoperatively of the possibility of this temporary postoperative problem. Long-term sensory loss can occur if the greater auricular nerve is transsected, with subsequent numbness of the upper portions of the ear.

Facial nerve damage is also a possibility during rhytidectomy. The nerve lies deep to the parotid fascia in the preauricular area but courses more superficially as the nerve terminates in the muscles of facial expression. For this reason, when elevating the skin flap, care should be taken in the elevation of the distal component of the flap, as it is during this portion of flap elevation that motor nerve injury can result. The marginal mandibular nerve, which has a superficial course as it runs over the angle of the mandible, is the most commonly injured branch. Damage to this nerve can result in permanent weakness at the corner of the mouth.

Another complication, termed "pixie ear," can result if undue tension is applied to the earlobe closure during surgery (Figure 30.21). Hypertrophic scar formation, yet another com-

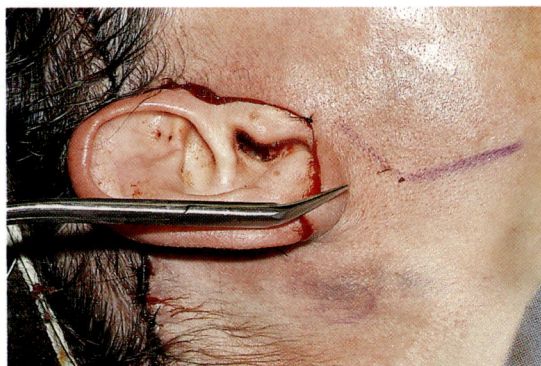

FIGURE 30.18 The position of the lobule is an important detail in completing the trimming of the flap. We prefer to drape the cervical skin over the lobule, and using the helix as a guide excise the skin until it can be inserted in a tension-free manner beneath the lobule.

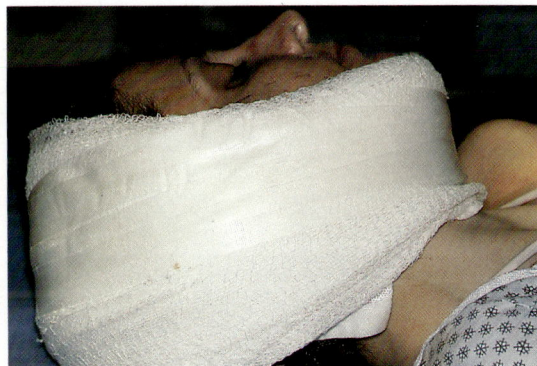

FIGURE 30.19 A compressive dressing is placed, with surgical drains exiting posteriorly.

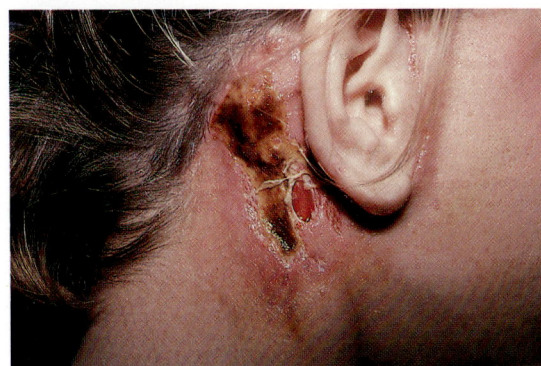

FIGURE 30.20 The sloughing of this patient's skin 2 weeks postoperatively is likely due to her heavy cigarette smoking during the perioperative period.

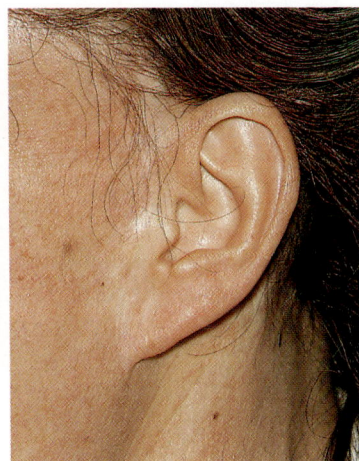

FIGURE 30.21 "Pixie ear" deformity is the result of an improper degree of tension at the lobule.

plication, can be seen particularly in individuals who have a tendency toward making such scars. Patients should be screened carefully, prior to surgery, for such a tendency and should be informed preoperatively of their risk for this complication. Lastly, infection is a rare complication of facelift surgery, partially because of the rich vascular nature of

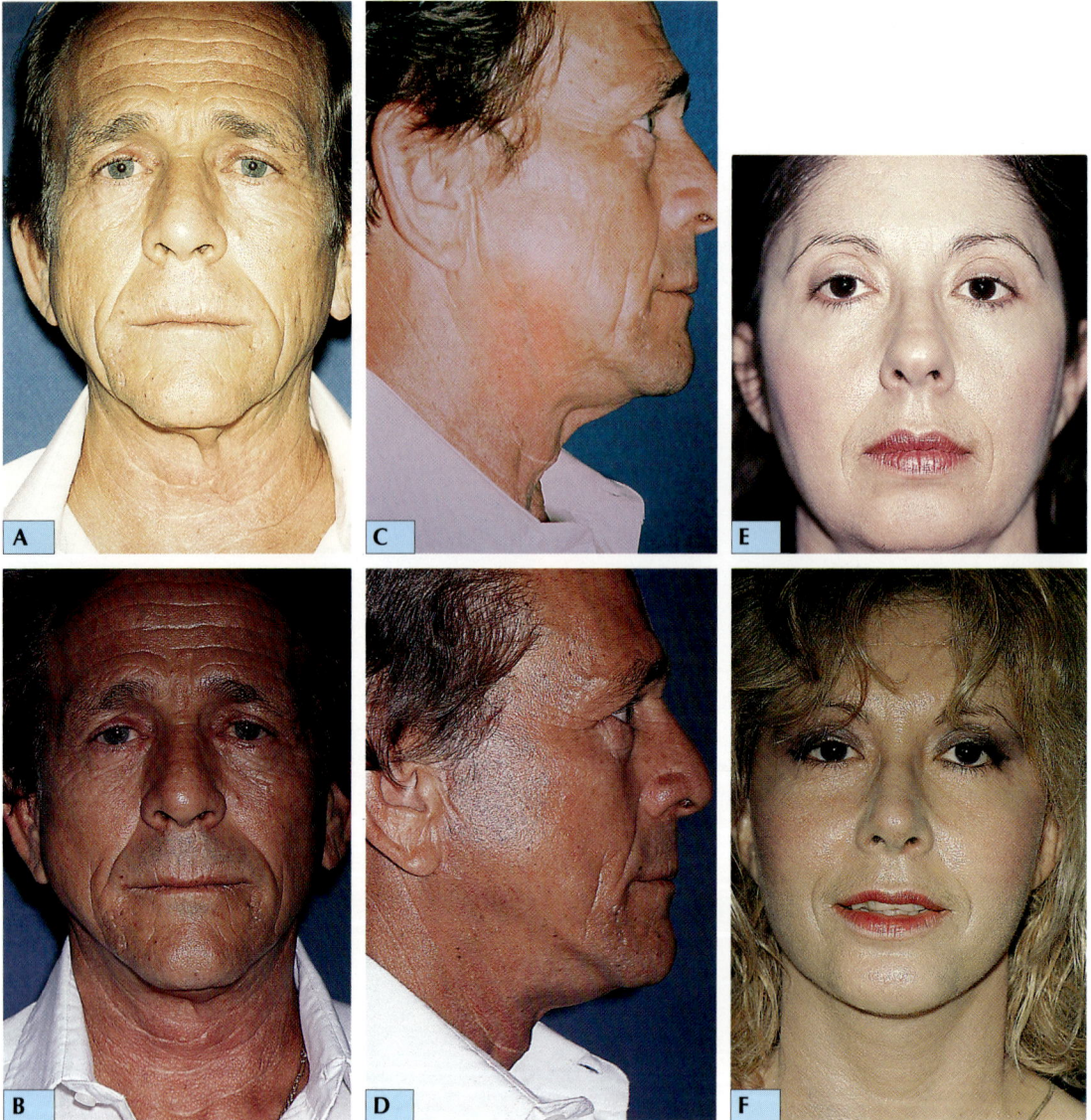

FIGURE 30.22 (A–L) Preoperative and postoperative photographs of patients who have undergone successful rhytidectomies.

the tissues in the head and neck region. Furthermore, antibiotics are routinely administered in the intraoperative and postoperative periods.

"Before and after" photographs from several patients illustrate typical rhytidectomy results (Figure 30.22A–L).

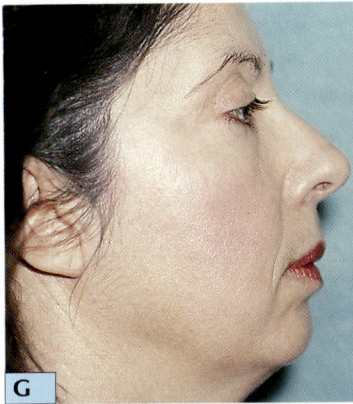

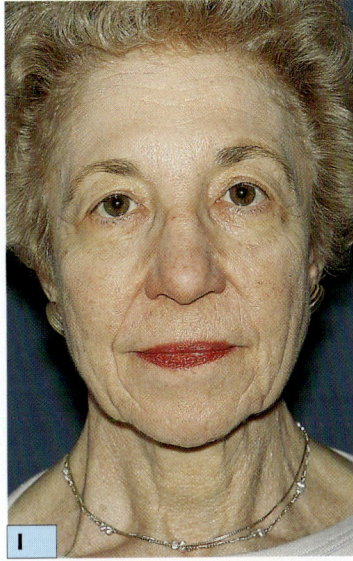

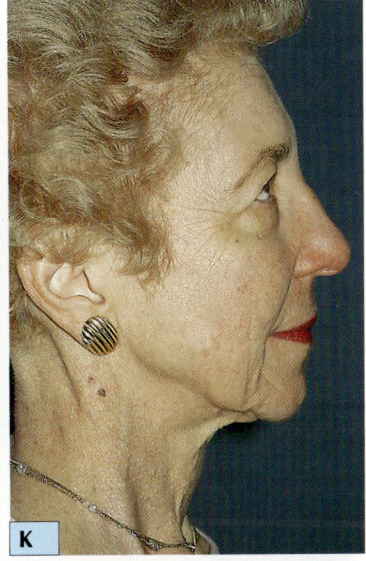

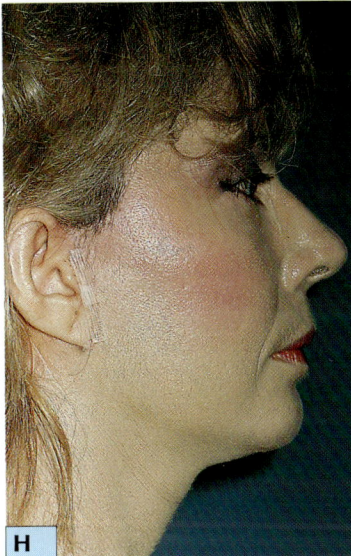

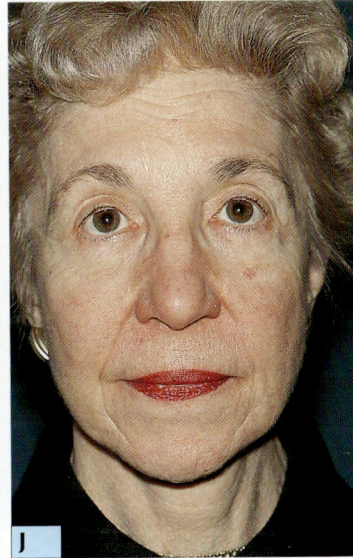

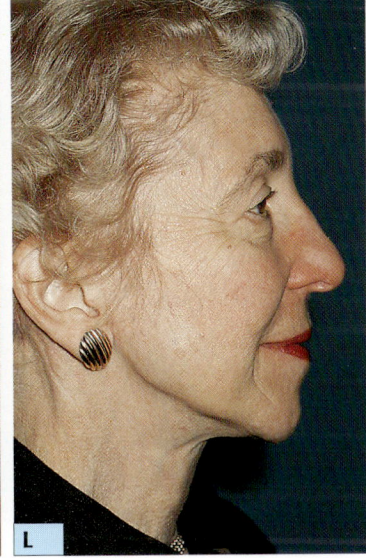

SUGGESTIONS FOR FURTHER READING

Anderson JR. The tuck-up operation. A new technique of secondary rhytidectomy. Arch Otolaryngol. 1975;1:739-760.

Hollander MM. Rhytidectomy: anatomical, physiological and surgical considerations. Plast Reconstr Surg. 1957;20(3):218-231.

Johnson CM Jr, Adamson PA, Anderson JR. The face-lift incision. Arch Otolaryngol. 1984;110:371-373.

Johnson CM Jr, Toriumi DM. Open Structure Rhinoplasty. Philadelphia, Pa: WB Saunders Co;1990.

Kamer FM. Sequential rhytidectomy and the two stage concept. Otolaryngol Clin North Am. Symposium on the Aging Face. 1980; 13(2):305-320.

Leist FD, Masson JK, Erick JB. A review of 324 rhytidectomies emphasizing complications and patient dissatisfaction. Plast Reconstr Surg. 1977;59(4):525-529.

McCollough EG, Perkins SW, Langsdon PR. SASMAS suspension rhytidectomy. Arch Otolaryngol Head Neck Surg. 1989;115: 228-234.

Rees TD. Aesthetic Plastic Surgery. Philadelphia, Pa: WB Saunders Co;1980.

Webster RC. Facelift, parts I to V. Head Neck Surg. 1983;5:525-534 and 1983/1984;6:590-596,696-702,780-792.

Webster RC. Male and female face-lift incisions. Arch Otolaryngol. 1982;108:299-302.

chapter 31

BLEPHAROPLASTY

Upper and lower eyelid blepharoplasty is frequently performed on patients with blepharochalasis, a condition in which the skin of the eyelid becomes thin and atrophic and is characterized by extreme laxity, with an associated decrease in visual fields. Indications for aesthetic blepharoplasty include excessive eyelid skin and muscle, brow ptosis, protrusion of fatty compartments against a weakened orbital septum, and transverse bulging of the orbicularis oculi muscle, near the ciliary margin. Many of these changes are characteristics of the normal facial aging process (Figure 31.1).

Important structures in eyelid function are the orbicularis oculi muscle, the orbital septum, the eyelid fatty compartments, and the lacrimal gland. The location of these structures, as well as their anatomic relationships, is important in the surgical correction of the aging eyelid (Figure 31.2).

PREOPERATIVE PLANNING

Preoperative evaluation for blepharoplasty includes a thorough ophthalmologic examination, including visual field assessment, ophthalmoscopic examination, and testing for tear production. Preoperative instructions to the patient are the same as those for rhytidectomy (see Chapter 30) and include the avoidance of aspirin for 3 weeks prior to surgery. Upper and lower eyelid blepharoplasties may be performed in an outpatient facility or in a hospital ambulatory setting.

ANESTHESIA

Upper and lower eyelid blepharoplasties are performed utilizing intravenous sedation, supplemented by a local soft-tissue infiltrate of 1% lidocaine with epinephrine 1:100,000.

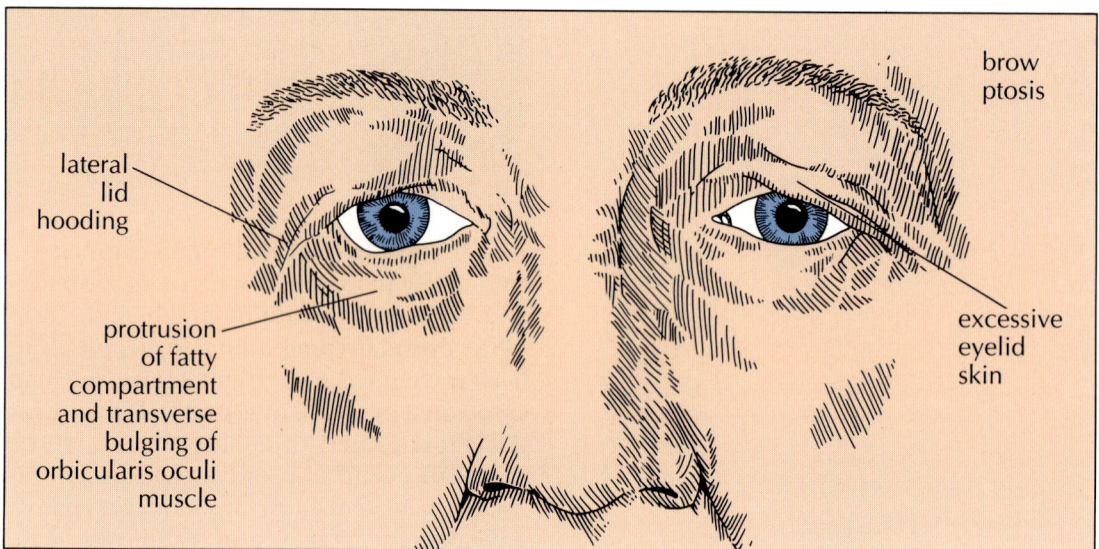

FIGURE 31.1 Schematic drawing showing eyelid changes characteristic of normal facial aging.

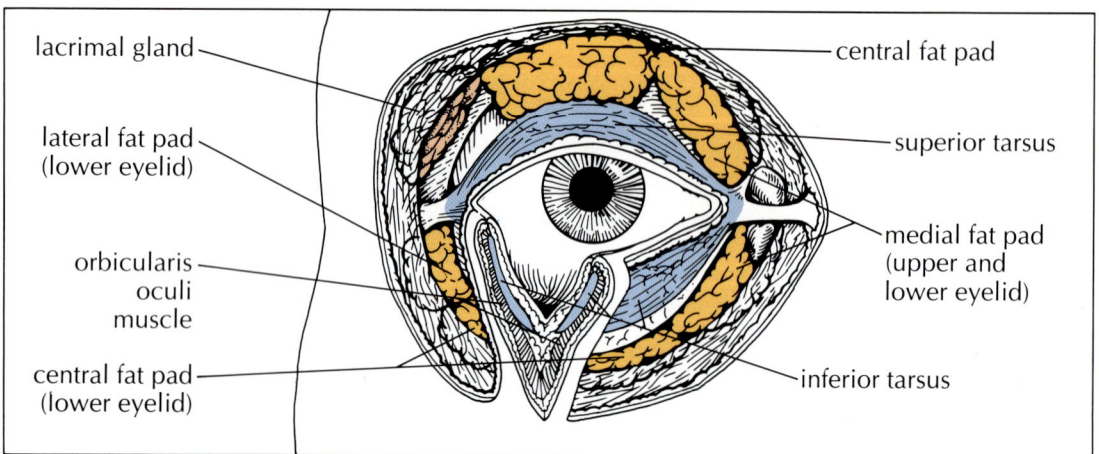

FIGURE 31.2 Schematic drawing showing the anatomic structures important in aesthetic eyelid surgery.

Sedation techniques are the same as those for rhytidectomy (see Chapter 30). The surgical incision is marked prior to injection of local anesthetic to ensure proper placement of the incision on natural eyelid creases.

OPERATIVE PROCEDURE

UPPER EYELID BLEPHAROPLASTY

A gently sloping elliptical incision is planned (Figure 31.3), which begins approximately 1 mm superior to the margin of the upper tarsal plate and is carried to a width of 4 to 6 mm depending on the individual patient's needs. The incision should course laterally into a naturally occurring skin fold. If both upper and lower eyelid blepharoplasties are planned, the incisions for the two procedures should be no closer than 4 mm (Figure 31.4).

The incision is begun using a #15 knife blade and is carried to its full extent across the upper eyelid (Figure 31.5A,B). A 3-mm section of orbicularis oculi muscle should then be excised across the full extent of the surgical site. Hemostasis is obtained using a bipolar cautery. The orbital septum underlying the orbicularis oculi muscle must be

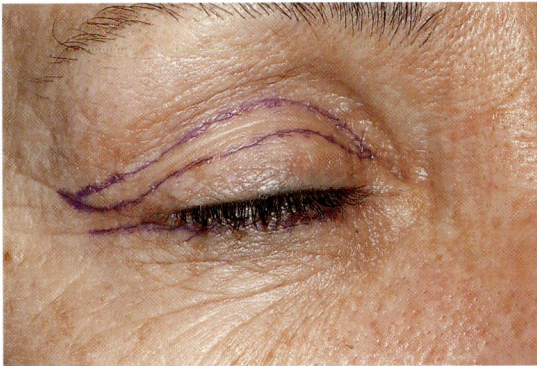

FIGURE 31.3 The incision for upper eyelid blepharoplasty begins at the margin of the upper tarsal plate and extends in a gently sloping ellipse to a width of 4 to 6 mm.

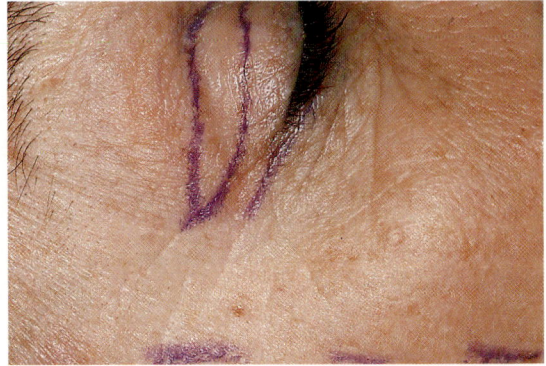

FIGURE 31.4 If upper and lower eyelid blepharoplasties are planned, there should be a gap of at least 4 mm between the incision sites. The incision lines should be incorporated into natural skin folds and should follow the curvature of the eye.

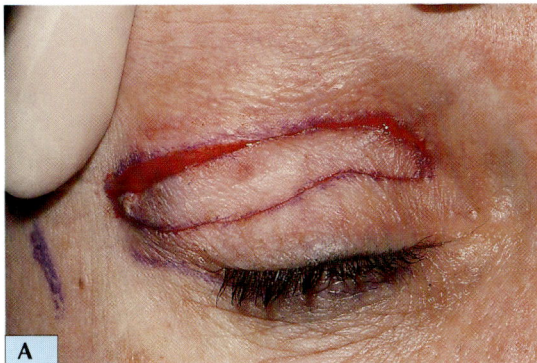

A

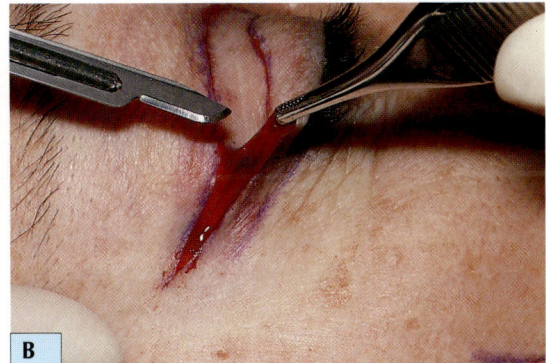

B

FIGURE 31.5 (A,B) A #15 knife blade and Brown-Adson forceps are used to score the incision and to excise the excessive upper eyelid skin.

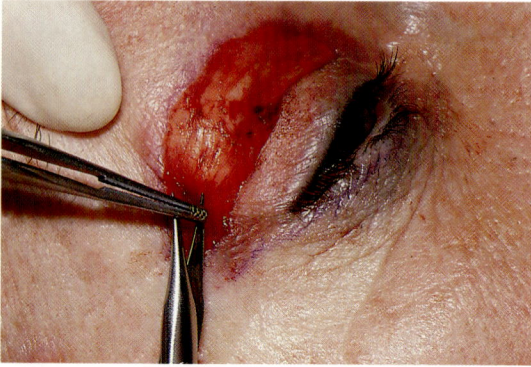

FIGURE 31.6 Beginning laterally, the orbital septum is excised across the full extent of the upper eyelid.

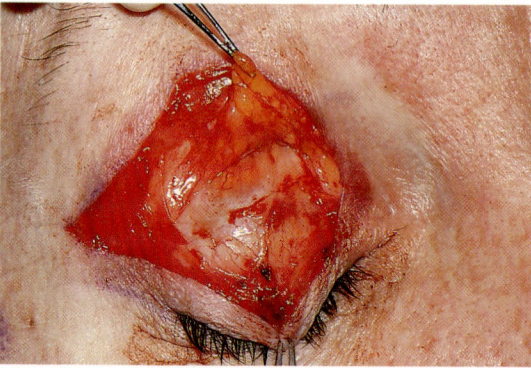

FIGURE 31.7 After the orbital septum is opened, the medial and central fat pads are gently teased free of surrounding soft tissue with careful avoidance of the lacrimal gland, which lies laterally in the wound.

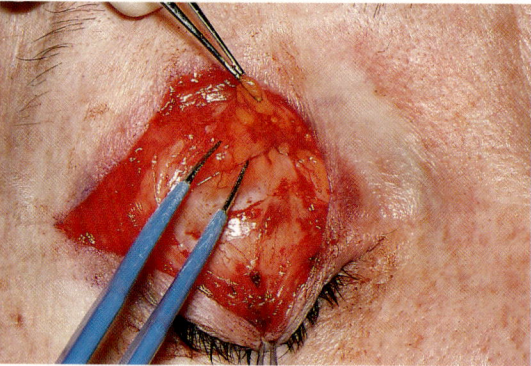

FIGURE 31.8 The fat pads are gently retracted and cauterized at their base with bipolar current to ensure adequate hemostasis.

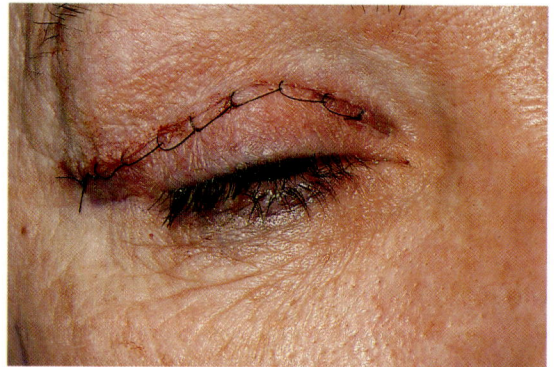

FIGURE 31.9 Final closure utilizes 6-0 silk, with a running locked suture technique. Subcutaneous sutures are not used. A 1- to 2-mm area of orbital exposure is acceptable at the completion of surgery.

excised as well, and should be entered in a linear fashion across the full extent of the eyelid incision (Figure 31.6).

The medial and central fat pads are then gently teased free, with care taken to ensure that they have no traction, as this can lead to retrobulbar hematoma formation (Figure 31.7). Bipolar current is used to cauterize the base of the fat pads to ensure adequate hemostasis, after which the fat pads are excised (Figure 31.8). Following hemostasis and thorough irrigation of the wound, 6-0 silk is used to suture the wound externally, using a running locked suture technique. There are no subcutaneous sutures used in this closure (Figure 31.9). Finally, the eyelid should be checked for adequate closure, allowing a 1- to 2-mm exposure.

LOWER EYELID BLEPHAROPLASTY

For lower eyelid blepharoplasty, the incision is placed in a natural, subciliary crease (Figure 31.10). After the area is anesthetized locally, along the lines of the incision and under the lower eyelid (Figure 31.11), the incision is begun medially using a #15 knife blade and is continued laterally to approximately 4 to 6 mm lateral to the lateral canthus (Figure 31.12A,B). Using sharp dissecting scissors, a skin–muscle flap is elevated in the lateral aspect. To achieve an avascular plane,

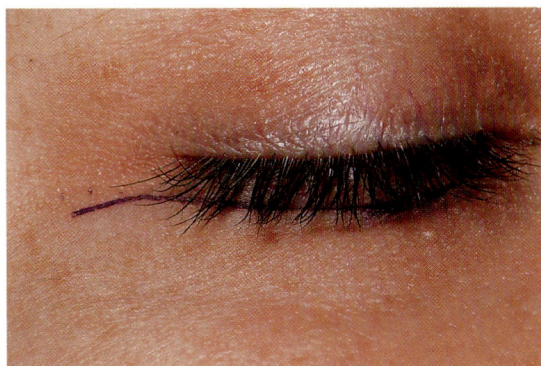

FIGURE 31.10 The incision for lower eyelid blepharoplasty is placed in a natural subciliary crease, with a 4- to 6-mm extension beyond the lateral canthus.

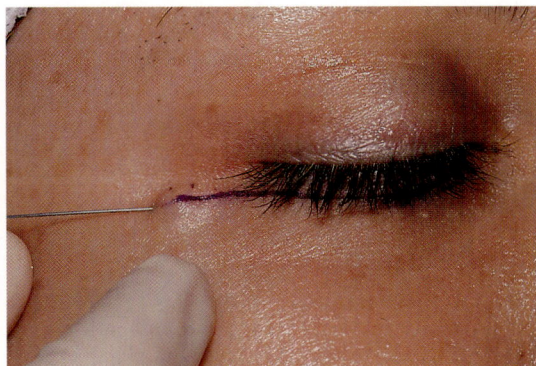

FIGURE 31.11 Anesthetic is injected locally after the incision has been planned, and relies on a local field block.

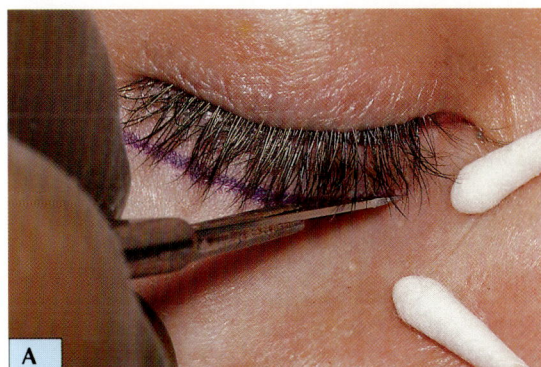

A

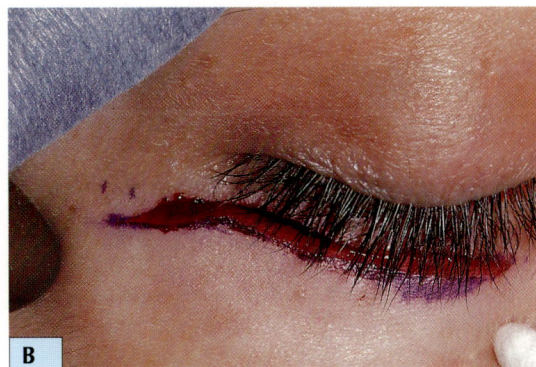

B

FIGURE 31.12 (A,B) The subciliary incision is begun medially with a #15 knife blade and is carried laterally into a natural malar crease.

gentle downward pressure is applied over the malar eminence and the lateral edge of the skin–muscle flap is retracted superiorly. Dissection between the orbicularis oculi muscle and the orbital septum is thereby facilitated (Figure 31.13A,B).

After hemostasis has been obtained, identification of the orbital septum is important as the orbital fat pads lie just beneath it (Figure 31.14). Next, 4-0 silk sutures are placed in the superior aspect of the incision to retract the eyelid and to expose the fat pads (Figure 31.15). Following adequate upward retraction, the orbital septum is then entered and excised across the full extent of the lower eyelid, with identification of the medial, central, and lateral fat pads (Figure 31.16A,B). After meticulous hemostasis is again obtained using bipolar cautery, the fat pads are injected at their base with 1% lidocaine with epinephrine (Figure 31.17) and they are cauterized at their base using bipolar current (Figure 31.18). The fat pads are then excised at their base, with care taken to avoid excessive retraction (Figure 31.19).

The skin is then redraped laterally in a

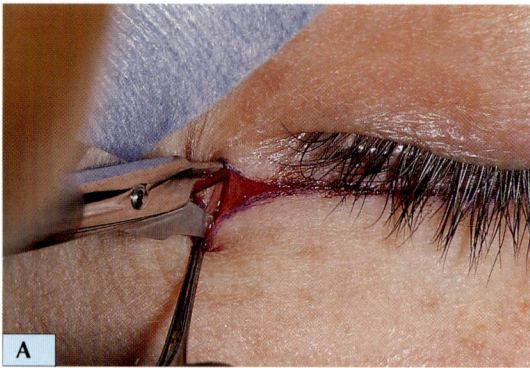

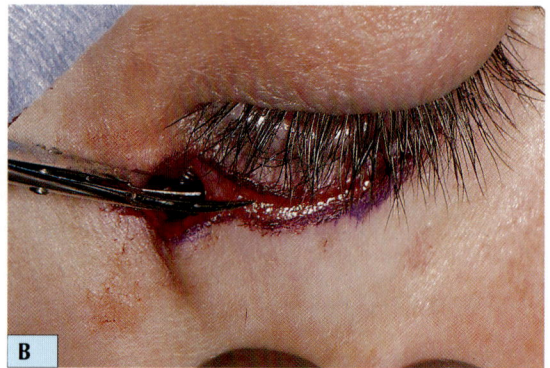

FIGURE 31.13 (A,B) Sharp dissecting scissors are used to establish a skin–muscle flap in the lateral aspect of the dissection and a surgical plane is developed between the orbicularis oculi muscle and the orbital septum.

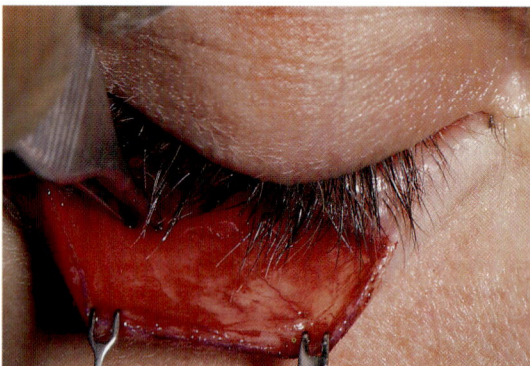

FIGURE 31.14 The orbital septum should be identified beneath the orbicularis oculi muscle so that adequate exposure of the lower eyelid fat pads is obtained.

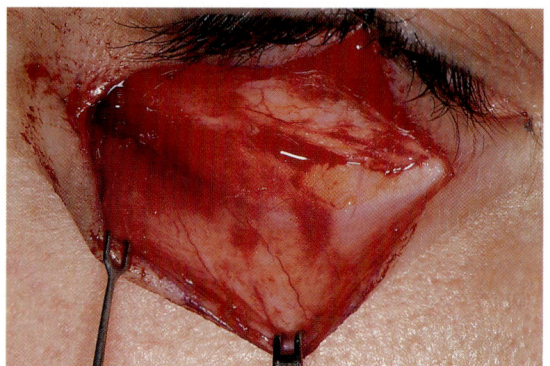

FIGURE 31.15 Sutures of 4-0 silk are placed below the ciliary margin and are retracted superiorly to highlight the location of the orbital fat pads.

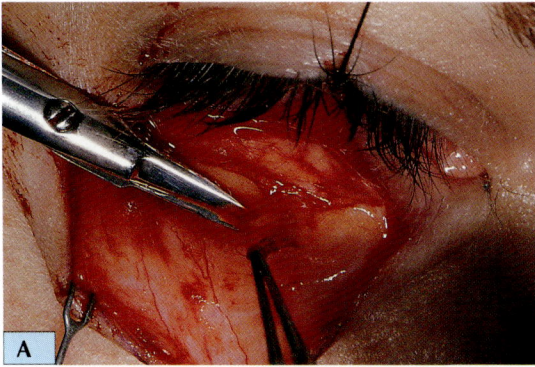

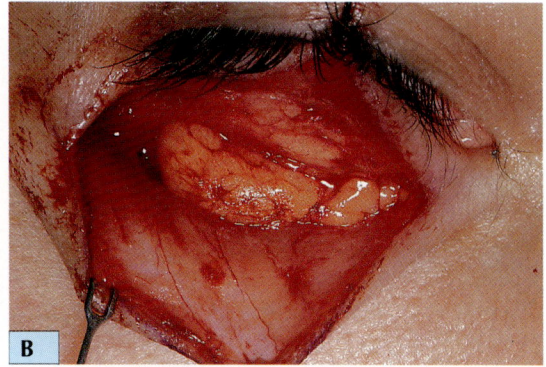

FIGURE 31.16 (A) The orbital septum is excised across the full extent of the three fat pad components. **(B)** The medial, central, and lateral fat pads are identified. In some cases, the central and lateral fat pads are confluent.

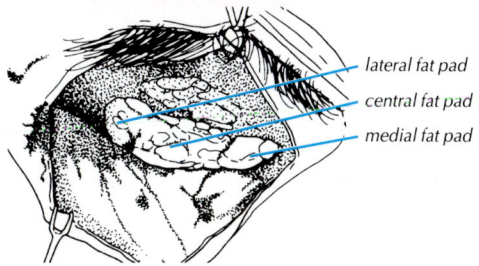

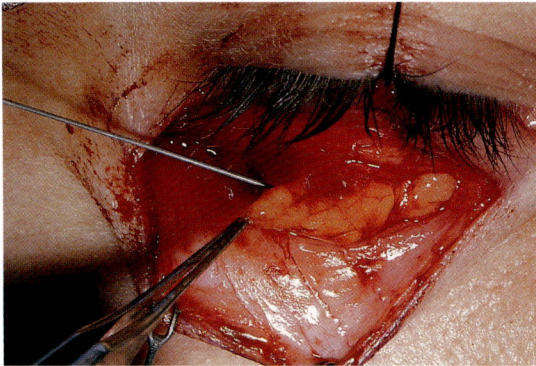

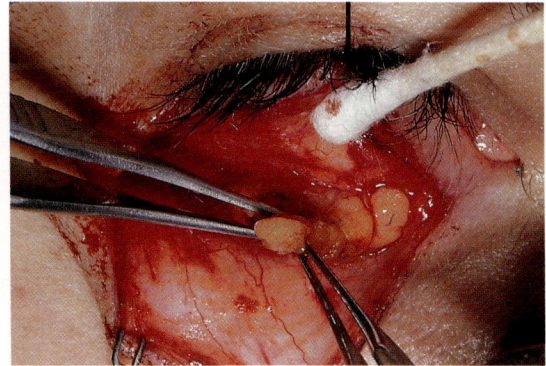

lateral fat pad
central fat pad
medial fat pad

FIGURE 31.17 After adequate hemostasis has been obtained, the fat pads are injected at their base with 1% lidocaine with epinephrine.

FIGURE 31.18 The base of the fat pads is cauterized prior to their excision.

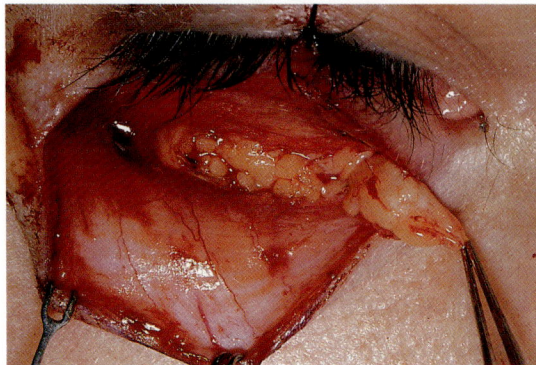

FIGURE 31.19 The fat pads are excised at their base with care taken to avoid excessive retraction.

horizontal orientation, to ensure proper lower eyelid tone, thereby avoiding downward tension on the eyelid margin (Figure 31.20). The skin is initially tailored laterally (Figure 31.21) and the orbicularis oculi muscle is stabilized using 5-0 Mersilene suture to suspend the muscle to the lateral orbital rim. Minimal excision of the lower eyelid skin underlying the ciliary margin is performed (Figure 31.22), keeping in mind that since the primary skin excision is lateral to the canthus, minimal excision in this area reduces the possibility of ectropion. The wound is then closed with 6-0 interrupted silk suture, which should be left in place for 3 to 5 days (Figure 31.23).

POSTOPERATIVE MANAGEMENT

Patients are taken to the recovery room and observed for 3 to 5 hours. Cold saline compresses are placed on the eyes to control swelling. Postoperatively, patients are treated with oral analgesics and antibiotics. If stable, they are discharged to be seen again in 3 to 5 days, at which time the sutures may be removed. The use of makeup is avoided for 7 to 10 days postoperatively and rigorous exercise is avoided for 1 week. Aspirin should not be taken for 2 weeks following surgery.

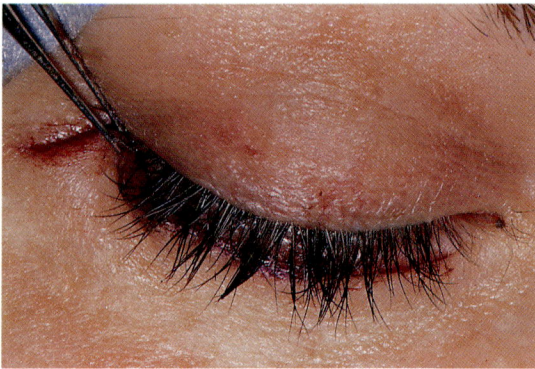

FIGURE 31.20 Redraping of the skin–muscle flap is initiated in the lateral aspect and relies on horizontal tension to minimize the risk of postoperative ectropion.

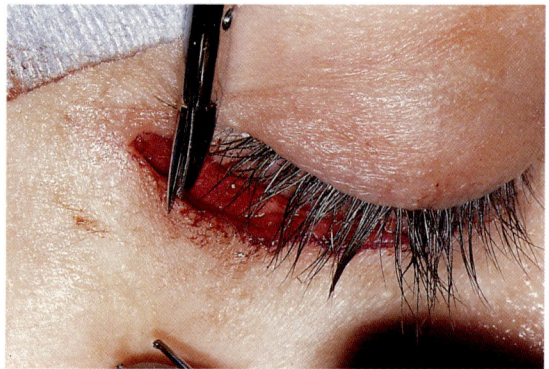

FIGURE 31.21 The skin is tailored laterally, with the majority of lower skin excision occurring beyond the lateral canthus.

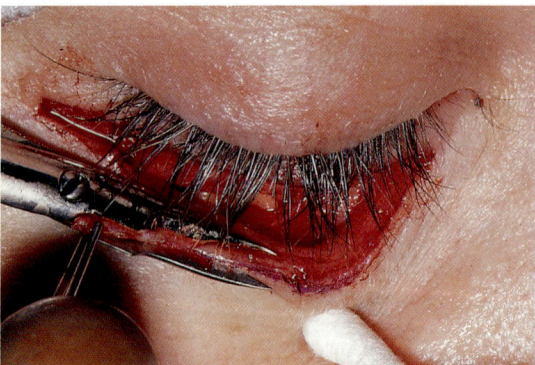

FIGURE 31.22 Minimal excision of the skin below the ciliary margin is carried out.

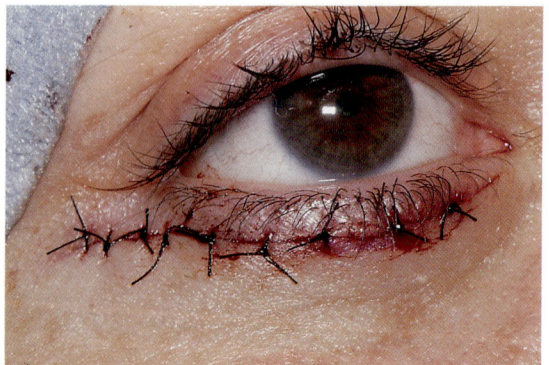

FIGURE 31.23 The surgical site is closed with 6-0 interrupted silk suture and a light application of bacitracin ointment is used to seal the wound.

COMPLICATIONS

The immediate complications of eyelid surgery include eyelid hematomas, retrobulbar hematomas, eyelid infections, and ocular mobility dysfunction. The prevention of both eyelid and retrobulbar hematomas is dependent on meticulous hemostasis at the time of surgical closure of the wound. Retrobulbar hematomas, in particular, can be caused by aggressive retraction of the orbital fat pads. Postoperative infections of the periocular area are unusual but when they occur should be treated with appropriate antibiotic therapy in combination with warm compresses. Ocular mobility dysfunction can occur if there is inadvertent injury to any of the orbicularis rectus muscles. In particular, the inferior oblique muscle is at risk during lower eyelid surgery.

Delayed complications include postsurgical ectropion and dry eye. Both of these complications occur in patients in whom excessive lower eyelid laxity and borderline dry eye syndrome would be identified at the preoperative ophthalmologic consult.

CASE STUDIES

A 34-year-old woman presented for elective lower eyelid blepharoplasty with laxity of the orbital septum and protrusion of fat pads in all three quadrants (Figure 31.24A–C). Postoperative photographs illustrate the result (Figure 31.25A–C).

A 58-year-old woman presented for

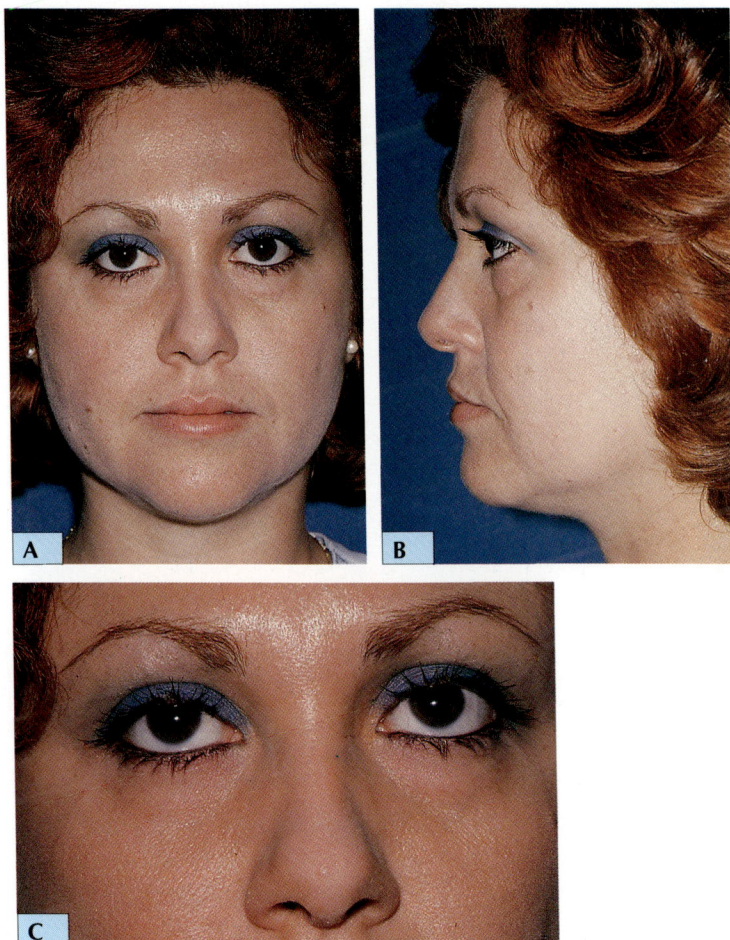

FIGURE 31.24 (A–C) Preoperative photographs of a 34-year-old woman who presented with laxity of the orbital septum and protrusion of the medial, central, and lateral fat pads.

elective rhytidectomy and upper and lower eyelid blepharoplasty. Physical examination showed upper eyelid hooding associated with excessive skin laxity. The lower eyelids exhibited a lack of tone and fine rhytids (Figure 31.26A–C). Postoperative photographs illustrate the result (Figure 31.27 A–E).

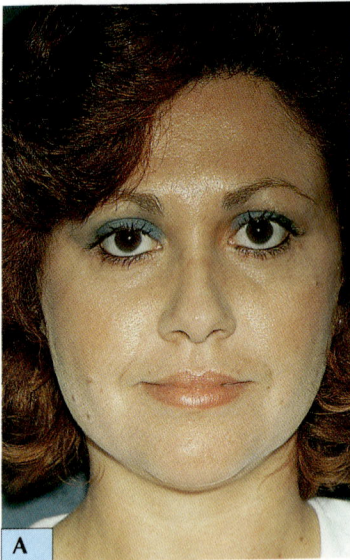

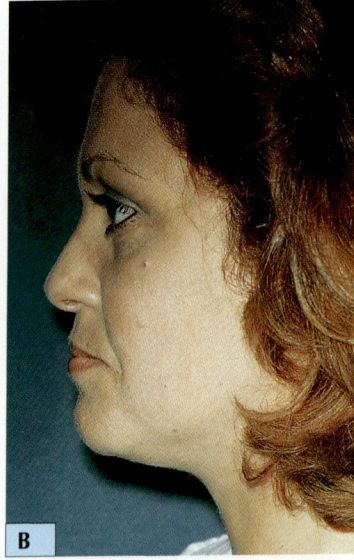

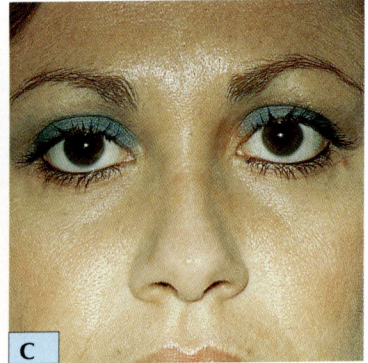

FIGURE 31.25 (A–C) Postoperative photographs illustrate the result following lower eyelid blepharoplasty.

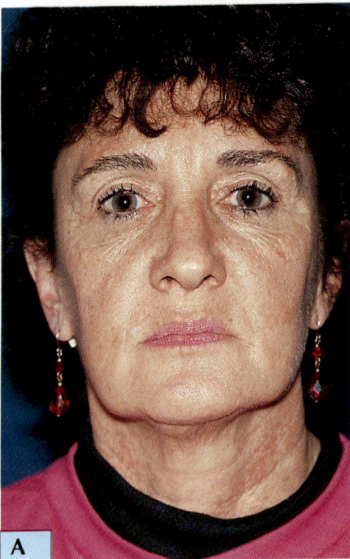

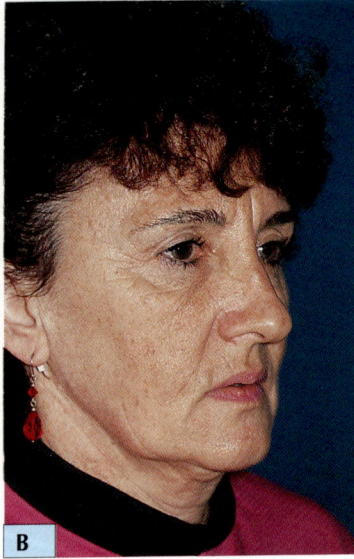

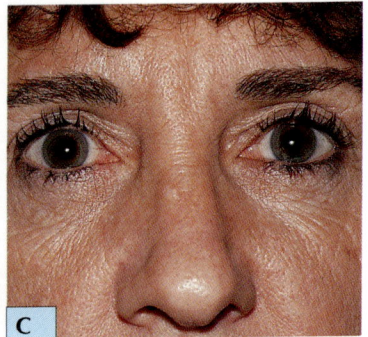

FIGURE 31.26 (A–C) Preoperative photographs of a 58-year-old woman who presented for upper and lower eyelid blepharoplasty associated with facelift.

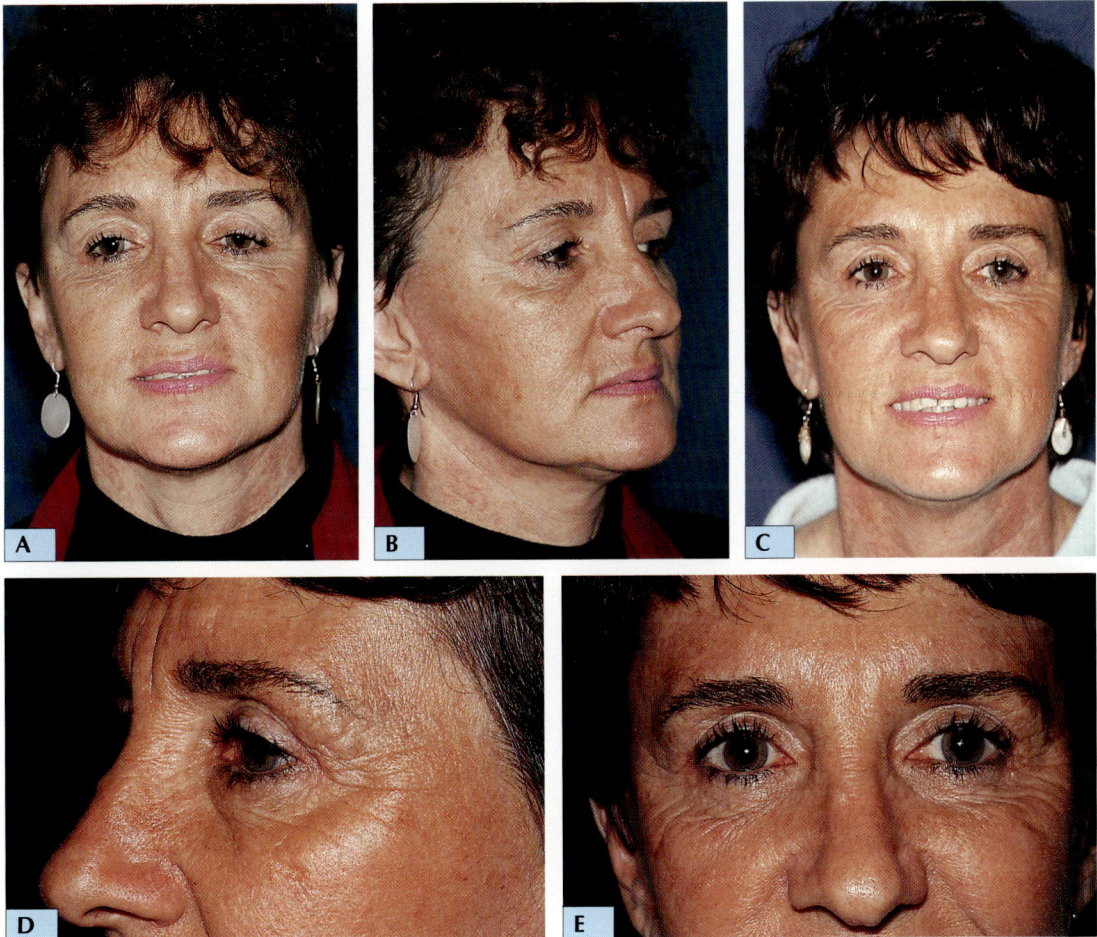

FIGURE 31.27 (A–E) Postoperative photographs illustrate the result at 1 year.

SUGGESTIONS FOR FURTHER READING

Beekhuis GJ. Blepharoplasty. Otolaryngol Clin North Am. Symposium on the Aging Face. 1980;13(2):225-236.

Holt JE, Holt GR. Blepharoplasty: indications in preoperative assessment. Arch Otolaryngol Head Neck Surg. 1985;111:394-397.

Hugo N. Anatomy of blepharoplasty. Plast Reconstr Surg. 1984;53:381-383.

Rees TD. Aesthetic Plastic Surgery. Philadelphia, Pa: WB Saunders Co;1980:459-525.

Wolfley DE. Blepharoplasty, the ophthalmologist's view. Otolaryngol Clin North Am. Symposium on the Aging Face. 1980;13(2):237-263.

chapter 32

LIP RECONSTRUCTION

The upper and lower lips are the most common site of origin for squamous cell carcinoma of the oral cavity. The lips represent the anterior boundary of the oral pharynx and additionally function dynamically in speech, facial expression, and deglutition. This combination of functional requirements makes the aesthetic reconstruction of lip defects challenging for the reconstructive surgeon.

ANATOMY

The orbicularis oris is a circular muscle extending circumferentially around the lips. Its function is to contract the lips in deglutition and speech and to provide muscular tone for the maintenance of oral competence. The orbicularis oris and buccinator muscles form a continuous functional ring with the pharyngeal constrictors. Disruption in the continuity of any of the elements of this ring results in decreased oral compression and competence (Figure 32.1). Additionally, it is important to recognize that the muscles of the midface including the zygomaticus major and minor, the depressor anguli oris, and the depressor labii inferioris attach to the orbicularis oris muscle and to the perioral skin, thereby regulating the function and position of the lips and oral commissure.

Motor nerve innervation of the lips is primarily from the buccal and marginal mandibular divisions of the facial nerve. The infraorbital and mental branches of the trigeminal nerve constitute the primary sensory innervation. The blood supply is from branches of the facial artery and from the superior and inferior labial arteries. Venous drainage of the area is from the facial vein; lymphatic drainage is through the submental and submaxillary lymph nodes (Figure 32.2).

PRINCIPLES OF RECONSTRUCTION

The primary goals of lip reconstruction include the preservation of sensation, the maintenance of oral competence, vermilion border continuity, sufficient oral access, adequate lip cosmesis, and when possible the convenience of a one-stage reconstructive procedure. Techniques of lip reconstruction should provide for reconstruction in three layers: skin, muscle, and mucosa. The gingivolabial sulcus should be maintained where possible, as it is important in normal lip function and movement as well as to those patients who wear dentures. Other important considerations include the establishment of lip symmetry, commissure competence, preservation of the philtrum, and adequate tissue match in terms of color and texture.

As a general rule, split-thickness skin grafts are to be avoided in the labial area as contracture of the graft tends to displace the vermilion border. Similarly, the mobility of the area makes full-thickness skin grafting unreliable.

PREOPERATIVE CONSIDERATIONS

When possible, a preoperative consultation with the patient undergoing lip resection is important so that proper understanding is achieved regarding the limitations of the reconstructive component of the treatment. The potential for disruption of oral compe-

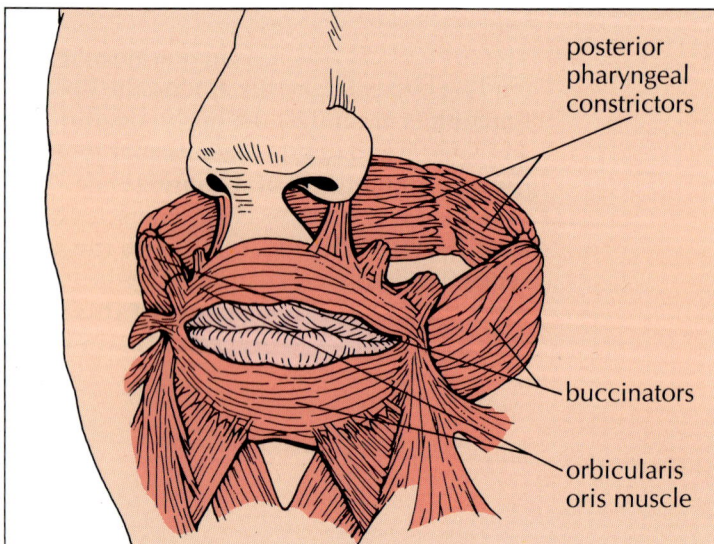

FIGURE 32.1 The oral commissure is suspended by the orbicularis oris anterior muscle in continuity with the buccinators and the posterior pharyngeal constrictors. Disruption in the continuity of this ring can lead to oral incompetence.

posterior pharyngeal constrictors

buccinators

orbicularis oris muscle

tence and tone, loss of lip sensation, and distortion of lip cosmesis all should be topics for discussion between the patient and surgeon before removal of the lesion. In addition, careful instruction to the patient as to the potential for extensive lip soft-tissue and muscular defects in the process of tumor removal must be given.

As a general rule, full-thickness lip reconstructions are performed under general anesthesia utilizing endonasal intubation in an inpatient setting. For cutaneous and mucosal reconstructions, surgery is normally performed in an outpatient setting with the patient placed under local anesthesia.

STRATEGY OF RECONSTRUCTION

Skin defects of the upper lip must take into account that the nasal alar base, as well as the oral commissure, must not be distorted by the reconstruction. The technique we use for defects of the lateral third of the upper lip is the perialar crescent advancement flap. This flap relies on the principle that in most individuals excessive soft-tissue and skin can be found in the midfacial cheek area. By mobilization of the subcutaneous tissue and skin and careful direction of the tension horizontally, few of the important structures in the

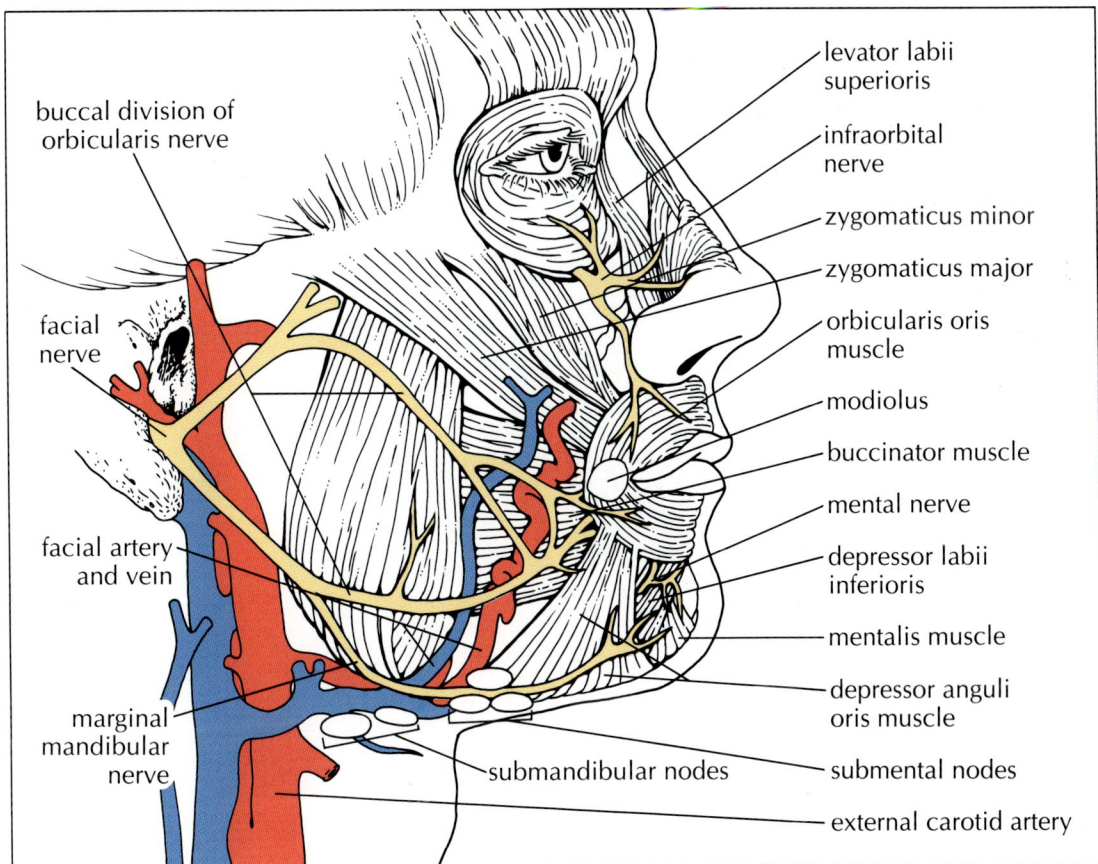

FIGURE 32.2 Muscular, vascular, and neural anatomy of the lips.

midfacial region are distorted, ie, the nasal base and vermilion border are not displaced superiorly. The blood supply to this flap is based on random perforators from the facial artery and vein.

Potential pitfalls in the design and execution of the perialar crescent advancement flap include overambitious closure with associated distortion of the nasal base and alar area and/or downward displacement of the lower eyelid (iatrogenic ectropion). In each case in which this flap is utilized, the primary concern is avoidance of distortion of the vermilion border of the lip (Figure 32.3A–D). This anatomic landmark can be maintained by meticulous attention to wound closure with the surgeon insisting on horizontally directed wound tension (see Figure 32.3C).

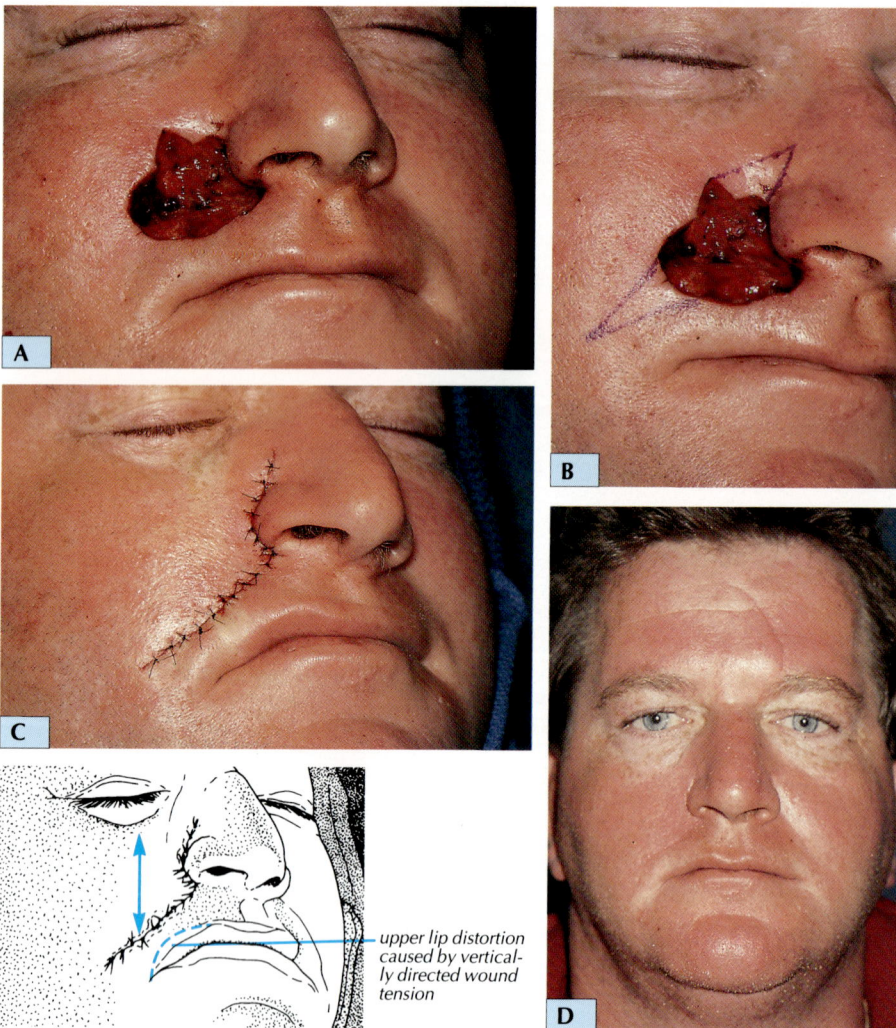

upper lip distortion caused by vertically directed wound tension

FIGURE 32.3 (A) Patient following Mohs' excision of a basal cell carcinoma of the upper lip. **(B)** A perialar crescent advancement flap is designed with the superior limb along the nasal base and the inferior limb extending into the nasolabial crease. **(C)** Closure uses 3-0 PDS subcutaneously and 5-0 nylon externally. Wide undermining using Metzenbaum scissors is necessary to avoid distortion of the upper lip vermilion border and nasal base. **(D)** Result at 6 months.

In addition, if the continuity of the orbicularis oris muscle is disrupted by the soft-tissue defect, the free edges of the muscle must be reapproximated, repaired, and sutured with a long-term absorbable suture, such as 3-0 PDS. With repair of this muscle defect, oral competence is maintained.

Skin defects of the upper lip that lie more medially can be reconstructed using a two-stage nasolabial flap. This flap uses as its donor area the cheek, which normally has adequate tissue reserve to allow for primary donor site closure (Figure 32.4). The flap is raised in a subcutaneous plane, relies on a random cutaneous blood supply, and is best based superiorly for upper lip reconstruction.

The advantages of this flap include the fact that the distortions of ill-directed tension are eliminated, thereby avoiding the potential complication of free-margin distortion. The flap can be an answer to specific defects, in particular those that lie adjacent to or involve the philtrum. Its disadvantages are the obvious need for a two-stage reconstruc-

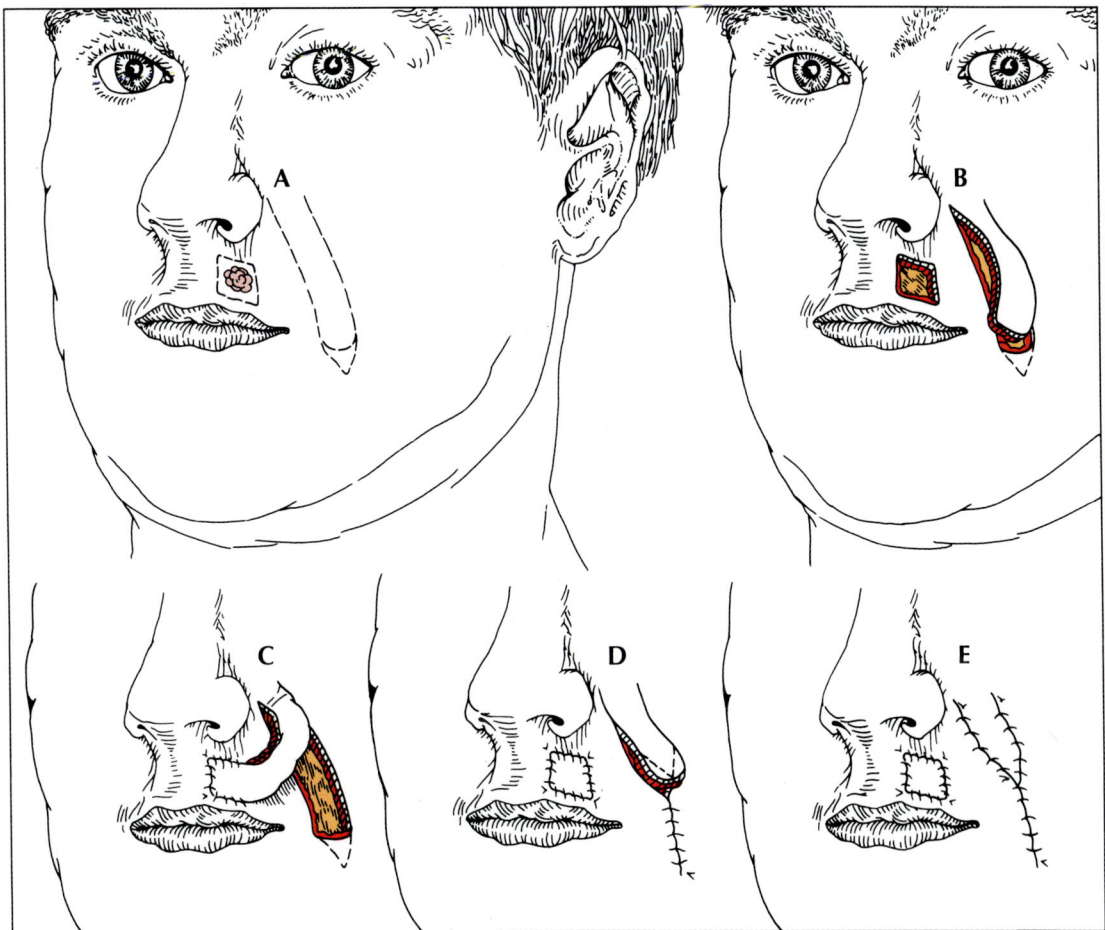

FIGURE 32.4 Schematic drawing illustrating the two-stage nasolabial flap. (A) These flaps can be useful in the reconstruction of sizeable cutaneous defects of the central upper lip. (B) The donor skin is harvested from the cheek and is centered over the nasolabial crease. (C) The flap is transposed medially and sutured into position to close the defect. The donor site is closed primarily. (D) The flap is maintained for 14 days and is then released. (E) The proximal portion of the flap can then be returned to the cheek or discarded, depending on the amount of distortion created by the donor site closure.

tive procedure and the unpredictable nature of the blood supply to the transferred tissue. Particular caution should be taken in patients who are heavy cigarette smokers, as the reliability of the flap is compromised in such patients.

Full-thickness defects of the upper and lower lip are managed according to the percentage of lip involved in tumor resection. Defects measuring less than one third of the lip can be closed primarily, utilizing a three-layer closure that carefully aligns muscular, cutaneous, and mucosal layers. When possible, primary closure should be performed as it provides the best results in terms of function and cosmesis (Figure 32.5A–D). Functionally, it reestablishes the continuity of the oral sphincter and the orbicularis oris muscle and cosmetically it reconstitutes the vermilion border and lip mucosa. In addition, full return of lip sensation and movement can be expected in most cases.

Defects measuring one third to two thirds of the upper or lower lip can be closed with an Abbe flap, a Gillies fan flap, or a Karapandzic flap. Abbe flaps can be used when the defect involves the medial portion of the upper or lower lip and includes a portion of lip that is approximately one half the size of the surgical defect. The lower lip is normally lax and can donate up to one quarter of its length for reconstruction. The great advantage of the Abbe flap is that it provides immediate replacement of normal lip muscu-

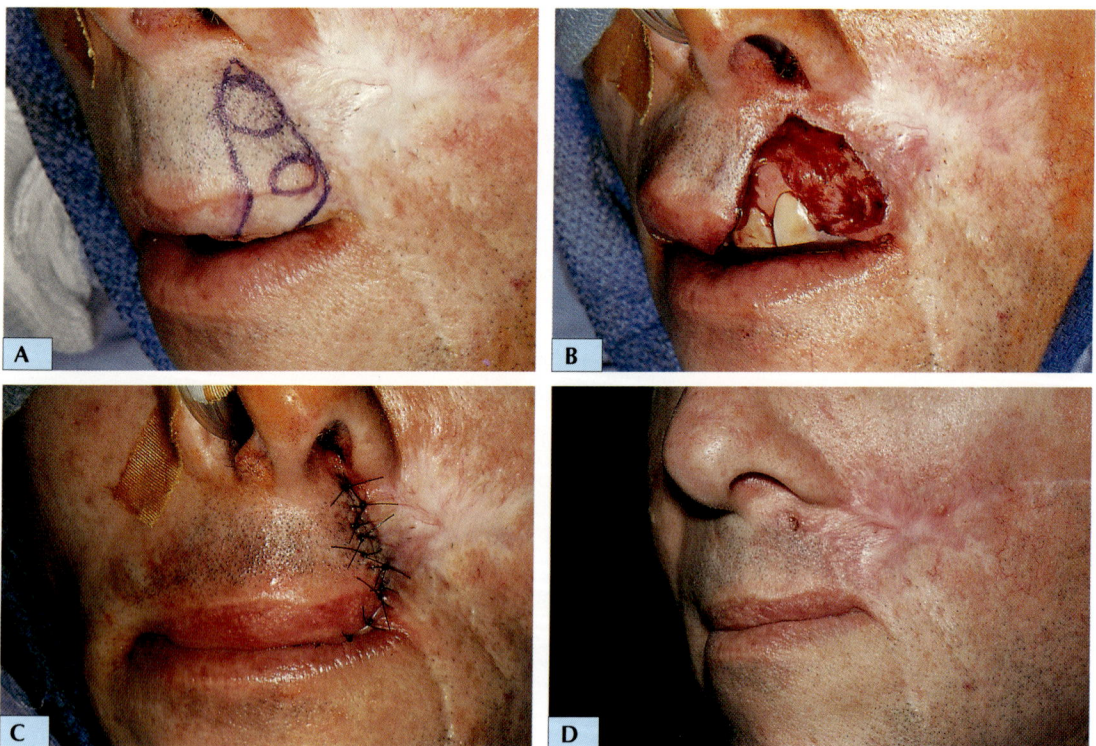

FIGURE 32.5 (A) A 36-year-old man with recurrent basal cell carcinoma of the upper lip and oral commissure presents with two satellite recurrent lesions of the upper lip. Full-thickness wedge excision is performed with an inset designed at the vermilion border to ensure adequate vermilion-to-vermilion contact. **(B)** Full-thickness defect of the upper lip measuring 3.5 cm at the lip margin. **(C)** Appearance immediately following careful three-layer closure of the mucosa, the orbicularis oris muscle, and lip skin. **(D)** Result at 3 months.

lature, skin, and mucosa. In addition to this, the flap incorporates a reliable blood supply based on the labial artery and therefore can be used in clinical situations in which the recipient-site defect is compromised. Its disadvantage lies in the challenge of proper flap design and execution as well as in its two-stage requirement.

The first stage involves proper orientation and design of the flap, with capturing of the arterial supply from the labial artery. This is followed by a 10- to 14-day period during which the transferred tissue reestablishes local vascularization. At the end of this period, the vascular pedicle undergoes a tourniquet test in which a rubber band is placed around the vascular pedicle for 5 minutes,

constricting the labial artery and indicating whether adequate neovascularization has occurred. If the tissue maintains its perfusion the second stage of reconstruction is performed, including amputation of the vascular pedicle and soft-tissue tailoring to reestablish vermilion continuity (Figure 32.6A–D).

The Gillies fan flap was developed to reconstruct shallow, rectangular defects of the lower lip that involve more than one half of the lip. A fan-shaped flap is designed from the contralateral lip and cheek and relies on the labial vessels for its blood supply. The primary problems encountered with this flap include obligatory microstomia, reduced sensation of the lower lip, and in many cases a poor match of mucosal height when the wide

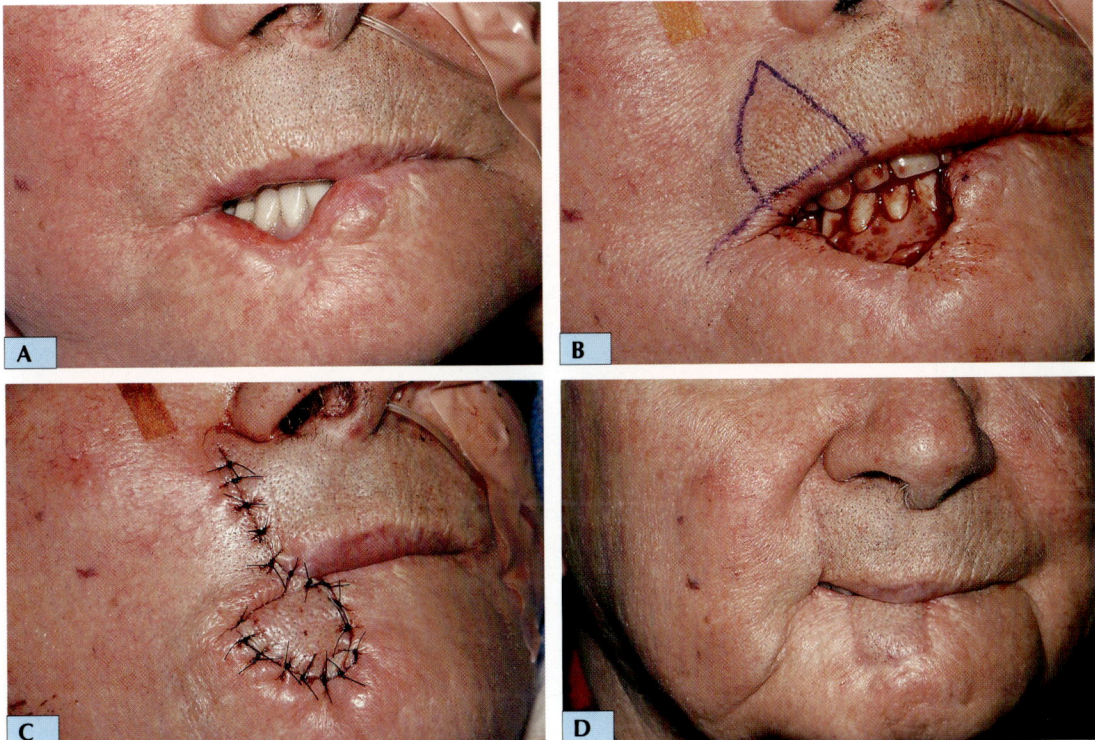

FIGURE 32.6 (A) Patient with full-thickness oral defect following primary excision and radiation therapy for squamous cell carcinoma of the lower lip. Primary complaints included drooling, poorly fitting dentures, and cosmetic defect. **(B)** An Abbe flap is designed after the cutaneous edges of the defect are excised. The flap is based on the labial artery. **(C)** The Abbe flap is transferred and suture stabilized into the lower lip. **(D)** Result at 6 months, with restoration of oral continuity.

central lip mucosa is lateralized to abut the narrower mucosa in the region of the oral commissure (Figure 32.7A–E). The secondary defect in the cheek can be adequately closed relying on the normal laxity of the cheek skin.

Recently, the Karapandzic neurovascular fan flap has become a popular option for reconstruction of full-thickness defects that lie in the one-third to two-thirds range of the lip (Figures 32.8A–H and 32.9A–C). The principle of this flap involves the movement of adjacent lip and cheek flaps to reconstruct

the defect. The adjacent lip flaps are designed to be of equal height to the lip defect to be reconstructed, thereby ensuring that adequate height of the reconstructed lip is maintained.

An additional design advantage to this flap is its incorporation of a neurovascular pedicle bilaterally from the cheeks, so that a reliable blood supply is captured and orbicularis oris muscle function is maintained. In addition, lower lip sensation is preserved in those cases in which the mental nerves are not affected by the disease process. The naso-

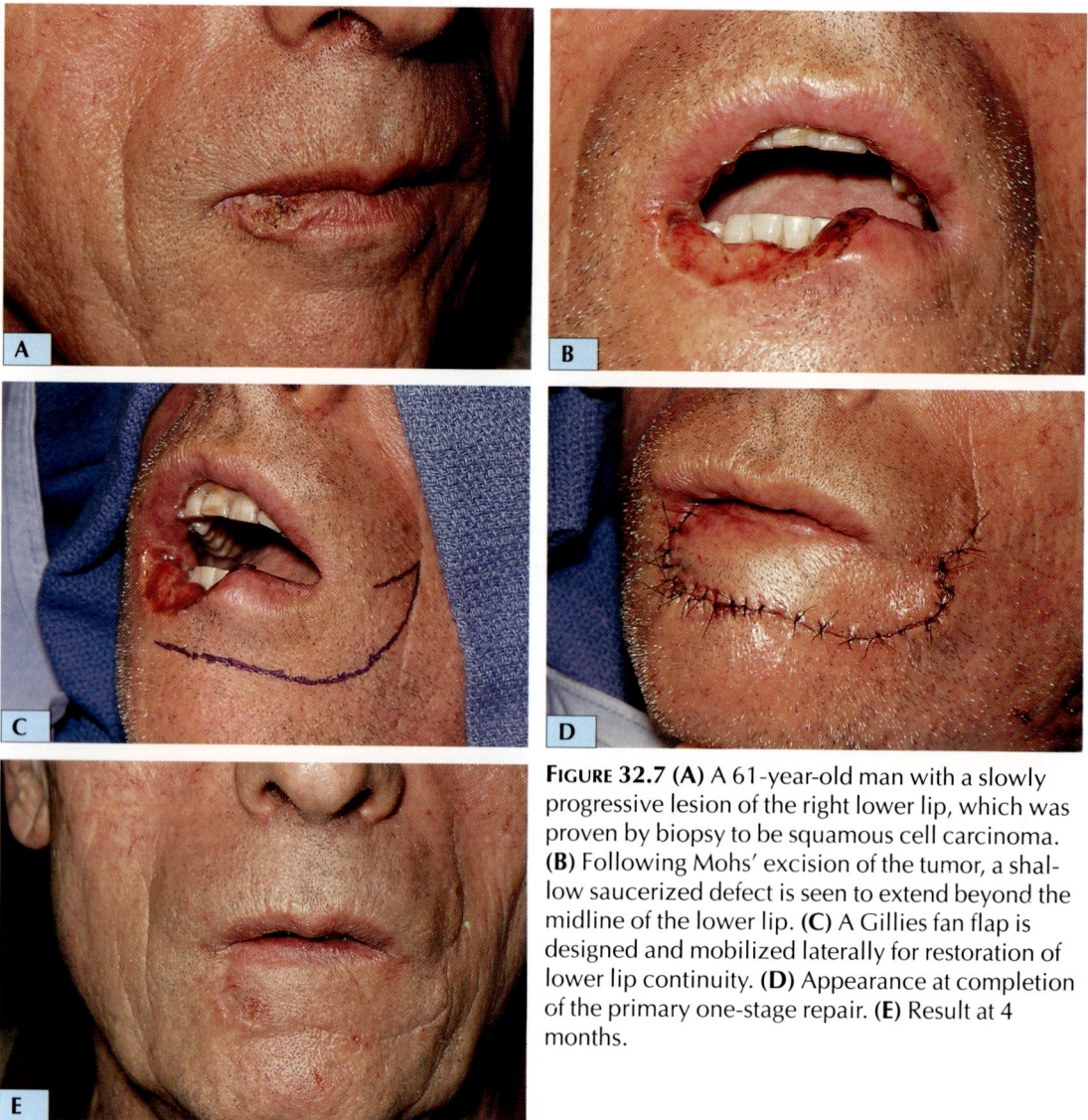

FIGURE 32.7 (A) A 61-year-old man with a slowly progressive lesion of the right lower lip, which was proven by biopsy to be squamous cell carcinoma. **(B)** Following Mohs' excision of the tumor, a shallow saucerized defect is seen to extend beyond the midline of the lower lip. **(C)** A Gillies fan flap is designed and mobilized laterally for restoration of lower lip continuity. **(D)** Appearance at completion of the primary one-stage repair. **(E)** Result at 4 months.

labial grooves are used laterally to camouflage the incisions utilized for tissue advancement. The primary disadvantage to the Karapandzic flap is the unavoidable occurrence of microstomia, which results in a relative dis-

crepancy between the upper and lower lips as seen in profile. In some cases, microstomia can be severe enough to require a secondary commissurotomy.

Total full-thickness reconstruction of

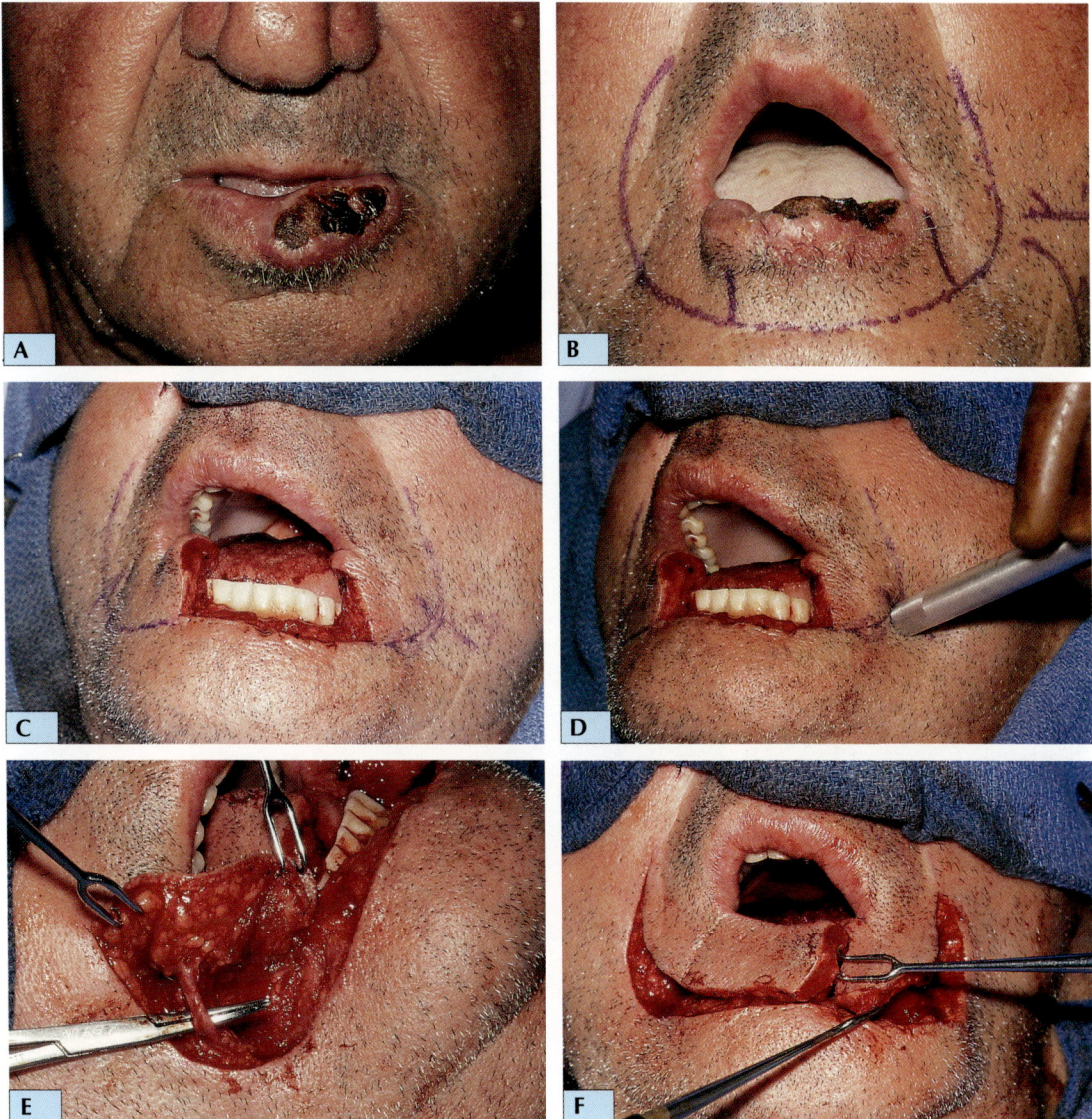

FIGURE 32.8 (A) A 71-year-old man with a fungating lesion of the lower lip, proven by biopsy to be squamous cell carcinoma. **(B)** A Karapandzic neurovascular fan flap is designed with consideration given to the neurovascular supply that enters from the lateral cheek. The superior extent of the flap approximates the nasolabial grooves. **(C)** Excision

of the primary tumor with the resultant defect measuring 4.5 x 4.0 cm. **(D)** Doppler ultrasonography is performed to identify the vascular supply. **(E)** The neurovascular pedicle is isolated and preserved. **(F)** Bilateral flaps of orbicularis oris, lip mucosa, and skin are mobilized to restore lip continuity.

(continued on next page)

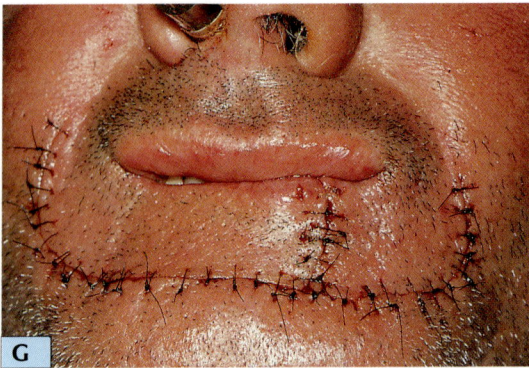

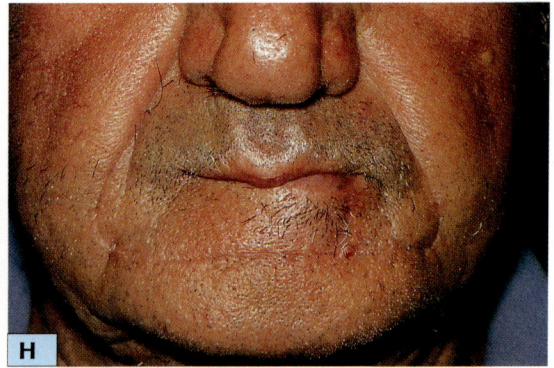

FIGURE 32.8 (G) Appearance at the time of immediate three-layer closure with careful attention given to reapproximation of the mucosa, the orbicularis oris muscle, and the external lip skin. **(H)** Appearance at 4 months, with preservation of motor and sensory function.

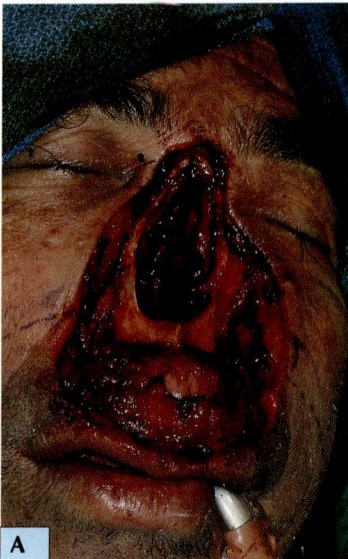

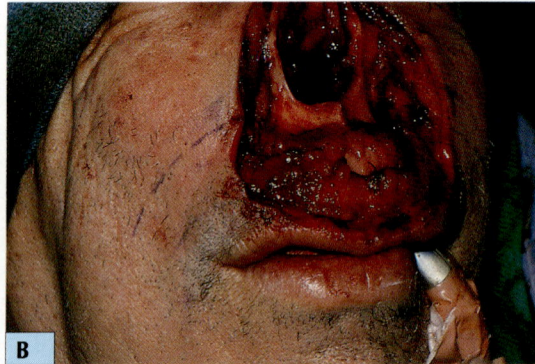

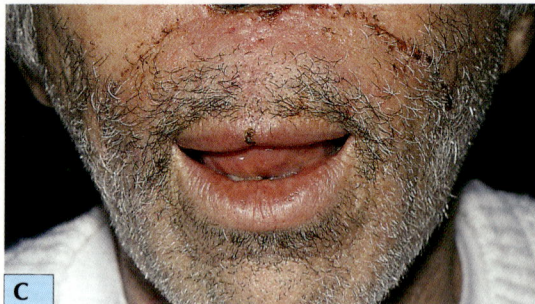

FIGURE 32.9 (A) Patient with surgical defect following resection of a recurrent squamous cell carcinoma of the upper lip and nose. **(B)** The upper lip was reconstructed using a reverse Karapandzic flap, which by design is a mirror image of the traditional Karapandzic flap. Its main advantage is utilization of the nasolabial groove with bilateral advancement flaps and preservation of sensation and motor function. **(C)** Result at 4 weeks. The primary disadvantage of this flap is obligatory microstomia.

the lip represents a difficult problem with no easy solution. Traditional techniques for reconstruction have included the bilateral fan flap and the Webster cheek advancement flap, both of which result in a lack of tissue in the lower lip and a relatively bulky upper lip. In addition, both of these techniques result in a deficit in sensation and in reduced functional capacity of the oral sphincter.

Our preferred method for total lip reconstruction utilizes an extended nasolabial myocutaneous flap, incorporating anterior tongue mucosa for vermilion border and mucosal reconstruction. The nasolabial myocutaneous flap is designed so that the width of the flap fulfills the vertical height require-ments of the lip defect. Additional design features require that the facial artery be included in the flap, which is ensured by Doppler location of the artery prior to tissue mobilization. The flap is based inferiorly and is raised in a plane so that facial muscles, facial artery, and facial skin all are components of the tissue to be transferred. The flap is then rotated 90° with the requirement that a 2- to 3-cm section at the base of the flap be de-epithelized so that complete tissue transfer can be accomplished (Figure 32.10A–D).

Commissure defects must be reconstructed to avoid the long-term complications of secondary wound contracture, lip asymmetry, oral incompetence, and drooling. Many

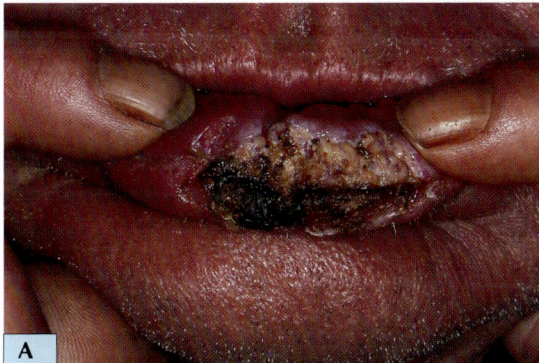

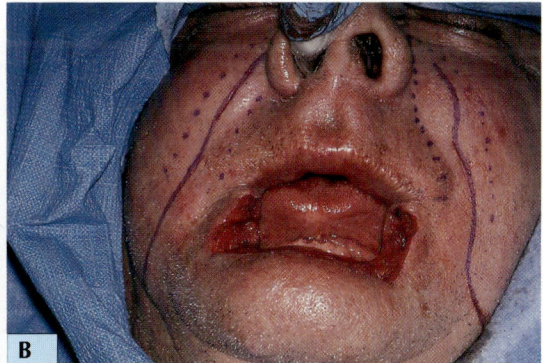

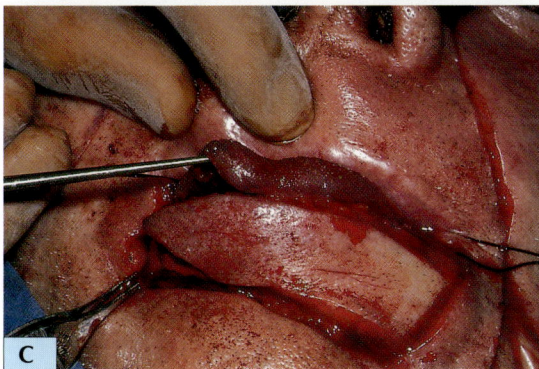

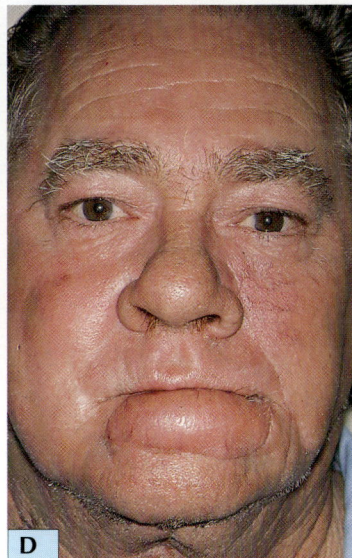

FIGURE 32.10 (A) Patient with a lesion of the lower lip that required total lower lip excision. (B) Surgical defect with the design of a large nasolabial flap for primary reconstruction. (C) The flap is transposed, with an anterior tongue flap used to reconstruct the lower lip mucosa. The tongue flap is released at 2 weeks. (D) Result at 6 months.

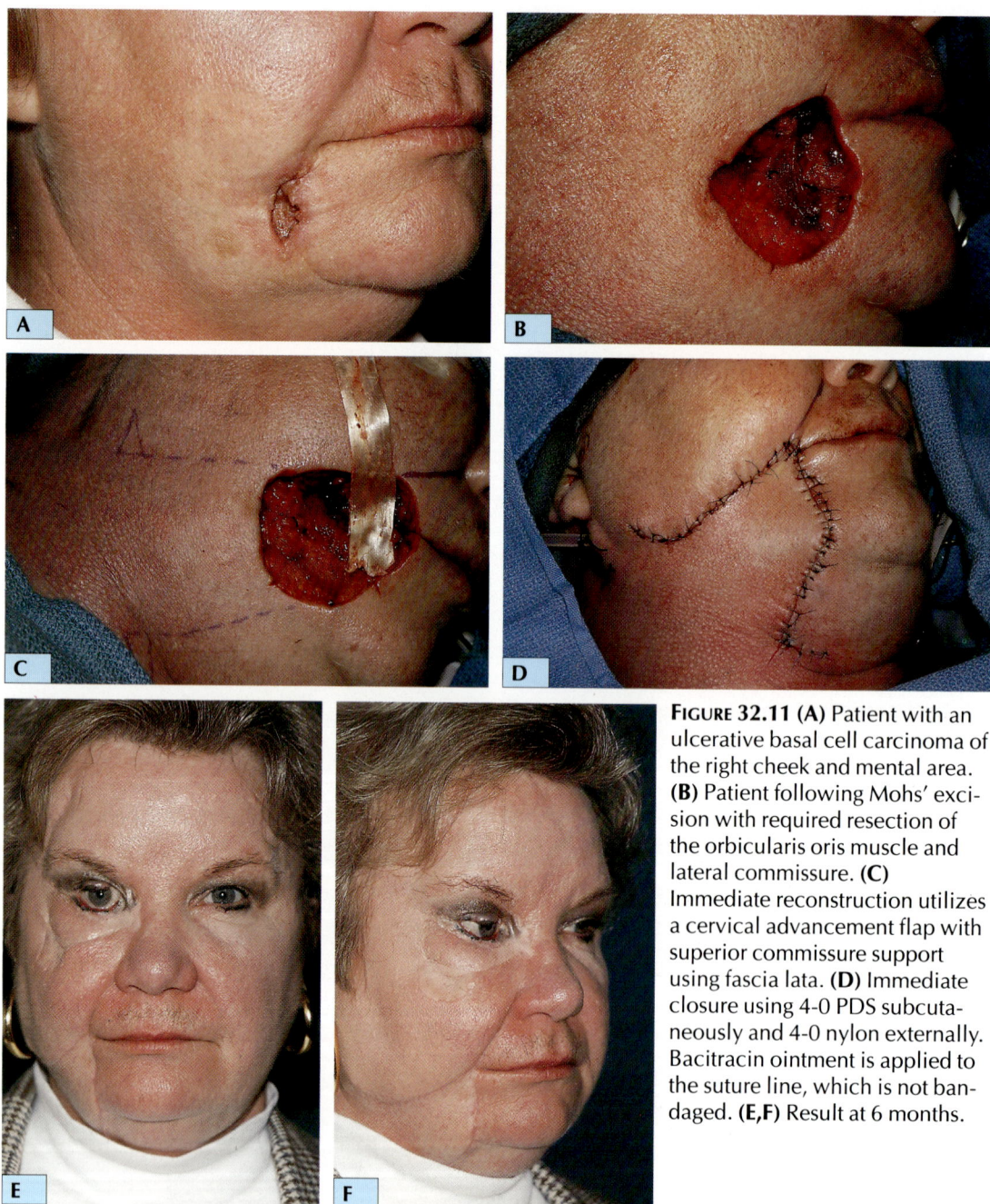

FIGURE 32.11 (A) Patient with an ulcerative basal cell carcinoma of the right cheek and mental area. **(B)** Patient following Mohs' excision with required resection of the orbicularis oris muscle and lateral commissure. **(C)** Immediate reconstruction utilizes a cervical advancement flap with superior commissure support using fascia lata. **(D)** Immediate closure using 4-0 PDS subcutaneously and 4-0 nylon externally. Bacitracin ointment is applied to the suture line, which is not bandaged. **(E,F)** Result at 6 months.

techniques have been utilized for correction of this problem, including double rhomboid flaps and Mustardé cervical rotation flaps. We have found the greatest success utilizing a direct cervical advancement flap in which the width-to-length ratio can be increased if the facial artery and vein are captured within the flap design. An additional advantage to this flap is that its superior limb can be designed to mimic the nasolabial crease.

In cases where extensive loss of the orbicularis oris muscle is encountered in the region of the commissure, superior support may be necessary through the use of autogenous fascia lata suspended from the zygomatic facial region to the orbicularis oris muscle (Figure 32.11A–F).

POSTOPERATIVE CARE

Postoperatively, general rules can be applied to patients who undergo major local tissue transfer for lip reconstruction. Occlusive dressings are to be avoided so that the flaps can be carefully monitored for early evidence of ischemia. Patients also are instructed as to the strict avoidance of cigarette smoking, which has been shown to induce ischemic tissue changes. Local antibiotic ointments are used during the first postoperative week and patients are placed on a soft diet and instructed to limit oral communication and excessive oral movement. These measures are designed to ensure that adequate time has elapsed to allow for orbicularis oris muscle, mucosal, and cutaneous healing.

SUGGESTIONS FOR FURTHER READING

Jackson I. Local Flaps in Head and Neck Reconstruction. St Louis, Mo: C V Mosby Co; 1985.

McGregor I. Reconstruction of the lower lip. Br J Plast Surg. 1983;30:40-47.

Meyer R. New concepts in lower lip reconstruction. Head Neck Surg. 1982;4:240-245.

Renner GJ. Reconstruction of the lip. Otolaryngol Clin North Am. 1990;23:975-990.

Renner GJ: Carcinoma of the lip. In: Gates GA, ed. Current Therapy in Otolaryngologic Head and Neck Surgery. 4th ed. Philadelphia, Pa: BC Decker Inc;1990.

Schater ME. Lip surgery. Clin Plast Surg. 1984;11:569-790.

Wilson J. Reconstruction of the lower lip. Head Neck Surg. 1981;4:29-44.

Yarington CT. Reconstruction following lip resection. Otolaryngol Clin North Am. 1983;16:407-421.

chapter 33

AURICULAR RECONSTRUCTION

Acquired auricular deformities present the surgeon with a wide variety of reconstructive challenges. Although most such deformities occur as a result of skin cancers and are almost always partial defects, accurate reconstruction is nevertheless a challenge due to the delicacy of the ear and the complexity of its convolutions and depressions. The goals of auricular reconstruction are to produce a normal-appearing and normal-feeling ear, which is symmetrical to the contralateral ear and in proper relationship to the periauricular skin and scalp. These goals must be met while also trying to preserve the postauricular sulcus.

The anatomy of the auricle and its three-dimensional detail are important factors in the planning of the reconstruction. The normal auricle is composed of lateral and medial cutaneous surfaces and a central cartilaginous framework. The conchal bowl, antihelix, and antitragus represent the most medial units of the cartilage complex and the helix and the lobule make up the lateral structures (Figure 33.1).

Adding to the challenge of auricular reconstruction is the ear's limited and inconsistent vascularity. Posteriorly, the arterial supply to the auricle is from the postauricular artery (a division of the external carotid artery) and anteriorly from branches of the superficial temporal artery. Venous drainage occurs via the postauricular vein into the external jugular system and also by way of the superficial temporal and retromandibular veins. The auricle is innervated by the great auricular nerve (C2-C3), the auriculotemporal nerve (V3), and the lesser occipital nerve (Figure 33.2).

SURGICAL TREATMENT OF ACQUIRED AURICULAR DEFECTS

PREOPERATIVE PLANNING

A number of factors must be considered in the preoperative planning that occurs prior to reconstruction of the defect. As auricular cartilage is very supple, contractile forces may distort the ear if attention is not paid to pri-mary closure. The tension on local tissue also must be considered. Because the vascularity of the ear is limited, great care must be taken to avoid the creation of scars or the utilization of contracted or scarred local auricular or periauricular skin, which has a limited potential for three-dimensional expansion. Essential scars on or behind the reconstructed ear are acceptable, whereas scars in the preauricular area or on the lateral surface of the auricle should be minimized.

Hair-bearing scalp, which is in close proximity to the auricle, often must be factored into the reconstructive plan so that hair-bearing skin is not used in the definitive reconstruction. A thorough understanding of average auricular dimensions and proportions also is important in planning the reconstruction, although the most important element is utilization of the patient's contralateral auricle as a template for the size and anatomic detail necessary for accurate reconstruction of the defect (Figure 33.3).

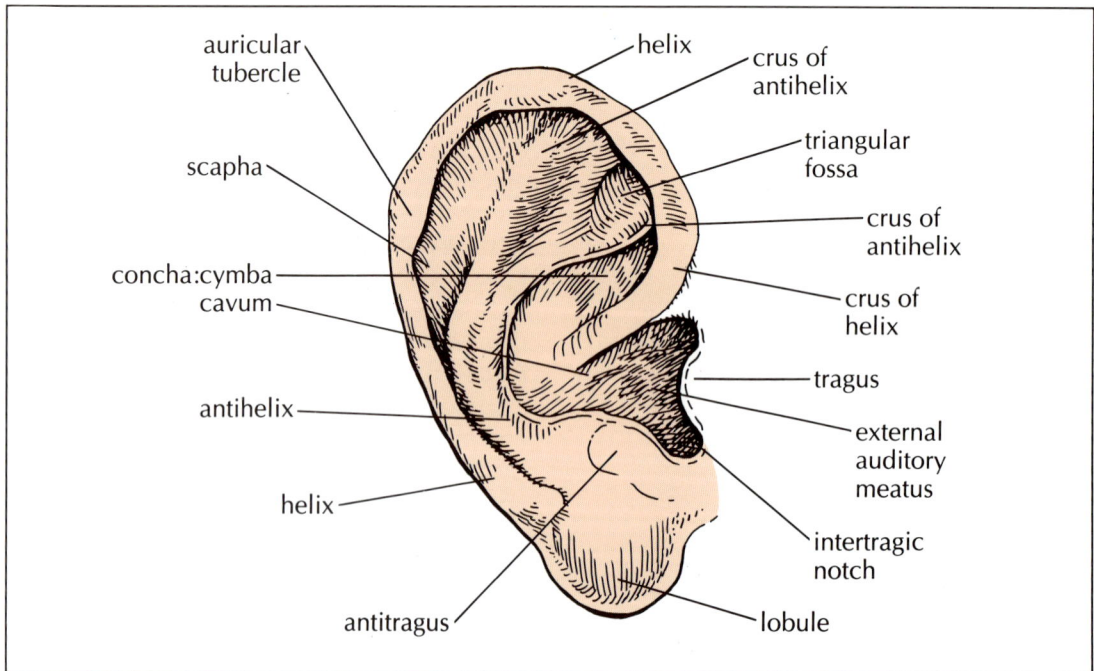

FIGURE 33.1 Schematic drawing showing the basic anatomy of the auricle.

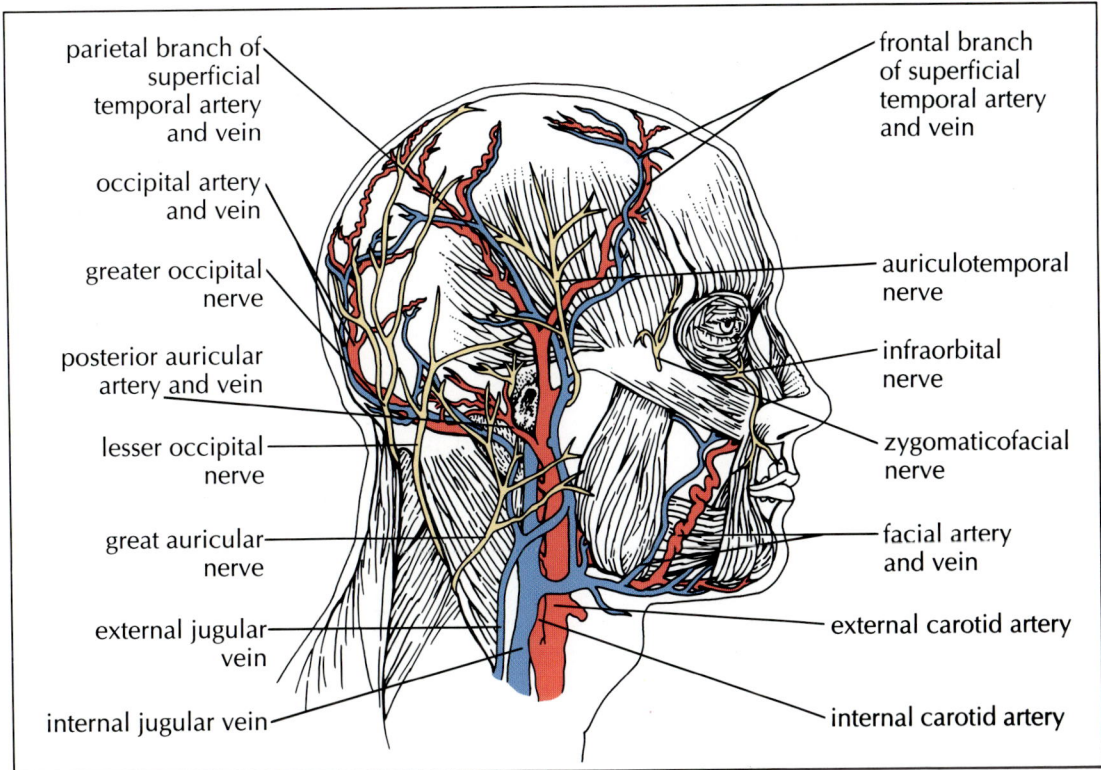

FIGURE 33.2 Schematic drawing showing the vascular and neural anatomy of the auricular and facial region.

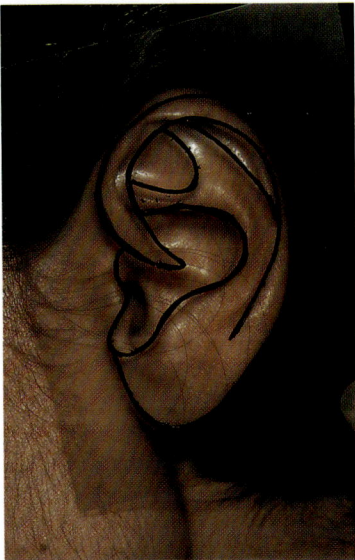

FIGURE 33.3 Accurate auricular reconstruction is dependent on a detailed x-ray template pattern, which is drawn from the contralateral ear and is used in the sculpting of autogenous costal cartilage.

PATIENT PREPARATION

The most important aspect of patient preparation prior to reconstruction of an auricular defect is clarification for the patient of the limitations of the reconstruction and the anticipated time frame for results. Specifically, the patient must be informed that a delay of at least 2 to 6 months can be expected, due to persistent postsurgical edema and pro-longed loss of definition of the detailed auricular convolutions. A complete review of the surgical plan should be undertaken, as well as the preparation of accurate templates in those cases in which they are needed.

Minor local flaps can be performed in an outpatient setting under local anesthesia whereas larger defects requiring major tissue mobilization are performed under general

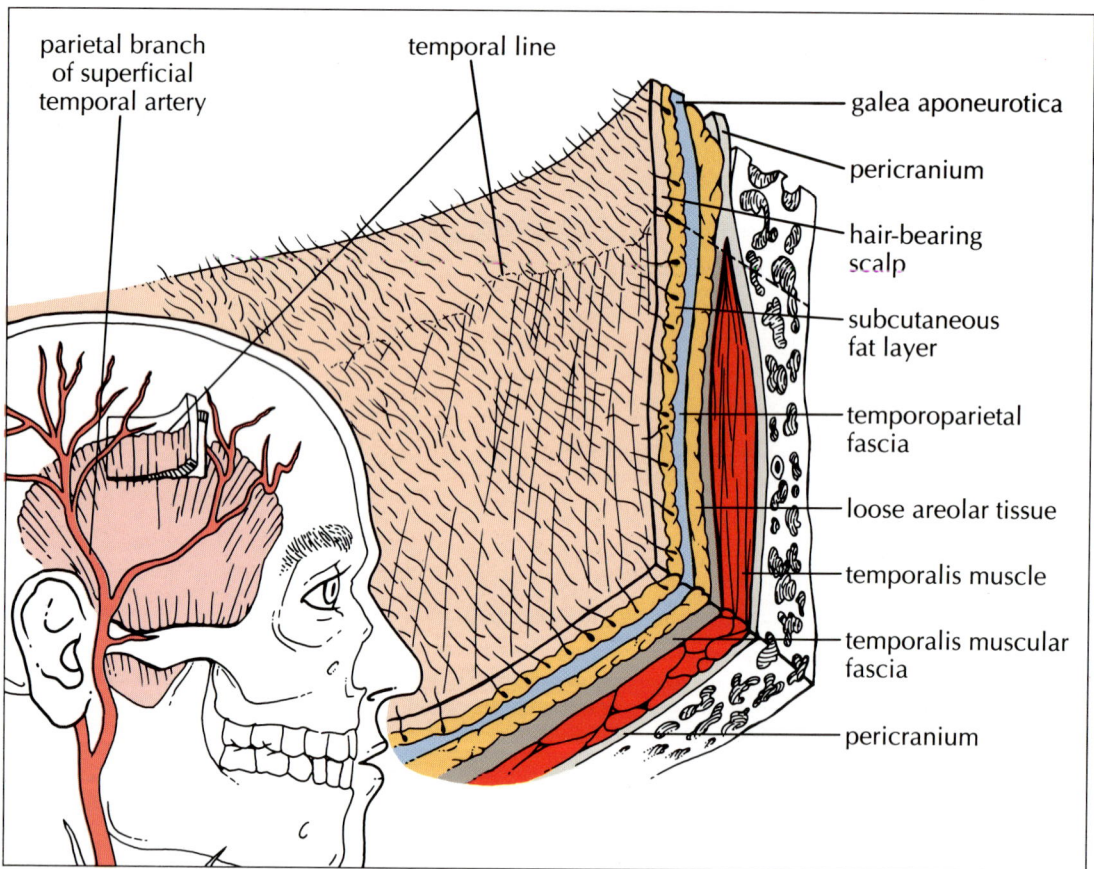

FIGURE 33.4 Schematic drawing showing the five-layer composition of the temporoparietal region. The temporoparietal fascia lies in a central position between two pairs of tissue layers below the temporal line. The temporoparietal fascia becomes the galea aponeurotica superior to the temporal line. Lateral tissue planes include subcutaneous fat and hair-bearing scalp. Medial tissue planes consist of loose areolar tissue and temporalis muscular fascia. The temporalis muscle itself is enveloped by the temporalis muscular fascia and the pericranium below the temporal line. These two layers converge at the temporal line to become the pericranium overlying the calvarium.

anesthesia. The use of suction drains also necessitates the use of general anesthesia, with hospitalization overnight.

FLAP REPAIR

The soft-tissue transfer options in auricular reconstruction are varied and appropriate selection depends on the specific auricular defect with which the surgeon is faced. Because of the wide range of potential defects encountered, many methods have been utilized, including helical advancement flaps, simple advancement flaps, and two-stage reconstruction utilizing postauricular skin in addition to free-tissue transfer. Auricular defects can be categorized as full-thickness defects, skin-coverage defects, partial defects, and defects of the upper, middle, or lower third of the auricle. The reconstructive options of each can be systematized based on the particular skin flap utilized.

TEMPOROPARIETAL FASCIAL FLAP

Ideally, the coverage for the framework of any auricular reconstruction should be thin, vascular, non–hair-bearing skin that is well matched for color and is available locally. For cutaneous defects measuring greater than one third of the auricle, which are beyond the limits of the available postauricular non–hair-bearing skin, regional flaps must be considered. The temporoparietal fascial flap is ideally suited for coverage of such defects. In addition, the donor site is well hidden in hair-bearing scalp.

The flap is harvested in the temporoparietal scalp region and allows for a quantity of fascial flap tissue in the range of 14 x 12 cm that will readily support a split-thickness skin graft. The flap is highly vascular, has a long vascular pedicle, and is maneuvered easily to a wide range of anatomic locations. Blood supply to the temporoparietal fascia is by way of the superficial temporal artery and vein. The temporal artery branches from the external carotid artery and becomes superficial in the pretragal area.

Anatomically, the temporoparietal area consists of five layers (Figure 33.4). The third layer, the temporoparietal fascia, extends inferiorly as the superficial temporal fascia and continues superiorly as the galea aponeurotica. The temporoparietal fascia should not be confused with the fascial layers surrounding the temporalis muscle itself. The latter passes deep through the zygomatic arch to insert on the coronary process of the mandible while the former attaches to the arch. The temporoparietal fascia, on average, measures 2 to 3 mm in thickness in the parietal area.

Since the scalp has its own abundant vascular network, there is little danger of skin loss or impairment of hair growth in the area if the hair follicles of the scalp are not damaged in the dissection. Nonetheless, care should be taken to dissect the temporoparietal flap in the anatomic plane that respects the hair follicles, which is that just medial to the subcutaneous layer of the scalp.

The deep layer of the dissection is begun in a natural plane between the temporoparietal fascia and the true muscular fascia of the temporalis muscle. Unlike the lateral plane of dissection, the medial plane is a natural ana-

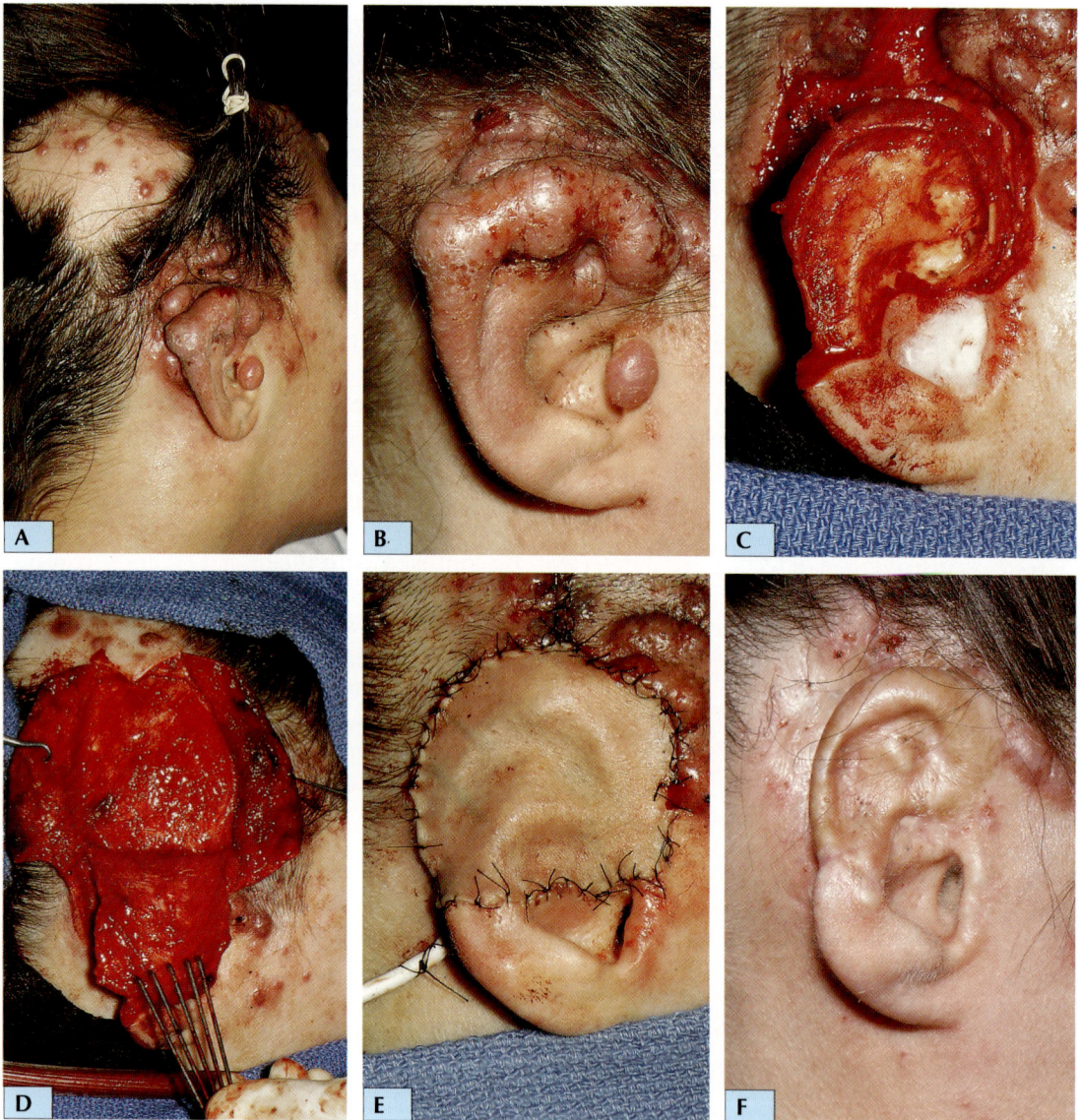

FIGURE 33.5 (A) Patient with angiolymphoid hyperplasia with eosinophilia, a locally aggressive but benign dermal tumor. **(B)** Because of the recurrent infection and cellulitis caused by this tumor, surgical excision was advised. **(C)** The auricular cartilage was not involved and therefore was spared. **(D,E)** Using a temporoparietal fascial flap, the cartilage was covered and a split-thickness skin graft was applied. **(F)** The postoperative result is seen at 1 year.

tomic plane that can be elevated easily. The flap can then be transposed to reach the periauricular area to be reconstructed (Figure 33.5A–F).

POSTAURICULAR MYOCUTANEOUS FLAP

For a full-thickness defect of the auricle, the donor tissue must employ its own vascular supply to ensure reliable tissue transfer. In our experience the postauricular myocutaneous flap, based on the postauricular artery and vein, fulfills this criterion. The flap incorporates the postauricular artery and vein, a postauricular skin paddle, and the postauricular muscle. The flap can be elevated and folded on itself for the reconstruction of full-thickness defects of the middle and upper thirds of the auricle (Figure 33.6A–D).

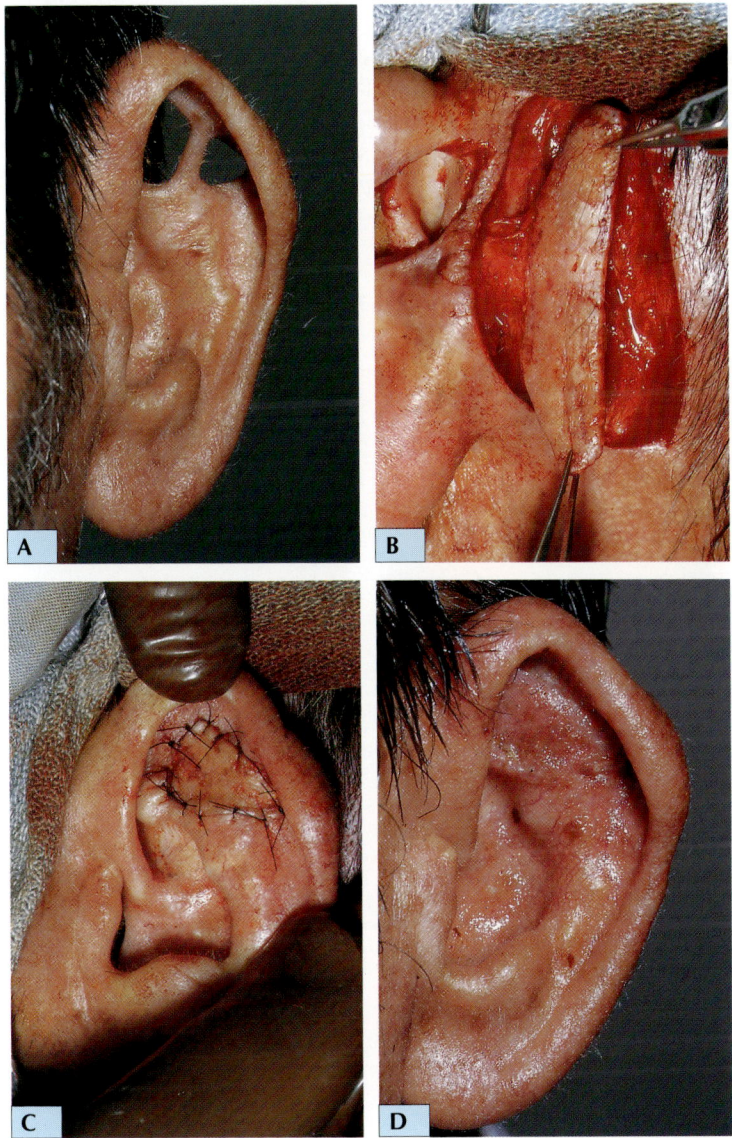

FIGURE 33.6 (A) A 55-year-old man is seen 1 year following full-thickness resection of a basal cell carcinoma of the upper one third of the auricle. (B) A one-stage reconstruction utilizes a postauricular myocutaneous flap based on the postauricular artery, incorporating a postauricular cutaneous paddle and postauricular muscle. (C) Medial and lateral cutaneous repair is performed by folding the myocutaneous paddle on itself and suture stabilizing the flap into position using 4-0 nylon. (D) The result of the repair is seen at 6 weeks.

CLASSIFICATION OF DEFECTS ACCORDING TO LOCATION

As a rule, acquired auricular defects are classified according to their location on or around the ear. Following tumor therapy, the reconstructive plan should be influenced by the nature of the excisional defect and by the presence or absence of an irradiated field.

PREAURICULAR DEFECTS

Preauricular defects following excision of cutaneous tumors, especially basal cell carcinomas, are common. Prior to the time of initial resection and reconstruction, the clinical function of the facial nerve should be determined and well documented, as lesions in this area commonly affect facial nerve func-

tion. Lesions not involving the tragus, conchal bowl, or root of the helix can be reconstructed through the use of simple cheek advancement flaps, with soft-tissue closure designed to emulate the preauricular crease (Figure 33.7A,B). In addition to simple cheek advancement flaps, larger defects in the preauricular area lend themselves to bilateral V-Y advancement flap closure. Advantages to the use of this flap in the preauricular area include an abundant blood supply, single-stage reconstruction, a good cutaneous color match, and continuity of the donor site with the defect that is being reconstructed. The design of the bilateral flap should be as wide as the defect. Of particular advantage is the fact that hair-bearing scalp may be appropriately mobilized to produce a satisfactory result (Figure 33.8A–D).

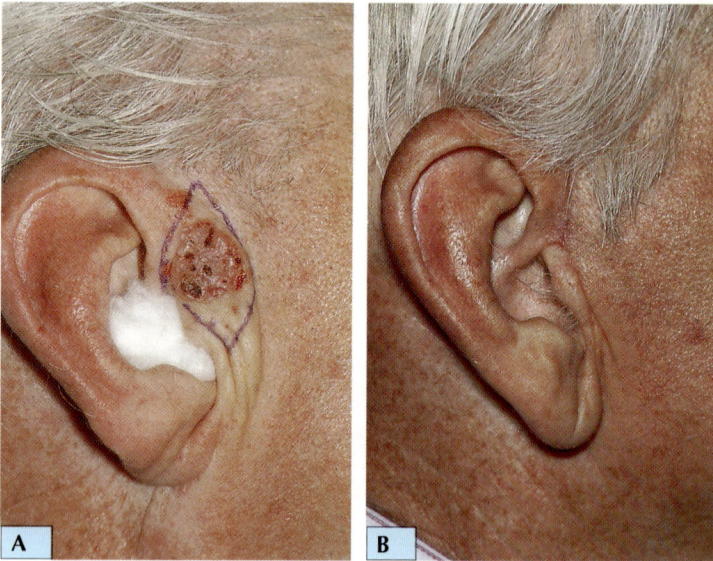

A

B

FIGURE 33.7 (A) A 62-year-old man is seen with a 3 x 3-cm basal cell carcinoma of the preauricular region, excised by Mohs' technique. (B) Result at 3 months, following cheek advancement flap repair.

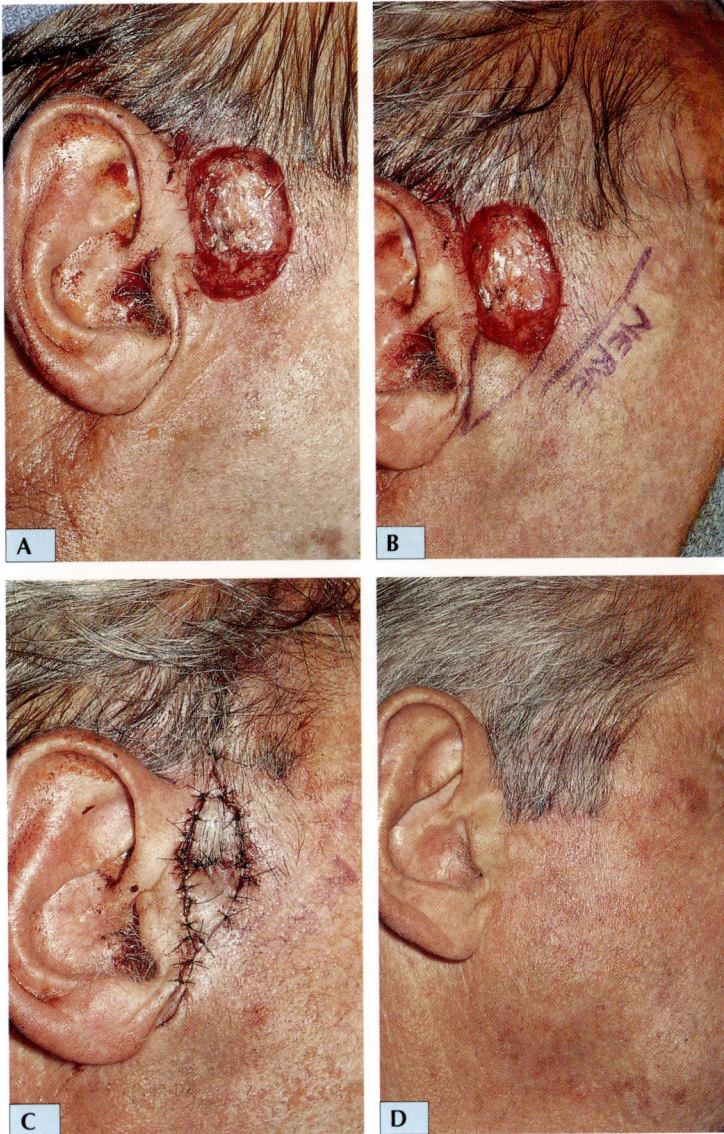

FIGURE 33.8 (A) A 58-year-old man is seen following Mohs' excision of a basal cell carcinoma of the preauricular region. **(B)** Bilateral V-Y advancement flaps are designed for superior and inferior reconstruction of the defect. **(C)** Immediate closure. **(D)** Postoperative result at 3 months with accurate restoration of the temporal hairline.

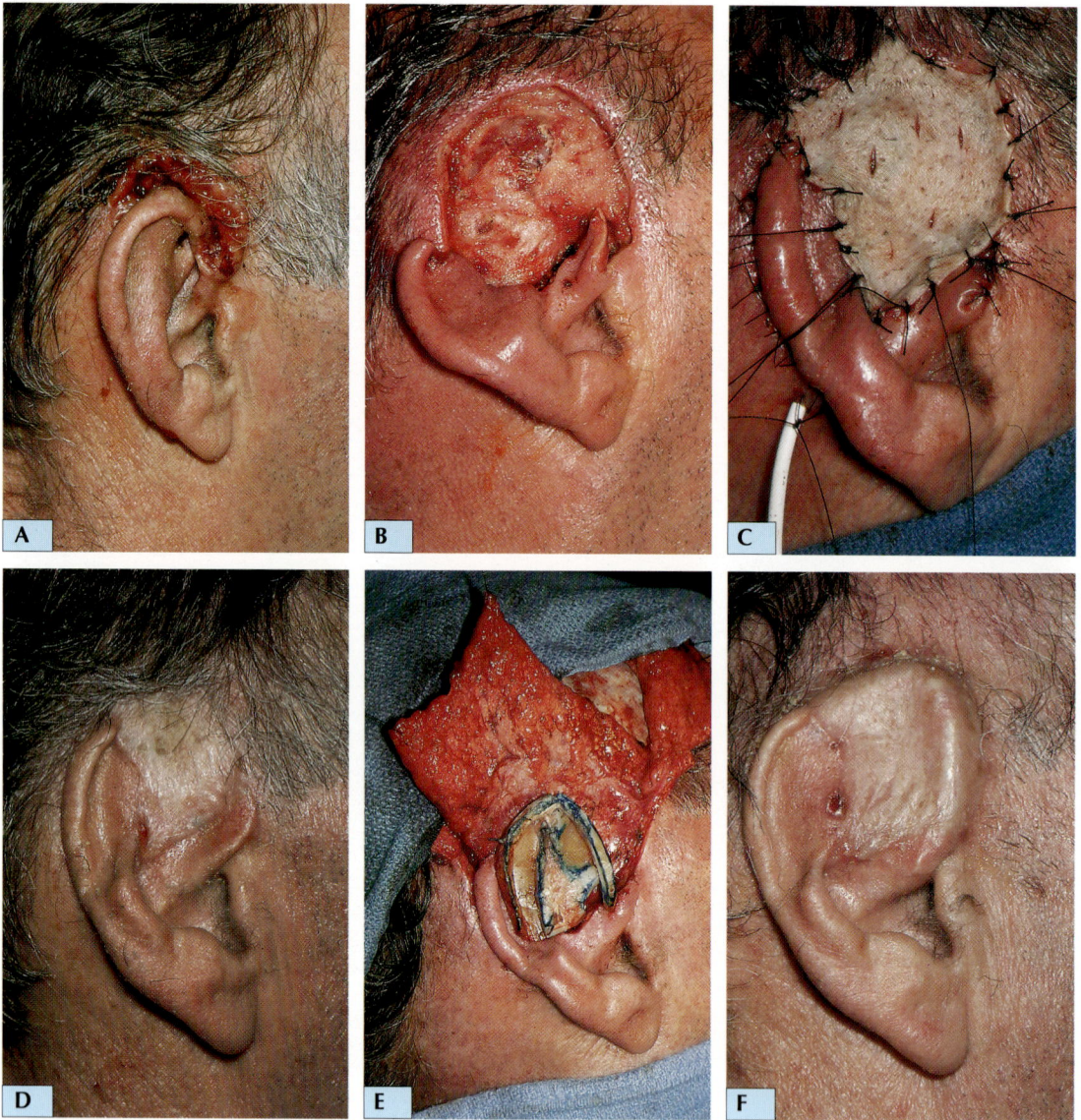

FIGURE 33.9 (A) A 55-year-old man is seen with extensive basal cell carcinoma of the upper auricle. **(B)** The lesion is excised utilizing Mohs' technique. **(C)** The primary reconstruction utilizes a split-thickness skin graft to ensure ease of postoperative monitoring of local recurrence. **(D)** Appearance at 1 year. **(E)** Secondary reconstruction utilizes the temporoparietal fascial flap and an autogenous costal cartilage framework. **(F)** Result at 3 months.

UPPER-THIRD AURICULAR DEFECTS

Although the upper third of the auricle can be concealed by hair, it is functionally important in the wearing of eyeglasses. Two basic techniques have been used for the correction of defects in this area: the helical advancement flap and the autogenous costochondral cartilage graft with temporoparietal fascial flap coverage (Figure 33.9A–F). Additionally, anterior skin defects of the upper and middle thirds of the auricle can be managed by rotation flaps with the incision hidden in the scapha (Figure 33.10A–C).

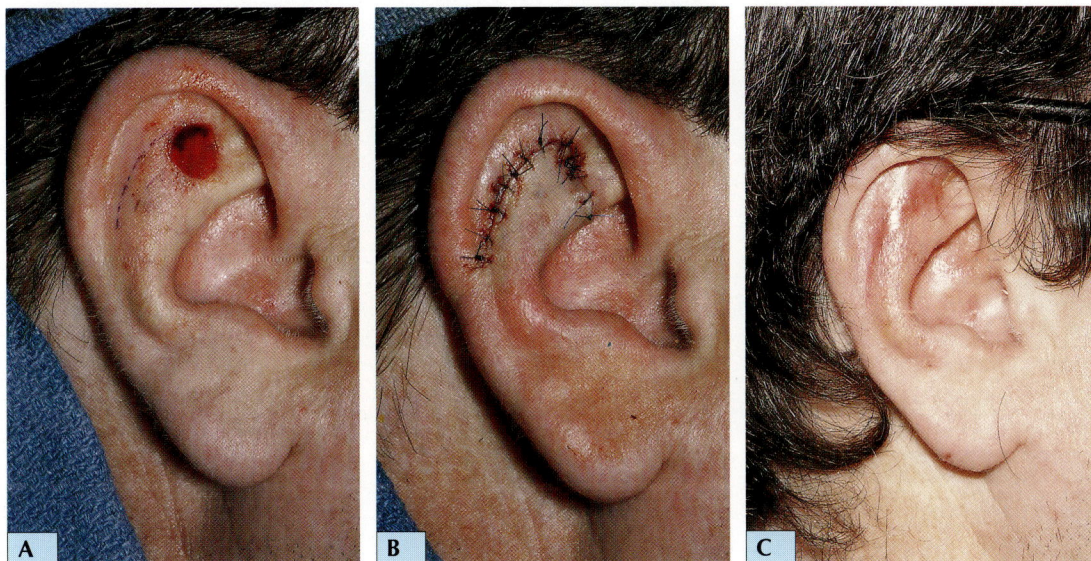

FIGURE 33.10 (A) A 28-year-old man is seen following Mohs' excision of a basal cell carcinoma of the triangular fossa. **(B)** An advancement rotation flap is elevated and mobilized to provide immediate coverage of the exposed cartilage. The incision is planned so that the long limb of the flap resides within the scapha. **(C)** Postoperative result seen at 4 months.

MIDDLE-THIRD AURICULAR DEFECTS

The absence of tissue in the middle third of the auricle is quite noticeable. Simple defects can be closed by advancement flaps or through the utilization of techniques described earlier for the correction of defects of the upper third of the ear. Conchal bowl defects lie within the middle one third of the auricle and when reconstruction of this area is called for, full-thickness skin grafts have been utilized with success (Figure 33.11 A–D). More complex defects requiring cutaneous and cartilaginous reconstruction have been managed successfully by a two-stage technique that utilizes postauricular non–hair-bearing skin and autogenous cartilage (Figure 33.12A–F).

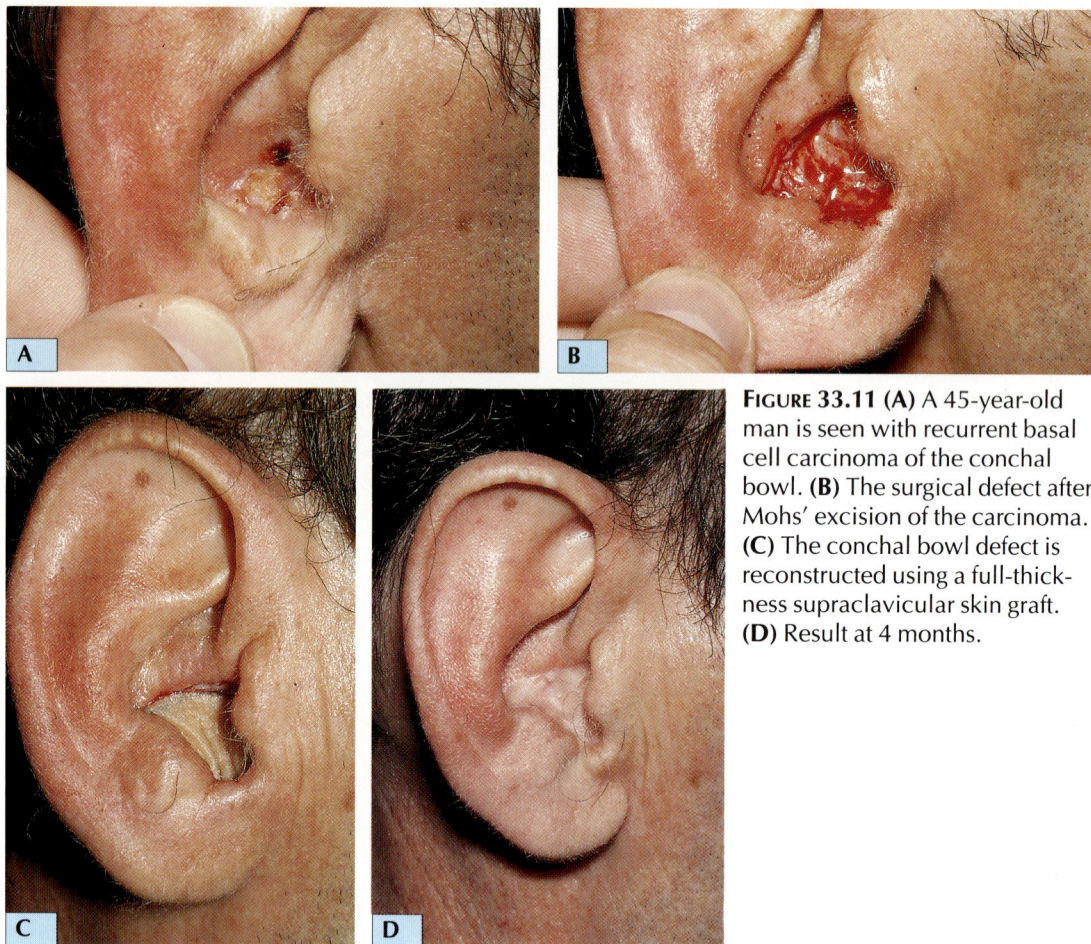

FIGURE 33.11 **(A)** A 45-year-old man is seen with recurrent basal cell carcinoma of the conchal bowl. **(B)** The surgical defect after Mohs' excision of the carcinoma. **(C)** The conchal bowl defect is reconstructed using a full-thickness supraclavicular skin graft. **(D)** Result at 4 months.

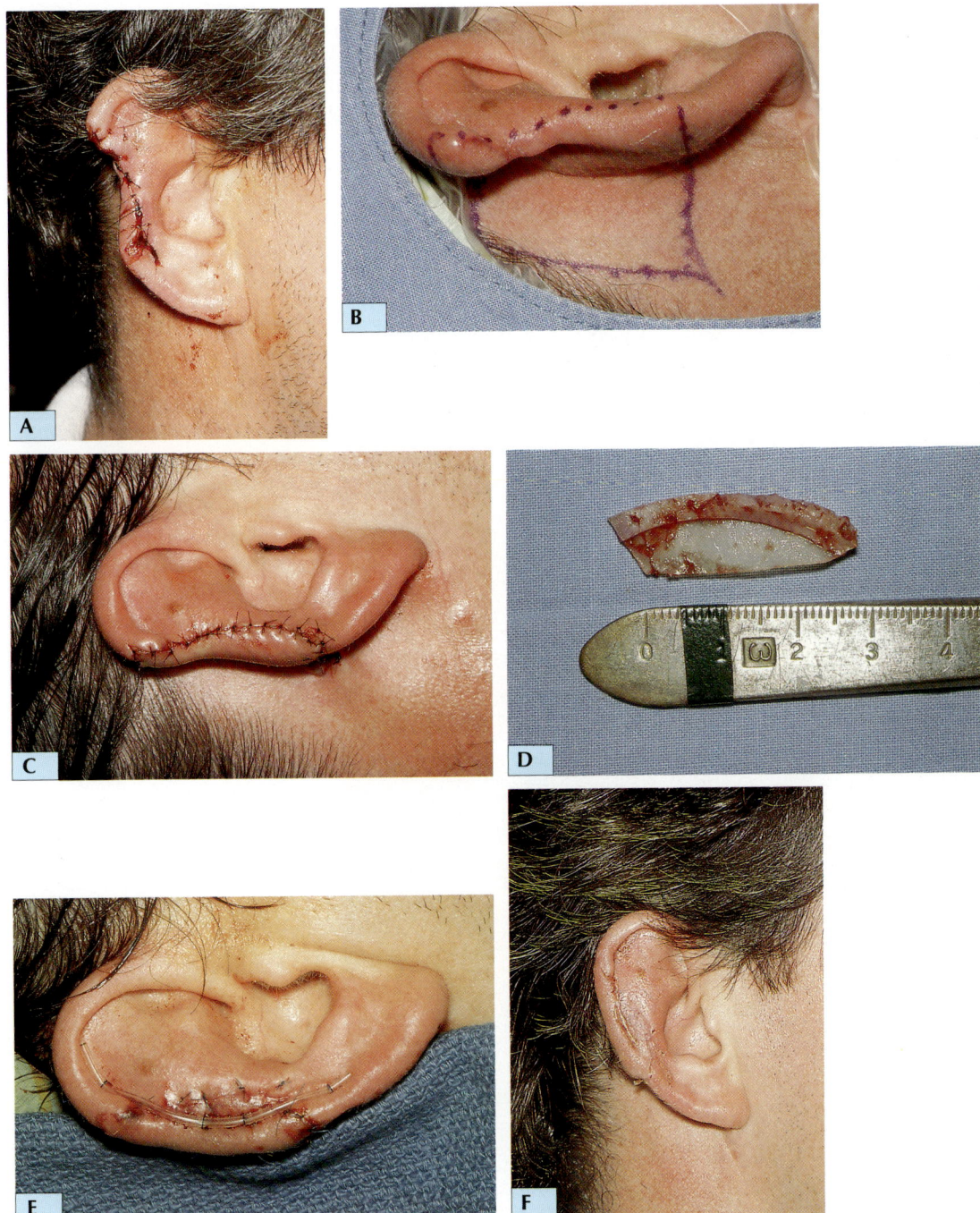

FIGURE 33.12 (A) A 26-year-old man is seen 3 days following a human bite to the middle one third of the auricle. **(B)** Six weeks following injury, the patient has presented for reconstruction using a two-stage postauricular cutaneous flap with excision of scarred tissue at the margin of the auricular defect. **(C)** The flap is sutured into place at the completion of the first stage. **(D)** After 14 days, autogenous nasal septal cartilage is harvested and sculpted to recreate the helical rim. **(E)** The postauricular flap is released, the autogenous septal cartilage framework is embedded between the cutaneous leaves of the flap, and Silastic tubing is utilized to bolster the helical rim. **(F)** Result of the reconstruction at 6 months.

LOWER-THIRD AURICULAR DEFECTS

Reconstruction of the lower one third of the auricle and of the lobule presents a challenge in that the repair must include cartilage-containing techniques to provide the necessary support for successful long-term results. Our preferred method for a lobule reconstruction utilizes conchal cartilage in a two-stage procedure. Initially, the cartilage is embedded in a cutaneous pocket in the postauricular skin. Then, 6 to 8 weeks later, the composite carti-

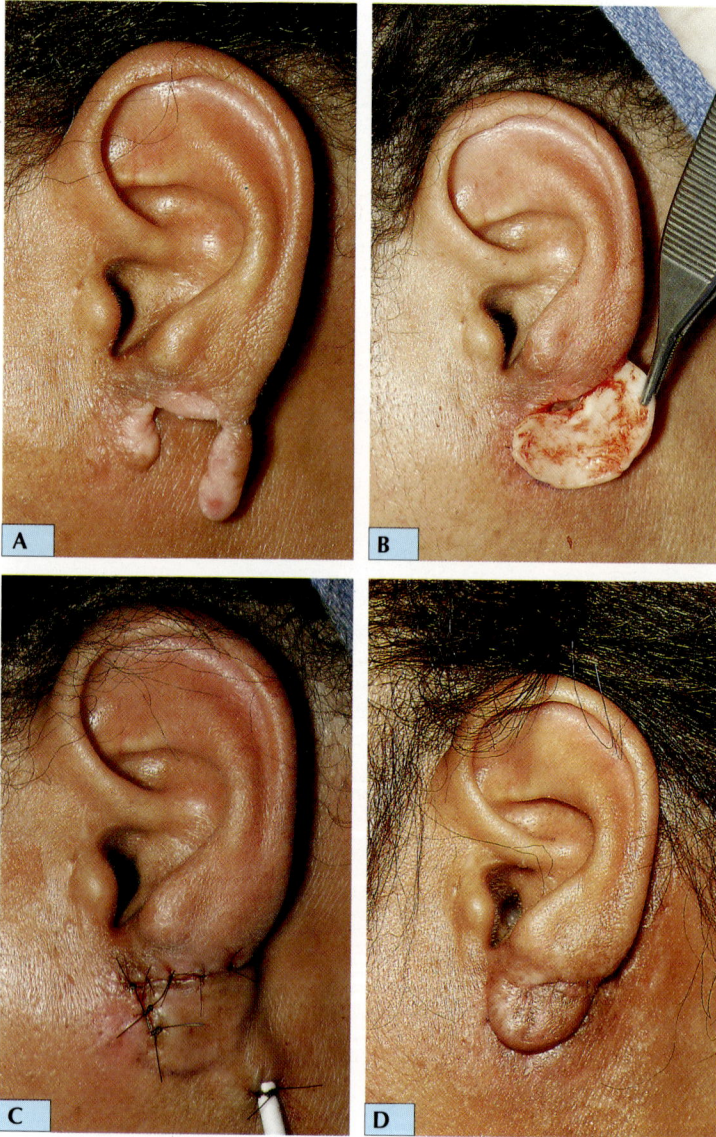

FIGURE 33.13 (A) A 42-year-old woman is seen 3 months following a traumatic lobular laceration. (B) First-stage reconstruction of the lobular defect utilizes autogenous conchal cartilage from the contralateral ear. (C) The conchal cartilage is tailored and placed in a subcutaneous pocket for a period of 3 weeks. (D) The result at 2 months after release of the cartilage and split-thickness skin-graft repair of the medial surface of the lobule.

lage-skin graft is elevated and the area of the medial lobule is covered with a split-thickness skin graft (Figure 33.13A–D).

"Pixie ear" deformity, a commonly encountered defect of the lower one third of the auricle, occurs as a result of rhytidectomy. Pixie ears can be corrected by the design and utilization of a mini-facelift incision around the tragus, lobule, and postauricular sulcus and with advancement of the cervical skin to ensure proper orientation of the auricular lobule (Figure 33.14A–D).

POSTOPERATIVE CARE AND COMPLICATIONS

A broad range of complications can result from auricular reconstructive surgery. However, the primary complications include hematoma formation, chondritis and/or cellulitis,

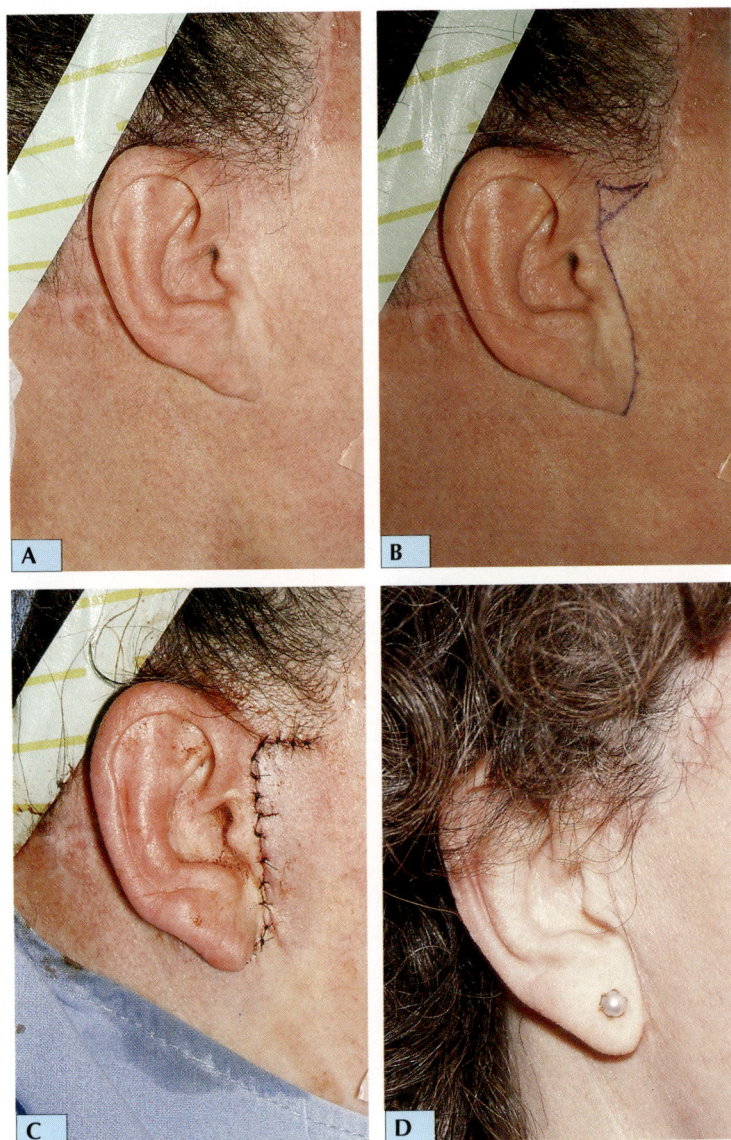

FIGURE 33.14 (A) A 52-year-old woman is seen 1 year following rhytidectomy, with the chief complaint of alteration in the position and orientation of the lobule (pixie ear deformity). (B) Release of the lobular attachment is accomplished by use of cheek and cervical advancement flaps in combination with Burow's triangles in the preauricular and postauricular areas. (C) Immediate postoperative result with successful detachment of the lobule. (D) Result at 4 months.

and tissue necrosis. Hematomas generally occur within the first 24 to 48 hours following the operative procedure and their risk is reduced by careful preoperative instructions to the patient concerning the use of aspirin and aspirin-containing products. Additionally, suction drains are applied for 24 to 48 hours in any situation in which extensive soft-tissue undermining or mobilization is necessary. The auricular reconstruction is also secured by a mastoid type of pressure dressing for 24 to 48 hours. These precautions reduce the risk of hematoma formation, thereby placing the patient at reduced risk for infection and cartilage distortion.

Chondritis/cellulitis is a known complication of auricular reconstruction and for this reason our patients are given intraoperative intravenous antibiotics and are required to maintain a regimen of broad-spectrum oral antibiotics for 2 weeks following surgery to minimize the risk of local infection. In situations in which cartilage grafts are placed into compromised local soft tissue, the risk of pressure necrosis is increased. Careful analysis of the capacity of the local tissue should preclude the placement of three-dimensional cartilage frameworks under two-dimensional skin that is compromised by local scar tissue or infection.

SUGGESTIONS FOR FURTHER READING

Brent B. Reconstruction of the Auricle. In: McCarthy JG, ed. Plastic Surgery. The Face. Part 2. Philadelphia, Pa: WB Saunders Co; 1990;3: 2094-2152.

Brent B, ed. The Artistry of Reconstructive Surgery. St Louis, Mo: C V Mosby Co; 1987.

Brent B, Byrd HS. Secondary ear reconstruction with cartilage grafts covered by axial, random and free flaps of temporoparietal fascia. Plast Reconstr Surg. 1983;72:141-151.

Jackson IT. Local Flaps in Head and Neck Reconstruction. St Louis, Mo: C V Mosby Co; 1985.

Masson JK. A simple island flap for reconstruction of concha-helix defects. Br J Plast Surg. 1972;25:399-403.

chapter 34

CULTURED EPIDERMAL AUTOGRAFTS

Since sustaining the earliest thermal burns, humans have sought a substitute to replace damaged, lost skin. The ideal skin substitute should prevent water and protein loss, protect the organism from trauma, prohibit the entry of bacteria, and be durable and long-lived. For small wounds, replacement skin can be harvested from one part of the body and grafted onto another, as in the case of split-thickness and full-thickness skin grafts. For large wounds, however, adequate healthy skin may be lacking and skin must be obtained from other sources such as cadavers, pigs, and human donors. While such xenografts and allografts can provide adequate initial coverage for large wounds, they cannot provide permanent wound coverage because of rejection. In addition, because of the possible transmission of lethal viruses, human allograft tissue is of limited desirability.

In 1975 Howard Green and James Rheinwald at Massachusetts Institute of Technology serially cultured human keratinocytes, which up to then had been difficult to cultivate. They supported their cultures with irradiated 3T3 cells. The addition of epidermal growth factor and other culture medium additives to stimulate growth enabled them to produce large sheets of viable epidermis in culture. The next step was to see if these sheets would take in vivo to produce real skin. The cells were then used to cover wounds in athymic mice, resulting in the production of durable human epidermis. Through use of this technique, a 1-cm² piece of skin could be expanded 10,000 times in culture. The application of these cells to cover large burn wounds was obvious.

In 1980 the first such human autologous grafts, termed cultured epidermal autografts (CEA), were successfully transplanted onto two burn patients. Later, in 1984, the use of CEA proved critically important when two young boys sustained burns covering 95% of

FIGURE 34.1
INDICATIONS FOR USE OF CEA

1. Patients with multiple lesions that require grafting

2. Patients lacking donor sites

3. Patients who are elderly and intolerant of a second procedure or a second surgical site

4. Patients in whom there is a need to limit anesthesia, either by amount (for local) or duration (for general)

5. Patients who have experienced previous graft failure

6. Patients in whom there is a need to enhance second-intention healing

their bodies. With little unburned skin available, a 2-cm² biopsy was taken from the axilla of each boy, and the skin samples were then cultured to provide autografts that enabled coverage of 50% of each boy's body surface.

INDICATIONS FOR USE

In addition to the earliest application of CEA to burn patients who have extensive open wounds and markedly decreased donor sites, uses have been found for other patients who lack donor sites, such as those with extensive skin diseases like psoriasis. These patients may have multiply recurrent skin cancers or leg ulcers and can be treated successfully with CEA. Similarly, a debilitated patient requiring a large skin graft may be put at risk for a chronic decubitus wound at the donor site, which the use of CEA will prevent.

Elderly patients also may be found to fare better with CEA, as one surgical site rather than two is created resulting in decreased morbidity. These indications are summarized in Figure 34.1.

PREPARATORY STEPS

CELL CULTURE TIMETABLE

To begin a cell culture, a 1- to 2-cm² full-thickness biopsy is obtained using sterile technique. Protected sites in burn patients usually are found in the axilla, groin, abdomen, and postauricular sulcus. In an outpatient setting, the axilla and postauricular sulcus are the sites most readily accessible (Figure 34.2). Immediately after removal, the piece of tissue is dropped into a transport culture medium (Figure 34.3) and the biopsy site is closed primarily or allowed to heal by second intention.

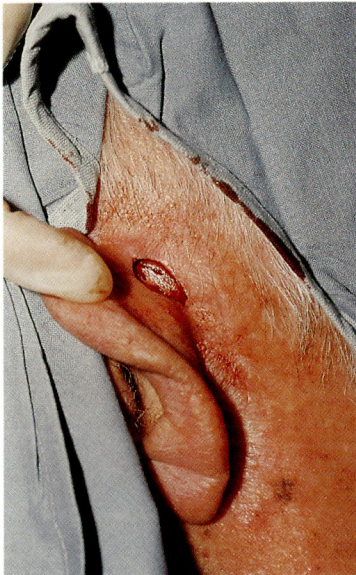

FIGURE 34.2
After sterile preparation and draping, a scalpel is used to create an elliptical biopsy, 1 cm², down to the subcutaneous fat. As a donor site, the postauricular sulcus is easily reached, heals well, and leaves no visible scar. It also yields skin that is relatively free of sun damage.

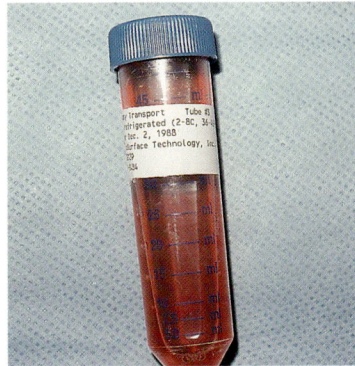

FIGURE 34.3
The transport culture medium is supplied in small plastic vials that can be maintained up to 60 days by refrigeration.

The tissue is then transported to the laboratory where the epithelium is gently teased off the dermis with scissors and is dropped into trypsin, where it disaggregates to form a single-cell-layer suspension. Aliquots of the suspension are then plated in flasks and allowed to grow. Each cell forms individual colonies, which coalesce in approximately 11 days to form a confluent sheet of undifferentiated epithelial cells. The cells are then re-plated in other flasks to form secondary cultures (Figure 34.4).

Each sheet of cells is then detached from the flask with the protease, Dispase (Figure 34.5), following which it contracts to form a graft of approximately 25 cm^2. To enable handling of the epithelium, which is a diaphanous, slightly pink, gelatinous struc-

ture, it is attached with metal surgical clips to a piece of petrolatum gauze. The gauze is then placed in a petri dish containing transport medium (Figure 34.6) and it is brought to the patient's side in a cooled, sealed chamber. The grafts are viable for 24 hours from the moment they are removed from the flasks with Dispase.

PATIENT SELECTION AND PREPARATION

In addition to burns, two areas of immediate applicability of CEA for the cutaneous surgeon are (1) following removal of a large skin lesion requiring a graft, and (2) for coverage of an existing skin ulcer. Removal of a large skin cancer or nevus is usually an

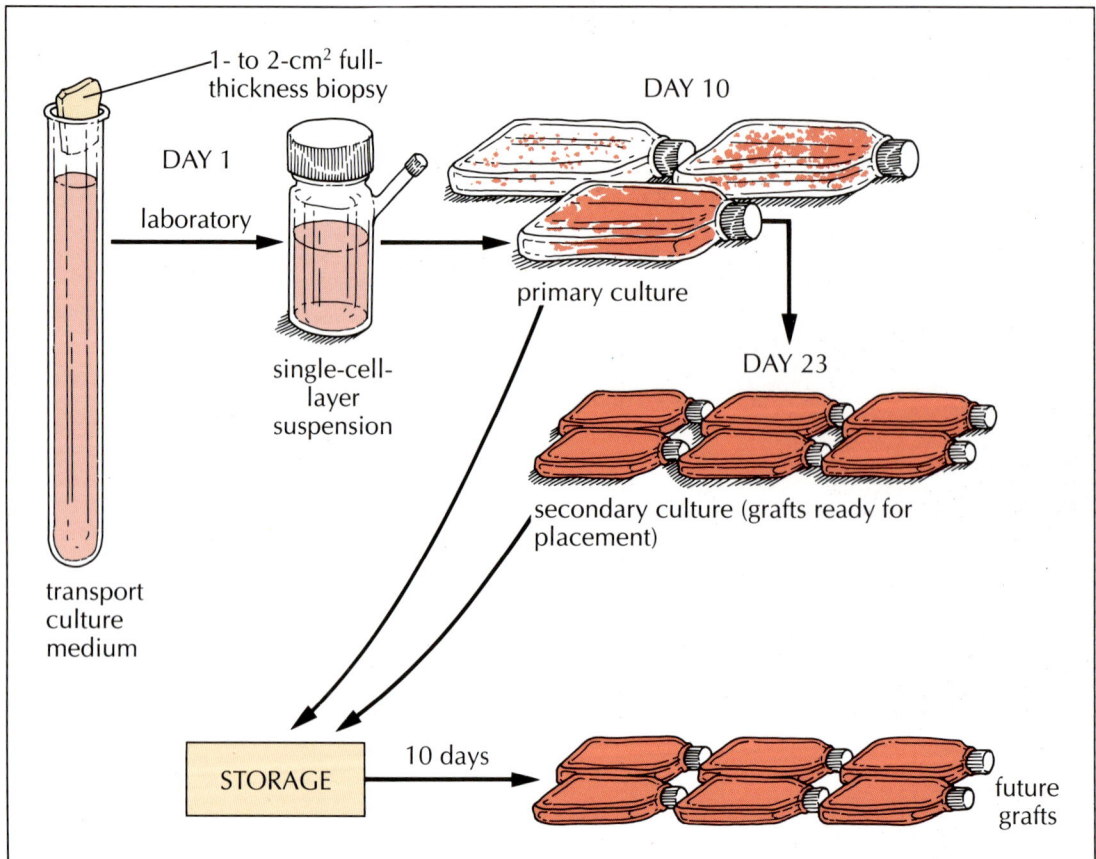

FIGURE 34.4 Schematic diagram showing a timetable for growth of the cultures.

anticipated event. Therefore, at the time of initial consultation a determination can be made as to whether coverage of the defect with CEA is feasible. Figure 34.7 summarizes the advantages of this technique. Its main disadvantage is that wounds replaced by CEA contract just like those replaced by split-thickness skin grafts. Therefore, in situations in which a split-thickness skin graft would be inappropriate, as for example in the periorbital area, a CEA would be equally inappropriate.

To determine the length of time between the biopsy and production of the first available grafts, a timetable can be consulted (see Figure 34.4). The biopsy can be performed on the day of consultation, after which a surgical appointment can be scheduled appropriately. There is no specific preoperative preparation for the CEA patient with a large skin lesion.

In the case of a leg ulcer, specific preoperative considerations do exist. Since the grafts may be sensitive to topical antibacterial

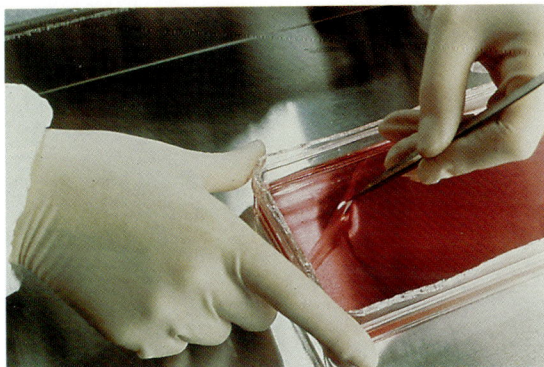

FIGURE 34.5 The final confluent layer of keratinocytes is seen as it is lifted from its flask. *(Courtesy of Biosurface Technology Institute.)*

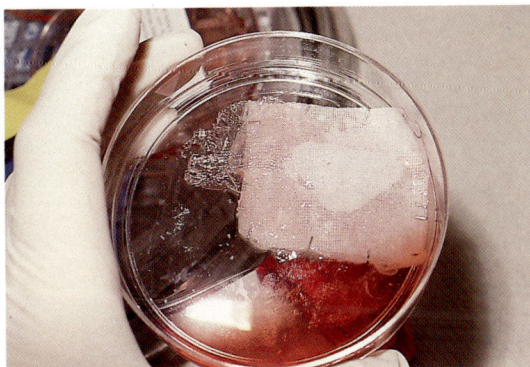

FIGURE 34.6 To the left of the piece of gauze is a reflective pink diaphanous layer of keratinocytes. It is floating in the red liquid medium, which has accumulated at the bottom of the petri dish.

FIGURE 34.7
ADVANTAGES OF CEA

1. Briefness of procedure

2. Only one assistant needed

3. No need for donor or second surgical site

4. No need for special equipment

5. No need for local anesthesia

6. Availability of cells for subsequent procedures at other sites or in case of graft failure

7. Surgery performed on an outpatient basis

preparations, all wound care other than sterile water and gauze should be discontinued at least 3 days prior to grafting. Moist-to-dry, moist-to-moist, or dry dressings may be used depending on the individual ulcer. In addition, bleeding should be minimal at the time of graft placement. Therefore, 1 to 3 days prior to surgery, the ulcer should be debrided to prepare it for grafting. At the same time, the wound should be cultured and oral antibiotic therapy should be initiated.

Last, but of equal importance, is a preoperative assessment of the patient's degree of cooperation. Considering the delicacy of CEA or of any graft, conditions must be maximized for success. In the case of a leg wound, patients need to be advised preoperatively of the need to avoid weight-bearing in the postoperative period. They also need to be assessed for their willingness to keep the leg elevated, to take their prescribed antibiotics, to follow the necessary wound care regimen, and to return

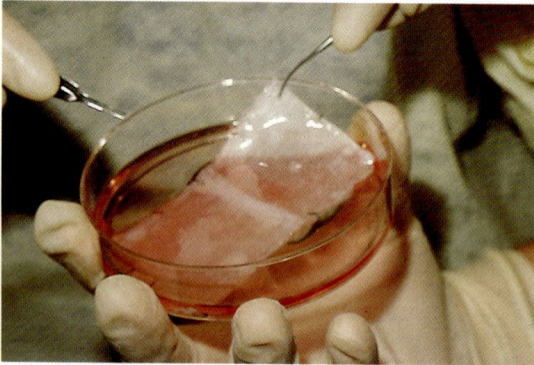

FIGURE 34.8 The petri dish is held by an assistant as the graft is slid gently out of it. Because the cells will drape over the edges of the gauze if it is held vertically, it should be maintained in a horizontal position.

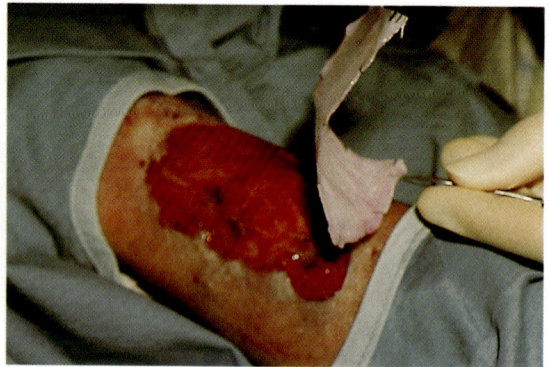

FIGURE 34.9 The side of the graft that was facing upward is now placed directly on the wound bed, thus leaving the gauze on top.

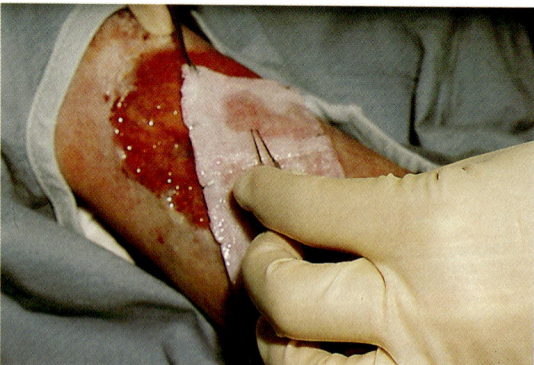

FIGURE 34.10 Once in position, the grafts must be left in place. Here, they are seen being gently pressed down to adhere to the wound surface.

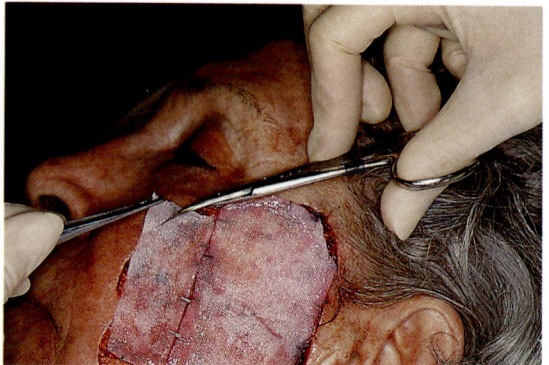

FIGURE 34.11 Trimming to fit. Sharp scissors should be used to avoid any trauma to the graft.

for follow-up visits to assess wound healing.

PROCEDURE

Once the defect has been created or the ulcer or wound has been prepared, the cultured cells can be placed on it. The grafts are sterile and must be handled as such. To remove each graft from its petri dish, it should be lifted gently with toothed forceps, taking hold of the gauze backing along with the graft to avoid tearing of the thin epidermal sheet (Figure 34.8). Since the cells float on top of the piece of gauze, the gauze must be flipped so that the cells are placed directly in contact with the wound bed and the gauze is

on top of the cells (Figure 34.9). If several grafts are needed, they should be placed to provide minimal overlap. Once in place, the cells should not be moved, as shearing forces will disrupt them (Figure 34.10).

The graft is then trimmed to fit the size and shape of the defect (Figure 34.11). Trimming also may be done prior to graft placement, by using a template or by estimating the necessary size. No anesthesia of the wound bed is necessary for placement of the graft.

Following graft placement, the wound is covered (Figure 34.12) with a nonadherent permeable membrane dressing placed directly on top of the gauze backing (Figure 34.13). Bridal veil gauze also may be used

FIGURE 34.12
INITIAL WOUND COVERAGE

1st layer: CEA with gauze backing

2nd layer: Nonadherent Exu-dry inner layer or bridal veil gauze

3rd layer: Molded petrolatum gauze

4th layer: Exu-dry or layers of gauze

5th layer: Kerlix

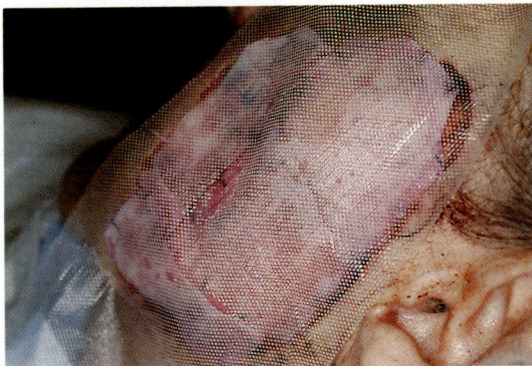

FIGURE 34.13 Wound with inner layer of Exu-dry dressing. This layer allows the wound to breathe and the exudate to pass, without adhering to the grafts once the dressing is removed.

(Figure 34.14). Synthetic wound coverings are not recommended as they are too occlusive and allow bacterial growth. A second layer of dressing follows, consisting of petrolatum-impregnated gauze molded to the wound (Figure 34.15). A third layer consists of Exu-dry held in place by Kerlix. Additional layers of gauze and/or Kerlix are used to protect the wound and to absorb the exudate (Figure 34.16A,B). Also in the immediate postoperative period, oral antibiotic coverage is initiated if it was not started previously, and it is usually maintained until the area has healed.

POSTOPERATIVE CARE

Proper wound care is crucial in the postoperative period. Since CEA wounds can be rather exudative, the outer layers of the bandage, down to the vaseline gauze, at first may need to be changed by the patient on a daily basis if they become saturated. The advantages of using Exu-dry in the dressing are as follows: (1) the patient has only one uncomplicated layer to identify and change, thus minimizing the chances of tampering with or moving the vaseline gauze or grafts; (2) it is highly absorptive and thus decreases the frequency of dressing changes; and (3) it

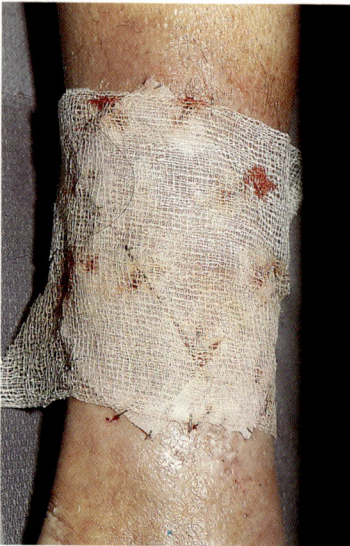

FIGURE 34.14 Bridal veil gauze. This thin layer of gauze will adhere to the wound slightly, although it is nonabsorbent.

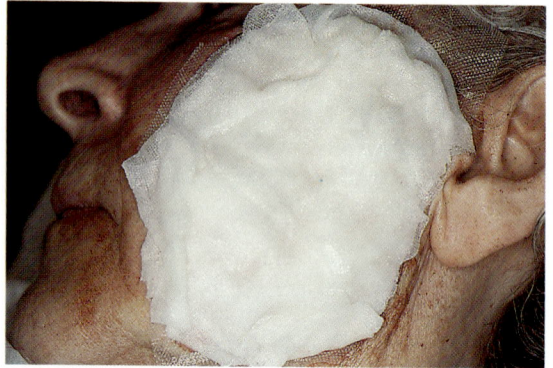

FIGURE 34.15 The moistened gauze provides an environment that will prevent desiccation of the wound, is nonadherent, and will cushion the area.

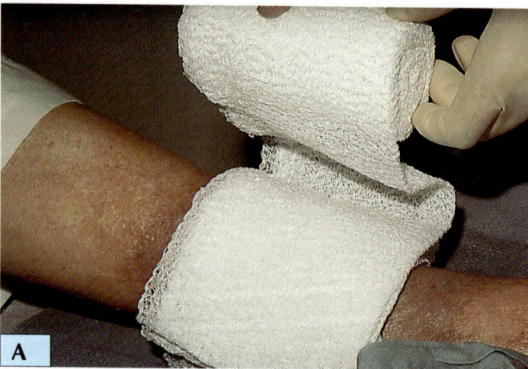

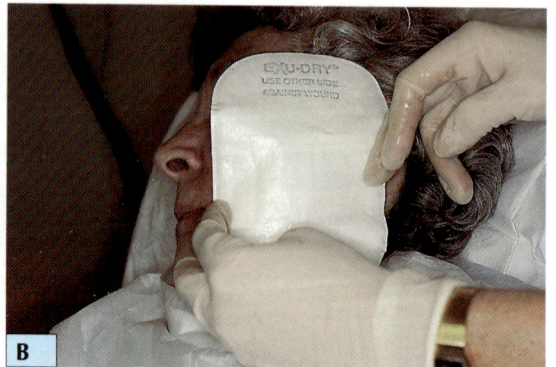

FIGURE 34.16 (A) This is a standard bandage made from several layers of Kerlix, heaped up by folding each layer back on itself for absorption and protec- tion. The bandage is then wrapped around the area to secure the dressings in place. (B) A single layer of Exu-dry serves the same purpose.

is nonadherent and cushions the area (Figure 34.17).

After 8 to 10 days, the entire dressing is removed down to the grafts and an opaqueness may be seen covering the wound (Figure 34.18). The wound also may continue to be somewhat exudative. Wound care at this point consists of cleansing with sterile water and daily replacement of vaseline gauze or just Exu-dry, depending on the dryness of the grafts.

RESULTS

Ideally, when the dressings are first removed, the wound should be covered by epithelium, as may be seen in medium-sized wounds or in wounds located on nondependent or nontraumatized parts of the body (Figure 34.19). For wounds located elsewhere, the wound at first is covered by a thin, diaphanous, dull, membrane-like structure, as seen in Figure 34.18. This gradually develops into durable, cosmetically accept-

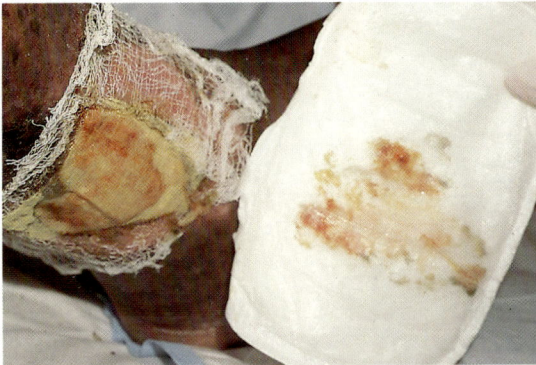

FIGURE 34.17 The Exu-dry has absorbed the exudate. Also seen covering the wound is bridal veil gauze and the petrolatum gauze.

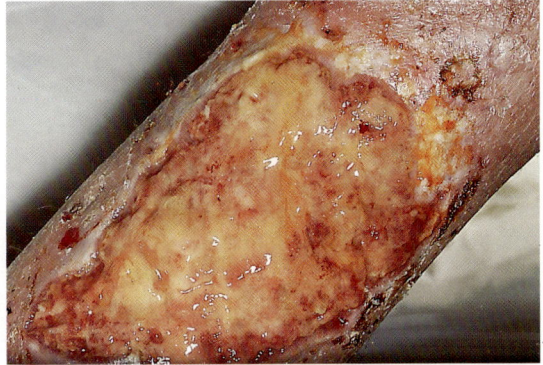

FIGURE 34.18 At first glance, this ulcer looks unchanged. On closer inspection, a thin film can be seen overlying the wound bed.

FIGURE 34.19 This forehead was grafted following removal of a skin lesion. Because of prior trauma to the area, wounds had healed poorly before the use of CEA. Following removal of the dressing, a slightly erythematous epithelium is seen to cover the defect site completely.

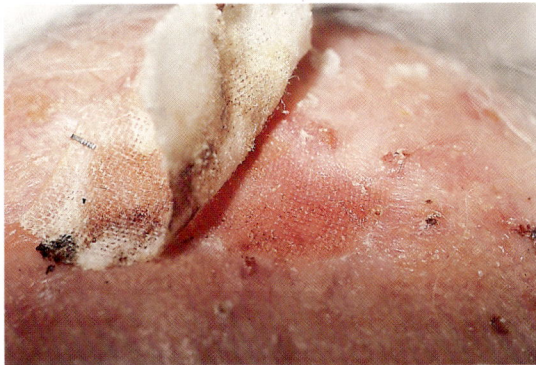

able skin. Nonhealing ulcers of 5 years' duration may heal in 6 weeks with a CEA (Figure 34.20A,B) while large wounds, such as those resulting from removal of a skin cancer, may heal in 10 weeks (Figure 34.21 A,B). Finally, if the grafted cells do not take, the laboratory can have fresh grafts available in 10 days.

FUTURE APPLICATIONS

CEA technology is advancing rapidly, such that cultured grafts will soon become viable in their petri dish transports for 48 to 72 hours. Additional developments may enable freezing of CEA so that sheets of epithelium may be stored at the physician's office and

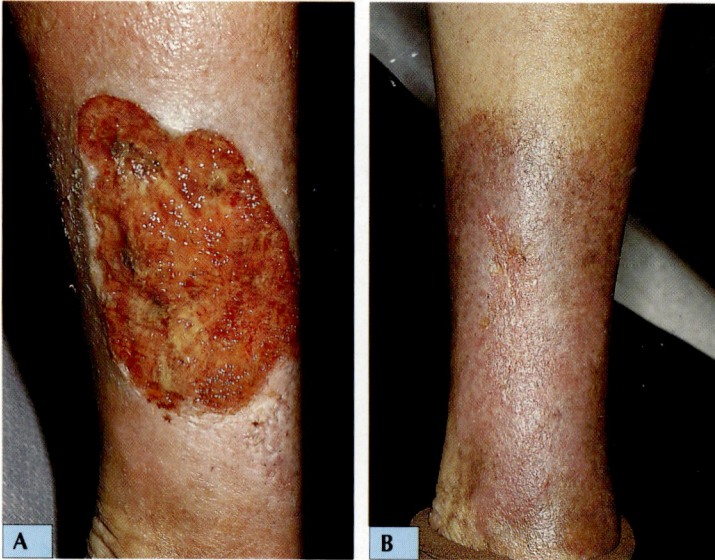

FIGURE 34.20 (A) This nonhealing ulcer of several years' duration had failed medical treatment, split-thickness skin grafting, and pinch grafting. (B) Following CEA transplantation, the ulcer healed in 6 weeks, and has remained healed for over 2 years.

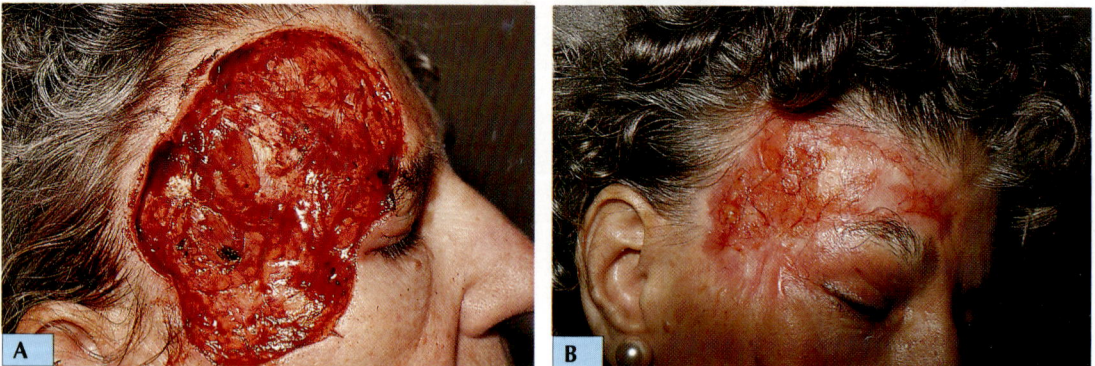

FIGURE 34.21 (A) A large defect after removal of a basal cell carcinoma. Following the procedure, the patient was fatigued and had received large amounts of anesthetic. Placement of the CEA took 10 minutes without the need for additional lidocaine. (B) After 10 weeks, the wound has healed.

used if the patient returns with a new ulcer or with a partially healed previous one. Also under way is the development of dermal grafts with or without epithelium. Neonatal foreskin cultured keratinocyte grafts are being tested and their combination with or without CEA or dermis is an exciting prospect. They might be available for any patient who presents with a skin defect.

A new era has arrived where we can replace damaged skin with its ideal substitute, namely, autologous human skin. It has all the properties necessary to protect the organism and make it viable, and it can be processed and placed with little insult to the donor or recipient. An almost unlimited supply is available for repeated grafting of the same site, for grafting to other sites, or for new lesions. The future can only make this useful tool more accessible and more promising in its applicability.

SUGGESTIONS FOR FURTHER READING

Falabella R, Escobar C, Borrero I. Transplantation of in vitro cultured epidermis-bearing melanocytes for repigmenting vitiligo. J Am Acad Dermatol. 1989;21:257-264.

Gallico G, O'Connor NE, Compton CC, et al. Permanent coverage of large burn wounds with autologous cultured human epithelium. N Engl J Med. 1984;311:448-451.

Green H, Kehinde O, Thomas J. Growth of cultured human epidermal cells into multiple epithelia suitable for grafting. Proc Natl Acad Sci U S A. 1979;76:5665-5668.

Hefton JM, Caldwell D, Biozes DG, et al. Grafting of skin ulcers with cultured autologous epidermal cells. J Am Acad Dermatol. 1986;14:399-405.

Phillips T, Kehinde O, Green H, Gilchrest BA. Treatment of skin ulcers with cultured epidermal allografts. J Am Acad Dermatol. 1989;21:191-199.